THIRD EDITION

# Community Nutrition

## Planning Health Promotion and Disease Prevention

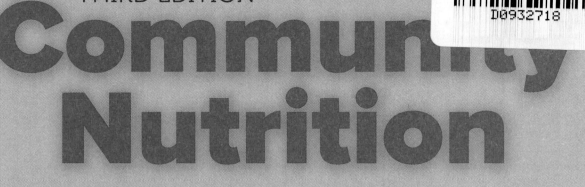

**Nweze Eunice Nnakwe, PhD, RDN, LDN, CFCS**

Professor, Department of Family and Consumer Services
Illinois State University

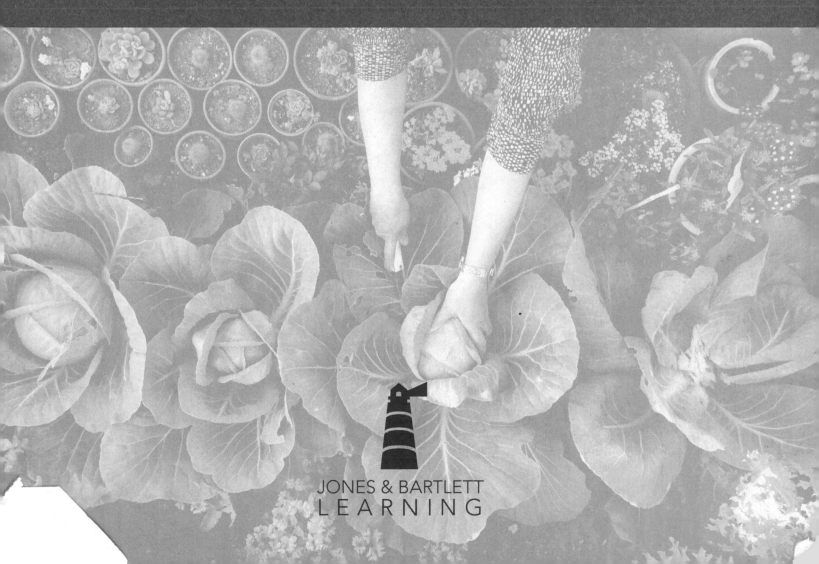

JONES & BARTLETT
LEARNING

*World Headquarters*
Jones & Bartlett Learning
5 Wall Street
Burlington, MA 01803
978-443-5000
info@jblearning.com
www.jblearning.com

Jones & Bartlett Learning books and products are available through most bookstores and online booksellers. To contact Jones & Bartlett Learning directly, call 800-832-0034, fax 978-443-8000, or visit our website, www.jblearning.com.

Substantial discounts on bulk quantities of Jones & Bartlett Learning publications are available to corporations, professional associations, and other qualified organizations. For details and specific discount information, contact the special sales department at Jones & Bartlett Learning via the above contact information or send an email to specialsales@jblearning.com.

34828-6

**Production Credits**

VP, Executive Publisher: David D. Cella
Publisher: Cathy L. Esperti
Acquisitions Editor: Sean Fabery
Associate Editor: Taylor Maurice
Director of Production: Jenny L. Corriveau
Director of Vendor Management: Amy Rose
Vendor Manager: Juna Abrams
Director of Marketing: Andrea DeFronzo
VP, Manufacturing and Inventory Control: Therese Connell

Composition: S4Carlisle Publishing Services
Project Management: S4Carlisle Publishing Services
Cover Design: Kristin E. Parker
Director of Rights & Media: Joanna Gallant
Rights & Media Specialist: Merideth Tumasz
Media Development Editor: Shannon Sheehan
Cover Image: © alyfromuk2us/Getty Images
Printing and Binding: Edwards Brothers Malloy
Cover Printing: Edwards Brothers Malloy

**Library of Congress Cataloging-in-Publication Data**
Names: Nnakwe, Nweze Eunice, author.
Title: Community nutrition : planning health promotion and disease prevention / Nweze Eunice Nnakwe.
Description: Third edition. | Burlington, MA : Jones & Bartlett Learning, [2018] | Includes bibliographical references and index.
Identifiers: LCCN 2017015568 | ISBN 9781284108323
Subjects: | MESH: Community Health Services | Nutritional Physiological Phenomena | Health Promotion--methods | Health Planning--methods | Nutrition Policy | United States
Classification: LCC TX354 | NLM QU 145 | DDC 363.8/560973--dc23 LC record available at https://lccn.loc.gov/2017015568

6048

Printed in the United States of America
21  20  19  18  17      10 9 8 7 6 5 4 3 2 1

## Dedication

*This book is dedicated to God, who makes all things feasible.*

*To my beloved, vivacious sister Beatrice: You were a blessing to everyone you met, and your beautiful smile and caring nature will be greatly missed.*

*To my brother in-law Titus: You were an invisible Angel who loved unconditionally.*

*May both of you who departed in 2016 rest in divine, perfect peace.*

# Brief Contents

# Contents

## Chapter 4   U.S. Nutrition Monitoring and Food Assistance Programs ...... 105

## Chapter 5   Cultural Influences and Public Health Nutrition .............. 143

## Chapter 6   Public Policy and Nutrition ..... 181

## Chapter 7   Public Health Nutrition: An International Perspective ... 209

## PART II Nutrition Interventions for Vulnerable Populations    229

### Chapter 8   Nutrition During Pregnancy and Infancy . . . . . . . . . . . . . . . . . 231

### Chapter 9   Nutrition in Childhood and Adolescence . . . . . . . . . . . . . . 281

### Chapter 10   Adulthood: Special Health Issues . . . . . . . . . . . . . . . . . . . . . 319

## Chapter 11 Promoting Health and Preventing Disease in Older Persons................ 359

## PART III Delivering Successful Nutrition Services    389

## Chapter 12 Principles of Planning Effective Community Nutrition Programs........... 391

## Chapter 13 Theories and Models for Health Promotion and Changing Nutrition Behavior ........... 413

## Chapter 14 Acquiring Grantsmanship Skills ...................... 429

# Preface

Community Nutrition: Planning Health Promotion and Disease Prevention, Third Edition provides nutrition students, community nurses, and health educators with the knowledge, skills, tools, and evidence-based approaches they need to promote health and prevent diseases. This *Third Edition* continues to reinforce core nutrition concepts and presents the tools and skills needed to enter the health professions. It takes a public health and community-based care approach rather than the business and hospital-based care perspective used by most other books in this area. This text considers the increased comprehensive approach of practitioners providing community-based services that emphasize primary, secondary, and tertiary prevention, and it reflects the latest direction in public health and community nutrition.

## ▶ Organization of This Text

This book is divided into three parts.

Part I provides an overview of community and public health nutrition landscapes and lays the foundation for primary, secondary, and tertiary prevention. Chapter 1 begins with a discussion of various community approaches to health promotion and disease prevention, and it details the Nutrition Care Process and Model (NCPM), a tool nutritionists use to communicate nutrition activities within the profession and among a variety of other healthcare professions. Chapter 2 discusses nutrition screening and assessment methods, including diet assessment methods, and contains comprehensive information and tools students can use to assess their clients. Chapter 3 describes the nuts and bolts of nutritional epidemiology and research methods and provides community and public health nutritionists with a step-by-step method of implementing different stages of the research process. Chapter 4 provides students with the most current information on the U.S. nutrition monitoring and food assistance programs for at-risk populations. It also provides a detailed description of the "working poor" and explains how to evaluate food insecurity. Chapter 5 addresses cultural influences and public health nutrition, providing community nutritionists with multiple ways of acquiring cultural competency and identifying barriers to effective multicultural health promotion and disease prevention programs. This chapter highlights dietary patterns of different cultural groups in the United States, including current nutrition practices and health-related issues. Chapter 6 provides strategies that can be used to develop public policy and discusses how dietitians can become involved in the policy process. Chapter 7 provides an overview of world hunger and food insecurity and discusses the role of women in the prevention of food insecurity and current nutrition issues. It also discusses chronic health conditions in developing and developed countries and equips nutritionists with the tools to provide nutrition intervention during emergency relief periods. In addition, it includes nutrition education and counseling for those with HIV/AIDS.

Part II focuses on the knowledge and intervention skills needed to promote health and prevent disease throughout the life cycle. Chapter 8 discusses nutrition during pregnancy and infancy and provides community nutritionists with information regarding nutrition care during these stages of life. It also covers important changes that must occur during the period of lactogenesis. Chapter 9 describes current nutrition trends and factors that contribute to overweight and obesity in childhood and adolescence. Screening and diagnosis tools for eating disorders are included in this edition. Chapter 10 focuses on special health issues in adulthood and challenges community and public health nutritionists to integrate evidence-based intervention strategies into their nutrition programs. It also equips community nutritionists with the knowledge and tools to address such chronic health conditions as cardiovascular disease, obesity, cancer, and osteoporosis. Chapter 11 discusses health promotion and disease prevention in older persons and provides multiple nutrition screening initiative tools for community and public health nutritionists to use in the nutrition care process.

Part III focuses on the skills, knowledge, and tools community nutritionists need to design effective nutrition and health promotion programs. This section applies the information presented in Parts I and II while discussing the principles of planning successful community nutrition programs. Chapter 12 focuses on program planning and the tools for planning an effective nutrition program.

Chapter 13 presents several research-based theoretical frameworks to guide nutrition education. It discusses steps for translating theory into research-oriented educational strategies and presents practical activities that nutritionists can use to conduct nutrition education. Chapter 14 addresses the process of grantsmanship and lays the foundation for writing and implementing grant proposals. Chapter 15 focuses on ethics and nutrition practices. It includes a code of ethics for the profession of dietetics. Chapter 16 discusses the principles of nutrition education. It presents the procedural model for designing research-based educational programs and strategies that provide valuable nutrition education throughout the life span. Chapter 17 focuses on marketing nutrition programs and the role of the food industry in food choice, including how advertising affects childhood obesity. Chapter 18 discusses the U.S. healthcare system.

The comprehensive coverage in *Community Nutrition: Planning Health Promotion and Disease Prevention, Third Edition* makes it an essential resource for community nutrition courses and a useful reference tool. It provides pertinent statistics on national health objectives and discusses both traditional concepts and current and emerging nutrition issues. Real-world examples throughout the text explain nutritional concepts and present the reader with an application of these important topics. The book presents concise information and provides helpful activities so the reader can consider important issues without receiving a great deal of unnecessary information.

## ▶ Key Features of This Text

This text includes a variety of features that help students and other healthcare professionals prepare and provide effective nutrition intervention to different groups in the community:

- **Learning Objectives** emphasize key concepts to help students focus on what they need to learn.
- **Boxes** highlight important points in each chapter.
- **Successful Community Strategies** discuss effective intervention programs and provide examples of research-based best practices for each chapter.
- **Chapter Summaries** highlight important concepts for each chapter.
- **Critical Thinking Activities** incorporate a variety of cognitive skills such as synthesizing, analyzing, applying, and evaluating information. The activities help students develop expertise and provide them with the opportunity to understand and evaluate health information and then apply the concepts in community settings.

- **Case Studies** provide students the opportunity to apply what they have learned in each chapter.
- **Think About It** questions and scenarios in each chapter emphasize active learning and content integration and keep students engaged. Answers to the Think About It questions are provided at the end of each chapter.

## ▶ New to the *Third Edition*

The *Third Edition* has been thoroughly updated to reflect the latest research in the fields of community and public health nutrition. Highlights include the following:

### Chapter 1
- Presents *Healthy People 2020* focus areas
- Updates content relating to the Healthy People Progress Report
- Incorporates the most recent Millennium Development Goals Progress Report

### Chapter 2
- Incorporates an introduction to program planning
- Adds emphasis on using a collaborative approach for conducting a needs assessment
- Discusses steps for identifying target populations

### Chapter 3
- Incorporates discussion of community audits and "ground truthing"
- Includes general rules for writing survey questions, including nine steps for the development of a questionnaire
- Features a new "Successful Community Strategies" box focused on a NHANES study describing perceptions of child weight status among American children

### Chapter 4
- Features revised table presenting the different costs of USDA food plans
- Includes updated statistics on poverty food insecurity in the United States
- Incorporates updated DHHS poverty guidelines

### Chapter 5
- Includes new section discussing Caucasian American food patterns, nutrition practices, and health-related issues

## Chapter 6

- Includes new information about the ability of RDNs to order diets in hospitals
- Incorporates discussion of the 2014 Farm Bill, whose initiatives contribute to improving the nation's health

## Chapter 7

- Features updated statistics regarding urbanization and maternal mortality rates in the developing world, as well as HIV/AIDS prevalence in women and children
- Updates discussion of global rehydration projects
- Features a new "Successful Community Strategies" box focused on efforts to fight malnutrition in Senegal and Madagascar

## Chapter 8

- Documents the Healthy People 2020 Maternal and Infant Health Objectives

## Chapter 9

- Documents the Healthy People 2020 Objectives Related to Children and Adolescents
- Includes updated annual eligibility guidelines for federal child nutrition programs, as well as current basic cash reimbursement rates for school lunches
- Features the Healthy Eating Index components and standards for scoring

## Chapter 10

- Incorporates updated statistics for chronic health conditions
- Documents Healthy People 2020 Objectives for Adults
- Includes discussion of the World Heart Federation's nine antiobesity initiatives
- Features a new "Successful Community Strategies" box focused on a Healthy Heart Program conducted in New York

## Chapter 11

- Includes updated longevity statistics
- Features a new "Successful Community Strategies" box focused on the Eat Better and Move More program

## Chapter 12

- Describes the "A to E" method of writing objectives, also noting words to use and avoid when writing objectives

## Chapter 13

- Features an additional example of a nutrition program utilizing the Social Learning Theory
- Includes an enhanced discussion of how behavioral models can provide positive nutrition messages

## Chapter 16

- Incorporates updated communication guidelines for educational interactions

## Chapter 18

- Includes updated statistics regarding healthcare coverage, Social Security spending, and Medicare spending

# ▶ Supplemental Resources

## For Instructors

Comprehensive online teaching resources are available to instructors adopting this *Third Edition*, including the following:

- Test Bank
- Slides in PowerPoint format
- Instructor's Manual, including annotated lecture outlines
- Answer Key for Case Study questions

## For Students

Robust study tools are available online for students, including the following:

- An Interactive eBook that contains Knowledge Check questions tied to every major heading in the text
- Interactive Flashcards that allow students to test their knowledge of key terms
- Slides in PowerPoint format that empower the student to review key chapter content

# Acknowledgments

The author's writing is one small part of the work involved in development and production of a text. Many people worked dexterously with a shared goal to produce a visually appealing, error-free, up-to-date, high-quality textbook. I would like to acknowledge the dedication and hard work of these individuals; without them this project would never have been realized.

A heartfelt thanks to Sean Fabery, Taylor Maurice, and Merideth Tumasz for their unwavering support and significant contributions, performing an astonishing job of keeping a very complex procedure progressing smoothly. Furthermore, Jones & Bartlett Learning is progressive in integrating technology with print materials for learning; the excellent web-based materials that are a part of *Community Nutrition* could not have been developed without this type of technical support.

A special thanks to my graduate students and the administrative assistants for their contributions to the preparation of this text and to my undergraduate students for their constructive feedback.

Finally, many community and public health instructors and researchers contributed significantly to the revision of this book. I am very grateful to the following reviewers who contributed their expertise and valuable direction to the development of this text:

- Bryce Abbey, PhD, University of Nebraska—Kearney
- Dorothy Chen Maynard, PhD, RD, FAND, California State University—San Bernardino
- Teresa Drake, PhD, RD, CHES, Bradley University
- Pamela E. Galasso, RDN, CDN, Gateway Community College
- Rachael Martin, MS, RDN, CED
- Tonia Reinhard, MS, RD, FAND, Wayne State University
- Derrick L. Sauls, PhD, Saint Augustine's University
- Vidya Sharma, MA, RD, LD, CDE, University of the Incarnate Word

- Jyotsna Sharman, PhD, MBA, RDN, Radford University
- Ahondju Umadjela Holmes, MS, RD/LD, Langston University
- Crystal Wynn, PhD, MPH, RD, Virginia State University

and the following experts who reviewed the *Second Edition*:

- Malinda D. Cecil, MS, RD, LDN, University of Maryland Eastern Shore
- Lydia Chowa, DrPH, RD, California State University
- Jessica L. Garay, MS, RD, George Washington University
- Cary Kreutzer, MPH, RD, California State University, Northridge
- Lisa Martin, MA, RD, CDE, Winthrop University
- Draughon McPherson, MEd, RD, LD, Delta State University
- Willie M. Singleton, MS, RD, Wayne County Community College
- Najat Yahia, PhD, LD, Central Michigan University

and the following experts who reviewed the *First Edition*:

- Mclanic Tracy Burns, PhD, RD, Eastern Illinois University
- Katherine L. Cason, PhD, RD, Clemson University
- Nancy Cotugna, PhD, RD, University of Delaware
- Lynn Duerr, PhD, RD, CD, Indiana State University
- Erin Francort, RD, Idaho State University
- Jeanne Florini, MS, RD, LD, St. Louis Community College at Florissant Valley
- Carol Friesen, PhD, RD, Ball State University
- Nancy Harris, MS, RD, LDN, FADA, East Carolina University
- Mary Mitchell, PhD, RD, Ohio State University
- Martha L. Rew, MS, RD, LD, Texas Woman's University

Thanks to all of you.

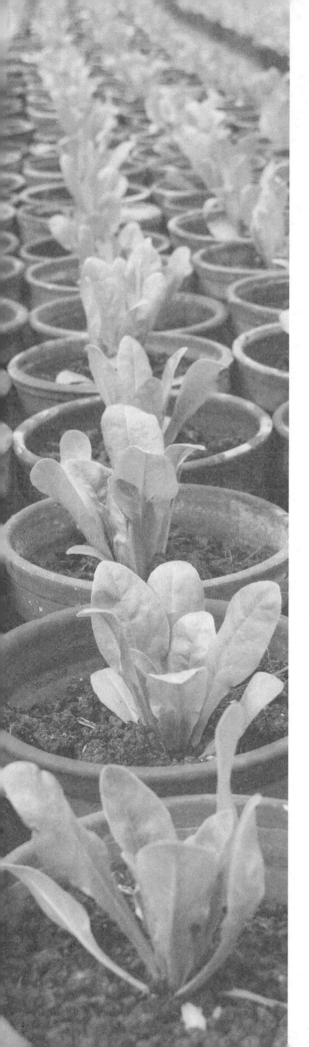

# PART I

# Overview of the Public Health Nutrition Landscape

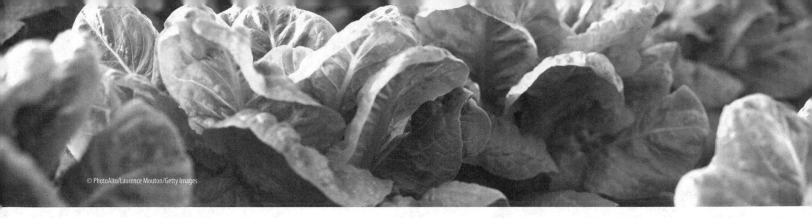

# CHAPTER 1

# Community Nutrition and Public Health

## CHAPTER OUTLINE

- Introduction
- The Concept of Community
- Public Health and Nutrition
- The Relationship Between Eating Behaviors and Chronic Diseases
- Reducing Risk Through Prevention
- Levels of Prevention
- Health Promotion
- Public and Community Health Objectives
- Canadian Health Promotion Objectives
- Historical U.S. National Health Objectives
- Healthy People in Healthy Communities
- Knowledge and Skills of Public Health and Community Nutritionists
- Places of Employment for Public Health and Community Nutritionists
- Ethics and Community Nutrition Professionals
- Preventive Nutrition
- Nutrition Care Process: Evidence-Based Practice
- The Cooperative Extension System

## LEARNING OBJECTIVES

- Define public health and community nutrition.
- Discuss the relationship between diet and diseases.
- List current nutrition- and diet-related public health problems.
- Explain primary, secondary, and tertiary prevention.
- Outline the educational requirements, practice settings, roles, and responsibilities of community and public health nutritionists.

*(continues)*

- Define the terms *Registered Dietitian (RD)* and *public health nutrition.*
- Discuss the role of Healthy People Objectives in health promotion and disease prevention.
- Explain the importance of the Academy of Nutrition and Dietetics Code of Ethics.
- Discuss the different steps of the Nutrition Care Process of the Academy of Nutrition and Dietetics.

## ▶ Introduction

**Community nutrition** is a modern and comprehensive profession that includes, but is not limited to, public health nutrition, dietetics and nutrition education, and medical nutrition therapy.[1] Community nutrition aims to improve the health of those people within a defined community. It deals with a variety of food and nutrition issues related to individuals, families, groups within the community, and special groups who have a common link such as place of residence, language, culture, or health issues.[2] An example of a successful community nutrition program using a special group was conducted in the city of Baltimore and six Maryland counties simultaneously. Over 2-year period, a multifaceted intervention program was carried out at 16 Special Supplemental Nutrition Program for Women, Infants, and Children (WIC) sites to increase fruit and vegetable consumption among the women. After 1 year of this intervention program[2] the amount of fruits and vegetable consumed increased. Changes in consumption were related to the number of nutrition sessions the participants attended.[2] There is an increasing need to focus on community in **health promotion** and disease prevention because behavior is highly influenced by the environment in which people live. Local values, norms, and behavior patterns have a significant effect on shaping an individual's attitudes and behaviors.[3,4] The increasing movement toward using a community approach requires community **nutritionists** to become more visible and vocal leaders of community health. However, before community nutritionists can participate in nutrition and healthcare planning, they must be knowledgeable about the concept of community as a client.

## ▶ The Concept of Community

The concept of **community** varies widely. The World Health Organization (WHO) defines community as "a social group determined by geographic boundaries and/or common values and interests."[5] Community members know and interact with one another; function within a particular social structure; and show and create norms, values, and social institutions.[6] Suburbs and other areas surrounding the legal limits of a city are also an integral part of that city's total community.[7]

A second definition of community is demographic and involves viewing the community as a subgroup of the population, such as people of a particular age, gender, social class, or race.[8] A community also can be defined on the basis of a common interest or goal. A collection of people, even if they are scattered geographically, can have a common interest that binds its members. This is called a common-interest community.[9] Many successful prevention and health promotion efforts, including improved services and increased community awareness of specific problems, have resulted from the work of common-interest communities. The following are some examples of common-interest communities[9]:

- Members of a national professional organization (e.g., Academy of Nutrition and Dietetics (formerly known as American Dietetic Association), American Medical Association, Federation of American Societies for Experimental Biology, African American Career Women, National Association of Asian American Professionals, American Public Health Association)
- Members of churches
- Disabled individuals scattered throughout a large city
- Individuals with a specific health condition (e.g., diabetes, hypertension, breast cancer, and mental illness)
- Teenage mothers
- Homebound elderly persons

Community nutrition and dietetics professionals are also members of a community and are public health agency professionals who provide nutrition services that emphasize community health promotion and disease prevention. They deal with the needs of individuals through primary, secondary, and tertiary preventions (which will be discussed in detail later in this chapter).

- **Primary prevention** involves designing activities to prevent a problem or disease before it occurs.
- **Secondary prevention** involves planning activities related to early diagnosis and treatment, including screening for diseases.

■ **Tertiary prevention** consists of designing activities to treat a disease state or injury and prevent it from progressing further.[10]

Community nutrition and dietetics professionals establish links with other professionals involved in a wide range of education and human services, such as childcare agencies, social work agencies, services for older persons, high schools, colleges and universities, homeless shelters, and community-based epidemiologic research.

▶ ## Public Health and Nutrition

**Public health** is defined as "the science and art of preventing disease, prolonging life, and promoting health and efficiency through organized community efforts, so organizing these benefits as to enable every citizen to realize his/her birthright of health and longevity."[11] It has been viewed as the scientific diagnosis and treatment of the community. In this vision, the community, instead of the individual, is seen as the patient. When the focus is on the community, patterns and processes begin to emerge and combine to form a unified whole.[12] Using this approach avoids focusing on risks and diseases; instead, the focus is on the community's strengths and resilience. Community strengths can be physiological, psychological, social, or spiritual. They include such factors as education, coping skills, support systems, knowledge, communication skills, nutrition, coherent belief systems, fitness, ability to develop a supportive environment, and self-care skills.[3]

Community nutritionists can utilize any of the community strengths to increase the nutrition knowledge of the community members, which can subsequently reduce medical care costs and improve quality of life.[13-16] The negative consequences of nutrition-related problems include malnutrition and chronic health conditions such as obesity, cardiovascular disease, cancer, and diabetes mellitus.[17,18] In addition, these conditions contribute significantly to the world's burden of morbidity, incapacity, and mortality, despite the tremendous amount of biological knowledge accumulated over the years.[18] The WHO estimated that prevention of the major nutrition-related risk factors (high fat, sodium, and sugar intake; cigarette smoking; inactivity; poor dietary behavior; and alcohol abuse) could translate into a gain of 5 years of disability-free life expectancy.[19,20]

A community and **public health nutrition** approach will make it possible to reverse the course of major nutrition problems.[21,22] Dietetics professionals can take the lead in prevention programming because their training as counselors and educators provides skills that make them important members of the public health profession.

Public health nutrition was developed in the United States in response to societal events and changes to the following situations[1,23,24]:

■ Infant mortality
■ Access to healthcare
■ Epidemics of communicable disease
■ Poor hygiene and sanitation
■ Malnutrition
■ Agriculture and changes in food production
■ Economic depression, wars, and civil rights issues
■ Aging of the population
■ Behavior-related problems or lifestyle (poor dietary practices, alcohol abuse, inactivity, and cigarette smoking)
■ Chronic diseases (obesity, heart disease, diabetes mellitus, mental health, cancer, osteoporosis, and hypertension)
■ Poverty and immigration
■ Preschool and after-school childcare and school-based meals
■ Ebola virus
■ Zika virus

▶ ## The Relationship Between Eating Behaviors and Chronic Diseases

As evidenced by an introductory review of the literature and research in the area of eating behavior and chronic disease, the relationship between eating behaviors and chronic diseases is significant and affects individuals and communities greatly.[25] **TABLE 1-1** shows dietary factors linked to some of the most common chronic diseases. It is important to note that dietary factors overlap with multiple problems and are applicable to many of the health conditions listed.

The *Surgeon General's Report on Nutrition and Health*, government agencies, and nonprofit health and scientific organizations have provided comprehensive analyses of the relationships among diet, lifestyle, and major chronic diseases.[26-28] Health conditions such as coronary heart disease, stroke, cancer, and diabetes are still the leading causes of death and disability in the United States and globally, and changes in current dietary practices could produce substantial health gains.

There have been concerns about the eating patterns of the U.S. population since the 1980s. Health policy makers have linked several dietary-related factors to chronic diseases, such as heart disease, cancer, birth defects, and osteoporosis, among the U.S. population

**TABLE 1-1** Some Possible Health Problems Linked with Dietary Habits

| Beneficial Behavior | Risk for Heart Disease | Risk for Some Cancers | Risk for Diabetes | Risk for Obesity | Risk for Osteoporosis | Risk for Birth Defects | Risk for High Blood Pressure | Risk for Anemia |
|---|---|---|---|---|---|---|---|---|
| Eat foods lower in total fat, saturated fat, and cholesterol | ✓ | ✓ | ✓ | ✓ | | | ✓ | |
| Eat foods lower in calories; balance caloric intake with physical activity | ✓ | ✓ | ✓ | ✓ | | | ✓ | |
| Drink alcohol in moderation | ✓ | ✓ | | | | | | |
| Eat less cured and smoked foods | | ✓ | | | | | | |
| Prepare foods with less salt | ✓ | | | | | | ✓ | |
| Eat foods high in calcium and vitamin D | ✓ | | | | ✓ | | ✓ | |
| Eat foods high in iron | ✓ | ✓ | | | | | | ✓ |
| Eat foods high in folic acid | ✓ | ✓ | ✓ | | | ✓ | | ✓ |
| Eat foods high in antioxidants | ✓ | ✓ | ✓ | | ✓ | ✓ | | |
| Eat foods high in soluble and insoluble fiber | ✓ | ✓ | ✓ | ✓ | | ✓ | ✓ | ✓ |
| Eat foods high in omega-3 fatty acids | | ✓ | ✓ | | | ✓ | | |
| Breastfeed infants | | | | | | | | |

and that of other industrialized countries.[25,29] This link between diet and disease has led to the publication of guidelines to promote healthier eating habits. The National Academy of Sciences, the U.S. Department of Health and Human Services, and the U.S. Surgeon General have published the majority of these guidelines, which are discussed later in this chapter.[11,12,30,31]

In addition to dietary intake, many other factors contribute to chronic diseases, such as genetic factors and lifestyle factors (e.g., cigarette smoking).[31] Medical geneticists working on the Human Genome Project, a major international initiative to decipher the 3-billion-unit code of DNA in the 80,000 to 100,000 genes found in humans, have already identified genes associated with many chronic diseases, such as breast, colon, and prostate cancers; severe obesity; and diabetes.[32–35]

Programs to promote health and longevity start with examining the major causes of death and disability. The top causes of death according to the National Center for Health Statistics and Global Statistics and the WHO's 2012 and 2015 data are presented in **BOXES 1-1** and **1-2**.[36,37]

The public health approach to prevention understands that the reduction of risk for individuals with average risk profiles might be small or negligible. However,

---

**BOX 1-1**  The 10 Leading Causes of Death in the United States

1. Heart disease
2. Cancer
3. Chronic lower respiratory tract disease
4. Accidents (unintentional injuries)
5. Stroke (cerebrovascular disease)
6. Alzheimer's disease
7. Diabetes
8. Influenza and pneumonia
9. Nephritis, nephrotic syndrome, and nephrosis
10. Intentional self-harm (suicide)

Reproduced from: National Center for Health Statistics. Leading causes of death. http://www.cdc.gov/nchs/fastats/leading-causes-of-death.htm. Accessed March 2, 2016.

---

**BOX 1-2**  The 10 Leading Causes of Death Worldwide

1. Ischemic heart disease
2. Cerebrovascular disease
3. Acute lower respiratory tract infections
4. HIV and AIDS
5. Chronic obstructive pulmonary disease
6. Diarrheal diseases
7. Tuberculosis
8. Malaria
9. Cancer of the trachea, bronchus, or lung
10. Road traffic accidents

Data from: World Health Organization (WHO). The top 10 causes of death. http://www.who.int/mediacentre/factsheets/fs310/en/index.html. Accessed March 2, 2016.

---

high-risk persons need special attention through primary, secondary, and tertiary preventions. Although it may not eliminate a disease for people who are genetically inclined to it, good primary prevention strategies could reduce the severity of the disease.[38]

## ▸ Reducing Risk Through Prevention

Prevention is important in public health as well as community nutrition practice. The three important parts of prevention are personal, community-based, and systems-based.[6] Each part has a different role and focus. Establishing an overall effective community nutrition practice involves correctly using and combining each part.

Personal prevention involves people at the individual level—for instance, educating and supporting a breastfeeding mother to promote the health of her infant.

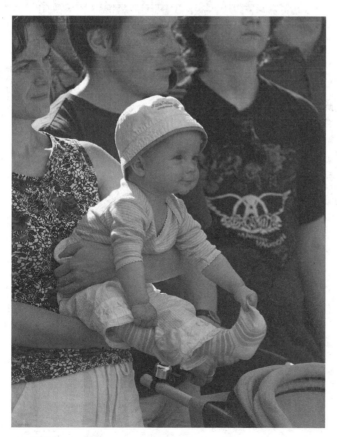

Public speaking is a great way to pass along nutrition information.

© Dariush M./ShutterStock, Inc.

Community-based prevention targets groups—for example, public campaigns for low-fat diets to decrease the incidences of obesity and heart disease.[39,40]

Systems-based prevention deals with changing policies and laws to achieve the objectives of prevention practice, such as laws regarding childhood immunization, food labels, food safety, and sanitation.

One part of systems-based prevention deals with socioeconomic status, which affects health through environmental or behavioral factors. The socioeconomic model hypothesizes that poor families do not have the economic, social, or community resources needed to be in good health. For instance, poverty affects children's well-being by influencing health and nutrition, the home environment, and neighborhood conditions.[41,42] The combined effects of poverty provide the foundation for a cycle of poverty and hopelessness among family members, who in turn engage in risky health behaviors, such as substance abuse, smoking, and poor dietary habits, that can result in obesity and nutrition-related chronic diseases.

Socioeconomic models have been used to develop policies and disease prevention strategies, such as the Mackenbach model, that can be used as a basis for developing policies and intervention strategies. **FIGURE 1-1** presents the link between socioeconomic status and health-related problems triggered and maintained by two processes (selective and causative) that are active during different periods of life.[43] The selective process is represented by childhood health, which determines adult health as well as socioeconomic position. The

causative process represents three groups of risk factors (lifestyle, structural or environmental, and psychosocial stress–related factors), which are intermediaries between socioeconomic position and health problems. The model also acknowledges that childhood environment and cultural and psychological factors contribute to inequalities in health through both selection and causation. Health inequalities become self-perpetuating through a cycle of inadequate childhood health, adult socioeconomic position, and incidence of health problems at adult ages.[43]

# ▶ Levels of Prevention

Each part of prevention itself has three levels. *Primary prevention* is an early intervention focused on controlling risk factors or preventing diseases before they happen, thus reducing their incidence. Examples of primary prevention include fortifying milk with vitamin D to prevent rickets in children, fortifying infant formula with iron to prevent anemia, and fluoridating public water supplies to prevent dental decay. *Secondary prevention* includes identifying disease early (before clinical signs and symptoms manifest) through screening. Timely intervention is provided to deter the disease process and prevent disability that may be caused by the disease. For instance, providing **nutrition education** on the importance of reducing dietary cholesterol, saturated fat, and caloric intake and increasing dietary fiber to individuals with high blood cholesterol is a secondary

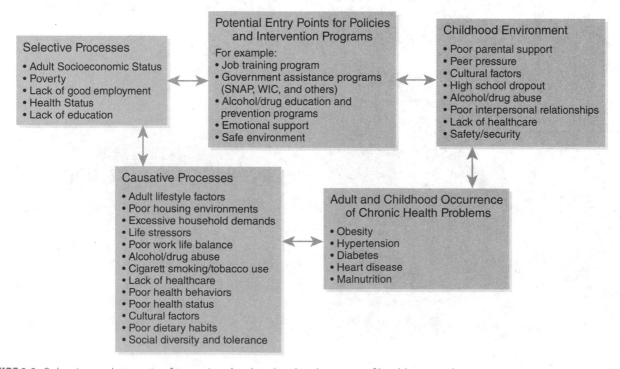

**FIGURE 1-1** Selective and causative factors involved in the development of health inequalities in society.
Modified from: Mackenbach J, Bakker M. *Reducing inequalities in health: A European perspective.* London: Routledge; 2002:18.

intervention to prevent the complications of heart disease.[15,44–46] *Tertiary prevention* is intervention to reduce the severity of diagnosed health conditions to prevent or delay disability and death. For example, providing education programs for persons recently diagnosed with hypertension is an intervention to prevent disability and additional health problems.[47] **FIGURE 1-2** presents the three levels of prevention and intervention approaches.

**FIGURE 1-3** shows that a natural progression of a disease starts at the induction or initiation period. It also shows the relationship between disease progression and level of intervention. Early intervention (primary prevention) can reduce disease progression in its early stages. For example, for bacterial infections (such as *Escherichia coli*), the incubation period is an early stage of disease development in which individuals are not yet feeling the infection's effects. Also, an intervention such as a structured daily physical activity can slow weight gain and prevent obesity. Latency or dormancy is a similar early period when a disease (e.g., cardiovascular

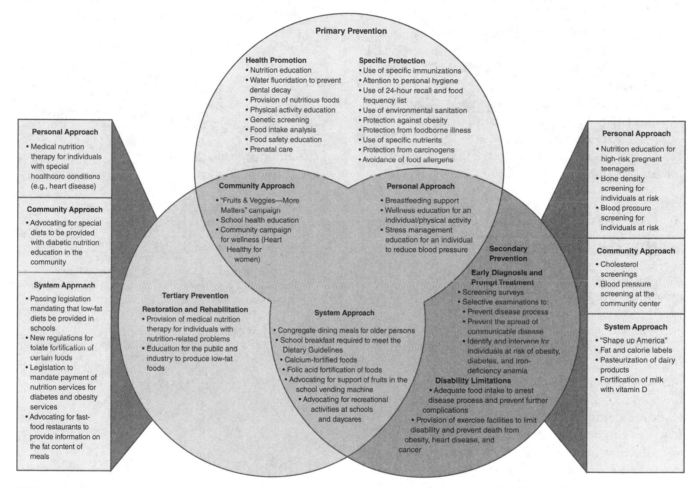

**FIGURE 1-2** The three levels of prevention and intervention approaches.

Adapted from: Mandle CL. *Health Promotion Throughout the Lifespan.* 5th ed. St. Louis, MO: Mosby; 2002. Public Health Nutrition Practice Group, 1995; and Owen AL, Splett PL, Owen GM. *Nutrition in the Community.* 4th ed. New York, NY: McGraw-Hill; 1999.

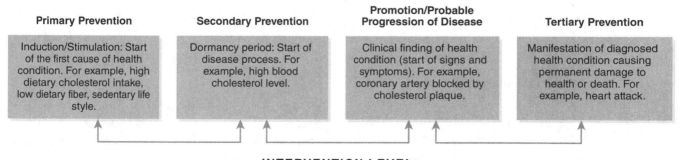

**INTERVENTION LEVEL**

**FIGURE 1-3** Levels of epidemiologic research: a conceptual elaboration.

Modified from: Kleinbaum DG, Kupper LL. *Epidemiologic Research: Principles and Quantitative Methods Solution Manual.* New York, NY: Van Nostrand Reinhold. Reprinted with permission of John Wiley & Sons; 1982:22.

disease) has the potential of being expressed. Secondary prevention, such as blood pressure screening, will detect clinical symptoms and can help prevent the progression of a disease. The expression period is when the disease has occurred. At this point an intervention (tertiary prevention) is provided to reduce the severity of the disease or prevent death; for example, a person could reduce dietary fat intake to manage heart disease.[1]

## ▶ Health Promotion

Health promotion is another major concept important to community and public health nutrition. Health promotion can be defined as the process of enabling people to increase control over the determinants of good health and subsequently improve their health.[24] Two strategies that can be used to design a health promotion campaign to reduce risk are presented in **TABLE 1-2**, and the advantages and disadvantages of these strategies are presented in **BOX 1-3**.

## ▶ Public and Community Health Objectives

Around the world, health promotion has proved to be an effective strategy for improving health and preventing chronic health conditions. Health promotion approaches can change lifestyles and have an impact on the social, economic, and environmental conditions that determine health.[47] The WHO is the leader in promoting health and preventing diseases throughout the world. In 1978, the WHO and the United Nations Children's Fund (UNICEF) held a conference at Alma-Ata, Union of Soviet Socialist Republics (USSR), and declared that health is more than the absence of disease; the attainment of the highest possible level of health is a vital worldwide social goal. In 1981, the Alma-Ata Declaration prompted the development of the Global Strategy for Health for All by the Year 2000. The major themes were as follows[48]:

- Equity in health
- Health promotion
- Enhancing preventive activity in primary healthcare settings
- Cooperation among government, community, and the private sector
- Increasing community participation

The Alma-Ata Declaration provided a good theoretical base and an ethical or moral imperative for developing a primary healthcare approach, but the framework for action was not clear. The WHO, in collaboration with

---

**BOX 1-3** Advantages and Disadvantages of Population and Individual Health Promotion Strategies

### Advantages
*Population Approach*
- The population approach may instigate a behavior change that may become the norm and create conditions that make it easier for any individual to change. For example, if everyone is urged to reduce fat and saturated fat intake, this increases the incentive for the food industry to develop and market products that are low in fat and/or saturated fat, such as low-fat milk, which makes it easier to adopt a low-fat diet.
- The population approach is likely to save more lives and prevent more illness than the individual approach when the risk factors are widely diffused throughout the community.

*Individual Approach*
- Using the individual approach, people at high risk are specifically targeted and the intervention is provided on time. More attention is given to ensuring that individuals with chronic disease are following necessary, strict dietary programs.
- Using the individual approach reduces the costs associated with screening an entire population and releases health professionals to attend to the community's other healthcare needs.

### Disadvantages
*Population Approach*
- This approach requires mass change and may not be needed by the entire population.
- It may not be cost-effective and may inconvenience people.

*Individual Approach*
- With the individual approach, screening may not be universal and thus some high-risk individuals may not be identified.

Data from: Webb G. *Nutrition: A Health Promotion Approach*. 2nd ed. New York, NY: Arnold; 2002.

---

other organizations, subsequently co-sponsored international conferences on health promotion, which are presented in **TABLE 1-3**.

In 2000, the global community made a commitment, known as the Millennium Development Goals (MDGs), to eliminate extreme poverty and hunger and improve the health of the world's poorest people within 15 years. The eight goals agreed upon by the 191 United Nations member nations were to be achieved by 2015, and the outcomes are shown in **TABLE 1-4**.[51]

**TABLE 1-2** Strategies for Designing a Health Promotion Campaign

|  | Concept | Benefit | Example |
|---|---|---|---|
| Population | Instruction is directed at the entire population (national, local community, schools, and neighborhoods) with messages and programs aimed at reducing behavioral risk factors, such as poor eating habits or physical inactivity. | Members of the community may lower their risk by a small percentage, thereby reducing new cases of chronic health conditions and mortality. | A nutritionist changing the eating patterns of families and advocating for fluoridation of the water supply—rather than screening all postmenopausal women for bone loss or hiring dentists to treat every child and adolescent—may reduce the risk for osteoporosis and dental decay.<br><br>Instruction about reducing sodium intake may reduce a population's mean systolic blood pressure by 3 percent, which will decrease the number of people in the high-risk group by 25 percent if high risk for systolic blood pressure is considered to begin at 140 mm Hg.<br><br>If excess body weight is 92 kg/202 pounds, reducing the population's mean weight by 1 kg/2.2 pounds (approximately 1 percent) will cut the number of overweight people by 25 percent.<br><br>Instruction could be provided to engage in regular physical activity and reduce excess calorie consumption.<br><br>If everyone is encouraged to consume high-calcium and/or low-fat food products and then food industries develop and market these food products, this will subsequently prevent osteoporosis and obesity.<br><br>The Fruits & Veggies—More Matters campaign is an example of a population approach to health promotion. |
| Individual | The nutritionist focuses on identifying individuals at risk, and the intervention is directed specifically at these "high-risk" individuals. | This method may be more beneficial when the risk conditions are highly restricted, such as with preschool children who were exposed to foods containing lead. | Intervention could be limited to persons with family histories of heart disease, and these people could be taught about reducing fat intake and increasing physical activities to reduce the potential of experiencing heart disease.<br><br>Nutrition intervention could be limited to the children of adult alcoholics, individuals with a family history of diabetes, and low-income pregnant women participating in the Special Supplemental Nutrition Program for Women, Infants, and Children (WIC), which may translate to risk reduction. |

Data from: Webb G. *Nutrition: A Health Promotion Approach*. 2nd ed. New York, NY: Arnold; 2002.

**TABLE 1-3** The Sequence and Outcome of International Conferences on Health Promotion[49,50]

| Year | Title | City, Country | Health Promotion Outcomes |
|------|-------|---------------|---------------------------|
| 1986 | First International Conference on Health Promotion | Ottawa, Canada | ▪ Build healthy public policy<br>▪ Create supportive environments<br>▪ Develop personal skills<br>▪ Strengthen community action<br>▪ Reorient health services |
| 1988 | Second International Conference on Healthy Public Policy | Adelaide, Australia | ▪ A call for action: Health promotion in developing countries |
| 1991 | Third International Conference on Health Promotion | Sundsvall, Sweden | ▪ Addressed the issue of millions of people who are living in extreme poverty and deprivation in degraded environments that threaten their health, making the goal of Health for All by the Year 2000 very difficult to achieve |
| 1997 | Fourth International Conference on Health Promotion | Jakarta, Indonesia | ▪ Leading health promotion into the 21st century<br>▪ The first to be held in a developing country and the first to involve the private sector in supporting health promotion<br>▪ Reflected on what had been learned about effective health promotion, reexamined determinants of health, and identified the directions and strategies required to address the challenges of promoting health in the 21st century<br>▪ Five priorities for health promotion in the 21st century were:<br>  • Promote social responsibility for health<br>  • Increase investments for health development<br>  • Consolidate and expand partnerships for health<br>  • Increase community capacity and empower the individual<br>  • Secure an infrastructure for health promotion |
| 2000 | Fifth Global Conference on Health Promotion | Mexico City, Mexico | ▪ Discussed how health promotion addressing the social determinants of health can help improve the lives of economically and socially disadvantaged populations |
| 2005 | Sixth Global Conference on Health Promotion | Bangkok, Thailand | ▪ Identified actions, commitments, and pledges required to address the determinants of health in a globalized world through health promotion<br>▪ The WHO indicated that the workplace has been established as one of the priority settings for health promotion into the 21st century because it influences physical, mental, economic, and social well-being and offers an ideal setting and infrastructure to support the promotion of health for a large audience. For example, in a review of comprehensive health promotion and disease management programs at the worksite, Pelletier[98] reported positive clinical and cost results. |

**TABLE 1-4** The Millennium Development Goals Progress Report[51]

| Goal | Progress |
| --- | --- |
| To eradicate extreme poverty and hunger | It was reported that poverty reduced significantly in 2015 to 836 million from 1.9 billion. |
| To achieve universal primary education | The progress report showed that primary school enrollment increased in 2015 from 83 percent to 91 percent. |
| To promote gender equality and empower women | Though gender inequality and discrimination against women continues, there was a slight increase in paid employment not including agricultural from 35 percent to 41 percent. |
| To reduce child mortality | Report shows that global mortality rate for children less than 5 years old reduced significantly from 12.7 to 6 million. |
| To improve maternal health | In 2015, the ratio of maternal mortality rate reduced by 45 percent; however globally maternal mortality rate continues to be high. |
| To combat HIV and AIDS, malaria, and other diseases | It was reported that newly diagnosed HIV infections decreased from estimated 3.5 million cases to 2.1 million.<br>The rate of malaria reduced by approximately 37 percent and mortality rate by 58 percent.<br>Report shows that tuberculosis mortality rate reduced by 45 percent and the prevalence rate by 41 percent between 1999 and 2013. |
| To ensure environmental sustainability | It was reported that ninety eight percent of ozone-depleting substances was eradicated in 1990. |
| To develop a global partnership for development | Report shows that imports from developing to developed countries were permitted duty free, which increased from 65 to 79 percent. |

Source: United Nations Organization. The Millennium Development Goals Report 2015 Summary. 2016. http://www.un.org/millenniumgoals/2015_MDG_Report/pdf/MDG%202015%20 Summary%20web_english.pdf. Accessed February 24, 2016.

# ▶ Canadian Health Promotion Objectives

In Canada, preventable chronic diseases such as cardiovascular diseases, cancer, and type 2 diabetes have increased, causing a push for more health promotion at worksites to reduce the incidence of these conditions. These chronic diseases have common risk factors, including physical inactivity, poor dietary habits, and the use of tobacco.[52] In addition, environmental factors such as personal health practices, income, employment, education, geographic isolation, and social exclusion contribute to these chronic diseases.[53] In 2002, Canada's federal, provincial, and territorial governments expressed the need for a pan-Canadian healthy living approach. Therefore, an extensive consultation process, including a national symposium, was organized to develop a Healthy Living Strategy. The target for the pan-Canadian Healthy Living Strategy was to obtain a 20 percent increase in the proportion of Canadians who are physically active, eat healthily, and are at healthy body weights. The targets of the Healthy Living Strategy are as follows[52,54,55]:

- *Healthy eating:* Proportion of children (ages 12 to 17) who reported they consumed fruit or vegetables at least five times per day showed no improvement, 45.5% from 2011 to 2012 and 43.9% in 2013.
- *Physical activity:* Proportion of children and youth (ages 5 to 17) who met physical activity guidelines by accumulating at least 60 minutes of moderate to vigorous physical activity per day increased from 4.4% to 9.3% between 2012 and 2013.
- *Healthy weights:* Proportion of children (ages 5 to 17 years) who are overweight (measured body mass index [BMI]), WHO cutoffs decreased from 19.8% to 18.6% in 2015.

- The objectives of the overall Healthy Living Strategy are[54]:
  - Increased prevalence of healthy weights—achieved through healthy means among Canadians
  - Increased levels of regular physical activity among Canadians
  - Improved healthy eating practices and activity levels among Canadians, particularly infants, children, and youth
  - Increased access to affordable healthy food choices, appropriate physical activity facilities, and opportunities for at-risk and vulnerable communities
  - Improved infrastructure and neighborhood design that supports opportunities for healthy eating and physical activity
  - Reduced health disparities

A progress report in 2005 showed 50 percent of Canadians ages 18 years or older reported that they were at least moderately active. Results also revealed that 42 percent of Canadians ages 18 or older reported that they consumed fruits and vegetables five or more times per day. In addition, the BMI of almost half (47.4 percent) of Canadian adults was in the normal range. The calculation is that by 2015, Canadians ages 18 or older would be accumulating at least 30 minutes a day of moderate physical activity, 50.4 percent would report that they consumed fruits and vegetables five or more times per day, and 56.88 percent would be in the normal BMI range.[56]

Reports such as the Lalonde Report (*A New Perspective on the Health of Canadians*, 1974), *Achieving Health for All* (1986), and the 1988 *Ottawa Charter on Health Promotion* have helped advance knowledge about the effect of people's lifestyles and socioeconomic circumstances on their health and well-being.[56]

# ▶ Historical U.S. National Health Objectives

In the United States, health promotion and disease prevention have been public health strategies since the late 1970s and health promotion at worksites is increasing. Interest in how dietary excesses and imbalances increase the risk for chronic diseases also began in the 1970s. In 1979, Healthy People: The Surgeon General's Report on Health Promotion and Disease Prevention provided nutritional goals for reducing premature deaths and preserving older adult independence. This publication also directed attention toward environmental and behavioral changes that Americans might make to reduce risks for morbidity and mortality.[26] The 1980 report Promoting Health/Preventing Disease: Objectives for the Nation

contained 226 objectives and provided the foundation for a national prevention agenda. It included 17 specific, quantifiable objectives in nutrition designed to reduce risks and prevent illness and death by 1990.[56] The objectives were grouped into the categories of improvement in health status, reduction of risks to health, increased awareness, improved and expanded preventive health services, and improved surveillance.[57] This effort was moderately successful. Three of the four mortality-related goals were met or exceeded. Specifically, the infant and adult mortality goals were met, and the childhood mortality target was significantly exceeded. The mortality goal for adolescents was not met due to high rates of both unintentional (motor vehicle accidents) and intentional (homicide) fatal injuries in this age group.[57]

The 1988 Surgeon General's Report on Nutrition and Health stimulated health promotion and disease prevention actions. Detailed information on dietary practices and health status was included in this report, which also included specific science-based health recommendations. It included implications for the individual and for future public health policy decisions. This report is still a useful reference and tool for nutrition-related health promotion.[26,30,58] In the late 1980s, the Public Health Service and a team of health educators and U.S. government officials analyzed the results of research studies, reports, and recommendations that summarized the health status of Americans. Subsequently, in 1991, these experts published their findings in a report called Healthy People 2000: The National Health Promotion and Disease Prevention Objectives. This document contained the following three general goals[21]:

- Increase the span of healthy life
- Reduce health disparities among Americans
- Achieving access to preventive services

The majority of the 27 nutrition objectives were either met or at least moved toward their year 2000 targets. However, for some objectives the progress was modest and for others there was movement away from the targets; for example, smoking during pregnancy increased among teenagers, with significant increases among African American and Puerto Rican teens. On the positive side, the prevalence of high blood cholesterol among people ages 20 to 74 years decreased to a level that met its target. Growth retardation among low-income children ages 5 years or younger exceeded its target, declining from 11 percent in 1987 to 8 percent in 1999. The percentage of elementary and secondary schools offering low-fat choices for breakfast and lunch increased noticeably, although by the end of the decade, only about one in five schools offered lunches that met goals for total fat and saturated fat content. Other nutrition objectives also showed improvement during the

1990s. The average fat intake among people age 2 years or older declined and the proportion of the population who consumed no more than 30 percent of calories from fat increased. The availability of reduced-fat processed foods increased to such an extent that the 2000 target was surpassed early in the decade. Informative nutrition labeling was found on more processed foods, fresh produce, and fresh seafood. Similar labeling of fresh meat and poultry, however, decreased.[59]

## ▶ Healthy People in Healthy Communities

A healthy community embraces the belief that health is more than merely an absence of disease. A healthy community includes those elements that enable people to maintain a high quality of life and productivity. For example, a healthy community offers access to healthcare services that focus on both treatment and prevention for all members of the community in a secure environment.[60]

### Healthy People 2010

The continued success of Healthy People 2000 encouraged the creation of a new set of objectives to be achieved by 2010. **Healthy People 2010** was designed to serve as a roadmap for improving the health of all people in the United States. It included national health promotion and disease prevention goals, objectives, and measures that served as a model for nutrition and health practitioners to develop their own goals and objectives and improve the health of everyone in the community.[35,61] Healthy People 2010 was designed to achieve the following two overarching goals[61]:

- Increase the quality and years of healthy life
- Eliminate health disparities. (A health disparity is a gap in the health status of different groups of people in which one group is healthier than the other group or groups.)

These two goals were supported by 467 objectives in 28 specific focus areas, including cancer; diabetes; nutrition and overweight; access to quality health services; food safety; maternal, infant, and child health; heart disease; and stroke. The focus areas are presented in **TABLE 1-5**.[46] The major challenge of Healthy People 2010 was balancing a broad set of health objectives with a smaller set of health priorities. Consequently, the 10 leading health indicators presented in **TABLE 1-6** served as a link to the original 467 objectives in Healthy People 2010 and have served as the foundation for many state and community health initiatives. They included national health promotion and disease prevention goals, objectives, and measures that helped serve as a model for nutrition and health

practitioners to develop their own goals and objectives to improve the health of everyone in the community.

The Leading Health Indicators reflected the major public health concerns in the United States and were chosen based on their ability to motivate action, the availability of data to measure their progress, and their relevance as broad public health issues. Furthermore, some states and communities used the Leading Health Indicators as a framework to plan programs directed at promoting health and preventing diseases.

### Healthy People Progress Report

An important part of Healthy People 2010 was assessing progress toward the targeted objectives. The first goal of Healthy People 2010 was to help individuals of all ages increase quality and years of healthy life. A review of the data shows that years of life measured in terms of life expectancy increased. However, significant gender, racial, and ethnic differences exist. Women continue to live longer than men. African American men and women are still behind Caucasian American men and women in

**TABLE 1-5** Healthy People 2010 Focus Areas[46]

1. Access to Quality Health Services
2. Arthritis, Osteoporosis, and Chronic Back Conditions
3. Cancer
4. Chronic Kidney Disease
5. Diabetes
6. Disability and Secondary Conditions
7. Educational and Community- Based Programs
8. Environmental Health
9. Family Planning
10. Food Safety
11. Health Communication
12. Heart Disease and Stroke
13. HIV
14. Immunization and Infectious Diseases
15. Injury and Violence Prevention
16. Maternal, Infant, and Child Health
17. Medical Product Safety
18. Mental Health and Mental Disorders
19. Nutrition and Overweight
20. Occupational Safety and Health
21. Oral Health
22. Physical Activity and Fitness
23. Public Health Infrastructure
24. Respiratory Diseases
25. Sexually Transmitted Diseases
26. Substance Abuse
27. Tobacco Use
28. Vision and Hearing

Source: U.S. Department of Health and Human Services, Healthy People 2010. http://www.health.gov/healthypeople/. Accessed February 20, 2017.

**TABLE 1-6**  The Objectives and Subobjectives Used to Track Progress Toward the Leading Health Indicators

| Objectives | Leading Health Indicators |
|---|---|
| **Physical Activity**<br>Objective 22-2 | Increase the proportion of adults who engage in moderate physical activity for at least 30 minutes per day 5 or more days per week or vigorous physical activity for at least 20 minutes per day 3 or more days per week. |
| Objective 22-7 | Increase the proportion of adolescents who engage in vigorous physical activity that promotes cardiorespiratory fitness 3 or more days per week for 20 or more minutes per occasion. |
| **Overweight and Obesity**<br>Objective 19-2 | Reduce the proportion of adults who are obese. |
| Objective 19-3c | Reduce the proportion of children and adolescents ages 6–19 who are overweight or obese. |
| **Tobacco Use**<br>Objective 27-1a | Reduce tobacco use by adults—cigarette smoking. |
| Objective 27-1b | Reduce tobacco use by adolescents—cigarette smoking. |
| **Substance Abuse**<br>Objective 26-10a | Increase the proportion of adolescents not using alcohol or any illicit drugs during the past 30 days. |
| Objective 26-10c | Reduce the proportion of adults using any illicit drug during the past 30 days. |
| Objective 26-11c | Reduce the proportion of persons ages 18 years or older engaging in binge drinking of alcoholic beverages. |
| **Responsible Sexual Behavior**<br>Objective 13-6 | Increase the proportion of sexually active persons who use condoms. |
| Objective 25-11 | Increase the proportion of adolescents who abstain from sexual intercourse or use condoms. |
| **Mental Health**<br>Objective 18-9b | Increase the proportion of adults ages 18 years or older with recognized depression who receive treatment. |
| **Injury and Violence**<br>Objective 15-5 | Reduce deaths caused by motor vehicle crashes. |
| Objective 15-32 | Reduce homicides. |
| **Environmental Quality**<br>Objective 8-1a | Reduce the proportion of persons exposed to air that does not meet the U.S. Environmental Protection Agency's health-based standards for harmful air pollutants—ozone. |
| Objective 27-10 | Reduce the proportion of nonsmokers exposed to environmental tobacco smoke. |
| **Immunization**<br>Objective 14-24 | Increase the proportion of young children and adolescents who receive all vaccines that have been recommended for universal administration for at least 5 years. |
| Objective 14-29a | Increase the proportion of noninstitutionalized adults who are vaccinated annually against influenza. |
| Objective 14-29b | Increase the proportion of noninstitutionalized adults who are ever vaccinated against pneumococcal disease. |

| TABLE 1-6 | The Objectives and Subobjectives Used to Track Progress Toward the Leading Health Indicators (continued) |
|---|---|
| **Objectives** | **Leading Health Indicators** |
| **Access to Health-care** | |
| Objective 1-1 | Increase the proportion of persons with health insurance. |
| Objective 1-4a | Increase the proportion of persons of all ages who have a specific source of ongoing care. |
| Objective 16-6a | Increase the proportion of pregnant women who receive early and adequate prenatal care beginning in the first trimester. |

Source: U.S. Department of Health and Human Services. http://www.health.gov/healthypeople/. Accessed March 04, 2016.

overall life expectancy, although the average number of years lived for African American men and women has increased. Although U.S. life expectancy has increased, the life expectancy in other developed countries is still higher.

The second national goal for Healthy People 2010 was the elimination of health disparities related to social disadvantage in the United States. Disparities in deaths and risk factors for death remain unchanged among Caucasian Americans and minorities in mortality, morbidity, health insurance coverage, and the use of health services.[62] According to national data from the period 2003 to 2006[63]:

- The proportion of young people ages 6 to 19 years who were overweight or obese was 17 percent, an increase from 11 percent.
- The age-adjusted proportion of adults ages 20 years or older whose weight was in the healthy range was 32 percent, a decrease from 42 percent; the 2010 target was 60 percent. This downward trend in healthy weight carries across all demographic groups for whom data were collected, including Mexican American, non-Hispanic black, and non-Hispanic white. The trend also prevails across genders and income levels.
- The age-adjusted proportion of adults ages 20 years or older who were obese (BMI of 30 or more) was 33 percent, with a baseline of 23 percent; the target was 15 percent. Increases in this proportion were evident in all racial and ethnic groups for whom data were collected, including Mexican Americans (rising from 29 percent to 35 percent over that period), African Americans (from 30 percent to 45 percent), and Caucasian Americans (from 22 percent to 32 percent).
- Overweight and obesity in children ages 6 to 11 years increased from 11 percent to 17 percent. In adolescents ages 12 to 19 years, the increase over the same period was from 11 percent to 18 percent. The proportion of children and adolescents who were overweight or obese increased for all racial and ethnic groups surveyed.

- The proportion of people age 2 years or older (age-adjusted) who ate at least two servings of fruit per day increased slightly from 39 percent to 40 percent. The target was 75 percent.
- There was little or no change in the proportion of the population meeting the criteria for vegetable intake of at least three daily servings, with at least one-third being dark green or orange.

Data on the achievement of past **Healthy People Objectives** are presented in **TABLE 1-7**.

## Healthy People 2020

As with earlier Healthy People initiatives, Healthy People 2020 is a national health agenda that communicates a vision and a strategy for improving the health of the U.S. population and achieving health equity for the next decade. Healthy People 2020 retains the practice of previous Healthy People initiatives of promoting and improving the health of every individual in the United States. Healthy People 2020 is designed to make health determinants a primary focus and healthcare a secondary focus.[63]

Health determinants are the variety of personal, social, economic, and environmental factors that determine the health status of individuals or populations. They are embedded in our social and physical environments. *Social determinants* include family, community, income, education, sex, race/ethnicity, geographic location, and access to healthcare, among others. *Physical determinants* include our natural and built environments, exposure to toxins (e.g., coal tar), manmade pollutants, or substandard housing.

The vision of Healthy People 2020 is a society in which all people live long, healthy lives. Its mission includes the following:

- Improve health through strengthening policy and practice
- Identify nationwide health improvement priorities

**TABLE 1-7** Recent Data on Achievement of Past Healthy People Objectives[63]

| Most Recent Data | Number of Objectives/ Targets | Achieved Target (%) | Progressed Toward Target (%) | Showed No Progress or Regressed from Target (%) | Data Unavailable (%) |
|---|---|---|---|---|---|
| 1990 Health Objectives (Final Review) NCHS, 1992 | 226 objectives, 266 targets* | 32 | 34 | 11 | 23 |
| Healthy People 2000[†] (Final Review) NCHS, 2001 | 319 | 21 | 41 | 17 | 10 |
| Healthy People 2010 (Midcourse Review) HHS, 2006[§] | 467 | 6 | 30 | 16 | 40[‡] |

* All percentages for the 1990 Health Objectives reflect attainment of the 266 measured targets.

† Percentages for Healthy People 2000 Objectives do not add up to 100 percent in this table because 11 percent of objectives (35) that showed mixed progress have been excluded.

‡ This percentage includes 28 objectives that were deleted, as well as 158 objectives that could not be assessed due to a lack of tracking data.

§ Percentages for Healthy People 2010 Objectives do not add up to 100 percent in this table because 12 percent of objectives (57 of 467) that showed mixed progress have been excluded.

Reproduced from: U.S. Department of Health and Human Services. The Secretary's Advisory Committee on National Health Promotion and Disease Prevention Objectives for 2020 October 28 2008.

- Increase public awareness and understanding of the determinants of health, disease, and disability and the opportunities for progress
- Provide measurable objectives and goals that can be used at the national, state, and local levels
- Engage multiple sectors to take actions that are driven by the best available evidence and knowledge
- Identify critical research and data collection needs

The overarching goals for Healthy People 2020 are as follows[63]:

- *Eliminate preventable disease, disability, injury, and premature death.* This goal supports health promotion and disease prevention for all U.S. populations, including those with or without evident health problems. It includes people with significant diseases or health conditions that cannot be prevented or cured with the application of current knowledge. Health promotion and disease prevention efforts can slow functional declines or improve a person's ability to live independently and participate in daily activities and community life.
- *Achieve health equity and eliminate health disparities.* This goal deals with important determinants of health disparities that can be influenced by institutional policies and practices. These include disparities in healthcare, but also in other health determinants, such as living and working conditions. Social policies related to education, income, transportation, and housing are powerful influences on health, because they affect factors such as the types of food one can buy, the quality of the housing and neighborhood where one can live, the quality of one's education, and one's access to good quality medical care.
- *Create social and physical environments that promote good health for all.* This goal advocates an ecological approach to health promotion. It suggests that health and health behaviors are determined by influences at multiple levels, including the personal (e.g., biological and psychological), organizational and institutional, environmental (e.g., social and physical), and policy levels. Policies that can improve the income of low-income persons and communities; for example, education, job opportunities, and improvements to public infrastructure may improve population health. Improving rewards for productive economic activity, whether by eliminating disparities in pay for equal work due to discrimination or by reducing taxes for earnings of low-income persons, could promote the economic well-being of vulnerable populations and thereby contribute to their health.
- *Promote healthy development and healthy behaviors at every stage of life.* This goal addresses human development across the life span because exposures in early life can be linked to outcomes in later life.

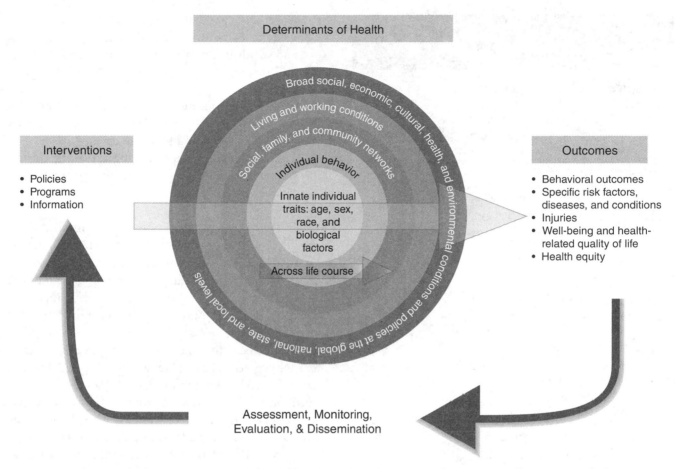

**FIGURE 1-4** Action model for achieving Healthy People 2020 Goals.

Reproduced from: U.S. Department of Health and Human Services.

It states that the prenatal and adult periods can be bridged by studying how early life factors (e.g., lack of prenatal care, gestational diabetes, and others) together with later life factors (e.g., lack of education, low income, etc.) contribute to health outcomes and identifying risk and preventive processes across the life course.[64]

**FIGURE 1-4** presents an action model to guide the achievement of the Healthy People 2020 goals. The Action Model[65] to Achieve Healthy People Goals represents the impact of interventions (e.g., policies, programs, and information) on determinants of health at multiple levels (e.g., individual; social, family, and community; living and working conditions; and broad social, economic, cultural, health, and environmental conditions) to improve outcomes. The results of such interventions can be demonstrated through assessment, monitoring, and evaluation. Through dissemination of evidence-based practices and best practices, these findings would feed back to intervention planning to enable the identification of effective prevention strategies in the future. A feedback loop of intervention, assessment, and dissemination of evidence and best practices would enable achievement of Healthy People 2020 goals. **TABLE 1-8** presents 2020 focus areas.

**TABLE 1-8** Healthy People 2020 Focus Areas

1. Access to Health Services
2. Adolescent Health
3. Arthritis, Osteoporosis and Chronic Back
4. Blood Disorders and Blood Safety
5. Cancer
6. Chronic Kidney Disease
7. Dementias, Including Alzheimer's Disease
8. Diabetes
9. Disability and Health
10. Early and Middle Childhood
11. Educational and Community-Based Programs
12. Environmental Health
13. Family Planning
14. Food Safety
15. Genomics
16. Global Health
17. Healthcare-Associated Infections
18. Health Communication and Health Information Technology
19. Health-Related Quality of Life and Well-Being
20. Hearing and Other Sensory or Communication Disorders

*(continues)*

**TABLE 1-8** Healthy People 2020 Focus Areas *(continued)*

21. Heart Disease and Stroke
22. HIV
23. Immunization and Infectious Disease
24. Injury and Violence Prevention
25. Lesbian, Gay, Bisexual, and Transgender Health
26. Maternal, Infant, and Child Health
27. Medical Product Safety
28. Mental Health and Mental Disorders
29. Nutrition and Weight Status
30. Occupational Health
31. Older Adults
32. Oral Health
33. Physical Activity
34. Preparedness
35. Public Health Infrastructure
36. Respiratory Diseases
37. Sexually Transmitted Diseases
38. Sleep Health
39. Social Determinants of Health
40. Substance Abuse
41. Tobacco Use
42. Vision

Source: U.S. Department of Health and Human Services, Healthy People 2020. http://www.cdc.gov/nchs/healthy_people/hp2020/hp2020_topic_areas.htm. Accessed March 4, 2016.

# Knowledge and Skills of Public Health and Community Nutritionists

In most instances, a community or public health nutritionist must be a member of an **interdisciplinary team** to provide an effective nutrition program. An interdisciplinary team is a collaboration among personnel representing different disciplines of public health workers (nurses, social workers, physicians, daycare workers, dietitians, and dietetic technicians). They use various approaches to diagnose and address public or community issues, including the following[23]:

- Using interventions that promote health and prevent communicable or chronic diseases by managing or controlling the community's environment
- Channeling funds and energy to problems that affect the lives of the largest numbers of people in a community
- Seeking unserved or underserved populations (due to income, age, ethnicity, heredity, or lifestyle) and those who are vulnerable to disease, hunger, or malnutrition

- Collaborating with the public, consumers, community leaders, legislators, policy makers, administrators, and health and human service professionals to assess and respond to community needs and consumer demands
- Monitoring the public or community's health in relation to public health objectives and continuously addressing current and future needs
- Planning, organizing, managing, directing, coordinating, and evaluating the nutrition component of health agency services

For community nutritionists to accomplish these actions, they need to acquire normal and clinical nutrition knowledge and be skilled in educating the public regarding changes in eating behavior. The minimum education requirements for a community nutritionist include a bachelor's degree in foods and nutrition or dietetics from an accredited college or university and a Master of Public Health degree with a major in nutrition or a Master of Science degree in applied human nutrition with a minor in public health or community health.[23] Some community nutrition positions require certification as a **Registered Dietitian (RD)** and/or an advanced degree in nutrition. Academic training includes knowledge of biostatistics and skill in collecting, analyzing, and reporting demographic, health, and food nutrition data.[66,67]

The community nutritionist must understand the epidemiology of health and disease patterns in the population as well as trends of diseases over a long period. He or she must be knowledgeable about the principles of health education, program planning, program **evaluation**, community organization, management, marketing, and policy formation.[68]

Marketing skills are very important because they help nutritionists know how to convey effective nutrition messages using a variety of media formats for their audiences. Community nutritionists must keep current with advances in research and food and nutrition sciences, and changing practices in public health service.[67]

In some situations, Dietetic Technicians, Registered (DTRs), are employed in the food service area, clinical settings, and community settings. They may assist the community nutritionist or RD in determining the community's nutritional needs and in providing community nutrition programs and services. At a minimum, DTRs must have an associate's degree from an approved educational program. After that, they must successfully complete a national examination administered by the Commission on Dietetic Registration (CDR).

Community and public health nutritionists provide a wide variety of nutrition services through government and nongovernment agencies at the local, state, national, and international levels.[23] In most cases, the activities require multitasking roles such as blood pressure screening, diet counseling, and medical nutrition therapy. At the international level, duties may include education on sanitation, water purification, and gardening.

## ▶ Places of Employment for Public Health and Community Nutritionists

Community and public health nutritionists work in official community settings or voluntary agencies to promote health, prevent disease, conduct epidemiological research, and provide both primary and secondary preventive care. The agencies include city, county, state, federal, and international agencies.[23] The following are examples of places where community and public health nutritionists may be employed:

### State, City, and County Level

- Cooperative extension services
- Home healthcare agencies
- Hospital outpatient nutrition education departments
- Local public health agencies
- Migrant worker health centers
- Native American health services
- Neighborhood or community health centers
- Nonprofit and for-profit private health agencies
- Universities, colleges, and medical schools
- Wellness programs

### National and Regional Level

- U.S. Food and Drug Administration (FDA)
- U.S. Department of Agriculture (USDA)
- U.S. Department of Health and Human Services (DHHS)

### International Level

- Food and Agriculture Organization of the United Nations (FAO)
- Pan American Health Organization (PAHO)
- United Nations (UN)
- UNICEF
- World Food Agency (WFA)
- Supermarket or grocery store
- WHO

## ▶ Ethics and Community Nutrition Professionals

Community and public health nutritionists must abide by the Academy of Nutrition and Dietetics (AND) ethical code, regardless of where they practice. **Ethics** is the study of the nature and justification of principles that guide human behaviors and are applied when moral problems arise.[8,69] The AND Ethics Committee is a joint committee of the Board of Directors, House of Delegates, and Commission on Dietetic Registration. Its purpose is to review, promote, and enforce the AND and Commission on Dietetic Registration Code of Ethics for the Profession of Dietetics (http://www.eatright.org/codeofethics). The committee is also responsible for educating members, credentialed practitioners, students, and the public about the ethical principles of the Code of Ethics. There are 19 principles in the code, which covers the diversity in the dietetic profession[70] (see Chapter 15).

In promoting health and preventing diseases, community and public health nutritionists have the responsibility to provide accurate and reliable information so their clients can make appropriate choices. They must interpret **evidence-based** scientific information without bias to enable the community or clients to make informed decisions. The nutritionist maintaining consistent ethical behavior will increase the level of the public, community, or client trust in the nutritionist's profession. In 2002, the ANDs' *Nutrition and You: Trends*[71] reported that a majority (51 to 55 percent) surveyed indicated that dietitians are a credible source on topics that included obesity, dietary supplements, food irradiation, and genetically modified foods. It is important that, as a profession, all nutritionists and dietitians continue to maintain this professionalism.

However, sometimes principles collide or do not resolve the moral conflict or dilemma. That is when the theory of moral virtues for healthcare professionals can be useful. This set of virtues was established by the American Board of Internal Medicine in 1984 as the definition of a virtuous clinician. The virtues include the following[72,73]:

- *Integrity:* Telling the truth, keeping promises, and being able to do what one claims to do. For example, a community nutritionist violated her integrity after a food safety workshop by providing a list of kosher meat shops to her Jewish clients that included her uncle's meat shop—with a discount of 25 percent—without informing them that his meat is not kosher. The Jewish clients did not know that her uncle owned the shop and that his meat is not kosher.
- *Respect:* Treating other people as having worth and involving them as partners in the clinical or educational encounter.
- *Compassion:* Being able and willing to experience suffering from the client's perspective and allowing that experience to guide the behavior of the healthcare provider and community nutritionist.

## ✎ Think About It

What ethical or moral violations has Eugene, a community nutritionist, committed?

Eugene read an article published in the *ADA TIMES* discussing Muslim dietary guidelines and the percentage of Muslim Americans born in the United States who observe the dietary practice of eating foods that are halal (permitted under Islamic law). The article also listed foods that are not halal. Eugene has to make a difficult decision about recommending foods that are high in vitamin $B_6$ and thiamin to vitamin-deficient Muslim teenage mothers who have recently arrived in the United States. Because pork is a good source of vitamin $B_6$ and thiamin, which can improve their nutritional status and reduce their deficiencies, he asked them to consume pork and products containing pork. Another reason for his recommendation is limited community resources and language barriers.

## ▶ Preventive Nutrition

**Preventive nutrition** can be defined as dietary practices and interventions directed toward a reduction in disease risk and/or improvement in health outcomes.[74] Preventive nutrition is an important strategy that works to prevent disease instead of treating the condition after it materializes. The U.S. government and other health agencies have taken actions to reduce the incidences of chronic diseases, such as recommending a reduction in saturated fat intake for cardiovascular disease prevention and inclusion of B vitamins, vitamins A and D, iron, and calcium in staple foods such as grain products, milk, and cereals to prevent nutrient-related health conditions.[75,76] These preventive nutrition strategies have been part of public health policy for many years and have been effective in preventing nutrition-related health conditions.[77,78] For example, there has been a decrease in cardiovascular disease mortality in the past 25 years due to the massive campaign to reduce fat intake and increase physical activity in the United States and most industrialized countries.[28,79]

Other concerns have prompted policy changes regarding prevention of chronic diseases. The high costs of medical care put economic pressure on both individuals and nations to prevent chronic diseases. The cost of cardiovascular diseases and stroke in the United States each year was estimated at $312.6 billion.[80] Estimates show that $22 billion per year could be saved in this disease category if preventive nutrition measures were fully implemented.[74]

Another disease category that could be significantly affected if prevention were emphasized more strongly is that of birth defects. Birth defects in infants are the leading cause of hospitalizations.[81] Research shows that the possibility of reducing infant morbidity and mortality through nutritional interventions becomes a tangible outcome when women who take a folic acid–containing multivitamin daily for at least 1 month before conception and during their pregnancies have

approximately a 50 percent decrease in neural tube defects.[81,82] This outcome alone is expected to save approximately $70 million annually.[74]

In addition, a decrease in medical care for breast-fed infants is the primary socioeconomic benefit of breastfeeding. Medicaid costs for infants breastfed by low-income mothers in Colorado were $175 lower than for infants who were fed formula.[83] In addition, breastfed infants are less likely to have any illness during the first year of life. It is reported that infants who were never breastfed required more care for lower respiratory tract illness, otitis media (ear infection), and gastrointestinal disease than infants breastfed for at least 3 months.[84]

The effectiveness of nutrition education is related to applicable use of behavior science theories and models (see Chapter 13). These models assist healthcare professionals to formulate an action plan that meets the needs and capabilities of the individuals making health behavior changes. The Health Belief Model (HBM) is one of the health education models (derived from behavior science theory) that has been successful in providing nutrition education.[85] One of the components of HBM is perceived benefits of health action.

For instance, a study was carried out to compare the effect of a nutritional educational program based on HBM with traditional education among pregnant women. The target population was pregnant women residing in Gonabad attending an urban healthcare centers for prenatal care. Of 1,388 pregnant women, 110 (HBM group: 54, control group: 56) were selected in the first stage of prenatal care (6th to 10th week). The interview based on HBM was performed in two sessions of nutritional education using live lecture and group discussions. In the control group, nutrition education during pregnancy was performed in healthcare centers without using the educational model. Posttest based on two sessions of nutritional education in a similar pattern to pretest was performed for HBM and control groups in the 38th to 40th weeks of pregnancy. Results shows no significant differences in nutritional behavior mean score before the intervention program. However, after intervention, there was a significant difference in HBM structure mean score compared with the control group and the highest increase in score was related to perceived benefits (15.13 increment). In addition, this study showed that nutritional education based on HBM for recommended weight gain during pregnancy was successful compared with traditional education.[85]

# Nutrition Care Process: Evidence-Based Practice

The AND plays a significant role in preventing nutrition-related diseases and improving health outcomes. One of the nutrition and health-related efforts of the AND was the establishment of the **Nutrition Care Process and Model (NCPM)**, presented in **FIGURE 1-5**. The NCPM is a systematic problem-solving method that food and nutrition professionals use to critically evaluate nutrition-related problems and make decisions regarding them.[86] It provides a consistent framework for food and nutrition professionals to use when delivering nutrition care and is designed for use with patients, clients, groups, and communities of all ages and conditions of health or disease.[87] It contains the following four separate but interrelated steps.

- Nutrition assessment
- Nutrition diagnosis (problems)
- Nutrition intervention
- Nutrition monitoring and evaluation

Each step informs the subsequent step. As new information is collected, a food and nutrition professional may revisit previous steps of the process to reassess, add, or revise nutrition diagnoses, modify interventions, or adjust goals and monitoring parameters. The outer ring of the NCPM influences how clients receive nutrition information. The practice setting reflects

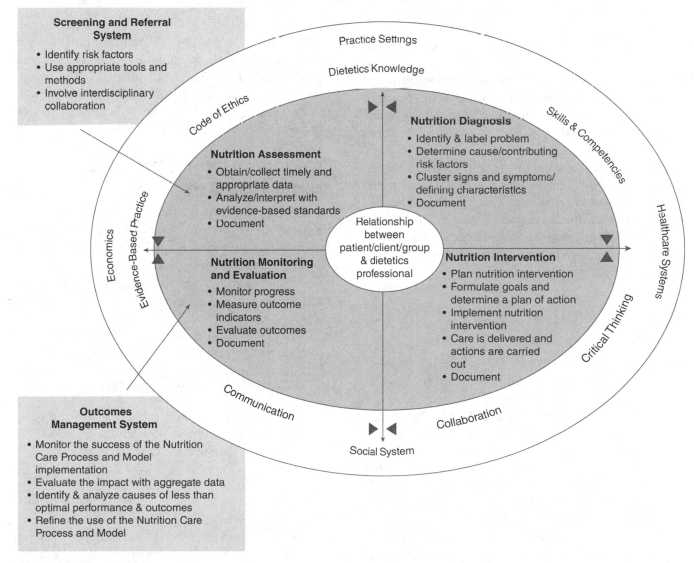

**FIGURE 1-5** The nutrition care process model.

rules and regulations governing practice, the age and health conditions of particular clients, and how a food and nutrition professional's time is allocated. The social system reflects clients' health-related knowledge, values, and the time devoted to improving nutritional health. The economic aspect incorporates resources allocated to nutrition care, including the value of a food and nutrition professional's time in the form of salary and reimbursement. The middle ring of the NCPM distinguishes the unique professional attributes of food and nutrition professionals from those in other professions. The inner ring illustrates the four steps of the NCPM. The central core of the model depicts the essential and collaborative partnership with clients. The model is intended to reflect the dynamic nature of relationships throughout the NCPM.

The AND developed a standardized language for the NCPM to describe the activities of RDs within each of the four steps. For example, the term for identifying and labeling clients with a nutrition diagnosis regarding nutrient intake could be *suboptimal vitamin intake* or *inadequate protein intake.*[88]

Community nutritionists and other dietetic professionals are very familiar with three aspects of the NCPM (nutrition assessment, **nutrition intervention**, and **nutrition monitoring and evaluation**). However, there is also a less well-defined aspect of nutrition care: **nutrition diagnosis**.[88] Each step will be explained in the following sections.

Community and public health nutritionists can use the NCPM to develop, plan, monitor, and implement high-quality nutrition services to their clients in the community. In this textbook, problem-based and critical thinking situations are presented in the form of case studies for each chapter, with blank NCPM charts provided in the student's manual.

## The Nutrition Care Process Step 1: Nutrition Assessment

Nutrition assessment is discussed in detail in Chapter 2. It involves the systematic gathering, verifying, and interpreting of data needed to identify nutrition-related problems, their causes, and their significance. Nutrition assessment involves initial data collection, but also continual reassessment and analysis of the client's status compared to specified criteria.[88] Nutrition assessment may include the following data sources when identifying nutrition-related problems: interviewing, community-based survey, epidemiological studies, observations, medical records, focus groups, key informants, community forum, and information gained from other healthcare providers or agencies. If a problem is identified, the community nutritionist can then label the problem and create a problem, etiology, and signs and symptoms (PES) statement in Step 2 of the NCPM (discussed next).

Critical thinking skills are very important for the selection, collection, and interpretation of relevant data. *Critical thinking* is the way individuals learn to assess and modify a situation before acting. A critical thinker is simultaneously problem solving and self-improving his or her thinking ability.[89] Critical thinking skills are required for good diagnostic reasoning and clinical judgment. Examples of critical thinking skills are as follows[88]:

- Determining appropriate data to collect about your clients
- Determining the need for additional information for your clients
- Selecting assessment tools and procedures that match the situation and alternative possibilities
- Applying assessment tools in valid and reliable ways
- Distinguishing relevant from irrelevant data
- Validating the data

In the development of the standardized nutrition diagnosis language, five domains of nutrition assessment were identified: food and nutrition-related history, biochemical data, anthropometric measurements, physical findings, and client history. **TABLE 1-9** presents the five domains of nutrition assessment.

## The Nutrition Care Process Step 2: Nutrition Diagnosis

Nutrition diagnosis is a critical step between nutrition assessment and nutrition intervention. The reason for this step is to identify and label specific nutrition problems that nutritionists can independently resolve or improve through nutrition intervention. The nutrition diagnosis is summarized into a structured sentence called a nutrition diagnosis statement or a PES statement.[88] The etiology and the signs and symptoms are determined during nutrition assessment. The standard phrases included in a nutrition diagnosis statement are "related to" and "evidenced by." The following is an example of a PES:

> A group of pregnant high school teenagers in a Midwestern city (target population) are obese and anemic (problem) *related to* frequent consumption of high-fat food and sugary drinks from vending machines plus low iron intake and physical inactivity (etiology) as *evidenced by* BMI between 27 and 30, hemoglobin level of less than 10 g/dl, and spoon-shaped fingernails, as well as vending machines in and around the high school containing high-fat chips and sugary soft drinks (signs and symptoms).

**TABLE 1-9** The Five Categories of Nutrition Assessment

| Food and Nutrition–Related History | Anthropometric Measurements | Biochemical Data, Medical Tests, and Procedures | Nutrition-Focused Physical Findings | Client History |
|---|---|---|---|---|
| Food and nutrient intake, food and nutrient administration, medication and herbal supplement use, knowledge and beliefs, food and supplies availability, physical activity, nutrition, and quality of life | Height and weight, body mass index, and growth pattern indices/percentile ranks, and weight history | Laboratory data (e.g., electrolytes, glucose) and tests (e.g., gastric emptying time, resting metabolic rate) | Physical appearance, muscle and fat wasting, swallow function, appetite, and affect | Personal, family social, medical, and health, history; treatments and complementary or alternative medicine use |

Nutrition assessment data (indicators) are compared to criteria and relevant norms and standards, for interpretation and decision making. These may be national, institutional, or regulatory norms and standards. Nutrition assessment findings are documented in nutrition diagnosis statements and nutrition intervention goal setting.

Source: Modified from International Dietetics and Nutrition Terminology. *International Dietetics and Nutrition Terminology (IDNT) Reference Manual: Standardized Language for the Nutrition Care Process*, 3rd ed. Chicago, IL: American Dietetic Association; 2011:13.

The community and public health nutritionist's PES statement needs to be clear and concise. It is important to define the main nutrition problem related to the community or clients. In some cases more than one problem may occur. It is practical to first address the most important and urgent problem. The nutritionist must ask critical thinking questions to clarify the nutrition diagnosis when he or she is specifying the diagnosis and writing the PES statement. The nutritionist can evaluate the PES statement using the following example[88]:

*P:* Can the nutritionist resolve or improve the nutrition diagnosis for this community, individual, group, or population?

*E:* Can the nutritionist evaluate what was used as the etiology to determine whether it is the root cause to address with a nutrition intervention to reduce the signs and symptoms?

*S:* Can measuring the signs and symptoms show that the problem is resolved or improved?

*PES overall:* Do the nutrition assessment data support a particular nutrition diagnosis with a typical etiology, signs, and symptoms?

The most distinctive feature of the NCPM is the nutrition diagnosis. The AND recognizes more than 60 nutrition diagnoses/problems, which have been given labels that are grouped into three domains: intake, clinical, and behavioral-environmental. Each domain represents unique characteristics that contribute to nutrition-related health conditions. Within each domain are classes and,

in some cases, subclasses of nutrition diagnosis.[88] The details of each are presented in **TABLE 1-10.**

# The Nutrition Care Process Step 3: Nutrition Intervention

The purpose of the nutrition intervention step of the NCPM is to take specific action that can resolve or improve the identified nutrition problem or diagnosis through nutrition assessment. The nutrition intervention consists of two components: planning and implementation.[88,90] The use of nutrition interventions is determined by the nutrition diagnosis and its cause[88]; for example, the nutritionist may educate a teenage mother on how to breastfeed her infant or iron-deficient pregnant women on how to select iron-rich foods.

The four categories of nutrition intervention strategies that nutritionists can use are as follows[88]:

- *Food and/or nutrient delivery:* This strategy/approach focuses on food and nutrient provision, in the form of meals and snacks, medical food supplements, feeding assistance, and enteral and parenteral nutrition. For example, the nutritionist could provide low-sodium meals to participants in a congregate meal program.
- *Nutrition education:* This strategy is a formal process that instructs or trains individuals in a skill or imparts knowledge to help clients voluntarily manage or modify choices and eating behavior to maintain or improve health. For example, a nutrition professor could instruct dietetic students who are providing nutrition services to athletes on how to

**TABLE 1-10** Categories of Nutrition Diagnostic Terminology, Examples, and Applications

| Domain | Class | Nutrition Diagnostic Terminology | Example | Application |
|---|---|---|---|---|
| *Intake:* Lists actual problems related to intake of energy, nutrients, fluids, or bioactive substances through oral diet or nutrition support (enteral or parenteral nutrition) | *Energy Balance:* Actual or estimated intake of energy (kilocalories [kcal]) | Excessive energy intake | Energy intake that exceeds energy expenditure established by reference standards or recommendations based on physiological needs | May not be an appropriate nutrition diagnosis when weight gain is desired. |
| | *Oral or Nutrition Support Intake:* Actual or estimated food and beverage intake from oral diet or nutrition support compared with client's goal | Inadequate oral food and beverage intake | Oral food and beverage intake that is less than established reference standards or recommendations based on physiological needs | May not be an appropriate nutrition diagnosis when the goal is weight loss, during end-of-life care, etc. |
| | *Fluid Intake:* Actual or estimated fluid intake compared with client's goal | Inadequate fluid intake | Lower intake of fluid-containing foods or substances compared to established reference standards or recommendations based on physiological needs | Whenever possible, nutrient intake data should be considered in combination with clinical, biochemical, and anthropometric information; medical diagnosis; clinical status; and/or other factors, as well as diet, to provide a valid assessment of nutritional status based on a totality of evidence (Dietary Reference Intakes). |
| | *Bioactive\* Substances Intake:* Actual or estimated intake of bioactive substances, including single or multiple functional food components, ingredients, dietary supplements, and alcohol | Inadequate bioactive substance intake | Lower intake of bioactive substances compared to reference standards or recommendations based on physiological needs | Bioactive substances are not included as part of the Dietary Reference Intakes; therefore, there are no established minimum requirements or Tolerable Upper Intake Levels. But, dietitians can assess whether estimated intakes are adequate or excessive using the client goal or nutrition prescription for comparison. |

| | | | |
|---|---|---|---|
| **Nutrient Intake:** Actual or estimated intake of specific nutrient groups or single nutrients compared with desired levels | Increased nutrient intake (specify) | Increased need for a specific nutrient compared to established reference standards or recommendations based on physiological needs | Whenever possible, nutrient intake data should be considered in combination with clinical, biochemical, and anthropometric information; medical diagnosis; clinical status; and/or other factors, as well as diet, to provide a valid assessment of nutritional status based on totality of the evidence (Dietary Reference Intakes). |
| **Subclass:** Fat and cholesterol | Inadequate fat intake | Lower fat substances compared to reference standards or recommendations based on physiological needs | May not be an appropriate nutrition diagnosis when the goal is weight loss or during end-of-life care. |
| **Subclass:** Protein | Inadequate protein intake | Lower intake of protein compared to reference standards or recommendations based on physiological needs | Whenever possible, nutrient intake data should be considered in combination with clinical, biochemical, and anthropometric information; medical diagnosis; clinical status; and/or other factors, as well as diet, to provide a valid assessment of nutritional status based on totality of the evidence (Dietary Reference Intakes). |
| **Subclass:** Carbohydrates and Fiber | Inadequate carbohydrate intake | Lower carbohydrate intake compared to reference standards or recommendations based on physiological need | Whenever possible, nutrient intake data should be considered in combination with clinical, biochemical, and anthropometric information; medical diagnosis; clinical status; and/or other factors, as well as diet, to provide a valid assessment of nutritional status based on totality of the evidence (Dietary Reference Intakes). |
| **Subclass:** Vitamins | Inadequate vitamin intake (specify) | Lower intake of vitamins compared to reference standards or recommendations based on physiological needs | Whenever possible, nutrient intake data should be considered in combination with clinical, biochemical, and anthropometric information; medical diagnosis; clinical status; and/or other factors, as well as diet, to provide a valid assessment of nutritional status based on totality of the evidence (Dietary Reference Intakes). |

*(continues)*

**TABLE 1-10**  Categories of Nutrition Diagnostic Terminology, Examples, and Applications *(continued)*

| Domain | Class | Nutrition Diagnostic Terminology | Example | Application |
|---|---|---|---|---|
| | **Subclass:** Minerals | Inadequate mineral intake (specify) | Lower intake of minerals compared to reference standards or recommendations based on physiological needs. | Whenever possible, nutrient intake data should be considered in combination with clinical, biochemical, and anthropometric information; medical diagnosis; clinical status; and/or other factors, as well as diet, to provide a valid assessment of nutritional status based on totality of the evidence (Dietary Reference Intakes). |
| **Clinical:** Nutritional findings/problems identified as related to medical or physical conditions | **Functional:** Change in physical or mechanical functioning that interferes with or prevents desired nutritional consequences | Impaired or difficult movement of food and liquid within the oral cavity to the stomach; breastfeeding difficulty | Motor causes (e.g., neurological or muscular disorders, such as cerebral palsy, stroke, and prematurity); altered suck, swallow, breathe patterns | Whenever possible, nutrient intake data should be considered in combination with clinical, biochemical, and anthropometric information; medical diagnosis; clinical status; and/or other factors, as well as diet, to provide a valid assessment of nutritional status based on totality of the evidence (Dietary Reference Intakes). |
| | **Biochemical:** Change in the capacity to metabolize nutrients as a result of medications, surgery, or as indicated by altered laboratory values | Changes due to body composition, medications, body system changes, or genetics or changes in ability to eliminate by-products of digestive and metabolic processes | Increased need for a specific nutrient compared to established reference standards or recommendations based on physiological needs | Whenever possible, nutrient intake data should be considered in combination with clinical, biochemical, and anthropometric information; medical diagnosis; clinical status; and/or other factors, as well as diet, to provide a valid assessment of nutritional status based on totality of the evidence (Dietary Reference Intakes). |
| | **Weight:** Chronic weight gain or changed weight status when compared with usual or desired body weight | Underweight | Low body weight compared to established reference standards or recommendations | May not be an appropriate nutrition diagnosis when changes in body weight are due to fluid. |

|  |  |  |
|---|---|---|
| ***Behavioral–Environmental:*** Includes nutritional findings or problems that relate to knowledge, attitudes/beliefs, physical environment, access to food, and food safety | ***Knowledge and Beliefs:*** Actual knowledge and beliefs as reported, observed, or documented | Harmful beliefs or attitudes about food or nutrition-related topics | Disordered eating pattern: Beliefs, attitudes, thoughts, and behaviors related to food, eating, and weight management, including classic eating disorders as well as less severe, similar conditions that negatively affect health | Whenever possible, nutrient intake data should be considered in combination with clinical, biochemical, and anthropometric information; medical diagnosis; clinical status; and/or other factors, as well as diet, to provide a valid assessment of nutritional status based on totality of the evidence (Dietary Reference Intakes). |
| | ***Physical Activity and Function:*** Actual physical activity, self-care, and quality of life problems as reported, observed, or documented | Impaired ability to prepare food or meals | Cognitive or physical impairment that prevents preparation of foods or fluids; for example, learning disabilities, neurological or sensory impairments, and/or dementia | Whenever possible, nutrient intake data should be considered in combination with clinical, biochemical, and anthropometric information; medical diagnosis; clinical status; and/or other factors, as well as diet, to provide a valid assessment of nutritional status based on totality of the evidence (Dietary Reference Intakes). |
| | ***Food Safety and Access:*** Actual problems with food access or food safety | Intake of unsafe food | Intake of food and/or fluids intentionally or unintentionally contaminated with toxins, poisonous products, infectious agents, microbial agents, additives, allergens, and/or agents of bioterrorism | Whenever possible, nutrient intake data should be considered in combination with clinical, biochemical, and anthropometric information; medical diagnosis; clinical status; and/or other factors, as well as diet, to provide a valid assessment of nutritional status based on totality of the evidence (Dietary Reference Intakes). |

Whenever possible, nutrient intake data should be considered in combination with clinical, biochemical, and anthropometric information; medical diagnosis; clinical status; and/or other factors, as well as diet, to provide a valid assessment of nutritional status based on totality of the evidence (Dietary Reference Intakes).

Data from: American Dietetic Association. *International Dietetics and Nutrition Terminology, International Dietetics and Nutrition Terminology (IDNT) Reference Manual: Standardized Language for the Nutrition Care Process*, 3rd ed. Chicago, IL: American Dietetic Association; 2011:36–37.

perform skinfold measurements and calculate the percentage of body fat.

- *Nutrition counseling:* This strategy is a supportive process, characterized by a collaborative counselor–client relationship that sets priorities, establishes goals, and creates individualized action plans that acknowledge and promote responsibility for self-care or group care. It treats an existing condition and promotes health. The nutritionist provides direction or advice pertaining to a decision or course of action. For example, the nutritionist could counsel clients with high blood cholesterol on how to select low cholesterol and high dietary fiber foods.
- *Coordination of nutrition care:* This strategy includes consultation with, referral to, or coordination of nutrition care with other healthcare providers, institutions, or agencies that can assist in treating or managing nutrition-related problems. For example, a nutritionist could refer a pregnant teenager to the WIC program.

The nutritionist needs to also apply his or her critical thinking skills to providing appropriate nutrition intervention, including the following[88]:

- Setting goals and prioritizing the nutrition diagnoses based on problem severity, safety, client's needs, likelihood that the nutrition intervention will have an impact on the problem, and client's perception of the importance of the intervention
- Defining the nutrition prescription or basic plan
- Making interdisciplinary connections by networking with other professionals such as community nurses, physicians in the community, and others
- Initiating behavioral and other nutrition interventions
- Matching nutrition intervention strategies with client needs, nutrition diagnoses, and client values
- Choosing from among alternatives to determine a course of action
- Specifying the time and frequency of care and nutrition program

## Planning the Nutrition Intervention

The process of program planning is discussed in Chapter 12. Community nutritionists need to use assessment data to establish the etiology and signs and symptoms of a nutrition problem (PES) and direct the nutrition intervention at the etiology or cause of the problem identified in the PES statement. For example, an obese teenager *related to* frequent consumption of a large portion of high-fat foods as *evidenced by* a 17-pound weight gain during the last 2 months plus consumption of 1,000 kcal/day more than the estimated needs. In this instance, the intervention would aim at lowering the total fat intake to not more than 30 percent of the

total calories per day plus daily physical activity for at least 30 minutes.

It is crucial that the nutritionist uses evidence-based information to plan the intervention program. **Evidence-based practice** involves using the highest quality of available information to make practice decisions.[88] The nutritionist using evidence-based information would combine his or her experience with a critical evaluation of primary and secondary sources to support the decision-making process. The AND's electronic Evidence Analysis Library (http://www.adaevidencelibrary.com) contains numerous documents that can support the steps of the NCPM. The AND Evidence-Based Nutrition Practice Guidelines are published in the National Guideline Clearinghouse at http://www.guideline.gov.

A **nutrition prescription** is an important part of planning in which the nutrition intervention is specified. It is the community or individualized recommended dietary intake of selected foods or nutrients based on current reference standards and dietary guidelines and the client's or community's health condition and nutrition diagnosis.[88] It is determined using the assessment data, the nutrition diagnosis statement (PES), current evidence, policies and procedures, and client values and preferences, which guide intervention design and monitoring and evaluation plans. The nutrition prescription either drives the selection of nutrition intervention or provides the framework within which the nutrition intervention is implemented. For example, a nutrition prescription for adult men and women attending a nutrition education program for the reduction of cardiovascular disease may be to limit the intake of saturated fat to less than 10 percent of energy intake, trans-fat to less than 1 percent of energy intake, and cholesterol to less than 300 mg/day by choosing lean meats and vegetables and increasing dietary fiber to 25 to 30 g/day. Another example of a nutrition prescription could be a DASH eating plan (the consumption of a diet rich in fruits, vegetables, and low-fat dairy products with a reduced content of saturated and total fat and reducing dietary sodium intake to less than 2.4 g of sodium or 6 g of sodium chloride) for elderly individuals enrolled in a nutrition education program for the reduction of hypertension. A third example is a nutrition prescription for pregnant women 19 to 30 years old participating in a nutrition education program to increase calcium and vitamin D intake to 1½ cups of low-fat milk with morning and afternoon snacks, 1 cup of low-fat milk for lunch, and ½ cup of yogurt with dinner (providing 1,000 mg of calcium and 5 mg of vitamin D from food). A nutrition prescription for breastfeeding mothers less than 18 years old for calcium intake could be 1,300 mg of calcium and 5 mg of vitamin D from food and supplements. Finally, the nutrition prescription for an intervention program focusing on obese men and women at a worksite may be to consume less than 30 percent of calories from fat and increase physical activity to 30 minutes a day, 5 days a week.

## Implementing the Nutrition Intervention

**Nutrition implementation** is the action phase of the nutrition intervention. The purpose of the nutrition implementation is mainly to correct the nutrition diagnosis, remove the etiology, or reduce the signs and symptoms of the problem. During the implementation of the program, the nutritionist will do the following[88]:

- Communicate the plan of nutrition care or program
- Carry out the plan of nutrition care or the nutrition program
- Continue data collection and modify the plan of care or program as needed

Characteristics that define quality implementation include the following:

- Individualize the interventions to the setting, community, and/or clients
- Collaborate with colleagues and healthcare professionals such as social workers and the local public health department
- Follow up and verify that implementation is occurring and needs are being addressed
- Revise strategies as changes in condition or response occurs

**TABLE 1-11** presents specific nutrition intervention areas, definitions, and applications.

## The Nutrition Care Process Step 4: Monitoring and Evaluation

The reason for the monitoring and evaluation (M and E) step is to determine whether the goals and expected outcomes were achieved and whether progress was attained in resolving the nutrition problem.[88] In this step, the nutritionist uses different related nutrition indicators to measure and evaluate the specific changes in the community or client's progress. He or she needs to compare the community or client's previous status and nutrition intervention goals to reference standards (national, institutional, and/or regulatory standards). The nutritionist can measure the outcome by collecting data on the appropriate nutrition indicators and providing evidence that there is a change in behavior or health status. This may include the client's ability to prepare food and meals, portion control, self-monitoring, social support, access to food, and physical activity.

The following is a summary of the three components of the nutrition monitoring and evaluation step:

**Monitor progress[88]:**

- Check the client's understanding of and compliance with nutrition intervention
- Determine whether the intervention is being implemented as prescribed
- Provide evidence that the nutrition intervention is (or is not) changing the client's behavior or status
- Identify other positive or negative outcomes
- Gather information indicating the reasons for lack of progress
- Support the conclusions with evidence

**Measure outcomes:**

- Select the nutrition care indicators to measure the desired outcomes
- Use standardized nutrition care indicators to increase the validity and reliability of the measurements of change

**Evaluate outcomes:**

- Compare monitoring data with the nutrition prescription, goal, or reference standard to assess progress and determine future action
- Evaluate the impact of the sum of all interventions on overall client health outcomes

The following are critical thinking questions that nutritionists can ask during the nutrition M and E step. Did the nutritionist[88]:

- Select appropriate indicators and measures?
- Use appropriate reference standards for comparison?
- Define where the community or clients are in terms of expected outcomes?
- Explain a variance from expected outcomes?
- Determine factors that help or deter progress?
- Decide between discharge and continuation of nutrition care?

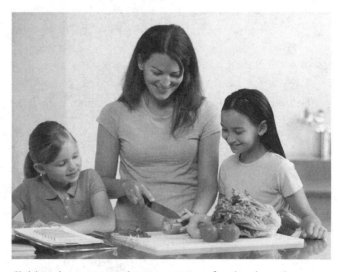

Children learn more about nutritious foods when they are involved in meal preparation.

© Artemis Gordon/ShutterStock, Inc.

**TABLE 1-11** Nutrition Intervention Domains, Definitions, and Applications

| Domains of Nutrition Interventions | Definition | Application |
|---|---|---|
| *Food and/or Nutrient Delivery* | An individualized approach for food and nutrient provision. | Direct food and/or nutrient needs to the PES in the community. |
| Meal and snacks | The nutritionist may provide meals and/or snacks. Meals are regular eating actions that include a variety of foods consisting of grains and/or starches, meat and/or meat alternatives, fruits and vegetables, and milk or milk products. A snack is food served between regular meals. | A nutritionist may use MyPlate food guidance and the Dietary Guidelines for Americans as a starting point in planning meals and snacks and to promote health and prevent diseases. |
| *Supplements* | Foods or nutrients that are not intended as a sole food item or a meal or diet but are intended to provide additional nutrients or to correct a deficiency. | The meal delivery could be in the form of supplements. Collaborate with other healthcare professionals (physicians, nurses, and others). |
| Enteral and parenteral nutrition | Enteral nutrition is provided through the gastrointestinal tract via a tube, catheter, or stoma that delivers nutrients distal to the oral cavity. Parenteral nutrition is provided intravenously (centrally or peripherally). | In a community setting (home healthcare), a dietitian may review changes in the intervention with the client(s) and/or caregivers and community nurse; may involve change of dressing. |
| Medical food supplements | Commercial or prepared food or beverages intended to supplement the nutrient intake in energy, protein, carbohydrates, fiber, and/or fat that may also contribute to vitamin and mineral intake. | A nutritionist may provide nutrition education and/or counseling to elderly individuals or children experiencing failure to thrive to increase protein, energy, and fat intake. |
| Vitamin and mineral supplements | A product that is intended to supplement vitamin or mineral intake. | A community nutritionist may recommend calcium supplements to women at a menopausal education program to reduce the occurrence of osteoporosis. |
| Bioactive substance supplement | Items that are intended to supplement bioactive substances (e.g., plant stanols and sterol esters, psyllium). | A community nutritionist may recommend an increase in the intake of psyllium to men and women with high blood cholesterol levels that are attempting to reduce cardiovascular diseases. |
| *Feeding Assistance* | Assistance in eating for the purpose of restoring the client's ability to eat independently, support adequate nutrient intake, and reduce the incidence of malnutrition, unplanned weight loss, and dehydration. | A community nutritionist may provide meals to elderly individuals who are homebound through the use of a Meals on Wheels program in the community. |
| *Feeding Environment* | Adjustment of the physical environment, temperature, convenience, and attractiveness of the location where food is served, which has an impact on food consumption. | A nutritionist may change the high-fat and sugary snacks in vending machines in and around the high schools in the community to include fruits and vegetables to promote health and prevent diseases. |

*(continues)*

| Domains of Nutrition Interventions | Definition | Application |
|---|---|---|
| ***Nutrition-Related Medication Management*** | Modification of a drug or herbal supplement to optimize a client's nutritional or health status. | A community nutritionist may discontinue a dangerous appetite suppressant drug being used by college students in the community. |
| ***Nutrition Education*** | A formal process to instruct or train clients in a skill or to impart knowledge to help clients voluntarily manage or modify food choices and eating behavior to maintain or improve health. | A WIC nutritionist may instruct breastfeeding mothers on how to use a breast milk pump and how to store the milk and prevent spoilage. |
| Initial/brief nutrition education | Instruction or training intended to build or reinforce basic nutrition-related knowledge, or to provide essential nutrition-related information until the client returns. | A community dietitian may provide nutrition education on how to reduce saturated fat intake to school-age children, college students, and low-income men and women. |
| Comprehensive nutrition education | Instruction or training intended to lead to in-depth nutrition-related knowledge and/or skills in given topics. | A WIC nutritionist may instruct low-income pregnant women on how to select iron-rich foods at the grocery store. |
| Nutrition counseling | A supportive process, characterized by a collaborative counselor–client relationship, intended to set priorities, establish goals, and create individualized action plans that acknowledge and promote responsibility for self-care to treat an existing condition and support health. | A community nutritionist may demonstrate how to prepare low-fat meals to older women at a community center to promote health and prevent disease. |
| ***Theoretical Basis and Approach*** | The theories or models used to design and implement an intervention. Theories and theoretical models consist of principles, constructs, and variables that offer systematic explanations of the human behavior change process. For example, Social Cognitive Theory introduces a construct called self-efficacy (confidence in one's ability to do a specific task), which influences the effort a client is willing to expend to achieve a goal. Detailed information about behavior change theories and models is presented in Chapter 13. | A community nutritionist may use games and brainstorming activities to educate elementary school children in how to increase their fruit and vegetable intake. |
| ***Coordination of Nutrition Care*** | Consultation with, referral to, or coordination of nutrition care with other healthcare providers, institutions, or agencies that can assist in treating or managing nutrition-related problems. | A community nutritionist in a local school district may refer pregnant teenagers to the WIC nutritionist, who also refers them to the community center or free clinic for prenatal care. |
| ***Coordination of Other Care During Nutrition Care*** | Facilitating services or interventions with other professionals or agencies on behalf of the client prior to discharge from nutrition care. | A WIC nutritionist may refer homeless individuals to a social worker, a public health nurse, and the Supplemental Nutrition Assistance Program for assistance. |

Data from: American Dietetic Association. *International Dietetics and Nutrition Terminology, International Dietetics and Nutrition Terminology (IDNT) Reference Manual: Standardized Language for the Nutrition Care Process.* 4th ed. Chicago, IL: American Dietetic Association; 2013:50-51.

## Nutrition Care Indicators

**Nutrition care indicators** are signs that can be observed and measured and are used to quantify the changes that occurred due to nutrition intervention. The indicators for nutrition monitoring should reflect the community or clients' nutrition diagnosis, etiology, and signs and symptoms. Nutrition care outcomes and indicators include factors that dietetics practitioners can use to make a direct impact on the problem, such as the following[88]:

- Food and nutrient intake; growth and body composition; change in food and nutrition-related knowledge, attitudes, and behaviors; and food access
- Laboratory values, such as HgbA1c, hematocrit, and serum cholesterol
- Functional capabilities, such as physical activity
- Client or community perception of nutrition care and results of nutrition program, such as nutrition quality of life, reduced serum cholesterol, or weight loss

## Examples of Monitoring and Evaluation in Community and Public Health

The following are some examples of a nutritionist performing monitoring and evaluation. A public health nutritionist could provide a nutrition and physical activity intervention program to fourth- and fifth-grade obese students after they completed a pretest questionnaire about their exercise and food habits. The nutrition diagnosis was high calorie intake *related to* frequent consumption of high fat from the fast foods served during school lunch and sugary snacks in the vending machines around the elementary school plus lack of physical activity, as *evidenced by* a BMI of 27 and estimated caloric intake of 600 calories per day more than estimated needs. The nutritionist prescribed 30 minutes of daily physical activity and six sessions of nutrition education to the children and two sessions to the parents. Also, homework was given to the parents to carry out with their children, which included exercising with their children and talking about healthy eating during dinner as a family. To monitor the outcome of the program, the parents and the children were asked to keep a 3-day food record, keep a daily log of their physical activity, and complete a posttest. The results of the posttest were compared to the pretest results.

Another example is an overweight 55-year-old woman with high blood cholesterol levels who participated in a community nutrition screening at a local clinic. She had a nutrition diagnosis of high fat intake *related to* daily consumption of high saturated and cholesterol foods, as *evidenced by* daily consumption of two scrambled eggs for breakfast and a half-pound hamburger 4 times a week, and a serum cholesterol level of 250 mg/dl. The nutritionist implemented a heart-healthy intervention with a nutrition prescription as follows: 25 g/day fiber intake (current is 15 g/day), 30 percent of total calories daily from fat, less than 10 percent of total calories daily from saturated fat, and reduce dietary cholesterol to less than 200 mg/day (current is estimated at 450 mg/day). The nutritionist monitored the intervention by asking the client to keep a record of her food intake and physical activity for 1 week.

Summing up, the NCPM is a tool nutritionists use to communicate nutrition activities within the profession and among a variety of other healthcare professionals.[88] The model provides a sequence of steps for dietitians to follow and lists essential components in each step of the process. It is helpful in documenting the impact the profession has on specific diagnoses and etiologies in patients/clients or populations. The four steps of the NCPM are nutrition assessment, nutrition diagnosis, nutrition intervention, and nutrition monitoring and evaluation. They are all essential in providing high-quality care to clients and in promoting health and preventing diseases using evidence-based strategies. The NCPM undergoes yearly review modifications. **TABLE 1-12** provides examples of nutrition diagnosis statements and dietary prescriptions.

## ▶ The Cooperative Extension System

The Cooperative Extension System (CES) is an agency under the U.S. Department of Agriculture. It provides educational programs that help individuals and families acquire life skills. The mission of the CES is to empower people through education using scientific, research-based information. Typically, land grant universities or colleges help carry out the CES's mission by providing their expertise to county and regional extension offices, which administer these programs. The colleges and universities help the public through informal, noncredit programs. The federal government provides support for the programs through the Cooperative State Research, Education, and Extension Service (CSREES). CSREES supports both universities and their local offices by annually distributing federal funding to supplement state and county programs.[90]

The Morrill Act of 1862 established land-grant universities to educate citizens in agriculture, home economics, mechanical arts, and other practical professions. In 1914,

**TABLE 1-12** Examples of Nutrition Diagnosis Statements (PES), Dietary Prescriptions, and Monitoring and Evaluation

| Diagnosis/Problem | Standard Phrase | Etiology/Cause | Standard Phrase | Signs and Symptoms | Dietary Prescription | Monitoring and Evaluation |
|---|---|---|---|---|---|---|
| | | | | | Using the established reference standards, the nutritionists may recommend | Select appropriate indicators, such as BMI, serum cholesterol level, Dietary Guidelines for Americans. |
| Overweight college students with excessive fat intake | Related to | Frequent consumption of fast-food meals | As evidenced by | 60 percent of students having a serum cholesterol level of 250 mg/dl and triglycerides of 165 mg/dl; 57 percent ate half-pound hamburgers and fries 4 times per week, and egg sandwich for breakfast daily. Ninety percent take walks twice per week for 20 minutes, and others do no exercise and smoke two packs of cigarettes a week. | Lifestyle modification: Increase exercise to 30 minutes daily, reduce energy intake, provide meal planning and portion size education, reduce fat intake to 30 percent of total calories, increase fiber intake to 25 or 30 g/day, and decrease dietary cholesterol to 200 mg/day. Refer cigarette smokers to the university health center for counseling. | |
| Obese high school students with excessive caloric intake | Related to | Frequent consumption of sugary drinks, candies, donuts, and fast food | As evidenced by | Assessments that show 35 percent of the students have a BMI of > 30, and 60 percent consumed 1,000 kcal/day more than estimated needs. | A caloric deficit of 500 to 1,000 kcal/day (energy level varies with the individual's size and activities), fat content of not more than 30 percent of total calories, and increasing exercise to 30 minutes daily. | BMI, Dietary Guidelines for Americans. |
| Anemic pregnant teenagers enrolled in a WIC program | Related to | Low iron and folate consumption | As evidenced by | An assessment showing Hb of 9 mg/dl, and daily intake of 600 kcal less than the recommended amount. | Increase caloric intake to meet their needs, increase the intake of iron (27 mg/day) and folate (600 µg/day), provide a list containing high-iron and high-folate foods. Vitamin and mineral supplement. | Hb levels, 3-day food records. |
| Malnourished children in a refugee camp | Related to | Lack of access to food due to political and economic constraints | As evidenced by | Edema of lower extremities, pluckable hair, thin and wasted appearance, low body temperature. | To avoid refeeding syndrome, provide high-calorie and high-protein intake gradually. Provide vitamin and mineral supplements. | Adequate weight and height gain, disappearance of edema of lower extremities. |
| Elderly women with osteoporosis enrolled in a congregate meal program | Related to | Less than recommended intake of dairy products and vitamin D, and lack of exercise | As evidenced by | Lactose intolerance, low bone density, <25(OH) D intake, lack of exposure to sunlight, and loss of height. | Increase calcium intake to 1,300 mg/day and vitamin D to 5 µg/day, include weight-bearing exercise for 20 minutes, 3–5 times a day. | 3-day food record, bone density measurement |

the Smith-Lever Act established a partnership between the USDA and land-grant universities. Currently, CES works in the following six major areas[90]:

- *4-H youth development:* Helps youth make life and career choices. At-risk youth participate in school retention and enrichment programs. They learn science, math, and social skills using hands-on projects and activities.
- *Agriculture:* Helps individuals learn new ways to improve their agricultural income through research-based management skills, resource management, controlling crop pests, soil testing, livestock production practices, and marketing.
- *Leadership development:* Trains extension professionals and volunteers to serve in leadership roles in the community and deliver programs in gardening, health and safety, and family and consumer issues.
- *Natural resources:* Provides educational programs in water quality, timber management, composting, lawn and waste management, and recycling to landowners and homeowners.

- *Family and consumer sciences:* Teaches families and individuals about nutrition, food preparation, positive childcare, family communication, financial management, and healthcare strategies so they can become healthy.
- *Community and economic development:* Helps local governments improve job creation and retention, small and medium-sized business development, effective and coordinated emergency response, solid waste disposal, tourism development, workforce education, and land use planning.

In addition, the Expanded Food and Nutrition Education Program (EFNEP) is a federally funded program designed specifically for nutrition education. The county extension home economists provide on-the-job training and supervise paraprofessionals and volunteers who teach low-income families and individuals about nutrition.[90] The Successful Evidence-Based Community Strategies features in this chapter discuss the successful Clemson University Cooperative Extension Nutrition Program on low-fat products and fat intake as well as a National Cancer Institute health promotion intervention program.

# Successful Community Strategies

## The National Cancer Institute's Health Promotion Intervention

Community and public health nutritionists can target worksites as a priority location for intervention efforts. An effective worksite nutrition program must include how to effectively communicate to clients how to choose and prepare foods that follow established dietary guidelines. One example of an effective worksite program is Working Well, which was a randomized worksite intervention trial. This 5-year study funded by the National Cancer Institute (NCI) tested the effectiveness of health promotion interventions directed at individual and organizational changes to reduce employee cancer risk in 57 matched pairs of worksites. Workers and worksites from a variety of geographic and industrial settings were utilized. Four project study centers, a coordinating center, and the NCI collaborated on common elements of design, data collection and analysis, and intervention standards for the common risk factor areas. The All Working Well study centers targeted nutrition and at least one other prevention component (e.g., smoking, cancer screening, occupational health, or physical activity). The study centers were Brown University School of Medicine and The Miriam Hospital (Rhode Island); the University of Florida; the University of Massachusetts Medical School and Dana-Farber Cancer Institute; and the University of Texas M.D. Anderson Cancer Center.

The Working Well intervention was based on a conceptual model that incorporated the following three important elements:

- The use of participatory strategies operated through a primary worksite contact and an employee advisory board
- An ecological approach targeting both individual behavior change and change in environmental and organizational structures
- The use of adult education and behavior change strategies in all aspects of intervention planning and delivery

The nutrition intervention messages are available in a summarized format at http://nutrition.jbpub.com/community nutrition. The messages were translated from nutrient terms into food terminology. They addressed groups of foods that contribute the highest amount of fat and fiber to the U.S. diet. All groups of foods were stated in positive terms.

The intervention was implemented in 114 worksites employing 37,291 workers who were engaged in a variety of businesses. In the fall of 1990, 20,801 respondents completed and returned a self-administered baseline survey. The worksite mean response rate was 71.6 percent. Responses to behavioral items regarding meat were used to measure meat preparation behaviors that could not be obtained from the food frequency questionnaire.

*(continues)*

## Successful Community Strategies *(continued)*

The intervention outcome showed that the average servings of fruits and vegetables per day were less than three in all study centers—2.7 in Florida, Massachusetts, and Rhode Island and 2.4 in Texas. Less than 30 percent of workers in Rhode Island and Massachusetts reported eating beans and lentils at least once per week, and 42 percent in Florida and 56 percent in Texas reported frequent bean and lentil consumption.

From 56 to 64 percent of workers reported eating high-fiber cereal at least half of the time they ate cereal, and 34 to 46 percent reported eating dark bread at least half of the time they ate bread.

The majority of workers reported eating chicken and fish that were not fried (55 to 84 percent), rarely eating visible meat fat (57 to 69 percent), and choosing lean meat (68 to 81 percent). On the other hand, avoiding the skin on chicken was reported less frequently (33 to 47 percent). Avoidance of meat fat was lower in Texas than in the other study sites for all four measures.

With regard to fat in dairy products, 65 to 71 percent drank low-fat or skim milk more than half the time they drank milk. Also, a smaller percentage, 42 to 64 percent, used low-fat cheese or low-fat frozen dairy products. The percentage who used low-fat dairy products other than milk was much higher in the Florida worksite than in worksites at the other study centers. Finally, 46 to 53 percent of subjects used low-fat salad dressing.

Modified from: Hunt MK, Stoddard AM. Measures of food choice behavior related to intervention messages in worksite health promotion. *J Nutr Educ.* 1997; 29:3-11.

## Successful Community Strategies

### The Clemson University Cooperative Extension Nutrition Program on Low-Fat Products and Fat Intake[91-97]

The percentage of calories from saturated and polyunsaturated fat and the amount of cholesterol in the diet are important determinants of the level of plasma cholesterol, a major contributor to heart disease risk. It is estimated on average that a 1 percent decrease in the intake of saturated fat results in a 2-mg/dl decrease in plasma cholesterol. This, in turn, can bring about a reduction in heart disease risk. High intake of dietary fat is also associated with an increased risk for developing cancer of the colon, prostate, and breast.

Programs that have demonstrated effective community interventions for a decrease in dietary fat include a program from Clemson University in South Carolina, which incorporated community nutrition classes, grocery store tours, speakers' bureaus, professional education classes, home study courses, and worksite nutrition education programs. This program focused on the impact of low-fat diets on serum cholesterol. The intervention community, compared with a control community, had a significant decrease in the intake of dietary fat (9 percent vs. 4 percent) and an increase in awareness of restaurant information (33 percent vs. 19 percent).

In South Carolina, 61 percent of adults were overweight or obese. From 1990 to 2002, the obesity rate among adults in South Carolina increased by 90 percent. The African American, Hispanic, and Native American populations in South Carolina had significantly high prevalence rates of obesity. Approximately 15 percent of South Carolina's high school students were at risk for becoming overweight, and approximately 11 percent were overweight. Data showed that less than 25 percent of all South Carolina's adults and only 18 percent of South Carolina's high school students ate the recommended five or more servings of fruits and vegetables each day. Obesity is associated with many health conditions, some of which include heart disease, stroke, and diabetes. These also make up the three major causes of death and disability in South Carolina. In South Carolina, medical expenditure due to obesity per year was $1.06 billion.

Clemson's extension agent provided low-fat programs at regional volunteer leader training, an assisted living facility, three community groups, and a summer youth camp. A low-fat nutrition education program was presented to 38 family and community project leaders at regional leader training. These project leaders taught the program to over 400 adult members in their four counties. In addition, the agent taught four 1-hour lessons emphasizing dietary guidelines to a senior group, two adult groups, and a group of young mothers of preschoolers. Also, a 3-hour workshop on nutritious snacks and Nutrition Facts labels was provided to 10 middle school youth. Thirty-two articles on low-fat ideas and nutrition tips were sent to 18 print media outlets in a three-county area (Richland, Lexington, and Fairfield). These print

*(continues)*

## *Successful Community Strategies* (continued)

media outlets reached a circulation of 473,000. The local Fairfield County newspaper (*Herald Independent*) published the nutrition articles 21 times from June 2004 to January 2005. Two Lexington County papers (*Twin-City News and Lexington County Chronicle* and *Dispatch-News*) published the nutrition articles 16 times from April 2004 to January 2005. These three newspapers had a circulation of 19,600 weekly. The state newspaper published three special interviews with the extension agent concerning nutrition information on a vegetable featured in their Life and Style food section. The newspaper had a circulation of 150,000 daily. The Focus on Family Matters quarterly newsletter published nine articles providing research-based nutrition information. The newsletter had a circulation of 1,000 in Lexington, Richland, and Fairfield counties. Nutrition recipe analyses on calories, carbohydrates, dietary fiber, sugar, fat, cholesterol, and sodium were published in the Cook's Corner column of *Living in South Carolina* magazine. The agent analyzed 45 recipes for 11 monthly columns. The magazine had a circulation statewide of 523,000 homes and businesses, with a readership of 1.2 million monthly.

At the end of the extension programs, 89 percent of participants surveyed said that the program had increased their nutrition knowledge. Approximately 72 percent said they would read the Nutrition Facts label on packaged foods. Seventy-five percent said they would reduce their intake of refined sugars. Approximately 78 percent said that they planned to control portion sizes and servings for each food group. Seventy percent said they would include 30 minutes of exercise per day. Sixty-five percent said they would include more whole grain breads and cereals in their diet. Eighty-seven percent said they would make one positive change as a result of the low-fat and healthy ideas programs.

## 🔍 CASE STUDY 1-1: Pregnant Teenagers and Dietary Habits

Beatrice is a community nutritionist (RD) who was employed to provide nutrition education programs to a group of pregnant teenagers attending high school in a Midwestern city of 200,000 people. The teenagers eat most of their meals on campus. Some participate in the school lunch program; others prefer purchasing foods from the vending machine located a few feet away from the cafeteria. Beatrice was asked to help improve the teenagers' nutrition and fitness status. Meetings with the teenagers revealed their opinions about food and physical activity. A 3-day dietary record and food frequency questionnaire were administered to the teenagers, and body measurements, such as height and weight for determining their BMI, were collected. She uncovered the following information:

- Analysis of the teenagers' food choices revealed a high fat intake of 39 percent of total calories.
- Thirty percent of the pregnant teens surveyed were obese (BMI of 30) and anemic, 40 percent were overweight (BMI of 27), and 30 percent were underweight (BMI of 16) and anemic.
- The average hemoglobin level was less than 10 g/dl and hematocrit was less than 35 percent.
- Ten percent of the teenagers had spoon-shaped fingernails on two or three fingers of both hands.
- In the vending machines in and around the high school, 80 percent of snacks were sugary or high-fat foods, such as chips, and they also contained soft drinks or other items with empty calories.
- Further analysis showed that the teen mothers' physical activity levels were inadequate.

The following plans reflect the program Beatrice devised after several meetings with the pregnant teenagers:

- Included fresh fruits and vegetables on every cafeteria menu. (These foods can offer vitamins, minerals, and fiber, as well as decrease the number of high fat items available.)
- Evaluated and found a place where they can perform physical activity and campaigned for needed changes.
- Established a place for physical activity around the teens' homes. (Inactivity is a major contributor to obesity.)
- Collaborated with the school food service director and the vending machine vendors to stock the vending machines with fruits and snacks low in fat and sugar, and to replace sugary soft drinks with fruit juices.

(continues)

## 🔍 CASE STUDY 1-1: Pregnant Teenagers and Dietary Habits *(continued)*

### Questions

1. Beatrice is a Registered Dietitian (RD). What are the educational requirements for becoming an RD?
2. Discuss the implications of the high-fat food consumption practices of these teenagers.
3. Some of the participants were anemic. What is the definition of anemia? Why is anemia a deleterious condition during pregnancy?
4. What is the current general physical activity recommendation for the individuals Beatrice is advising?
5. What are the disadvantages of drinking soft drinks (soda)?
6. Why does inactivity contribute to obesity? What are some of the effects of obesity on the health of individuals?
7. What are some of the primary prevention strategies Beatrice used to address the situation?
8. How could Beatrice improve the nutritional status of the students plus reduce their fat intake?
9. How can Beatrice increase the teens' physical activities?
10. In what kinds of settings do community nutritionists work?

Work in small groups or individually to discuss the case study and practice using the Nutrition Care Process chart provided on the companion website. You can also add other nutrition and health-related conditions or assessments to the case study to make the case study more challenging and interesting.

# Learning Portfolio

## Chapter Summary

- Community nutrition is a modern and comprehensive profession that includes, among other disciplines, public health, dietetics/nutrition education, and medical nutrition therapy.
- The World Health Organization (WHO) defined community as "a social group determined by geographic boundaries and/or common values and interests." Community members know and interact with one another; function within a particular social structure; and create norms, values, and social institutions.
- A community also can be defined on the basis of a common interest or goal. A collection of people, even if they are scattered geographically, can have a common interest that binds the members together.
- Community strengths can be physiological, psychological, social, or spiritual.
- Community nutrition and dietetics professionals are community and public health agency professionals who provide nutrition services that emphasize community health promotion and disease prevention.
- Public health has been viewed as the scientific diagnosis and treatment of the community. In this vision, the community, instead of the individual, is seen as the patient.

- In addition to dietary factors, two primary determinants of health status are genetics and lifestyle.
- Prevention is important in public health as well as in community nutrition practice. The three aspects of prevention are personal, community-based, and systems-based health.
- The three levels of prevention are primary, secondary, and tertiary prevention.
- Population and individual approaches are the two important strategies to choose from when designing a health promotion campaign aimed at risk reduction. The population approach directs instruction at the whole population or large sections of it, whereas the individual approach identifies those most at risk from the risk factor, and intervention is targeted specifically at these "high-risk" individuals.
- Health promotion can be defined as the process of enabling people to increase control over the determinants of good health and subsequently improve their health.
- In 1978, the WHO and UNICEF held a conference at Alma-Ata, USSR, and declared that health is more than the absence of disease and that the attainment of the highest possible level of health is a vital worldwide social goal.

- In Canada, chronic diseases have common risk factors, including physical inactivity, poor dietary habits, and the use of tobacco. Also, environmental factors such as personal health practices, income, employment, education, geographic isolation, and social exclusion.
- The Leading Health Indicators reflect the major public health concerns in the United States and were chosen based on their ability to motivate action, the availability of data to measure their progress, and their relevance as broad public health issues.
- The negative consequences of nutrition-related problems include malnutrition and chronic health conditions such as obesity, cardiovascular diseases, cancer, diabetes mellitus, and childhood deaths.
- Public health and community nutritionists carry out a wide variety of nutrition activities through various agencies at the local, state, national, and international levels. In most cases, the activities require multi-tasking roles such as blood pressure screening, diet counseling, and medical nutrition therapy.
- Preventive nutrition can be defined as dietary practices and interventions directed toward the reduction in disease risk and/or improvement in health outcomes.
- The Nutrition Care Process and Model (NCPM) contains four separate but interrelated and connected steps:
  - Nutrition assessment
  - Nutrition diagnosis (problems)
  - Nutrition intervention
  - Nutrition monitoring and evaluation
- The Cooperative Extension System (CES) is an agency under the U.S. Department of Agriculture. It provides educational programs that help individuals and families acquire life skills.

## Critical Thinking Activities

The working poor (defined as families whose earnings are less than twice the federal poverty level and in which the adults work an average of half time or more during the year[71]) are increasing in the current economy. Many public health programs may be eliminated or minimized, such as immunizations for all children and flu shots on demand for all people. Additionally, eligibility criteria for the WIC program may be altered.

- Divide into groups and provide each group a certain amount of money, for instance, $100,000. Then distribute the funds among the three levels of prevention (primary, secondary, and tertiary) and discuss the rationale behind the decisions. The table below presents examples of programs.

| Primary Prevention | Secondary Prevention | Tertiary Prevention |
| --- | --- | --- |
| Local Fruits and Veggies—More Matters campaign to schools | Worksite nutrition education for high-risk employees | Medical nutrition therapy for individuals with nutrition-related problems (e.g., heart disease) |
| School breakfast and lunch | Health Fair screening and referrals to primary care providers | |
| Breastfeeding support | | |
| Immunizations for all children | | |
| Prenatal care | | |

- Select four health issues from Table 1-1 and discuss the types of early intervention programs that can prevent the health conditions.
- Divide into groups and determine the locations for the WIC and Supplemental Nutrition Assistance (SNAP) programs in your community. Then, encourage teen mothers to enroll in these programs to obtain adequate prenatal care and nutrition counseling by giving them the addresses of the SNAP and WIC programs and the name of the WIC nutritionist.
- Collect and analyze a 3-day food record from a female high school student and compare the results with a female college student.
- Analyze a school lunch meal and determine the fat, protein, calcium, vitamin D, folic acid, iron, and fiber content.
- Provide a list of foods that are high in iron, calcium, and vitamin D.
- Provide a list of foods fortified with folic acid.
- Provide a list of foods low in saturated fat and cholesterol.

## Think About It

**Answer:** The nutritionist violated the moral virtue of respect. Identify other sources of these vitamins and other actions he could have taken to avoid this violation.

## Key Terms

**community:** A group of people who share a common geographic location, values, culture, or languages.
**community nutrition:** An area of nutrition that addresses the entire range of food and nutrition issues related to preventing disease and improving the health of individuals, families, and the community.
**ethics:** The study of the nature and justification of principles that guide human behaviors. They are applied when moral problems arise. Also the science of moral values and a code of principles and ideals that guides action.
**evaluation:** The systematic comparison of current program results/outcomes with previous status, interventions, goals, or a reference standard.
**evidence-based practice:** Using the highest quality available information to make practice decisions.
**health promotion:** The process of enabling people to increase control of and improve their health.
**Healthy People Objectives:** A tool to help a community create a vision for its future. It is designed to serve as a roadmap for improving the health of people in the United States.
**interdisciplinary team:** Collaborating personnel representing different disciplines (e.g., nurses, social workers, physicians, daycare workers, dietitians, and dietetic technicians).
**nutrition care indicators:** Signs that can be observed and measured; they are used to quantify the changes that occurred due to nutrition intervention.
**Nutrition Care Process and Model (NCPM):** A four-step approach to nutrition problem solving and care that is designed to guide and clarify the work of the nutritionist. It is a standardized process for providing nutrition care.
**nutrition counseling:** The nutritionist provides direction or advice pertaining to a decision or course of action.
**nutrition diagnosis:** Determining a nutrition problem that will be resolved with the dietitian's intervention.
**nutrition education:** A formal process that instructs or trains individuals in a nutrition-related skill.
**nutrition implementation:** The action phase of the nutrition intervention. The nutritionist carries out and communicates the plan of care/program to the clients.
**nutrition intervention:** A specific nutrition-related action that resolves a nutrition diagnosis and consists of two components: planning and implementation.
**nutrition monitoring and evaluation:** A procedure that determines whether the goals/expected outcomes were achieved and whether the nutrition intervention resolved the nutrition problem.
**nutrition prescription:** Recommended dietary intake of selected foods or nutrients for an individual or a community based on current reference standards and dietary guidelines and the client's or community's condition and nutrition diagnosis
**nutritionist:** A professional with academic credentials in nutrition; may also be a Registered Dietitian.
**preventive nutrition:** Dietary practices and interventions directed toward reducing disease risk and/or improving health outcomes.
**primary prevention:** Activities designed to prevent a problem or disease before it occurs.
**public health:** The science and art of preventing disease, prolonging life, developing policy, and promoting health through organized community effort.
**public health nutrition:** Focuses on the community and society as a whole and aims at optimal nutrition and health status. Public health nutritionist positions require dietetic registration by the Commission on Dietetic Registration and a graduate-level science degree that includes study of environmental sciences, health promotion, and disease prevention programs.
**Registered Dietitian (RD):** A dietitian meeting eligibility requirements (education, experience, and a credentialing examination) of the Commission on Dietetic Registration. Some RDs possess additional certifications in specialized areas of practice, such as diabetes, pediatrics, geriatrics, or renal nutrition.
**secondary prevention:** Activities related to early diagnosis and treatment, including screening for diseases.
**tertiary prevention:** Activities designed to treat a disease state or injury and to prevent it from further progression.

## References


1. Frank-Spohrer G. *Community Nutrition: Applying Epidemiology to Contemporary Practice.* 2nd ed. Sudbury, MA: Jones and Bartlet; 2008.
2. Havas S, Anliker J, Damron D, Langenberg P, et al. Final results of the Maryland WIC 5-A-Day Promotion Program. *AJPH.* 2015;88(8):1161-1167.
3. Goodman R, Wandersman A, Chinman M, Imm P, et al. An ecological assessment of community-based interventions for prevention and health promotion: approaches to measuring community coalitions. *J Comm Psychol.* 1996;24(1):33-61.
4. Merzel C, D'Afflitti, J. Reconsidering community-based health promotion: promise, performance, and potential. *AJPH. 557-574.* 2003;93(4):557-574.
5. World Health Organization (WHO). *Diet, Nutrition and the Prevention of Chronic Diseases.* Geneva, Switzerland: WHO; 1990.

6. Hawe P. Capturing the meaning of community in community intervention evaluation: some contributions from community psychology. *Health Promot Int.* 1994;9(3):199-210.

7. Denver A. *Community Health Analysis: Global Awareness at the Local Level.* 2nd ed. Gaithersburg, MD: Aspen Publisher; 1991.

8. McKenzie JF, Pinger RR, Kotecki JE. *An Introduction to Community Health.* 4th ed. Sudbury, MA: Jones and Bartlett; 2002.

9. Allender JA, Spradley BW. *Community Health Nursing: Promoting and Protecting the Public's Health.* 6 ed. New York, NY: Lippncott Williams and Wilkins; 2005.

10. Stanhope M, Lancaster J. *Community and Public Health Nursing: Population-centered Health Care in the Community.* 9th ed. New York, NY: Elsever; 2015.

11. Winslow C. *The Untitled Field of Public Health.* Vol 2. Chicago, IL: Modern Medicine; 1920.

12. Dossey B, Keegan L. *Holistic Nursing Practice.* 7th ed. Sudbury, MA: Jones & Bartlett Learning; 2016.

13. Finkelstein EA, Ruhm CJ, Kosa KM. Economic causes and consequences of obesity. *Annu Rev Public Health.* 2005;26:239-257.

14. Nedra K, Christensen E, Williams P, Pfister R. Cost savings and clinical effectiveness of an extension service diabetes program. *Diabetes Spectr.* 2004;17(171):171-175.

15. Qureshi AI, Suri MF, Kirmani JF. The relative impact of inadequate primary and secondary prevention on cardiovascular mortality in the United States. *Stroke.* 2004;35(10):2346-2350.

16. Guthrie JJ. Evaluating the effects of the Dietary Guidelines for Americans on consumer behavior and health: methodological challenges. *J Am Diet Assoc.* 2003;103(12):S42-S49.

17. Richardson RA, Cotton JW, Mark OR. Diet and colorectal cancer risk: Impact of a nutrition education leaflet. *J Hum Nutr Diet.* 2004;17(6):576.

18. Beaudry M, Hamelin AM, Delisle H. Public nutrition: an emerging paradigm. *Can J Public Health.* 2004;95(5):375-377.

19. World Health Organization (WHO). *Health and Welfare Canada and Canadian Public Health Association Ottawa Charter for Health Promotion.* Geneva, Switzerland: WHO; 1986.

20. World Health Organization (WHO); Pena M, Bacallao J, eds. *Obesity and Poverty: A New Public Health Challenge.* Washington, DC: WHO; 2000.

21. U.S. Department of Health and Human Services (DHHS). *Healthy People 2010: Understanding and Improving Health.* 2nd ed. Washington DC: DHHS; 2000.

22. U.S. Department of Health and Human Services (DHHS). *The Surgeon General's Call to Action to Prevent and Decrease Overweight and Obesity.* Rockville, MD: DHHS; 2001.

23. Kaufman M. *Nutrition in Promoting the Public's Health: Strategies, Principles, and Practice.* Sudbury, MA: Jones and Bartlett; 2007.

24. Webb G. *Nutrition: A Health Promotion Approach.* 2nd ed. New York, NY: Arnold; 2002.

25. Millen BBE. Dietary patterns, smoking, and subclinical heart disease in women: opportunities for primary prevention from the Framingham Nutrition Studies. *J Am Diet Assoc.* 2004;104(2):208-214.

26. U.S. Department of Health and Human Services, Public Health Service (DHHS, PHS). *The Surgeon General's report on nutrition and health.* Washington, DC: DHHS, PHS; 1988.

27. U.S. Department of Agriculture USDOA. Dietary guideline for Americans. 2010. http://www.healthierus.gov/dietaryguidelines/. Accessed June 20, 2005.

28. American Heart Association (AHA). Healthy lifestyle diet and nutrition. 2004. http://www.heart.org/HEARTORG/. Accessed March 2, 2016.

29. Tulchinsky TTH. Food fortification and risk group supplementation are vital parts of a comprehensive nutrition policy for prevention of chronic diseases. *Eur J Public Health.* 2004;14(3):226-228.

30. U.S. Department of Health and Human Services (DHHS). *The Surgeon General's report on nutrition and health.* PHS Publication No. 88-50210. Washington, DC: DHHS; 1988.

31. Bauman AE. Updating the evidence that physical activity is good for health: an epidemiological review 2000-2003. *J Sci Med Sport.* 2004;7(1):6-19.

32. Mulleln B, Cupples A, Franz M, Gagnon D. Diet and heart disease risk factors in adult American men and women: The Framingham Offspring-Spouse Nutrition Studies. *Int J Epidemiol.* 1993;22(6):1014-1025.

33. Willam M. *Nutrition for Health, Fitness and Sport.* 8th ed. St. Louis MO: McGraw-Hill; 2012.

34. Berdanier CD, Dwyer JT, Feldman EB. *Handbook of Nutrition and Good.* 2nd ed. New York, NY: CRC Press; 2007.

35. Roche HHM. Dietary lipids and gene expression. *Transactions.* 2004;32(Pt):999-1002.

36. U.S. Department of Health and Human Services (DHHS). Leading causes of death. 2015. http://www.cdc.gov/nchs/fastats/leading-causes-of-death.htm. Accessed March 2, 2016.

37. World Health Organization (WHO). The top ten leading causes of death. 2015. https://africacheck.org/factsheets/factsheet-the-leading-causes-of-death-in-africa/.

38. Vanden HJ. Diet, fatty acids, and regulation of genes important for heart disease. *Curr Atheroscler Rep.* 2004;6(6):432-440.

39. Skidmore PM, Yarnell JW. The obesity epidemic: Prospects for prevention. *QJM.* 2004;97(12):817-825.

40. Bautista-Castaño I, Doreste J, Serra-Majem L. Effectiveness of interventions in the prevention of childhood obesity. *Eur J Epidemiol.* 2004;19(7): 617-622.

41. Nies MA, McEwen M. *Community Health Nursing: Promoting the Health of Population.* 3rd ed. London, UK: Saunders; 2001.

42. Gakidou E, Oza S, Vidal Fuertes C, Li A, et al. Improving child survival through environmental and nutritional interventions. *JAMA.* 2007; 298:1876-1887.

43. Mackenbach J, Bakker M, eds. *Reducing Inequalities in Health: "A European Perspective".* London, UK: Routledge; 2002.

44. Stoddard AM. Cardiovascular disease risk reduction: The Massachusetts WISEWOMAN project. *J Womens health.* 2004;13(5):539-546.

45. Cheng CC. Cholesterol-lowering effect of the Food for Heart Nutrition Education Program. *J Am Diet Assoc.* 2004;104(12):1868-1872.

46. Pereira C, Carrazedo J, Colugnati F. Nutrition education in public elementary schools of São Paulo, Brazil: The Reducing Risks of Illness and Death in Adulthood Project. *Rev Nutr.* 2006;19(3):1-11.

47. Bemelmans WJE, Broer J, Hulshof KFAM, Siero FW, et al. Long-term effects of nutritional group education for persons at high cardiovascular risk. *Eur J Public Health.* 2004;14(3):240-245.

48. World Health Organization (WHO). Declaration of Alma-Ata, International Conference on Primary Health Care. 1978. http://www.who.int/publications/almaata_declaration_en.pdf. Accessed March 4, 2016.

49. World Health Organization (WHO). Global Conference on Health Promotion. http://www.who.int/healthpromotion/conferences/en/. Accessed March 4, 2016.

50. World Health Organization (WHO). Milestones in health promotion statements from global conferences. http://www.who.int/healthpromotion/Milestones_Health_Promotion_05022010.pdf. Accessed March 4, 2016.

51. United Nations Organization. The millennium development goals report 2015: Summary. 2016. http://www.un.org/millenniumgoals/2015_MDG_Report/pdf/MDG%202015%20Summary%20web_english.pdf. Accessed February 24, 2016.

52. Ready EA, Butcher JE, Dear JB. Canada's physical activity guide recommendations are a low benchmark for Manitoba adults. *Appl Physiol Nutr Metab.* 2009;34(2):172-181.

53. Public Health Agency of Canada (PHAC). Health living. http://www.phac-aspc.gc.ca/hp-ps/hl-mvs/index-eng.php. Accessed March 4, 2016.

54. Health Canada. A federal report on comparable health indicators. 2006. http://www.hc-sc.gc.ca/hcs-sss/pubs/system-regime/2006-fed-comp-indicat/index-eng.php. Accessed March 4, 2016.

55. Health Canada. Map of active physical activity index in Canada (both males and females). http://www.hc-sc.gc.ca/fn-an/surveill/atlas/map-carte/index-eng.php. Accessed March 04, 2016.

56. Health Canada. Nutrition for health: An agenda for action. https://books.google.com/books?id=0CIibtW7WscC&pg=PA273&lpg=PA273&dq=canada+nutrition+agenda&source=bl&ots=nb4PvQB6Oj&sig=SIOoVFbVVLhaz0qxQLJDYP3HMng&hl=en&sa=X&ved=0ahUKEwjCwK_1uqjLAhXDmIMKHUr_CkUQ6AEITzAI#v=onepage&q=canada%20nutrition%20agenda&f=false. Accessed March 4, 2016.

57. U.S. Department of Health and Human Services, PHS (DHHS, PHS). Healthy People 2000: National health promotion and disease prevention objectives. PHS 91-50213. Washington, DC: DHHS, PHS.

58. U.S. Department of Health and Human Services, Public Health Service (DHHS, PHS). Healthy People 2000: National health promotion and disease prevention objectives. PHS Publication 91-50212. Washington, DC: U.S. Government Printing Office; 1991.

59. U.S. Department of Health and Human Services, PHS (DHHS, PHS). Healthy People 2000: National health promotion and disease prevention objectives—Final review. http://www.cdc.gov/nchs/data/hp2000/hp2k01.pdf. Accessed March 4, 2016.

60. U.S. Department of Health and Human Services (DHHS). Health people progress reviews. http://www.cdc.gov/nchs/healthy_people/hp2000/reviews/family.htm. Accessed March 4, 2016.

61. U.S. Department of Health and Human Services (DHHS). *Healthy People in Healthy Communities: A Community Planning Guide Using Healthy People 2010.* Washington, DC: Government Printing Office; 2000.

62. Mollar MT. *Summary Measures of Popularion Health: Report of Findings on Methodological and Data Issues.* Hyattsville, MD: National Center for Health Statistics; 2003.

63. U.S. Department of Health and Human Services (DHHS). The Secretary's Advisory Committee on National Health Promotion and Disease Prevention objectives for 2020. https://www .healthypeople.gov/2020/About-Healthy-People. Accessed March 4, 2016.

64. Lynch J, Smith GD. A life course approach to chronic disease epidemiology. *Annu Rev Publ Health.* 2005;26:1-35.

65. Institute of Medicine. *The future of public health.* Washington, DC: National Academy Press; 1998.

66. Winterfeldt EA, Ebro LL. *Dietetics: Practice and Future Trends.* Sudbury, MA: Jones and Bartlett; 2005.

67. Dodds JM, Laraia BA, Carbone ET. Development of a master's in public health nutrition degree program using distance education. *J Am Diet Assoc.* 2003;103(5):602-607.

68. Johnson DB, Eaton DL, Wahl PW, Gleason C. Public health nutrition practice in the United Sates. *J Am Diet Assoc.* 2001;101(5):529-534.

69. American Dietetic Association, Commission on Dietetic. Registration code of ethics for the profession of dietetics and process for consideration of ethics issues. *J Am Diet Assoc.* 2009;109:1461-1467.

70. American Dietetic Association. Code of ethics for the profession of dietetics *J Am Diet Assoc.* 1999;99(1):109-113.

71. The American Dietetic Association. Nutrition and you: 2008 trend survey. http://www.eatright.org. Accessed March 4, 2016.

72. O'Sullivan J, Potter RL, Heller L. Position of the American Dietetic Association: ethical and legal issues in nutrition, hydration, and feeding. *J Am Diet Assoc.* 2002;102(5):716-726.

73. American Board of Internal Medicine. *Project Professionalism.* Philadelphia PA: American College of Physicians; 1995.

74. Bendich A. *Preventive Nutrition: The Comprehensive Guide for Health Professionals.* New York, NY: Humana Press; 2005.

75. Reddy K, Katan, M. Diet nutrition and the prevention of hypertension and cardiovascular diseases. *Health Nutr.* 2007;7(1A):167-186.

76. Dietrich M, Brown CJ, Block G. The effect of folate fortification of cereal-grain products on blood folate status, dietary folate intake, and dietary folate sources among adult non-supplement users in the United States. *J Am Coll Nutr.* 2005; 24(4):266-274.

77. Shepherd SSK. Consumer information gap on behavioral aspects of dietary change. *J Nutr Educ Behav.* 2004;36(3):113.

78. Cohen SS. Special action groups for policy change and infrastructure support to foster healthier communities on the Arizona-Mexico border. *Public Health Rep.* 2004;119(1):40-47.

79. Thom T, Haase N, Rosamond W, Howard VJ. Heart disease and stroke statistics—2006 update: A report from the American Heart Association Statistics Committee and Stroke Statistics Subcommittee. AHA Statistical Update. *Circulation.* http://www .circulationaha.org. Accessed March 8, 2011.

80. Go AS, Mozaffarian D, Roger VL, Benjamin EJ, et al. Heart disease and stroke statistics—2013 update: a report from the American Heart Association. *Circulation.* 2013;127(1):e6-e245.

81. Mosley BB. Folic acid and the decline in neural tube defects in Arkansas. *J Arkansas Med Soc.* 2007;103(10):247-250.

82. Canfield MA, Anderson JL, Waller DK. Recommendations and reports. *MMWR Morb Mortal Wkly Rep.* 2002;51(RR-13):16-19.

83. Splett PL, Montgomery DL. *The Economic Benefits of Breastfeeding on Infant in the WIC Program Twelve-Month Follow-Up Study.* Washington, DC: Food and Consumer Service, U.S. Department of Agriculture; 1998.

84. Cattaneo A, Ronfani L, Burmaz T, Quintero-Romero S, et al. Infant feeding and cost of health care: a cohort study. *Acta Paediatr.* 2006;95:540-546.

85. Whitehead D, Russell G. How effective are health education programmers: resistance, reactance, rationality and risk? Recommendation for affection practice. *Int J Nurs Stud* 2003;41:163-172.

86. Lacey K, Pritchett E. Nutrition care process and model: ADA adopts road map to quality care and outcomes management. *J Am Diet Assoc.* 2003;103:1061-1071.

87. Association AD. Nutrition care process and model: the 2008 update. *J Am Diet Assoc.* 2008;108(7 pt 1): 1113-1117.

88. Academy of Nutrition and Dietetics (AND). *International Dietetics and Nutritional Terminology (IDNT) Reference Manual: Standard Language for the Nutrition Care Process.* 4th ed. Chicago IL: AND; 2013.

89. Jarvis C. *Physical Examination and Health Assessment.* 5th ed. St. Louis, MO: Saunders; 2008.

90. U.S. Department Department of Agriculture. Cooperative State Research Education and Extension Office. http://www.csrees.usda.gov/. Accessed March 4, 2016.

91. Lupo BH. Lowfat products and nutrition success story. 2005. http://www.clemson.edu/lexington/Accomp133.htm. Accessed March 4, 2016.

92. Pieterse Z, Jerling JC, Oosthuizen W, Kruger HS, et al. Substitution of high monounsaturated fatty acid avocado for mixed dietary fats during an energy-restricted diet: effects on weight loss, serum lipids, fibrinogen, and vascular function. *Nutrition*. 2005;1(21):67-75.

93. Constant JJ. The role of eggs, margarines and fish oils in the nutritional management of coronary artery disease and strokes. *Keio J Med*. 2004;53(3):131-136.

94. Washington State. Washington State risk and protective factors: Nutrition. 2005. http://depts.washington.edu/commnutr/wadocs/wadocs-nutrition.htm. Accessed March 4, 2016.

95. Newman VA. Achieving substantial changes in eating behavior among women previously treated for breast cancer-an overview of the intervention. *J Am Diet Assoc*. 2005;105(3):382-391.

96. Zazpe I, Sanchez-Tainta A, Estruch R, Lamuela-Raventos R. A large randomized individual and group intervention conducted by registered dietitians increased adherence to mediterranean-type diets: The PREDIMED Study. *J Am Diet Assoc*. 2008;108:1134-1144.

97. Kazis R, Miller MS, eds. *Low-Wage Workers in the New Economy*. Washington DC: The Urban Institute Press; 2001.

98. Pelletier K. A review and analysis of the clinical and cost-effectiveness studies on comprehensive health and disease management programs at the worksite: Update VI 2000-2004. *J Occup Environ Med*. 2005;47(10):1051-1058.

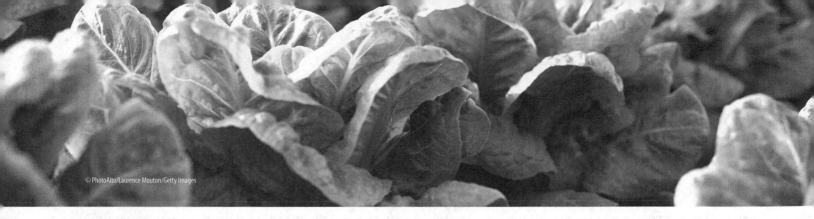

# CHAPTER 2

# Nutrition Screening and Assessment

## CHAPTER OUTLINE

- Introduction
- The Purpose of Community Nutrition Assessment
- Identifying Target Populations
- Historical Development of Nutrition Assessment
- Community Needs Assessment
- The Purpose of Assessment
- Screening for Assessment
- Nutritional Needs Assessment
- Different Methods and Tools for Assessing Nutrition Status
- How to Analyze Dietary Intake Data
- Food Consumption at the National and Household Levels
- Screening for Community Health
- The Purpose of Assessment

## LEARNING OBJECTIVES

- Define screening and assessment.
- Discuss the historical perspective of nutritional assessment.
- Define community nutrition assessment.
- List the needs assessment techniques.
- Explain the different methods of assessing nutritional status.
- Describe the various methods of dietary assessment and their advantages and disadvantages.
- Identify the appropriate dietary assessment tool for research purposes.

# ▶ Introduction

**Community assessment** is the process of critically thinking about a community by getting to know and understanding the community as a client.[1] Community assessment helps identify community needs, clarify problems, and identify strengths and resources. **Community nutrition assessment** is an attempt to evaluate the **nutritional status** of individuals or populations through measurement of food and nutrient intake and evaluation of nutrition-related health indicators.[2] The U.S. Department of Health and Human Services (DHHS) defines nutritional **assessment** as "the measurement of indicators of dietary status and nutrition-related health status to identify the possible occurrence, nature, and extent of impaired nutritional status," which can range from deficiency to toxicity.[3]

The type of information that can be collected during the community health assessment process includes statistical community profiles, qualitative data on the experiences of the community or population, and local resources and assets.[4] There are groups in every community that are interested in nutrition, including churches; healthcare institutions; government agencies; breastfeeding support groups; Head Start; schools and universities; parents; wellness programs; hospitals; doctors, nurses, and other healthcare professionals; the elderly; and international agencies.[5] A thoughtful compilation of assets prevents the assessment from becoming a log of morbidity and mortality statistics.

# ▶ The Purpose of Community Nutrition Assessment

Community assessment is a very important component of community nutrition practice. The purpose of a broad community nutrition assessment is to reveal the important nutrition-related needs in the community while finding opportunities for intervention. In order to accomplish this goal, data on the problems and their determinants are needed. A nutrition assessment of the community uses nutrition status measures acquired from **anthropometric**, biochemical, clinical, and dietary intake data, as well as epidemiological information.[6]

Measures of nutrition determinants, such as socioeconomic factors or the consequences, are used in applied settings (e.g., low-income pregnant mother participating in the WIC program) at the individual level or at the population level (e.g., setting policy, program evaluation, and nutritional surveillance). When discussing the latter applications, these nutritional variables are referred to as nutrition "indicators."[7] Nutrition indicators are used to screen, diagnose, and evaluate interventions in individuals and in populations. They can be used to make national and subnational comparisons and describe trends over time, identify populations at risk, target interventions, make policy decisions about resource allocation, monitor progress in achieving goals, and evaluate the impact of interventions.[8] In some cases, more than one nutrition indicator may be required in a nutritional needs assessment because there is no single best indicator for a nutrition-related problem.[7] For example, main indicators for marasmus (protein–calorie malnutrition) in children residing in a refugee camp may consist of weight-for-length below the 5th percentile, serum albumin less than 3.5 g/dl, painless pluckable hair, triceps skinfold less than 90 percent of standard, and mid-arm muscle circumference less than 90 percent of standard, plus vitamin and mineral deficiencies.

Community assessment is recognized as an important function of public health because it plays a primary role in promoting the health of communities.[9,10] Therefore, a comprehensive community assessment is needed to identify the health problems in the community and address the cause of the problems. A community nutrition assessment needs to do the following[1]:

- Identify the health of individuals within the community
- Identify the health of the community itself
- Determine the characteristics, resources, and needs of the community
- Work with community members on issues that arise
- Address not only individuals' behaviors, but also applicable environmental variables

Another aspect of assessment is program planning; it requires developing a doable plan. Program planning uses a timeline for achieving objectives, using resources, and assigning responsibilities (see Chapter 16 for details about program planning). The information gained from the needs and resource assessment is the basis for the plan.[11] Program planning is a multistep process that starts with the identification of the nutrition and health issue and development of an evaluation plan. Although specific steps may vary, they usually include a feedback loop, with findings from program evaluation being used for program improvement. The types of steps that are used in program planning are, but are not limited to, the following[12]:

- Identify primary health issues in your community
- After identifying the main health and nutrition issues in the community, develop measurable procedure and outcome objectives to assess progress in addressing these health issues

- Select effective interventions to help achieve these objectives
- Implement selected interventions
- Evaluate selected interventions based on objectives; use this information to improve program

Community assessment is used by many health and human service agencies, public and private agency planners, and businesses (market research).[5] It is the most cost-effective way to collect data because it uses existing vital statistics that are accessible, seeks the opinions of targeted group members and local health experts, and makes observations. Most of these data may not be specific to nutrition and diet; hence, the community or public health nutritionists needs to relate the available data to nutrition and diet issues. The nutritionist can focus on data associated with conditions that relate to nutrition, such as the number of infants with low birth weights, the number of low-income families who cannot purchase adequate food, or the number of elderly individuals who cannot participate in the Peace Meal Program (a senior nutrition program that offers mid-day meals to people ages 60 or older). Also, the rates of infant mortality, heart disease, and cancer can reveal whether the incidence of these problems is abnormally high in the community.[13]

An excellent way of gaining insight into the needs and priorities of a community is to collaborate with the community members. This is mainly beneficial when the effort is to reach vulnerable or underserved populations. It is advantageous for nutritionists to use the inside knowledge of community members in identifying mutually beneficial opportunities for the greatest impact that enables greater acceptability of the program within the community. The identified partners collaborate, review, and analyze the data leading to the development of nutrition and health improvement.[14] An example of a successful collaborative program was carried out with 19 houses of worship in the Central New Jersey area. There is great racial and ethnic diversity among these houses of worship, representing various faiths and denominations. Body & Soul: A Celebration of Healthy Living and Eating (B&S) is an evidence-based program developed by the National Cancer Institute in collaboration with the American Cancer Society, the University of North Carolina, and the University of Michigan. A Celebration of Healthy Living and Eating was created using a three-phase model to 1) educate lay members on nutrition and physical activity, 2) provide sustainable change through the development of physical activity programming, and 3) increase access to local produce through collaborations with community partners. The purpose of the program was 1) to establish a comprehensive program to improve nutrition and physical activity among people who attend houses of worship and 2) enhance the network of partners working with Rutgers Cancer Institute of New Jersey to provide community education. This collaborative case study included the successes and challenges through the development and recruitment periods of the program. This information was also used to inform future program activities.[15]

In addition, the nutritionist can use his or her knowledge of average household incomes; of the proportion of families participating in the Supplemental Nutrition Assistance Program (formerly the Food Stamp Program), soup kitchens, school breakfasts, school lunches, and food banks; and of the age distribution of the group to identify important nutrition concerns and issues.

Also, the aim of community needs assessment is to acquire information about the health and nutritional status of the target population. Therefore, targeting means limiting the nutrition intervention to the selected groups that are deemed most in need of those improvements (e.g., children younger than 5 years of age or pregnant or lactating mothers).[16]

## Identifying Target Populations

The process of targeting requires steps of decision making during the design and implementation of an effective food and nutrition program. Each step consists of gathering information and analyzing the food and nutrition situation. The steps in identifying target populations includes, but are not limited to, the following[16]:

1. Assessing the scale of the food and nutrition problems and their causes in the general population
2. Identifying the population groups most at nutrition risk
3. Generating problems list and prioritizing the situations according to the severity of the problems, the population groups affected, and/or the availability of resources

After completing the assessment, the data analysis will reveal the target community, available health and nutrition resources, and nutrition needs of the identified target population. A well-targeted nutrition program has the possibility of delivering a positive nutrition outcome in a more cost-effective way than an identical program that is poorly targeted. For example, providing foods high in calories and protein to children younger than 5 years in a developing country or iron-fortified food to pregnant women enrolled in WIC programs in rural communities will be more cost-effective than feeding all the children or pregnant women in the community.

# ▶ Historical Development of Nutrition Assessment

Nutrition assessment is a constant and evolving process. In 1932, the Health Organization of the League of Nations (HOLN) held its first conference to discuss the physical, clinical, and physiological aspects of nutrition assessment. This conference motivated the publication of the procedures needed for conducting nutrition surveys.[17] Subsequently, the monograph published by the Technical Commission of Nutrition of the Health Organization (TCNHO) was the first organized dietary standards. About the same time, Bigwood's *Guiding Principles for Studies on the Nutrition of Populations* provided detailed procedures for conducting nutrition surveys.[18] The basic philosophy of nutrition assessment has remained the same over the years, but these initial methods have been revised.[19]

In the 1940s, under the auspices of the United Nations, the Food and Agriculture Organization (FAO) and the World Health Organization (WHO) were established. Representatives from each organization were selected to form a Joint Expert Committee on Nutrition. In 1949, these representatives compiled information on nutritional status, dietary patterns, food supplies, and the economics of particular populations and recommended the establishment of nutrition policies for each nation. In 1951, the Joint Commission of the WHO published a report that emphasized anthropometric, clinical, and dietary data, but it did not make recommendations or set standards.[19,20]

## Nutrition Assessment in the United States

Despite these international organizations' attention to nutritional assessment, the United States did not recognize malnutrition as a health problem until fairly recently. Before the 1960s, the incidence of malnutrition in the United States was not noticed because little or no attention was given to nutritional health. This changed after the National Center for Health Statistics (NCHS) conducted the Ten-State Nutrition Survey (TSNS) between 1968 and 1970, and the first National Health and Nutrition Examination Survey (NHANES) between 1971 and 1974. These surveys discovered evidence of clinical and subclinical malnutrition in individuals in different areas of the country.[19,21] Results showed that population groups that were at nutritional risk were also socially, economically, educationally, or medically deprived. Malnutrition was associated with poor growth, developmental disability, poor pregnancy outcomes, susceptibility to infectious diseases, delayed recovery from illness, and reduced life expectancy.

These studies' dietary, clinical, and biochemical data have been reexamined by factor analysis, which analyzed eating habits as a means of relating food intake to health. The data also were analyzed to see the relationship between the combination of foods the participants ate and the condition of their nutritional health, for both samples in total and for various age, sex, race, regional, and income groups. Results showed significant associations between certain eating patterns and the lack of clinical symptoms and biochemical deficiencies. The factor analysis showed that some eating patterns were evidently better or worse than others.[22] The authors concluded that this food eating pattern model is a useful tool for 1) examining the association between food consumption and the incidence of disease states, such as obesity, hypertension, cardiovascular disease, cancer, and periodontal disease, for various large-scale dietary-health surveys; 2) establishing food regulatory policies; 3) setting national dietary goals; and 4) educating the public on nutrition and health issues.[22]

NHANES II was conducted between 1976 and 1980, and it targeted noninstitutionalized persons from 6 months to 74 years old. It used a data collection method similar to the one used in NHANES I. The Hispanic Health and Nutrition Examination Survey (HHANES) was conducted between 1982 and 1984. It was designed to obtain data from physical examinations, anthropometric measurements, laboratory analyses, and diagnostic tests of Mexican Americans, Puerto Rican Americans, and Cuban Americans. Dietary intake was analyzed using a 24-hour recall and a food frequency questionnaire (FFQ). The targeted population was individuals ages 6 months through 74 years.[23,24]

The third NHANES survey was conducted between 1988 and 1994 using nationwide samples of approximately 40,000 noninstitutionalized persons, ages 2 months or older. To obtain reliable estimates, infants and young children (1 to 5 years) and older persons (60 years and older) were sampled at a higher rate. Dietary intake was assessed by a 24-hour recall and FFQ. The examination parts of the study were varied based on age. Infants 2 to 11 months old received a physician's examination, body measurements, and other assessments. A dietary interview was conducted with the child's caregiver or parent. Between the ages of 1 and 19 years, additional assessments were included, such as a dental examination, vision test, cognitive test, allergy skin test, and spirometry (a measurement of lung capacity). Individuals over the age of 20 years received these assessments in addition to an oral glucose tolerance test, bone density test, fitness test, electrocardiogram, and other tests.[25]

## Growth Charts

In 1977, the NCHS developed growth charts as a clinical tool for health professionals to determine whether a child's level of growth was adequate. The WHO also adopted the 1977 charts for international use. With more recent and comprehensive national data available, along with improved statistical procedures, the 1977 growth charts were revised and updated in 2000 by the Centers for Disease Control and Prevention (CDC) to make them a more valuable clinical tool for health professionals. Most of the data used to construct these charts came from the NHANES surveys, which has periodically collected height, weight, and other health information on the U.S. population.[25] The revised growth charts provide an improved tool for evaluating the growth of children in community, clinical, and research settings.

The **body mass index (BMI)** is a significant new feature of the revised growth charts. These BMI-for-age charts were created for use in place of the 1977 weight-for-stature charts. BMI, also called the Quetelet index, is the most commonly used approach to determine whether adults are overweight or obese and is also the recommended measure to determine whether children are overweight or underweight. The BMI growth charts can be used clinically beginning at 2 years of age, when an accurate stature can be obtained.[25] To establish the BMI of a client, measure his or her height without shoes and his or her weight with minimal clothing. Then use the following equation to calculate the BMI.[26] For example, to determine the BMI for an adult:

1. Divide the individual's weight (in pounds) by his or her height (in inches).
2. Divide the result again by the individual's height.
3. Multiply the result by 703.

*or*

Weight $= 170\,\text{lb} \div 2.2 = 77.3\,\text{kg}$
Height $= 5', 1'' \,(71\,\text{in}) \times 2.54 = 180.3\,\text{cm}\,(1.83\,\text{m})$
BMI $= 77.3 \div 1.83^2 = 23.1$

## ▶ Community Needs Assessment

A needs assessment measures the current situation of a particular group or community.[27] Conducting a needs assessment involves completing a series of tasks and clearly identifying the priority health-related needs of a well-defined target population. A survey must be designed to ask about the needs of the community or group. This can include a variety of issues such as food stores moving out of the area, food assistance agencies, ethnic or racial needs, the number of healthcare professionals in the area, access to healthcare, and so on. Assessing community members' initial awareness about nutrition and then supporting community nutrition needs and services is essential if changes in behavior, norms, and public policy are to be evaluated.[10,13,28] In addition, a community needs assessment survey can be conducted when community groups want to take action, influence policy, or make changes.[10]

**TABLE 2-1** presents a subjective data assessment grid that can be used to evaluate healthcare professionals' and other important community members' knowledge of nutrition, the perceived proper nutrition needs, and attitudes toward nutrition and health. It is used as a starting point for program planning that involves the stakeholders (community leaders) and as a basis for developing programs that respond to their perceived needs that they will adopt. These data, along with data that characterize the community's nutrition and health status, are needed to develop programs for healthier living conditions.[5,29]

Community needs assessment studies are an effective way to find out what people are thinking and how they feel. Although information from a needs assessment study is valuable and useful, the process of gathering the information is also valuable. Needs assessment studies allow community groups or sponsoring agencies to do the following[30]:

- Collect information about community attitudes and opinions regarding specific nutrition, health, and other issues
- Determine how the community prioritizes the issues
- Provide the community the opportunity to determine policies, goals, methods, and procedures for solving the problem
- Evaluate current programs and policies and available resources

**TABLES 2-2** and **2-3** present examples of secondary and demographic datasets that could be sources for a community needs assessment.

## Methods of Performing a Community Needs Assessment

There are various methods of effectively assessing a community's needs. Selecting the best method is essential because the community group or organization may use the information gathered to make decisions about allocating public or private resources, determining program elimination or addition, and the like. Needs assessments can reveal and document a community

**TABLE 2-1** Subjective Data: Community Nutrition Assessment

| | Perceived Nutrition Needs in the Community | | | Attitude Toward Nutrition Services | | | Knowledge of Nutrition | | |
|---|---|---|---|---|---|---|---|---|---|
| | List | | | + | 0 | + | + | 0 | + |
| Clients/patients | | | | | | | | | |
| Public | | | | | | | | | |
| Media | | | | | | | | | |
| Government officials | | | | | | | | | |
| Agency administrators | | | | | | | | | |
| Physicians/dentists | | | | | | | | | |
| Hospital administrators | | | | | | | | | |
| Nurses | | | | | | | | | |
| Health educators | | | | | | | | | |
| Nutritionists/dietitians | | | | | | | | | |
| Agency board members | | | | | | | | | |
| Principals/teachers | | | | | | | | | |
| Social workers | | | | | | | | | |
| Clergy | | | | | | | | | |

Key: + = positive, supportive attitude toward nutrition and health services; 0 — neutral or apathetic attitude toward nutrition; − = negative attitude toward nutrition.
Modified from: Kaufman M. *Nutrition in Public Health: A Handbook for Developing Programs and Services*. Rockville, MD: Aspen; 1990:52.

need and have the added benefit of involving the public in problem solving and goal setting.[31]

Five different approaches are used frequently for collecting new information on the needs of the community. Different approaches are appropriate for different needs. To determine which approach is appropriate, examine the situation and the purpose of the needs assessment, and review the advantages and disadvantages of the various approaches. Sometimes, an assessment may need a combination of two or more techniques to obtain an accurate result or a good picture of the community's needs. The following sections describe the five needs assessment techniques that community nutritionists can use to assess the community.[27,32]

## Existing Data Approach

The nutritionist can use existing statistical data, such as national vital statistics, to obtain information about the well-being of people. This approach uses descriptive statistics such as census data, labor surveys, income data, NHANES data for food consumption patterns, U.S. Department of Agriculture (USDA) data from the Food Stamp Program, and school and hospital information to prepare an assessment report for the community. The advantages of this approach are as follows:

- The data are available, are relatively inexpensive, and are faster to use than conducting an original study.

**TABLE 2-2** Secondary Datasets That Could Be Sources for a Community Needs Assessment

| Description | Sources/Websites |
|---|---|
| 2010 Census datasets | http://www.census.gov/2010census/ |
| Data warehouse for NCHS public use data files for:<br>■ National Health and Nutrition Examination Survey<br>■ National Health Care Survey<br>■ National Health Interview Survey<br>■ National Immunization Survey<br>■ Longitudinal Studies on Aging | http://www.cdc.gov/nchs/about/fact_sheets.htm |
| Youth Risk Behavior Surveillance System:<br>■ Monitors priority health risk behaviors that contribute markedly to the leading causes of death, disability, and social problems among youth and adults in the United States<br>■ Data files and documentation | http://www.cdc.gov/healthyYouth/yrbs |
| DataFerrett System:<br>■ Collaboration between NCHS and the Bureau of the Census to provide NCHS datasets in the Census's DataFerrett system<br>■ A unique data mining and extraction tool that allows you to select a data basket full of variables, recode those variables as needed, and then develop and customize tables and charts | http://dataferrett.census.gov/ |
| U.S. Department of Agriculture (Economic Research Service):<br>■ Early Childhood Longitudinal Survey's Food Security in the United States | https://www.ers.usda.gov/topics/food-nutrition-assistance/food-nutrition-assistance-research/extramural-research/national-data-sets.aspx |

Source: Edelstein S. *Nutrition in Public Health: A Handbook for Developing Programs and Services*. 2nd ed. Sudbury, MA: Jones and Bartlett; 2006.

**TABLE 2-3** Sources of Demographic and Health Statistics for the Community Needs Assessment

| Description/Type of Data | Website with Link to Statistical Information |
|---|---|
| Census data: American Community Survey:<br>■ Includes state and county data | http://www.census.gov/acs/www/ |
| National health statistics produced in report format by NCHS (2010)<br>■ Comprehensive report drawing from a variety of data sources | http://www.cdc.gov/nchs |
| FastStats A to Z:<br>■ Provides state-specific fertility and natality information (e.g., age and parity of mother, duration of pregnancy, percentage of mothers who get prenatal care, number of unmarried mothers, infant's birth weight, type of birth [e.g., single, twin]), infant morbidity and mortality statistics, and health and health risk behavior data | http://www.cdc.gov/nchs/fastats/map_page.htm |

*(continues)*

**TABLE 2-3** Sources of Demographic and Health Statistics for the Community Needs Assessment (*continued*)

| Description/Type of Data | Website with Link to Statistical Information |
|---|---|
| NHANES results | http://www.cdc.gov/nchs/nhanes.htm |
| Links to NCHS surveys related to health and healthcare | http://www.cdc.gov/nchs/default.htm |
| National Vital Statistics system:<br>■ Annual reports that present detailed vital statistics data, including natality, mortality, marriage, and divorce | http://www.cdc.gov/nchs/products/vsus.htm |
| The Behavioral Risk Factor Surveillance System (BRFSS):<br>■ The world's largest telephone survey; tracks health risks in the United States<br>■ Includes national and state statistics as well as statistics on selected metropolitan areas | http://www.cdc.gov/brfss |
| Youth Risk Behavior Surveillance System (YRBSS):<br>■ Developed in 1990 to monitor priority health risk behaviors that contribute markedly to the leading causes of death, disability, and social problems among youth and adults in the United States | http://www.cdc.gov/healthyYouth/yrbs |
| The Pediatric Nutrition Surveillance System (PedNSS) and the Pregnancy Nutrition Surveillance System (PNSS):<br>■ Program-based surveillance systems that monitor the nutritional status of low-income infants, children, and women in federally funded maternal and child health programs | http://www.cdc.gov/pednss |
| Data warehouse for NCHS data:<br>■ Includes links to detailed statistical tables on a variety of health topics | http://www.cdc.gov/nchs |
| U.S. Department of Agriculture:<br>■ International food consumption patterns | https://www.ers.usda.gov/data-products/international-food-consumption-patterns/ |
| U.S. Department of Agriculture: Economic Research Service | http://www.ers.usda.gov |
| U.S. Department of Agriculture: Food Stamp Program statistics | http://www.fns.usda.gov |
| U. S. Department of Agriculture: WIC Program statistics | http://www.fns.usda.gov/pd/wicmain.htm |
| U.S. Department of Agriculture: Food Security in the United States:<br>■ Links to a variety of statistics on food security | https://www.ers.usda.gov/data-products/food-security-in-the-united-states/ |

Source: Edelstein S. *Nutrition in Public Health: A Handbook for Developing Programs and Services.* 2nd ed. Sudbury, MA: Jones and Bartlett; 2006

- The nutritionist can benefit from the research of top experts in the field, which ensures high-quality data.
- The nutritionist will benefit from utilizing samples from larger populations.

The disadvantages include the following:

- The nutritionist must relate the data to a particular community's nutrition issues.
- Many surveys deal with national populations, so the nutritionist may experience difficulty finding data for a well-defined minority subgroup.
- There is the potential of manipulating the data in such a way that the validity and reliability of the original research is lessened.
- Some research may involve very large samples and difficult statistical packages.

## Survey Approach

This approach requires some training or experience in how to create and administer survey questionnaires (e.g., writing clear and precise questions). In this approach, data are collected through personal interviews, telephone surveys, hand-delivered questionnaires, or mailed questionnaires. The data are collected from a wide range of representative community residents about issues pertaining to their well-being and needs. Responses are generally representative of the whole community. The nutritionist should consider the following before deciding to use this approach for the needs assessment: 1) cost of implementation, 2) time needed for completion, 3) individuals' rate of refusal, and 4) the magnitude and type of training the supporting staff need to carry out the survey. Some of the advantages to this approach are as follows:

- The entire population may be surveyed.
- It provides an opportunity for many people to feel involved in the decision-making process.
- It works well in combination with other systematic needs assessment techniques.

Some of the disadvantages to this approach are as follows:

- It may be expensive.
- It requires a great deal of time and expertise to develop the survey, train interviewers or staff, conduct interviews, and analyze and interpret the results.

## Key Informant Approach

The key informant approach requires the nutritionist to first identify the key leaders, decision makers, and professionals in the community (e.g., school faculty and administrators, hospital administrators, church leaders, mayors, commissioners, physicians) who can identify accurately the priority needs and concerns of the community. The nutritionist needs to compile a list of the key informants' names and decide how to collect data from them. As with the survey approach, you will need to create a questionnaire for gathering the information. Key informants would complete the questionnaire or be interviewed to obtain their perception of the community's needs. The information is then analyzed and presented to the community. Some of the advantages of this approach are as follows:

- This technique can be combined effectively with other techniques.
- It is inexpensive.
- It allows continuous clarification of ideas and information.

Some of the disadvantages include the following:

- An additional approach is needed because these results do not represent the total community perspective.
- The information obtained from this technique may be biased.

## Community Forum

One or more public meetings are held, and the participants discuss the needs of the community. The nutritionist should create a list of questions to be used for the group discussion. All members of the community, including key informants, should be encouraged to attend and express their concerns about their well-being and perceived needs. Some of the advantages of this technique are as follows:

- It allows input from many individuals with different perspectives on the needs of the community.
- It provides an opportunity for all the community members to participate in the needs assessment.
- In-depth information can be collected.
- It can be combined effectively with other techniques.
- Some of the disadvantages include:
  - The information collected may be limited to those who agree to participate.
  - Only those who are more vocal will be heard if the forum is not well conducted.
  - It may generate more questions than answers.

## Focus Group Interview

This approach involves selecting and interviewing people for their particular skills, experiences, or positions. Group discussions are then used to obtain detailed information about a particular issue. The participants are asked to respond to a series of questions about a topic or an issue. It is more effective to divide the participants into groups of 8, 10, or 20 if a large number of participants are involved. Each group member is asked to write his or her ideas on a piece of paper; all of the ideas are then listed on a chart or board. Each idea is discussed, clarified, and evaluated by the group, and then each person assigns a priority to each idea, or ranks the ideas by silent ballot. The prioritized ideas are tallied, and the final group ideas are listed and discussed. Some of the advantages of this approach are as follows:

- It can be used to expand the data obtained from surveys or existing data.
- The data can be used to create surveys for future use.
- It provides an opportunity to clarify ideas.
- It stimulates critical thinking.

Some of the disadvantages include the following:

- It does not give everybody in the community the opportunity to provide ideas.
- It must be combined with another technique because data from this approach may not be enough to get a complete picture of the issues.

## A Framework for Performing an Assessment

One person can carry out a needs assessment survey, but generally the survey will be more useful if it is designed and carried out by a group of individuals. This is particularly true if no one working on it has special experience in the field. The WHO and other authors suggested the following nine-step framework that provides a useful guide for planning and conducting a needs assessment[30,33,34]:

1. Decide when to conduct the needs assessment and set up a committee that will motivate community members to become involved in the needs assessment. Then, develop a plan of action.
2. List important issues or needs of the community. Decide what information needs to be collected after reviewing available information.
3. Determine the target population to be surveyed and how the data will be collected.
4. Determine the availability of existing data and what information will need to be gathered using a survey. Determine the cost estimates and the time frame.
5. Identify and train the assessment team. Develop and pretest the questionnaire, and then randomly select a sample of the individuals to survey.

6. Collect the data.
7. Analyze the data.
8. Interpret the results to identify priority needs, possible intervention strategies, and resources.
9. Present the results of the needs assessment to all the stakeholders and the community

## ▶ The Purpose of Assessment

All persons should receive nutritional status assessments throughout their life cycle as well as during illness. Assessment determines nutritional status by analyzing clinical, dietary, and social history; anthropometric data; biochemical data; and drug–nutrient interactions. Different approaches, such as calculating an individual's BMI and anthropometric measurements, can be used to assess nutritional status in both healthy populations and the critically ill.

Assessment of dietary intake is very important to the work of improving the health of individuals, communities, and populations. Berdanier[9] stated that dietary intake data are used for the following three major purposes[9]:

1. Dietary assessment at the individual level can be used to determine the individual's dietary adequacy and dietary patterns and for educating and counseling the individual.
2. Dietary assessment is an essential component of research studies that determine the health of individuals and populations. For example, etiological studies assess dietary intake as an exposure for association with disease outcomes. Behavioral research assesses dietary intake to develop and test strategies that encourage adoption of healthful eating patterns.
3. Dietary assessment also is important in identifying national health priorities, identifying population subgroups at risk or in need of special assistance, determining the success of public health interventions in improving dietary patterns, and developing public health dietary recommendations at the population/national level.[9]

Dietitians and nutritionists are responsible for nutrition assessment in community, population, and clinical settings. Several factors must be considered when conducting a nutritional assessment of the population. These factors include, but are not limited to, cost, convenience, and invasiveness. However, it is important to use the most convenient assessment method that can correlate findings with clinical, anthropometric, dietary, biochemical, and ecological factors.[19]

# ▶ Screening for Community Health

So far, this chapter has focused on different methods of studying community nutritional problems and assessing health risks for communities and their populations. The nutritional assessment process includes screening and assessment, and the major purpose of both is to screen for nutritional risks and apply specific assessment techniques to determine an action plan.[9,13] **Screening** is an attempt to detect unrecognized or subclinical health conditions among individuals. Community screening tests are not intended to be diagnostic.[31] Their purpose is to identify individuals who have a high risk for having or developing a specific health condition so they can be referred for definitive diagnosis and treatment. It also identifies individuals who may actually have an illness.[7,35] Screening carries an ethical commitment to continue working with these individuals and provide them with access to diagnostic and treatment services.

## Reliability and Validity of Screening for Community Health

One major concern about screening methods is the accuracy of the information gathered. **Reliability** is the consistency or repeatability and reproducibility of test results or whether a testing instrument will measure nutrient intake the same way twice on the same client.[35,36] A screening instrument that produces the same result on two or more different occasions, even when administered by different investigators, is considered reliable. **Validity** is the ability of a test instrument to measure accurately what it is supposed to measure. For example, a validity study may compare the results from an FFQ to a more accurate but difficult method such as a food record.[36]

## Reliability and Validity

Test results may yield invalid or unreliable results due to inconsistent administration of the instrument. To reduce the possibility of human error, it is very important to train all the personnel who will administer the testing instrument. Additional strategies that can be used to enhance accuracy include making precise measurements and calibrating the instruments before administering the test. The validity and reliability of the test instruments also depend on the responses of the participants.[35] It is important to modify the instrument for a specific population. For instance, one study found that although FFQ assessments were useful for ranking adults' consumption of fruits and vegetables compared to dietary recall, they underestimated the prevalence of fruit and vegetable consumption among high school students.[36]

In addition, two major theoretical perspectives (cognitive and situational) have been proposed to explain the source of validity problems that may occur with some self-reported data. The cognitive perspective focuses on the mental processes associated with validity problems, with inaccuracies originating from comprehension, recall, and other cognitive operations present in self-reported data.[37] The situational perspective focuses on validity problems that arise from factors related to social desirability and interviewing conditions (e.g., the presence of others while responding to questions, respondents' perceptions of the level of privacy or confidentiality provided).[38] Many other factors affect the reliability and validity of dietary assessment questionnaires. These include, but are not limited to the following[38,39]:

- Degree of variability permitted by the instrument (convenience of recording food intake, external environment, portion sizes used, types of foods listed, etc.)
- Quality control of coding and keying
- Real dietary change in the time between the two administrations of the questionnaire
- Respondent characteristics (level of education, cultural background, age, etc.)
- Questionnaire design
- Qualifications of the interviewer
- Adequacy of the reference data

Thus, to improve the reliability and validity of the diet recall, it is important to use a standardized protocol that specifies exact techniques for interviewing, recording, and calculating results. The instrument should use standardized graduated food models to quantify foods and beverages consumed. Similarly, use probing questions to determine foods and beverages most commonly forgotten. It is also important to use a culturally appropriate survey instrument.

## Sensitivity and Specificity

Two other measurements of a test are its sensitivity and specificity. A screening method with high **sensitivity** means there are few false negatives. A sensitivity test is able to correctly identify and classify individuals within the population who are truly malnourished as confirmed by a test (a true positive). For example, screening individuals who are at risk for poor nutrition (e.g., those with low hemoglobin levels) and who qualify for a nutrition assistance program will yield a high sensitivity rate.[7,35] A screening method with high sensitivity means there are few false negatives. For example, if a sensitive *specificity - & few   malnourshed* (handwritten)

mammogram finds a suspicious lump in a woman's breast, the test is usually followed with a biopsy to determine whether the lump is indeed cancerous.

A screening method with high **specificity** has few false positive results. A specificity test is able to, for example, correctly identify individuals who are not malnourished within a population (true negative). For instance, when screening well-nourished individuals without risk factors for poor nutrition, the method identifies those who do not need the nutrition service.

Preferably, a screening test's sensitivity and specificity should be 100 percent. Sensitivity, or the true positive rate, is the complement of the false negative rate, and specificity, or the true negative rate, is the complement of the false positive rate. Therefore, as sensitivity increases, specificity decreases.

In practice, nutritionists must strive to seek a balance between sensitivity and specificity. Both sensitivity and specificity can be improved by adjusting the screening process (such as by adding another test). An example of this might be to include a screening test that uses oral glucose tolerance instead of a urinary glucose test to determine the body's ability to utilize glucose, or performing a screening test that uses phlebotomy to detect high blood cholesterol concentrations instead of just a finger prick cholesterol test.

## ▶ Nutritional Needs Assessment

Dietary assessment is the first step in identifying nutritional deficiency. Nutritional needs assessments are conducted using different methods to determine the nutritional status of individuals or the entire population, dietary intake, and possible dietary inadequacies. The main methods of assessing individuals' food consumption (discussed later in the chapter) are a 24-hour recall, a food diary or record, a dietary history, and an FFQ. These methods are based on the anthropometric, biochemical, clinical, and dietary (ABCD) measures presented in **TABLE 2-4**. They can be used either alone or combined with other methods for more effective results.

Other factors, sometimes called ecological factors, that may influence the nutrition status of individuals or populations include socioeconomic and demographic data, such as the following[30,31]:

- Household composition (e.g., single parent head of household, number of children)
- Education (e.g., literacy)
- Ethnicity
- Religion
- Cultural practices
- Income
- Employment status

**TABLE 2-4** The ABCDs of Nutrition Assessment

| Assessment Method | Reasons for Use |
|---|---|
| Anthropometric measures | Measure growth in children; shows changes in weight that can reflect diseases (e.g., obesity, cancer, or thyroid problems); monitors progress in fat loss |
| Biochemical tests | Measure blood, urine, and/or feces for nutrients or metabolites that indicate deficiencies, infection, or disease |
| Clinical and physical observations | Assesses change in skin color, health, hair texture, fingernail shape, eyes, etc. |
| Dietary intake | Evaluates diet for nutrient intake (e.g., fat; calcium; iron; vitamins D, A, and C; protein) or food eaten (e.g., number of servings of fruits and vegetables), as well as eating patterns |

Adapted from: Insel P, Turner RE, Ross D. *Nutrition*. 3rd ed. Sudbury, MA: Jones and Bartlett; 2007.

- Material and community resources (e.g., access to health and agricultural services, land ownership)
- Ready access to a good source of drinking water
- Household sanitation

Additional factors, including the cost of foods, the adequacy of food preparation equipment, the availability of food reserves, and the percentage of household income spent on certain foods such as meats, fruits and vegetables, and grains also may be collected.[31] Data on health and vital statistics also may be obtained, such as the following[40]:

- The proportion of children immunized against measles and other infectious diseases
- The proportion of infants born with a low birth weight
- The percentage of mothers who are breastfeeding
- The proportion of mothers who used drugs or other substances while pregnant
- Mortality and morbidity rates

The story of the Delta Nutrition Intervention Research Initiative is discussed in this chapter as a Successful Community Strategy.

# Different Methods and Tools for Assessing Nutrition Status

Nutrients play many roles in the body, so measures of nutritional status must include many factors. Often these factors are referred to as the ABCDs of nutrition assessment: anthropometric measurements, biochemical tests, clinical observations, and dietary intake (see Table 2-5, later).[26]

## Anthropometric Measurements and Body Composition

Anthropometric measurements are physical measurements of the body, such as height, stature (standing height), recumbent length, weight, circumferences (head, waist, etc.), skinfold thicknesses, or limb lengths and breadths (elbow, wrist, shoulder). They are useful indicators of health, development, and growth. Anthropometric measures can be used to evaluate nutritional status in cases of obesity and emaciation due to protein-energy malnutrition. They are also important in monitoring the effects of nutritional intervention for diseases, trauma, surgery, or malnutrition.[23]

### Weight

Weight is a critical measurement in nutrition assessment. It is used to assess children's growth, predict energy expenditure and protein needs, and determine body composition. Weight should be measured using a calibrated scale.

### Length

Length (also known as recumbent length) is obtained while the client is lying down. It is generally used for children younger than 24 months of age or for children between 2 and 3 years old who cannot stand up straight without assistance.[41,42] This measurement requires a special measuring device with a stationary headboard and movable footboard that are perpendicular to the backboard. The device's measuring scale (in millimeters or inches) should have its zero end at the edge of the headboard and allow the child's length to be read from the footboard.[43] The average recumbent length for a child of about 2 years is about 5 mm higher than standing height for the same child. Therefore, 5 mm needs to be added to a standing height value when recumbent length measurement is not used.[43] The procedure is as follows:

1. Two examiners are needed to position the client and ensure accurate and reliable measurements of length.
2. Place the client lying on his or her back with the head toward the fixed end of the board and the body parallel to the board's axis. It is important that the client's shoulders and buttocks rest against the surface of the board.
3. One examiner gently brings the crown of the client's head into contact with the fixed headboard and positions the head so that the **Frankfurt horizontal plane** is vertical.
4. The second examiner holds the subject's feet, without shoes, toes pointing upward, and keeping the client's knees straight. If the client is restless, only the left leg should be positioned for the measurement.
5. The second examiner brings the movable footboard to rest firmly against the client's heels.
6. One of the examiners takes the reading to the nearest millimeter (0.1 cm or ⅛ inch).

### ✍ Think About It

What types of assessments should a nutritionist encourage in the following situation? Maria, an 8-weeks postpartum mother, attended a nutrition education class that the WIC nutritionist was providing to breastfeeding mothers. After the education session she told the nutritionist that she is concerned about not producing enough breast milk because her baby cries a great deal and seems to be hungry most of the time and is not as plump as her friend's formula-fed baby. Maria has lost 20 pounds and currently weighs 170 pounds with a BMI of 27.2 kg/m².

She also complained of fatigue and assumed it may be due to the demands of caring for her infant. In addition, she resumed menstruating 6 weeks after giving birth. Sometimes she has small amounts of blood in her stool from hemorrhoids. When the nutritionist asked her about eating habits, she said that she avoids red meat because it is high in saturated fat. The nutritionist felt Maria may be lacking in iron.

### Height or Stature

Height, or stature, is measured for children starting at 2 to 3 years of age and for adults who are able to stand straight. It can be measured in many different ways,[36] including using digital devices that measure stature to 0.1 mm or ⅛ inch. First the **stadiometer** needs to be calibrated. The client needs to be barefoot and wearing light clothing. The procedure for measuring height is as follows:

1. Ask the client to stand erect with the head in the Frankfurt plane (looking straight ahead), with heels together, arms to the side, legs straight, shoulders relaxed, and buttocks and

scapulae (shoulder blades) in contact with the vertical surface of the stadiometer or wall. Arms need to be hanging loosely at the sides with palms facing the thighs (see **FIGURE 2-1**).

2. Ask the client to inhale deeply, hold the breath, and maintain an erect position.

3. Lower the headboard gently onto the highest point of the head (the crown) with enough pressure to compress the hair.

4. Keep your eyes level with the headboard to avoid **parallax errors**.

5. Read the measurement to the nearest 0.1 mm or ⅛ inch.

For obese individuals, estimate height from knee height (see the following section).

Another method of measuring height is by using a right-angle headboard and a measuring rod or non-stretchable tape fixed to a vertical surface. Scales with movable measuring rods are not recommended because they produce inaccurate measurements. The client should wear minimal clothing and should not wear shoes and socks; infants should wear only a diaper.

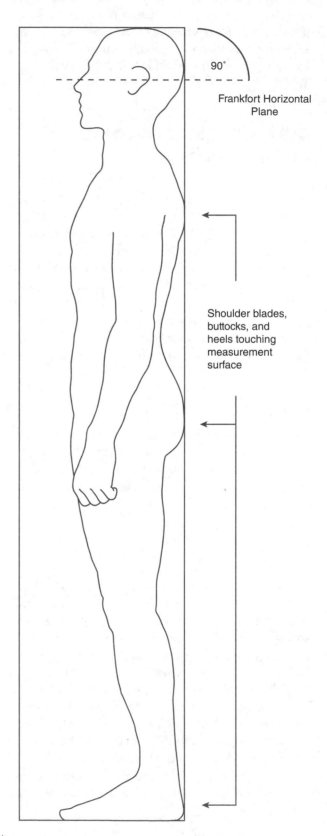

90°

Frankfort Horizontal Plane

Shoulder blades, buttocks, and heels touching measurement surface

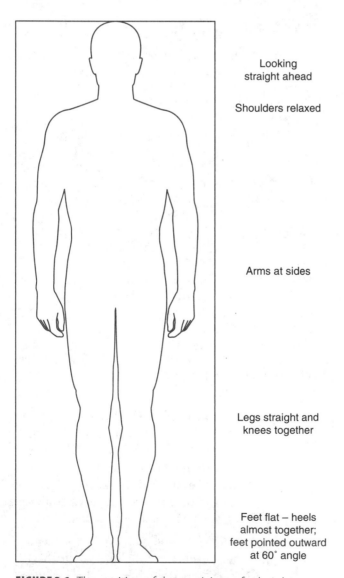

Looking straight ahead

Shoulders relaxed

Arms at sides

Legs straight and knees together

Feet flat – heels almost together; feet pointed outward at 60° angle

**FIGURE 2-1** The position of the participant for height measurement.

Reproduced from: Centers for Disease Control and Prevention, National Center for Health Prevention and Promotion. National Health and Nutrition Examination Survey III: Body Measurements Anthropometry. Atlanta, GA: Centers for Disease Control and Prevention, National Center for Health Prevention and Promotion; 2011.

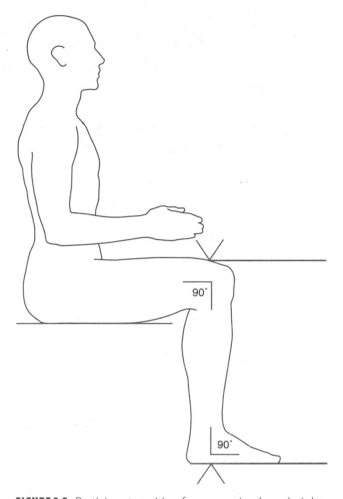

**FIGURE 2-2** Participant position for measuring knee height.

Reproduced from: Centers for Disease Control and Prevention, National Center for Health Prevention and Promotion (CDC, NCHPP). National Health and Nutrition Examination Survey III: Body Measurements Anthropometry. Atlanta, GA: Centers for Disease Control and Prevention, National Center for Health Prevention and Promotion; 2011.

## Knee Height for Nonambulatory Individuals

Knee height measurement is used for individuals who cannot stand or those with spinal curvature, paralysis, or other conditions limiting their ability to stand. It is also used for obese individuals. Knee height is highly correlated with stature. It is measured with a caliper consisting of an adjustable measuring stick with a blade attached to each end at a 90-degree angle. This can be purchased from a variety of sources online. The procedure for measuring knee height is as follows:

1. Take the measurements while the client is in the supine position (lying facing up).
2. Use a sliding caliper consisting of an adjustable measuring stick with a blade attached to each end at a 90-degree angle.
3. Take the measurement using the left leg.
4. Bend or position the knee at a 90-degree angle (see **FIGURE 2-2**).
5. Position one of the fixed blades under the heel of the left foot and the movable blade over the anterior surface of the left thigh.

6. Position the caliper shaft parallel to the fibula (the outside bone of the lower leg), over the lateral malleolus (the most prominent bony projection on the outer side of the left ankle), and just posterior to the head of the fibula.
7. Apply gentle pressure to the blades of the caliper to compress the tissues.[41,44,45] (Some knee-height calipers are equipped with a locking mechanism to retain the measurement after removing the caliper from the leg.)
8. Record the measurement to the nearest 0.1 cm. Two successive measurements should be made, and they should agree within 5 mm; the mean is then calculated.
9. Use the following formula to estimate stature from the knee height.[46,47] Research shows that the equations based on knee height predicted the client's stature to approximately 2.3 cm.[48]

There are separate knee-height equations for Caucasian American and African American men and women ages 60 to 80 years.[40,41]

Height (Caucasian American men, cm) = $(2.08 \times$ Knee height$) + 59.01$ (Stature)

Height (Caucasian American women, cm) = $(1.91 \times$ Knee height$) - (0.17 \times$ age$) + 75.00$ (Stature)

Height (African American men, cm) = $(1.37 \times$ Knee height$) + 95.79$ (Stature)

Height (African American women, cm) = $(1.96 \times$ Knee height$) + 58.72$ (Stature)

An alternative approach is estimating stature from either upper arm or lower arm length (see the following section).[49]

## Arm Span and Total Arm Length

Arm span measurement is also helpful as an alternative method of determining height. Arm span measurement may be used when actual height measurement is difficult to obtain. It is useful in situations such as children with cerebral palsy or scoliosis or the elderly with spinal curvature.[49] The following is the procedure for determining arm span. Two examiners are needed.[40,50]

1. It is easier to carry out the measurements against a flat wall to which is attached a fixed marker board at the zero end of a horizontal scale. A vertical movable arm should be attached to the scale.
2. Position the horizontal scale so it is just above the shoulders of the participant.
3. Ask the participant to stand with feet together and back against the wall.

4. Ask the participant to extend arms laterally (from the sides of the body) at shoulder height and outstretched maximally. The palms should be facing forward.

5. One examiner should stand at the fixed end of the scale, and the other examiner positions the movable arm and takes the readings.

6. Measure the distance from the tip of the middle finger on one hand to that on the other hand. Exclude the fingernails of both hands.

7. Take two readings for each measurement and record to the nearest 0.1 cm.[51]

Reliable measurements may be difficult for individuals with contractures or spinal deformities and those who are unable to fully extend their arms. Knee height may be used instead of arm span for individuals with major chest and spinal deformities because it provides a more valid estimate of maximum stature.[47]

## Frame Size

Frame size is calculated to determine the appropriate range of ideal body weight. The amount of bone, muscle, and fat are considered when determining appropriate weight. The classification of individuals on the basis of frame size was a common characteristic of the Metropolitan Life Insurance Company height–weight tables. The limitations of the Metropolitan height–weight tables were the inability to provide information on actual body composition and that the frame size classification may have depended on the participant's self-appraisal.[43,52] This led to the development of several techniques of determining frame size, including wrist circumference and elbow breadth.[53,54,55]

Therefore, as discussed earlier, BMI is a reliable approach for determining overweight and obesity, basically replacing the height–weight table. It is important to note that BMI does not differentiate between weight associated with muscle and weight associated with body fat. This website from the National Heart Lung and Blood Institute (http://www.nhlbi.nih.gov/guidelines /obesity/bmi_tbl.htm) presents a BMI for different heights and weights.

**Wrist Circumference.** The nutritionist can use wrist circumference to measure frame size. He or she needs to measure the right wrist circumference. The arm should be flexed at the elbow with the palm facing upward, and the hand muscles should be relaxed. The procedure is as follows[23]:

1. The measuring tape should be placed around the wrist crease just distal to (beyond) the

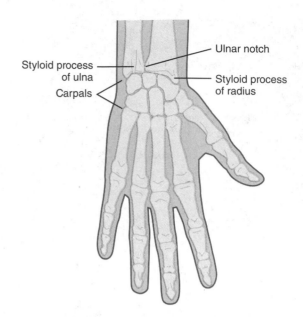

**FIGURE 2-3** Participant position for measuring wrist circumference.

Reproduced from: Centers for Disease Control and Prevention, National Center for Health Prevention and Promotion. National Health and Nutrition Examination Survey III: Body Measurements Anthropometry. Atlanta, GA: Centers for Disease Control and Prevention, National Center for Health Prevention and Promotion; 2011.

styloid processes of the radius and ulna (the two bony prominences at the wrist). Use a measuring tape that is not wider than 0.7 cm so it can fit into the depressions between the styloid processes and the bones of the hand (see **FIGURE 2-3**).

2. Place the tape perpendicular to the long axis of the forearm.

3. The tape should touch the skin, not squeeze the soft tissues.

4. Record the measurement to the nearest 0.1 cm.[56]

The formula for determining frame size from the ratio of body height to wrist circumference is as follows[57]:

$$R = H/C$$

R = Ratio of body height to wrist circumference
H = Body height in centimeters
C = Circumference of the right wrist in centimeters

### Frame Size Using *R* Value: Women

- Small > 10.9
- Medium 10.9 to 9.9
- Large < 9.9

### Frame Size Using *R* Value: Men

- Small > 10.4
- Medium 10.4 to 9.6
- Large < 9.6

**Elbow Breadth.** Elbow breadth also measures frame size. It is measured with the participant standing straight and the right upper arm extended forward perpendicular

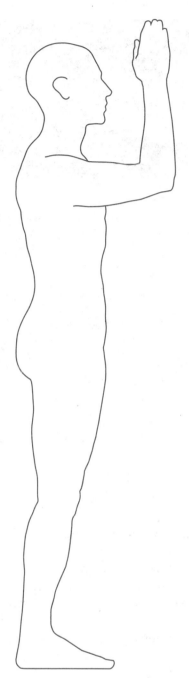

**FIGURE 2-4** Participant position for measuring elbow breadth.

Reproduced from: Centers for Disease Control and Prevention, National Center for Health Prevention and Promotion. National Health and Nutrition Examination Survey III: Body Measurements Anthropometry. Atlanta, GA: Centers for Disease Control and Prevention, National Center for Health Prevention and Promotion; 2011.

to the body, as shown in **FIGURE 2-4**.[54] The procedure for measurement is as follows:

1.  Ask the participant to raise the right arm and bend the elbow to a 90-degree angle, with fingers up and palm facing the participant.
2.  The nutritionist should feel for the widest bony width of the elbow and place the heads of a flat-blade sliding caliper at those points.
3.  Exert firm pressure to compress soft tissues.
4.  Read and record the measurement to the nearest 0.1 cm or ⅛ inch.[58]

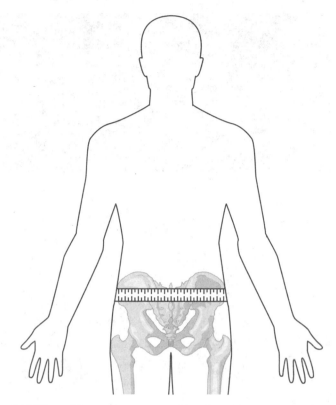

**FIGURE 2-5** Measuring tape position for waist circumference.

Reproduced from: Centers for Disease Control and Prevention, National Center for Health Prevention and Promotion. National Health and Nutrition Examination Survey III: Body Measurements Anthropometry. Atlanta, GA: Centers for Disease Control and Prevention, National Center for Health Prevention and Promotion; 2011.

## Waist Circumference

The most accurate method of measuring total abdominal fat is by using magnetic resonance imaging or computed tomography. But this technique is not easily available in a community setting. Waist circumference, however, is another way of assessing abdominal fat content, and it can be carried out in a community setting. It is a better predictor of total abdominal fat content than the waist-to-hip ratio.[59,60] Waist-to-hip ratio is calculated by dividing the waist circumference by the hip circumference. Waist circumference is measured around the smallest area below the rib cage and above the umbilicus, as shown in **FIGURE 2-5**.[53]

BMI and waist circumference significantly correlate with obesity and risk for chronic health conditions, and both measures should be used to classify overweight and obesity and to estimate disease risk[55] **TABLE 2-5** presents classifications of overweight and obesity and associated disease risk based on BMI. It is important to note that waist circumference has little predictive value for participants who have a BMI greater than 35 kg/m². For these people, waist circumference does not need to be measured; the cutoff points are 40 inches for men and 35 inches for women. Waist circumference may vary with race or ethnicity.[2,61] The waist circumference

**TABLE 2-5** Classifications of Overweight and Obesity by Body Mass Index and Waist Circumference and Associated Disease Risks

| | BMI (kg/m²) | Obesity Class | Disease Risk* Relative to Normal Weight and Waist Circumference | | | |
|---|---|---|---|---|---|---|
| | | | Men 102 cm (40 in) or less | Women 88 cm (35 in) or less | Men > 102 cm (40 in) | Women > 88 cm (35 in) |
| Underweight | < 18.5 | – | – | – | – | – |
| Normal | 18.5–24.9 | – | – | – | – | – |
| Overweight | 25.0–29.9 | | Increased | High | Increased | Increased |
| Obesity | 30.0–34.9 | I | High | Very high | Very high | Very high |
| | 35.0–39.9 | II | Very high | Very high | Very high | Very high |
| Extreme obesity | 40.0† | III | Extremely high | Extremely high | Extremely high | Extremely high |

* Disease risk for type 2 diabetes, hypertension, and cardiovascular disease.

† Increased waist circumference also can be a marker for increased risk, even in persons of normal weight.

Source: Adapted from National Heart, Lung, and Blood Institute. 1998 Clinical Guidelines on the Identification, Evaluation and Treatment of Overweight and Obesity in Adults. Washington, DC. http://www.nhlbi.nih.gov/health/public/heart/obesity/lose_wt/bmi_dis.htm. Accessed September 6, 2011.

cutoff points apply to all adult racial and ethnic groups in North America, although there are ethnic and age-related differences in regional body fat distribution that may influence the accuracy of waist circumference. For example, it has been reported that waist circumference is a better predictor than BMI of disease risk for persons of Asian descent. In older persons, waist circumference is more valuable at estimating obesity-related disease risk.[59,61] The procedure for measuring waist circumference is as follows [2,51]:

1. The participant should wear light clothing for easy access to the abdominal and waist area.
2. The participant needs to stand up straight, relax the abdominal muscles, place the arms at the side, and keep the feet together.
3. The nutritionist should locate the right iliac crest using the fingertips to gently feel for the highest point of the hip bone on the participant's right side.
4. Draw a short horizontal mark above the uppermost lateral border of the right iliac crest using a washable pen, then cross this with a vertical mark along the midaxillary line.

5. Place a flexible tape measure around the abdomen at the level of this marked point, about the level of the umbilicus (see Figure 2-5).
6. Snug the tape against the skin, but not so tight that it squeezes the skin.
7. Ask the participant to breathe normally and breathe out gently at the time of the measurement to prevent them from contracting their muscles or from holding their breath.
8. Take the reading and record to the nearest millimeter.
9. Repeat the measurement once or twice to ensure an accurate measurement was obtained.

## Hamwi Method for Ideal Body Weight

The Hamwi equation is another method of determining an individual's ideal body weight range. It was first published by George J. Hamwi in 1964. To calculate ideal body weight (IBW), also known as desirable body weight (DBW), the following formulas can be used for measurements in pounds and inches and kilograms and meters[62]:

■ Men: 106 pounds for the first 5 feet plus 6 pounds for every additional inch over 5 feet

- Women: 100 pounds for the first 5 feet plus 5 pounds for every inch thereafter

IBW in kilograms and meters:

- Men: 48.1 kg for each 1.52 m plus 0.9 kg for every centimeter above 1.52 m
- Women: 45.5 kg for each 1.52 m plus 1.1 kg for every centimeter above 1.52 m

For both the metric and nonmetric formulas, 10 percent can be added to or subtracted from the final value to accommodate variations in body frame size. Adjusting the ideal body weight for the obese patient is currently inconclusive. Adjustments can be made for spinal cord injuries. For paraplegia, subtract 5 percent to 10 percent from the IBW.[63] For quadriplegia, subtract 10 percent to 15 percent from the IBW. Nonambulatory persons and those with contractures, paralysis, or other conditions limiting their ability to stand will require an estimation of their height.

## Head Circumference

The anthropometric assessment of infants and young children includes head circumference. It is measured using a flexible tape measure, placed snugly around the head of the child (see **FIGURE 2-6**). Head circumference measures are useful indicators of normal growth and development during the rapid growth period from birth to 3 years.[25] Most assessments in the scientific and research communities use metric measurements.

## Skinfold Measurement

Skinfold measurement around different parts of the body can provide information about a person's percentage of body fat. The information obtained using this method can help determine the physical fitness of an individual or that person's risk for obesity. Skinfold data are collected using skinfold calipers (see **FIGURE 2-7**). The measurements can be compared to percentile tables for specific sex and age categories.

## National Center for Health Statistics' Percentiles for Physical Growth

The NCHS creates percentiles for physical growth charts that are standard for evaluating the physical growth of males and females from birth to 20 years. The standards are based on anthropometric measurements made on large, nationally representative samples of children in the United States. A single measurement is plotted on the percentile graph to determine how the child ranks in comparison to other children of the same age and sex in the United States. If the measurement is less than the 10th percentile, it should be checked for accuracy and compared with other types of assessment. Length for age less than the fifth percentile indicates chronic undernutrition. Weight for length less than the fifth percentile may reveal acute malnutrition.[25,64,65] Excessive weight for

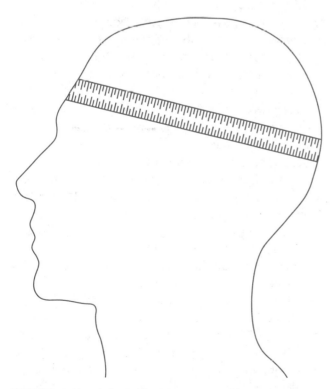

**FIGURE 2-6** Head circumference tape position.

Reproduced from: Centers for Disease Control and Prevention, National Center for Health Prevention and Promotion. National Health and Nutrition Examination Survey III: Body Measurements Anthropometry. Atlanta, GA: Centers for Disease Control and Prevention, National Center for Health Prevention and Promotion; 2011.

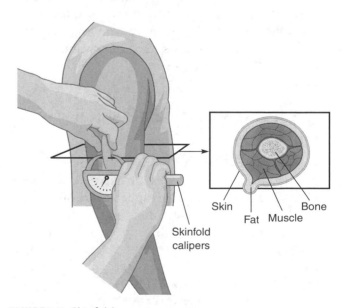

Skin  Fat  Muscle  Bone

Skinfold calipers

**FIGURE 2-7** Skinfold measurements.

Modified from: Gibson RS. *Principles of Nutritional Assessment.* 2nd ed. New York, NY: Oxford University Press; 2005.

**BOX 2-1** How to Plot Measurements on a Growth Chart

1. Choose the percentile chart based on age and gender.
2. Find the infant's weight in pounds or kilograms along the vertical axis of the chart.
3. Find the infant's age along the horizontal axis of the chart.
4. Ascertain and mark the chart where the age and weight lines intersect and record the percentile.

Visit for the growth charts: http://www.cdc.gov/nchs/data/series/sr_11/sr11_246.pdf. Accessed March 2, 2016.

length (above the 95th percentile) indicates obesity. Infants whose weight for length falls below the 5th percentile are classified as failure to thrive, and those below the 10th percentile are suspected for failure to thrive.[25,65,66] **BOX 2-1** provides instructions on how to plot the measures on a growth chart. The physical growth charts for girls and boys from birth to 20 years can be found at http://www.cdc.gov/growthcharts and an example with dot at Appendix B.

## Biochemical Tests and Data

Biochemical tests measure body fluids such as blood, urine, or feces. They are used mainly to detect subclinical deficiencies such as iron-deficiency anemia. They provide an objective means of determining nutritional status. They are also used to measure nutrients or the urinary excretion rate of nutrients or metabolites. **TABLE 2-6** presents examples of types of standard biochemical tests used in community and public health settings.

## Clinical Observations and Physical Examinations

Physical examinations are used to determine physical signs of nutrient deficiency or excess that developed over a long period (advanced stage of nutrient deficiency). A clinical nutrition examination would observe a person's hair, nails, skin, eyes, lips, mouth, muscles, and joints for specific signs.[2] For example, changes in hair color would suggest a protein deficiency. **TABLE 2-7** presents examples of generally used physical examination tests that use appearance as an indicator of nutrition status.

## Dietary Assessment Methods

Dietary information may confirm a lack or excess of a dietary constituent detected by anthropometric, biochemical, or clinical evaluations. There are primarily four ways to gather data on dietary intake: diet history, FFQ, food record or diaries, and 24-hour recall.

A **diet history** is any dietary assessment that asks clients to report about their past diet. It refers to the collection of the detailed make-up of meals (including preparation methods and foods eaten in combination), the intake frequency of various foods, and other risk factors such as the economic status of the client.[67] A trained interviewer typically completes this assessment. Many investigators now use the term *dietary history* to refer to the food frequency method of dietary assessment.

The **food frequency questionnaire (FFQ)** asks how often the respondent consumed specific foods or groups of foods for a specific period, instead of specific foods the respondents consumed daily.[68] Sometimes information about portion size, methods of cooking, or the combinations of foods eaten at meals is collected. **TABLE 2-8** presents a sample FFQ.

In **food records** or diaries, the respondent provides detailed information about daily eating habits. The respondent is usually asked to record all foods and beverages consumed during a defined period, typically over 3 to 7 consecutive days. The amount consumed may be measured using a scale or household measures (such as cups and tablespoons) or estimated using models, pictures, or no particular aid. The respondents normally become fatigued after several days of recording.[69] One of the disadvantages of dietary records includes incomplete records in the final days of a 7-day recording period. It may be more difficult for individuals with low socioeconomic status, recent immigrants, children, the poorly educated, and some elderly groups if they are required to respond on paper. Dictaphones, computer recording, and self-recording scales have been used to help respondents track their intake.[70]

As its name implies, a **24-hour recall** typically is administered for a 24-hour period. The respondents are asked to remember all foods and beverages they consumed in the past 24 hours (usually midnight to midnight). A trained staff member or a nutritionist typically collects these data by interview, self-administered questionnaire, or telephone.[71] Comprehensive population surveys normally use 24-hour recall as the main method of data collection. **TABLE 2-9** presents a sample of a 24-hour recall.

**TABLE 2-6** Biochemical Tests Used in Community and Public Health Settings

| Nutritional Indicators | Reference | Range Applications |
|---|---|---|
| Body protein status | Serum albumin: 3.5-5.0 g/dl (represents 50-60 percent total serum protein)<br>Other serum protein | High prevalence of children and pregnant women with abnormal blood protein levels is likely to be a public health problem of severe malnutrition.<br>■ Prevalence of stunting.<br>■ Prevalence of wasting.<br>■ Prevalence of kwashiorkor. |
| Iron status | Hemoglobin: Male, 14-17 g/dl; female, 12-15 g/dl; pregnant females, < 11 g/dl; newborns, 14-24 g/dl<br>Hematocrit: Male, 42-52 percent; female, 35-47 percent; pregnant females, < 33 percent; newborns, 44-64 percent<br>Others are serum ferritin, erythrocyte, protoporphyrin, and transferring saturation | ■ Prevalence of iron-deficiency anemia is likely to be a public health problem.<br>■ Proportion of children (of defined age and sex) and pregnant women with two or more abnormal iron indices (serum ferritin, erythrocyte, protoporphyrin, transferring saturation, and hemoglobin) plus abnormal hemoglobin. |
| Serum retinol | ≤ 0.70 mmol/L in children 6-71 months | ■ Vitamin A deficiency is a severe public health problem in developing countries.<br>■ Clinical indicator: Prevalence of maternal blindness more than 5 percent. |
| Iodine status | Median urinary iodine: ≤ 20 g/L based on ≥ 300 casual urine samples | ■ Severe risk for iodine deficiency disorders is likely to be a public health problem.<br>■ Clinical indicator: Proportion of children with total goiter rate more than 30 percent. |
| Blood lipids and lipoprotein status | Total serum cholesterol: < 200 mg/dl for ages 40-49 years; increases with age and lipoprotein levels:<br>LDL: < 100 mg/dl<br>HDL: 40-59 mg/dl<br>Triglycerides: < 150 mg/dl | ■ Proportion of men and women with abnormal blood cholesterol and lipoprotein levels (very-low-density lipoprotein [VLDL], low-density lipoprotein [LDL], and high-density lipoprotein [HDL]).<br>■ Coronary heart disease risk is likely to be a public health problem. |
| Lead status | 40 mg/L (normally much lower in children) | ■ Prevalence of abnormal blood lead levels is likely to be a public health problem.<br>■ A high proportion of children with abnormal levels is a severe public health problem. |
| Blood glucose | 70-99 mg/dl (tested after fasting) | ■ Diabetes mellitus is likely to be a public health problem. |

Modified from: Gibson RS. *Principles of Nutritional Assessment*. 2nd ed. New York, NY: Oxford University Press; 2005.

**TABLE 2-7** Physical Examination Tests That Use General Appearance as an Indicator of Nutrition Status[33,49,48]

| Physical Appearance | Normal | Abnormal | Nutrient Deficiencies | Could Indicate |
|---|---|---|---|---|
| Demeanor | Alert, responsive    Positive outlook | Lethargic    Negative attitude (irritable, etc.)    Sleep disturbances    Impaired coordination | Calories, protein, iron, fat, pantothenic acid | Poverty, malnutrition, hunger, and food insecurity |
| Weight | Reasonable for build    Appropriate weight for height and height for age | Underweight    Overweight, obese | Calories, fat, protein    Excessive intake of calories, lack of physical activity | Malnutrition    Overnutrition |
| Hair | Glossy, full, firmly rooted Uniform color | Dull, sparse Easily or painlessly plucked Thin, lackluster, dyspigmentation | Protein, vitamin C, calories, biotin, vitamin A toxicity | Socioeconomic factors (poverty and hunger) |
| Eyes | Bright, clear, shiny | Pale conjunctiva (dryness, thickening, and lack of luster of the bulbar conjunctiva of the exposed part of the eyeball)    Redness, dryness    Bitot's spots (well-demarcated, superficially dry, white-gray foamy plaques usually located lateral to the cornea in both eyes)    Keratomalacia (softening of cornea) | Vitamin A, thiamin, vitamin E, vitamin $B_{12}$, copper, toxicity | Lack of adequate fruit, vegetable, and grain products intakes |
| Lips | Smooth | Chapped, red, swollen    Angular stomatitis (lesions and fissuring at the corners of the mouth) | Riboflavin, niacin, biotin, vitamins $B_1$, $B_2$, $B_6$, $B_{12}$, and C | Inadequate fruit and vegetable intakes |
| Tongue | Deep red    Slightly rough | Bright red or purple    Swollen (edema) or shrunken    Geographic tongue (irregularly distributed patchy areas of atrophy of epithelium, etiology unknown) | Vitamin C, protein, riboflavin, and niacin | Lack of protein, fruits, and vegetables |
| Teeth | Bright, painless | Cavities    Painful, mottled, chipped, or missing | Calcium, vitamin D, fluoride | Inadequate intake of dairy product, fortified milk, fruits, and vegetables |
| Gums | Pink, firm | Spongy, bleeding, receding    Swelling of gingival tissue between teeth, which may bleed with slight pressure | Vitamin C | Lack of citrus fruits intake and cigarette smoking |

| Physical Appearance | Normal | Abnormal | Nutrient Deficiencies | Could Indicate |
|---|---|---|---|---|
| Skin | Clear, smooth, firm<br>Slightly moist | Rashes, swelling<br>Light or dark spots<br>Dry, follicular hyperkeratosis (hypertrophy of the corneous layer of skin surrounding the hair follicles with formation of plaques)<br>Petechiae (small hemorrhagic spots in skin or mucous membranes) Pellagrous dermatosis (symmetrical, clearly demarcated, hyperpigmented areas of skin most commonly exposed to sunlight) | Zinc, vitamins B and $B_{12}$, protein, vitamin C, essential fatty acids, vitamin A, folate, beta carotene, carotenoids, vitamin A toxicity | Inadequate protein, fruit, and vegetable intakes |
| Nails | Pink, firm | Koilonychia (spoon-shaped deformity of fingernails of both hands in older children and adults), ridged spongy bases | Iron or selenium toxicity | Inadequate intake of meat, leafy vegetables, and grain products |
| Face | Smooth, clear of spots | Diffuse depigmentation (this occurs in people of African descent)<br>Pallor (anemia may exaggerate the appearance of the condition) | Severe protein–calorie malnutrition and iron deficiency | Inadequate intake of meat, nuts, and legumes |
| Mobility/ weak joints | Erect posture<br>Good muscle tone<br>Walks without pain or difficulty | Muscle wasting<br>Skeletal deformities<br>Loss of balance | Calcium, protein, vitamins A, $B_1$, $B_2$, and D.<br>Beading of ribs (symmetrical nodular enlargement of costochondral junctions in ribs) | Inadequate intake of meat, legumes, nuts, dairy products, fruits, and vegetables |

**TABLE 2-8** Food Frequency Questionnaire

*Below is a list of food items. Please indicate how often/frequently you consume each.*

| Foods | Examples | Serving Size | How Many Times | | | | |
|---|---|---|---|---|---|---|---|
| | | | Day | Week | Month | *Seldom | Never |
| Dark green vegetables<br>Dark yellow vegetables<br>Other green vegetables<br>Other vegetables | Spinach, pumpkin, broccoli, squash, carrots, sweet potatoes, kale, peas, corn, vegetable juice | 1 cup of raw romaine lettuce and spinach<br>½ cup of other vegetables<br>¾ cup vegetable juice | | | | | |

*(continues)*

**TABLE 2-8** Food Frequency Questionnaire (*continued*)

| Foods | Examples | Serving Size | How Many Times | | | | |
|---|---|---|---|---|---|---|---|
| | | | Day | Week | Month | *Seldom | Never |
| Wheat germ<br>Cereal<br>Pasta<br>Potato<br>Other grain<br>Pancakes | Whole wheat bread, bagel, cereals, rice, spaghetti, macaroni, crackers | 1 slice of bread<br>1 cup of ready-to-eat cereal<br>½ cup of cooked cereal<br>6 whole crackers | | | | | |
| Citrus fruit or juice<br>Other fruits<br>Tomatoes<br>Dried fruits | Apple, banana, grape, kiwi, blueberry, date, peach, pear, orange, apricot, fig, tomato, canned fruit juice | 1 medium piece of whole fruit<br>½ cup of berries<br>½ cup of chopped, cooked, or canned fruit<br>¾ cup of fruit juice | | | | | |
| Milk and milk products | Milk, yogurt, frozen yogurt, cheese, cottage cheese | 1 cup of milk or yogurt<br>½ cup frozen yogurt<br>⅓ cup cottage cheese | . | | | | |
| Oil<br>Margarine<br>Butter<br>Salad dressing<br>Bacon and sausage<br>Fried foods<br>Salt pork<br>Cream, sweet<br>Cream, sour | Canola oil, corn oil, cottonseed oil, olive oil, safflower oil, soybean oil, sunflower oil, shortening, stick margarine, tub margarine, mayonnaise | Most Americans consume enough oil in the foods they eat, such as nuts, fish, cooking oil, salad dressings | | | | | |
| Beef, hamburger<br>Pork, ham<br>Liver<br>Fish<br>Lunch meat<br>Franks<br>Pizza<br>Poultry<br>Eggs<br>Peanut butter<br>Dried peas/beans | Duck, goose, turkey, ground chicken and turkey, beef, lamb, pork, veal, black-eyed peas, chickpeas (garbanzo beans), lima beans (mature), navy beans, pinto beans, soy beans, split peas, tofu (bean curd made from soy beans), white beans, catfish, cod, flounder, haddock, halibut, herring, mackerel, pollock, salmon | 2 to 3 ounces of meat or fish<br>2 tablespoons peanut butter<br>½ cup dried peas/beans | | | | | |

| Foods | Examples | Serving Size | How Many Times | | | | |
|---|---|---|---|---|---|---|---|
| | | | **Day** | **Week** | **Month** | **\*Seldom** | **Never** |
| Nuts<br>Seeds<br>Sprouts | Almonds, cashews, hazelnuts (filberts), mixed nuts, pecans, pistachios, pumpkin seeds, sesame seeds, sunflower seeds, walnuts | ⅓ cup | | | | | |
| Candy<br>Pie, cake, cookies<br>Potato chips, pretzels, popcorn, etc.<br>Teas/sugar<br>Soda pop<br>Fruit punch<br>Wine<br>Beer<br>Hard liquor<br>Ice milk<br>Sherbet | Regular soft drinks, fruit drinks (such as fruit punch), brown sugar, corn syrup, high-fructose corn syrup, honey, fructose, fruit juice concentrates, candy | Calorie allowance is part of total estimated calorie needs, not in addition to total calorie needs | | | | | |
| Other foods not listed | | | | | | | |

\*Seldom (less than six times per year)

*Use These Tips for Estimating Serving Sizes:*

| | |
|---|---|
| Four dice | = 1 ounce of cheese |
| One deck of playing cards or the palm of a woman's hand | = 3 ounces of cooked meat |
| One golf ball | = 2 tablespoons |
| A computer mouse | = 1 small baked potato |
| A baseball | = 1 cup |

Modified from: Simko MD, Cowell C, Gilbride JA. *Nutrition Assessment: A Comprehensive Guide for Planning Intervention*. Rockville, MD: Aspen; 1984. Reprinted with permission.

# ▶ How to Analyze Dietary Intake Data

After the data have been collected, they should be reviewed to ensure completion. Then, analyze the data to determine the nutrient content and compare the results using dietary standards or other reference points. This can be completed using a nutrient analysis software program or online program, such https://www .choosemyplate.gov/. Computer programs automatically perform the math using large databases and do not require the nutritionist to look up foods in nutrient composition tables.[26]

## Comparison to Dietary Standards

The respondent's nutrient intake can be compared to dietary standards using the Recommended Dietary Allowances (RDA) or Adequate Intake (AI) values.

**TABLE 2-9** Sample 24-Hour Recall Form

Name:                                                          Date:
Day of Week of Recall:

| Place | Time | Food Items | Type and Preparation | Amount | Place eaten | Office Use Only | | |
|---|---|---|---|---|---|---|---|---|
| | | | | | | Food Code | Amount | Code |
| | A.M. | Breakfast | Fried, baked, boiled | | Home | | | |
| | A.M. | Snack | Toasted | | Restaurant | | | |
| | Mid-day | Lunch | Whole wheat | | Carried lunch | | | |
| | Afternoon | Snack | Fresh, frozen, canned | | School | | | |
| | P.M. | Supper | Creamed | | Senior center   Childcare center, etc. | | | |

Additional Questions:
Was intake unusual in any way? Yes No
If yes, why (in what way)?
Do you take vitamin or mineral supplements? Yes No
If yes, how many per day? Per week?
If yes, what kind (give brand name if known)?
Multivitamin
Iron
Ascorbic acid
Other (list)
Do you exercise:
If yes, how many times per week? For how long?

Source: Simko MD, Cowell C, Gilbride JA. *Nutrition Assessment: A Comprehensive Guide for Planning Intervention*. Rockville, MD: Aspen; 1984. Reprinted with permission.

# Successful Community Strategies

## The Delta Nutrition Intervention Research Initiative (NIRI)[72-77]

Information gathered from community-level nutritional assessment can be used to develop community-wide programs addressing specific problem areas, such as childhood obesity or iron-deficiency anemia. Nutrition programs should be integrated into community-based health programs.

The Lower Mississippi Delta Nutrition Intervention Research Initiative (Delta NIRI) provides an excellent example of how community assessment can be utilized to address important community nutrition problems. In response to the nutrition-related health problems in this region, the U.S. Congress directed the U.S. Department of Agriculture (USDA) Research Service to establish Delta NIRI. The purpose was to conduct a comprehensive assessment of rural communities, examine the perceptions of community key informants regarding nutrition and health problems, evaluate the contributors to the problems, and assess the resources in Lower Mississippi Delta (LMD) counties. An additional purpose was to promote capacity-building and sustainability at the community level.

The LMD area of Arkansas, Louisiana, and Mississippi is characterized by high rates of poverty, low education attainment, and food insecurity. Food insecurity, when people live with hunger and the fear of starvation, is two and a half times the national average in each of these states. There is a high prevalence of hypertension, diabetes, obesity, anemia, and heart disease, all of which are influenced by nutrition.

The participation of the key informants allowed scientists to evaluate and generate knowledge about nutrition and health needs, food habits, and food consumption in 36 counties in the LMD. An adult food questionnaire developed by Tufts Human Nutrition Research Center was used to determine the composition of the diet and nutritional needs of the diverse population. In addition, an FFQ developed by Baylor University scientists was used to survey children. Based on existing literature on disease prevalence in the region, it was assumed that key informants would report hypertension, obesity, and diabetes as among the most important health problems in their counties.

Key informants were individuals who, by virtue of their role or position, have knowledge of and access to the community. The assessment used a modified key informant approach to conduct in-person interviews with 490 key informants in 36 selected counties and parishes.

The Delta NIRI conducted a comprehensive rural community assessment through five surveys: key informant survey, Food of Our Delta survey (FOODS 2000), food store survey, focus groups, and a community resources assessment. In one of the surveys (FOODS 2000), more than 1,500 people were followed by an in-store survey conducted in 174 stores, supermarkets, small to medium grocery stores, and convenience stores that identified the problems of access to and quality of foods in this high health risk, low-income region. A series of three focus groups were held in nine counties and parishes to identify barriers to improving food choices, food security, and shopping practices. In addition, a questionnaire developed to obtain perceptions of nutrition and health problems was pretested, revised, and administered to key informants by personal interviews.

Preliminary results show that key informants identified resources available in their counties to address food and nutrition problems. Ninety percent or more of key informants identified food stamps, school lunches, Head Start, Elderly Nutrition Programs, and the Special Supplemental Nutrition Program for Women, Infants, and Children (WIC) as available resources. Key informants identified hypertension as the most important health problem in their counties. They also saw multiple factors as contributing to the problems, but rated individual-level factors (food choices, education, willingness to change, and health behavior) as more important than community-level factors (food and healthcare access and resources).

Results showed that 97 percent identified consumption of high-fat foods and 94 percent identified consumption of too much fast food as nutrition concerns in their counties. Poverty, a lack of education, and an unwillingness to change were seen as major contributors to these problems by 92 percent, 94 percent, and 94 percent of key informants, respectively. The informants ranked hypertension, teen pregnancy, drug addiction, and heart disease, in that order, as the most significant health problems. Lack of exercise, poor food choices, and inadequate health insurance were seen as major factors contributing to health problems by 98 percent, 95 percent, and 91 percent of key informants, respectively. Data from this key informant survey demonstrated that perceptions of nutrition and health problems reflected the values and concerns of the local community. These results will help guide future planning for interventions to improve the nutrition and health status of the Delta community.

A comparison of individual diets to RDA or AI values needs to be interpreted with caution because the RDAs are the nutrient intakes that are sufficient to meet the needs of nearly all individuals (about 97 percent) in an age and gender group. Also, it is important to know that AI is not a standard, but can be used as a guide for the nutrient intake of individuals and groups in situations in which no RDA for a nutrient has been established. AIs are based on observed or experimentally determined estimates of the average nutrient intake that appears to maintain a defined nutritional state in certain populations (e.g., normal circulating nutrient values or bone health).[78]

## Comparison to MyPlate

The respondent's food intake can be compared to My-Pyramid, a guide created by the USDA to help individuals plan healthy diets. (See Appendix D for the USDA MyPlate food guidance system and Appendix E for Canada's Food Guide for Healthy Eating.) A nutritionist can categorize the listed foods into the different groups on the pyramid to determine the number of servings or amounts the respondents ate.

## Comparison to Dietary Guidelines for Americans

A nutritionist also can compare the respondent's diet to the *Dietary Guidelines for Americans*, a guide about lifestyle behaviors that relate to nutritional health, such as choosing nutrient-dense foods and being more physically active. This evaluation shows whether the respondent's diet is high or low in saturated fat and sodium, whether they are consuming adequate amounts of fruits and vegetables, and whether they perform regular physical activity. The *Dietary Guidelines* are available at http://www.health.gov/dietaryguidelines.

It is most effective to use a combination of these three methods to determine dietary inadequacies. **TABLE 2-10** presents a generalized scheme for determining nutrient deficiency.

**TABLE 2-10** Scheme for Determining Nutritional Deficiency

| Depletion Stage | Method(s) Used |
| --- | --- |
| 1. Dietary inadequacy | Dietary |
| 2. Decreased level in reserve tissue store | Biochemical |
| 3. Decreased level in body fluids | Biochemical |
| 4. Decreased functional level in tissues | Anthropometric/biochemical |
| 5. Decreased activity of nutrient-dependent enzyme or mRNA for some proteins | Biochemical/molecular/genetic |
| 6. Functional change | Behavioral/physiological/Biochemical |
| 7. Clinical symptoms | Clinical/observation |
| 8. Anatomical sign | Clinical/physical/observation |

Reproduced from: Sahn DE, Lockwood R, Scrimshaw NS. *Methods for the Evaluation of the Impact of Food and Nutrition Programmes.* Tokyo, Japan: United Nations University; 1984. Reprinted with permission of United Nations University Press.

## ▶ Food Consumption at the National and Household Levels

The USDA Economic Research Service uses a food **balance sheet approach** to estimate the total amount of foods consumed annually by the U.S. civilian population. The foods that are available for consumption are assessed using national-, household-, or individual-level food consumption surveys. National and household levels of food consumption are discussed in the following sections. Individual-level food consumption has already been discussed.

### Measuring Food Consumption at the National Level

The national food consumption level is used to compare the available food supply among countries and to monitor trends over time within an individual country.[40] The method for assessing food availability for consumption nationally is based on food balance sheets. The data are typically presented on a per capita basis using population estimates, but do not provide information on the distribution of available food supplies within the country or how food intake of individuals varies within the population. Also, it is not a direct measure of actual food consumption, but estimates of food available for purchase by consumers through wholesale and retail markets. [40]

Food balance sheet approaches are an indirect way of estimating the amounts of food consumed by a country's population over a specified period. It provides data on the food available for consumption. It is calculated using beginning and ending inventories; figures on food production, imports, and exports; and adjustments for nonhuman food consumption (e.g., cattle feed, pet food, seeds, and industrial use). Food disappearance is another term used to describe food balance sheets, which is the amount of food that disappears from the food distribution system. Consumers purchase most of these foods at supermarkets, but a significant amount is lost due to spoilage and waste.[2] For example[79]:

**Available Commodity Supply** (Production + Imports + Beginning stocks)

minus

**Measurable Nonfood Use** (Farm inputs [feed and seed] + Industrial uses [e.g., sugar in the brewing industry] + Exports + Ending Stocks)

equals

**Total Annual Food Supply of a Commodity**

The following are some of the strengths and weaknesses of food balance sheets[2]:

**Strengths:**

- It provides a total idea of a country's food supplies.
- It shows food habits and dietary trends of the population.
- It can be used to design international nutrition policies; plan agricultural policies related to food production, distribution, and consumption; and develop food programs.
- It may provide data on a country's food consumption practices.

**Weaknesses:**

- The accuracy of data is questionable.
- It shows foods that are available for consumption but does not show foods that were consumed.
- It does not show how food was distributed in the country.
- It does not report foods that were wasted or spoiled.

Mean per capita annual amounts are calculated by dividing total disappearance of food by the country's population.[80] The method has been valuable for detecting trends in the amount of food that disappears from the food distribution system within a country over time and to approximate trends in food consumption. Also, it is useful for promoting agricultural production in various parts of the world, for formulating agricultural policies about food production and consumption, and for encouraging a more even distribution of food among different countries.[75]

## Food Consumption at the Household Level

Household food consumption is the food and beverages available for consumption by the household, family group, or institution. It is defined as the total amount of food available for consumption in the household, generally excluding food eaten away from home unless taken from home.[81] Methods of assessing household food consumption consider the per capita food consumption of the household. Alternatively, information on the age and sex of persons in the household, their physiological state and activity level, number of meals eaten at home and away from home, shopping practices, income, and other socioeconomic characteristics of the household members can be collected. With this information, food consumption per capita can be calculated in terms of income level, family size, region of the country, or other criteria. In some cases, consumption of certain food groups, characteristic of food patterns for specific socioeconomic groups or high in a specific nutrient (e.g., vitamin A or calcium), may be calculated.

This method does not provide specific information on individual food consumption within the household. Generally, no record is taken of edible food waste or food obtained outside the household food supply. Household food consumption data are not suitable for the analysis of the quality of diet in relation to nutrient recommendations.[40]

## Food Consumption at the Individual Level

As discussed earlier, determining food consumption at individual level involves balancing national surveys with smaller, ongoing surveys to evaluate foods eaten at home and away from home. The individual food account reveals actual food consumed and provides over 25 nutrient intakes such as total energy, protein, carbohydrates, total fat, carotenes, calcium, iron, folate, and sodium. The database generated from the national surveys has now expanded to include fatty acid, antioxidant, B-vitamin, and mineral intakes.[40,82] Some of the methods used to determine individual dietary intake and diet history are 24-hour recall, food records, and the FFQ. The use of 24-hour recall or food records is not enough to estimate an individual's usual intake because eating patterns vary between weekdays and weekends and across seasons.[83]

## Mapping Tools in Community Assessment

The U.S. Department of Agriculture's Agriculture Research Service (ARS) developed a resource called the Community Nutrition Mapping Project (CNMap) that includes easy-to-read tables and color-coded customized maps to help states measure whether a community is at risk for food insecurity or other nutritional problems. The CNMap combines and aggregates food and nutrition indicators to provide a snapshot of them at the state and national levels.

CNMap is divided into five major categories: nutrient intakes, healthy eating patterns, physical activity and body weight indicators, food security indicators, and demographics.[84] The CNMap combined 1994 to 1996 Continuing Survey of Food Intakes by Individuals (CSFII) data with a geographic information system (GIS) that captures, stores, manages, manipulates, analyzes, and displays a wide range of information, and presents data that are linked to locations.[85] This provides a picture of food and nutrition at the region and state level. Also, it is an online resource for checking a state's nutritional health.[86] GIS mapping provides a visual depiction of retail food availability within the overall context of residential areas and in relation to other public infrastructure, such as schools and roads. ARS Community Nutrition Research Group (CNRG) is conducting small studies in several communities to further develop the map and provide specific community-level data. State and regional maps related to food and nutrition can be found at http://www.ars.usda.gov/research/docs.htm?docid=12396.

One example of a CNMap project is the Behavioral Risk Factor Surveillance System (BRFSS), an ongoing telephone health survey system that tracks health conditions and risk behaviors in the United States yearly since 1984. It is also a state-based system of health surveys that collects information on health risk behaviors, preventive health practices, and healthcare access related to chronic disease and injury.[78] Data are collected monthly in all 50 states, the District of Columbia, Puerto Rico, the U.S. Virgin Islands, and Guam. For many states, the BRFSS is the only available source of timely, accurate data on health-related behaviors. The interactive mapping application is presented at donehttps://www.cdc.gov/brfss/data_tools.htm. These interactive features make it easy for healthcare professionals to chart prevalence data for a specific area, track prevalence trends, follow historical changes, or create prevalence maps comparing state and local data across the nation.[87]

Another example of a CNMap project is a list of the farmers' markets and local food markets that are an integral part of the urban/farm linkage. Farmers' markets allow consumers to have access to locally grown, farm-fresh produce and enable farmers to develop a personal relationship with their customers and cultivate consumer loyalty. Direct marketing of farm products through farmers' markets is an important sales outlet for agricultural producers nationwide.[83] **GIS mapping** is useful in increasing the selection of healthy food choices, especially for low-income individuals. For example, one research study investigated the factors that affect obesity in California low-income neighborhoods. The aim of the study was also, to update program planning, nutrition education, community

participation, investment of *resources strategies*, and the involvement of stakeholders, health leaders, and community members. The researchers trained 18 staff members in the local health departments on how to use an online GIS and conduct field surveys. GIS data were aggregated from 68 low-income neighborhoods of one or more census tracts. The researchers collected data from 473 grocery stores in 62 neighborhoods starting in 2007 to 2009. Surveys were used to collect data dealing with food stores, walkability within two blocks of stores, fast-food outlets, outdoor marketing, food banks, and emergency food outlets. In addition, alternative food sources, such as farm stands, community gardens, and community-supported agriculture, were collected. Results showed that there were no supermarkets within any of their census tract boundaries in 31 percent of the neighborhoods mapped. However, estimates by health department staff members showed that 74.2 percent of residents had access to a large grocery store within 1 mile. Results also showed that in small markets, 81 percent sold produce and 67.6 percent provided better options of four or more types of fresh vegetables. These findings indicate that underserved areas can be part of community efforts to promote and increase the consumption of fruits and vegetables and healthy eating behaviors.[88] Agricultural Marketing Service (AMS) maintains a current list of farmers' markets throughout the United States. The farmers market database is updated on an ongoing basis. Farmers market data can be obtained from the AMS website at http://www.ams.usda.gov/farmersmarkets/map.htm.

# Learning Portfolio

## Chapter Summary

- The ABCDs of nutrition assessment are anthropometric measurements, biochemical tests, clinical and physical observations, and dietary intake.
- The goals of screening are to identify individuals who are at nutritional risk and those who need further assessment.
- It is important to use the most convenient screening method, and it is also advisable to maintain accuracy and correlate findings with clinical, anthropometric, dietary, biochemical, and ecological factors.
- Preferably, all persons should have nutritional status assessments throughout their life cycle as well as during illness. Different approaches can be applied to the healthy population and to the critically ill.
- At the population level, assessment of dietary intake is necessary to identify national health priorities and

develop public health dietary recommendations. These assessments are used to determine the success of public health interventions in improving dietary patterns and to identify population subgroups at risk or in need of special assistance.

- Anthropometric measurements are physical measurements of the body including height, stature, recumbent length, weight, circumferences, skinfold thicknesses or limb length, weight, and circumferences (head, waist, etc.). They are indicators of health, development, and growth.
- One major concern about screening methods is the accuracy of the information gathered.
- Reliability refers to the consistency or repeatability of test results; validity refers to the ability of a test to measure what it is supposed to measure.
- A test with high sensitivity is able to correctly identify and classify individuals within the population

who are truly malnourished as confirmed by the test (a true positive).

- A screening method with high specificity has few false positives.

## Critical Thinking Activities

- With the consent of the participants (e.g., women, older persons, college students, high school students) in a week-long health fair in the community or another community health event, collect a 24-hour recall. Analyze the subjects' dietary intake using computer software. Immediately review a printout of the data collected, including nutrient totals if the system being used permits.

- Query the participants on whether the amount they consumed was typical; if not, identify the reason the amount consumed was unusually low or high.

- Make a list of the foods and amounts eaten from the 24-hour recall. Next to each food, list the MyPlate food group to which it belongs. In the next column, list the number of MyPlate servings or fractions of servings it provides. For mixed foods, list all ingredients separately and identify the food groups and serving sizes that apply.

- Are foods represented from each food group?
- Does the diet follow the *Dietary Guidelines for Americans*?
- Examine your own nutritional risk factors:
- What do you eat?
- How do you eat?
- What factors would affect the absorption and utilization of the nutrients you consume?
- Use your height and weight and determine if your BMI is in the healthy range.

## 🔍 CASE STUDY 2-1: Screening in Ethnically and Income Diverse School Children

Ayanna, a community nutritionist consulting at local grade schools, was asked to provide nutrition screening to the 5th-, 6th-, and 7th-grade students in a low-income and ethnically diverse school district as well as in a middle-income school with more Caucasian students. The overall objective was to screen students from the five lower and middle socioeconomic and culturally diverse schools who may not have access to nutrition screening and to evaluate the rate of obesity in these age groups. The nutritionist sent flyers to the parents or guardians through the students and posted flyers at the school cafeterias and at different bulletin boards within the schools. In addition, a total of five announcements were made through the intercom before class periods in all the schools. Information about the event was also included in the school's newsletter. Screenings were conducted after school hours on different days of the week for 2 weeks to accommodate the target group. Despite all recruiting efforts, the results indicated that the targeted group did not use the service as hoped, and the predominant individuals who accessed the service were Caucasian, middle-class, insured students. Results also showed that 13 percent of the students screened were overweight with a BMI of 28 and BMI for age in the 85th percentile, 20 percent were obese with a BMI over 30 and BMI for age in the 95th percentile, and 5 percent of non-Caucasian students were underweight with a BMI of less than 15 and BMI for age below the 5th percentile. Physical examination revealed mottled, chipped, and missing teeth and chapped, red, swollen lips in some of the students.

### Questions

1. What is the definition of a community nutrition assessment? What are the different tools and methods for measuring nutritional status in the community?
2. Describe how to calculate BMI. What is the BMI of an individual who weighs 155 pounds and is 5′, 4″ tall?
3. What are the BMI ranges for determining the susceptibility to obesity?
4. What is the definition of a diet history? Describe three different dietary assessment methods.
5. What are some factors that can affect the reliability and validity of the dietary assessment questionnaires that Ayanna must apply to her program?
6. Ayanna considered using physical examination tests that use general appearance as an indicator of nutritional status. List five physical examination tests she could use; discuss the nutrient deficiencies that may affect the physical appearance of her clients.
7. Discuss the advantages and disadvantages of the use of 24-hour recall and food frequency questionnaires.
8. As a nutritionist, Ayanna must know the ABCDs of nutritional assessment. Describe them.
9. List two biochemical tests that Ayanna could perform to measure protein and iron status, and discuss the consequences of inadequate intake of these nutrients.
10. Work in small groups or individually to discuss the case study and practice using the Nutrition Care Process chart provided on the companion website. You can also add other nutrition and health-related conditions or assessments to the case study to make the case study more challenging and interesting.

## Think About It

**Answer:** The assessments that the nutritionist may recommend are a dietary history and a blood biochemical test to determine her eating habits and blood iron status.

## Key Terms

**24-hour recall:** A method of dietary assessment in which the individual is asked to remember everything eaten during the past 24 hours.

**anthropometric:** The measurement of human body size, weight, and proportions.

**assessment:** Determining nutritional status by analyzing clinical, dietary, and social history; anthropometric data; biochemical data; and drug–nutrient interactions.

**balance sheet approach:** The most common method of estimating per capita food availability at the national level. Food exports, nonfood use (e.g., livestock feed, seeds, and industrial use), and year-end inventories are subtracted from data on beginning-year inventories, total food production, and imports to arrive at an estimate of per capita food availability.

**body mass index (BMI):** Weight (kg)/height (m$^2$); an index calculated by a ratio of height to weight, used as a measure of obesity.

**community assessment:** Is the process of getting to know and understanding the community as a client. It helps to identify community needs, clarify problems, and identify strengths and resources.

**community nutrition assessment:** An attempt to evaluate the nutritional status of individuals or populations through measurements of food and nutrient intake and evaluation of nutrition-related health indicators.

**diet history:** A detailed dietary assessment, which may include a 24-hour recall, food frequency questionnaire, and additional information such as weight history, previous diet changes, use of supplements, and food intolerances.

**food frequency questionnaire (FFQ):** A method of dietary assessment in which the questions relate to how often foods are consumed.

**food record:** A written record of the amounts of all foods and liquids consumed during a time period, usually 3 to 7 days; often includes information on time, place, and situation of eating.

**Frankfurt horizontal plane:** An imaginary plane intersecting the lowest point on the margin of the orbit (the bony socket of the eye) and the tragion (the notch above the tragus, the cartilaginous projection just anterior to the external opening of the ear). This plane should be horizontal with the head and in line with the spine.

**Geographic information system (GIS):** A computer system that captures, stores, manages, manipulates and displays a wide range of information, and presents data that are linked to locations.

**nutritional status:** A measurement of the extent to which an individual's physiologic needs for nutrients are being met.

**parallax error:** The apparent difference in the reading of a measurement scale (e.g., a skinfold caliper's needle) when viewed from various points not in a straight line with the eye.

**reliability:** The consistency or repeatability and reproducibility of test results.

**screening:** An effort to detect unrecognized health conditions among individuals.

**sensitivity:** The ability to correctly identify individuals or a proportion of persons with a disease or condition.

**specificity:** The ability to correctly identify individuals or a proportion of persons without a disease or condition, as confirmed by a test.

**stadiometer:** A device capable of measuring stature in children over 2 years of age and in adults in a standing position.

**validity:** The ability of the test instrument to measure what it is supposed to measure accurately.

## References

1. Stanhope M, Lancaster J. *Community and Public Health Nursing: Population-Centered Health Care in the Community.* 9th ed. New York, NY: Elsever; 2015.

2. Lee RD, Nieman DC. *Nutritional Assessment.* New York, NY: McGraw-Hill; 2012.

3. US Dept of Health and Human Services. *Nutrition Monitoring in the United States: An Updated Report on Nutrition Monitoring.* Washington, DC: US Government Printing Office; 1989.

4. Washington State. Washington State risk and protective factors: Nutrition. 2005. http://depts .washington.edu/commnutr/wadocs/wadocs -nutrition.htm. Accessed March 4, 2016.

5. Kaufman MK, ed. *Nutrition in Public Health: A Handbook for Developing Programs and Services.* Rockville, MD: Aspen; 1990.

6. Kaufman M. *Nutrition in Promoting the Public's Health: Strategies, Principles, and Practice.* Sudbury, MA: Jones and Bartlett; 2007.

7. Anderson E, McFarlane J. *Community as Partner: Theory and Practice in Nursing.* 3rd ed. Philadelphia, PA: Lippincott; 2010.

8. Habicht JP, Pelletier DL. The importance of context in choosing nutritional indicators. *J Nutr.* 1990;120:1519-1524.

9. Berdanier CD. *Handbook of Nutrition and Food.* New York, NY: CRC Press; 2002.

10. Washington State. Washington State risk and protective factors: Nutrition. http://depts.washington.edu/commnutr/assess/cna-intro.htm#value. Accessed March 8, 2016.

11. Centers for Disease Control and Prevention. Program planning. http://www.cdc.gov/cancer/nbccedp/pdf/trainpdfs/hb-progplan.pdf. Accessed March 8, 2016.

12. US Dept Health and Human Services. About the community guide. 2014. http://www.thecommunityguide.org/uses/program_planning.html. Accessed March 8, 2016.

13. Council on Practice Quality Management Committee. ADA's definitions for nutrition screening and nutrition assessment. *J Am Diet Assoc.* 1994;94:838-839.

14. Centers for Diseas Control and Prevention. Community health improvement (CHI) overview. http://www.cdc.gov/chinav/resources/additional/index.html. Accessed March 5, 2016.

15. Evans KR, Hudson SV. Engaging the community to improve nutrition and physical activity among houses of worship. *Prev Chronic Dis.* 2014;11:130270-130277.

16. Food and Agriculture Organization. Targeting for nutrition improvement. http://www.fao.org/docrep/004/y1329e/y1329e01.htm. Accessed March 4, 2016.

17. Caliendo MA. *Nutrition and the Food Crisis.* New York, NY: MacMillan; 1979.

18. Bigwood EJ. *Guiding Principles for Studies on the Nutrition of Populations.* Geneva, Switzerland: League of Nations; 1939.

19. Simko M, Cowell C, Gilbride JA. *Nutrition Assessment: A Comprehensive Guide for Planning Intervention.* Rockville, MD: Aspen; 1984.

20. Frankle RT, Owen AY. *Nutrition in the Community.* St. Louis, MO: C.V. Mosby; 1978.

21. Interdepartmental Committee on Nutrition for National Development. *Manual for Nutrition Surveys.* Washington, DC: Interdepartmental Committee on Nutrition for National Development; 1957.

22. Schwerin HS, Stanton JL, Riley AM, Schaefer AE, et al. Food eating patterns and health: a reexamination of the Ten-State and HANES I surveys. *Am J Clin Nutr.* 1981;34(4):568-580.

23. Ford EE, Giles WH. Changes in prevalence of nonfatal coronary heart disease in the United States from 1971-1994. *Ethnicity Dis.* 2003;13(1):85-93.

24. Murphy SS. Use of national survey data bases for nutrition research. *Clin Nutr.* 1987;6(5):208-218.

25. Centers for Disease Control and Prevention. *Growth Chart.* Atlanta, GA: Centers for Disease Control and Prevention; 2000.

26. Insel P, Turner E, Ross D. *2002 Update Nutrition.* Sudbury, MA: Jones and Bartlett; 2002.

27. Carter KA, Lionel J. *Conducting a Community Needs Assessment: Primary Data Collection Technique.* Gainesville, FL: Cooperative Extension Service, Institute of Food and Agricultural Sciences, University of Florida; 1992.

28. Sanders CCG. Extending the reach of public health nutrition: Training community practitioners in multilevel approaches. *J Womens Health.* 2004;13(5):589-597.

29. Frank GC. *Community Nutrition: Applying Epidemiology to Contemporary Practice.* Rockville, MD: Aspen; 2007.

30. Kettering C. Community needs assessment: Taking the pulse of your community. http://www.communitydevelopment.uiuc.edu/resources/factsheets/needpuls.html. Accessed March 8, 2016.

31. Todorovic V. Nutritional screening in the community: Developing strategies. *Br J Community Nurs.* 2004;11(9):464-470.

32. Iowa State University Extension. Needs assessment strategies for community groups and organization. 2005. http://www.extension.iastate.edu/communities/tools/assess/. Accessed March 18, 2016.

33. World Health Organization. Reproductive health during conflict and displacement: A guide for programme managers. 2000. http://www.who.int/reproductivehealth/publications/maternal_perinatal_health/RHR_00_13/en/. Accessed February 19, 2017.

34. Hodges BC, Videto DM. *Assessment and Planning in Health Programs.* Sudbury, MA: Jones and Bartlett; 2005.

35. Coulston A, Rock C, Monsen E. *Nutrition in the Prevention and Treatment of Disease.* New York, NY: Academic Press; 2001.

36. Field AE, Colditz GA, Fox MK, et al. Comparison of 4 questionnaires for assessment of fruit and vegetable intake. *Am J Public Health.* 1998;88:1216-1218.

37. Means B, Habina K, Swan GE, et al. *Cognitive Research on Response Error in Survey Questions on Smoking: Vital and Health Statistics,* Series 6, No. 2. DHHS Pub. No. PHS 92-1080. Washington, DC: US Government Printing Office; 1992.

38. Kant A, Block G, Schatzkin A, Ziegler, Nestle, M. Dietary diversity in the U.S. population NHANES II 1976-1980. *J Am Diet Assoc.* 1991;91:34-38.

39. Brener ND, Billy JO, Grady MA. Assessment of factors affecting the validity of self-reported

health-risk behavior among adolescents: Evidence from the scientific literature. *J Adolesc Health.* 2003;33(6):436-457.

40. Gibson RS. *Principles of Nutritional Assessment.* 2nd ed. Dunedin, New Zealand: Oxford University Press; 2005.

41. Chumlea W, Roche AF, Mukherjee D. *Nutritional Assessment of the Elderly Through Anthropometry.* Columbus, OH: Ross Laboratories; 1987.

42. Gordon C, Chumlea WC, Roche AF. Stature recumbent length and weight. In: Lohman T, Roche AF, Martorell R, eds. *Anthropometric Standardization Reference Manual.* Champaign, IL: Human Kinetics; 1988:29-34.

43. World Health Organization. *Physical Status: The Use and Interpretation of Anthropometry.* Geneva, Switzerland: World Health Organization; 1995.

44. Chumlea W. Methods of nutritional anthropometric assessment for special groups. In: Lohuman T, Roche AF, Martorell R, eds. *Anthropometric Standardization Reference Manual.* Champaign, IL: Human Kinetics; 1988:55-60.

45. Chumlea W, Roche AF. Assessment of the nutritional status of healthy and handicapped adults. In: Lohman T, Roche AF, Martorell R, eds. *Anthropometric Standardization Reference Manual.* Champaign, IL: Human Kinetics; 1988.

46. Prothro J, Rosenbloom CA. Physical measurements in an elderly black population: Knee height as the dominant indicator of stature. *J Gerontol.* 1993;48(1):M15-M18.

47. Zhang H, Hsu-Hage BH, Wahlqvist ML. The use of knee height to estimate maximum stature in elderly Chinese. *J Nutr Health Aging.* 1998;2(2):84-87.

48. Cockram D, Baumgartner RN. Evaluation of accuracy and reliability of calipers for measuring recumbent knee height in elderly people. *Am J Clin Nutr.* 1990;52(2):397-400.

49. Jarzem P, Gledhil RB. Predicting height from arm measurements. *J Pediatr Orthop.* 1993;13(6):761-765.

50. Mitchell C, Lipschitz DA. Arm length measurement as an alternative to height in the nutritional assessment of the elderly. *J Patenter Enteral Nutr.* 1982;6(3):226-229.

51. Lohman T, Roche AF, Martorell R. *Anthropometric Standardization Reference Manual.* Champaign, IL: Human Kinetics; 1988.

52. National Task Force on the Prevention and Treatment of Obesity. Overweight, obesity and health risk. *Arch Intern Med.* 2000;160:898-904.

53. Hammond K. Assessment: Dietary and clinical data. In: Mahan L, Escott-Stump S, eds. *Krause's Food, Nutrition and Diet Therapy.* 12th ed. Philadelphia, PA: Saunders; 2004:383-410.

54. Frisancho AR, Flegel PN. Elbow breadth as a measure of frame size for U.S. males and females. *Am J Clin Nutr* 1983;37(20):311-314.

55. Association AD. Evidence analysis library adult weight management guidelines. 2016. http://www.andeal.org/topic.cfm?cat=2798. Accessed February 19, 2017.

56. Callaway CW, Chumlea WC, Bouchard C. Circumferences. In: Lohman T, Roche AF, Martorell R, eds. *Anthropometric Standardization Reference Manual.* Champaign, IL: Human Kinetics; 1988.

57. Grant JP, Custer PB, Thurlow J. Current techniques of nutritional assessment. *Surg Clin North Am.* 1981;61:437-463.

58. Wilmore JH, Frisancho RA, Gordon CC. Body breadth equipment and measurement techniques. In: Lohman TG, Roche AF, Martorell R, eds. *Anthropometric Standardization Reference Manual.* Champaign, IL: Human Kinetics; 1998.

59. National Heart Lung and Blood Institute. Clinical guidelines on the identification evaluation and treatment of overweight and obesity in adults. 2003. https://www.ncbi.nlm.nih.gov/books/NBK2003/. Accessed February 19, 2017.

60. Wang Y, Rimm EB, Stampfer MJ, Willett WD, Hu FB. Comparison of abdominal adiposity and overall obesity in predicting risk of type 2 diabetes among men. *Am J Clin Nutr.* 2005;81:555-563.

61. National Institutes of Health. The practical guide to identification, evaluation and treatment of overweight and obesity in adults. 200; https://catalog.nhlbi.nih.gov/catalog/product/Clinical-Guidelines-on-the-Identification-Evaluation-and-Treatment-of-Overweight-and-Obesity-in-Adults-The-Evidence-Report/98-4083. Accessed February 19, 2017.

62. Hamwi G. Changing dietary concepts. In: Donowski TS, ed. *Diabetes Mellitus Diagnosis and Treatment.* New York, NY: American Diabetes Association; 1964:73-78.

63. Peiffer S, Blust P, Leyson JF. Nutritional assessment of the spinal cord injured patient. *J Am Diet Assoc.* 1981;78(5):501-505.

64. Aziz S, Asim D, Kehkashan P, et al. Anthropometric indices of middle socio-economic class school children in Karachi compared with NCHS standards: a pilot study. *J Pak Med Assoc.* 2006;56:264-267.

65. Boyle MA, Holben D. *Community Nutrition in Action: An Entrepreneurial Approach.* 4th ed. Belmont, CA: Thomson Wadsworth; 2013.

66. Sirotnak AP, Pataki C. Failure to Thrive. Available at http://emedicine.medscape.com/article/915575-overview. Accessed April 3, 2017.

67. Burke BS. The dietary history as a tool in research. *J Am Diet Assoc.* 1947;23:1041-1046.

68. Zulkifli SN, Yu SM. The food frequency method for dietary assessment. *J Am Diet Assoc.* 1992; 92(6):681-685.

69. Kretsch MJ, Fong AK. Validity and reproducibility of a new computerized dietary assessment method: Effects of gender and educational level. *Nutr Res.* 1993;13:133-146.

70. Lindquist CH, Cummings T, Goran MI. Use of tape-recorded food records in assessing children's dietary intake. *Obes Res.* 2000;8(1):2-11.

71. Casey PH, Goolsby SL, Lensing SY, Perloff BP, et al. The use of telephone interview methodology to obtain 24-hour dietary recalls. *J Am Diet Assoc.* 1999;99(11):1406-1411.

72. Berdanier CD, Feldman EB, Flatt WP, St Jeor ST. *Handbook of Nutrition and Food.* Boca Raton, FL: CRC Press; 2007.

73. Bogle M. Assessment of community nutrition and health needs in the Delta Nutrition Intervention Research Initiative. 1998. https://www.ars.usda.gov/research/publications/publication/?seqNo115=107940. Accessed February20, 2017.

74. Yadrick K, Horton J, Stuff J, et al. Perceptions of community nutrition ahd health needs in the lower Mississippi Delta: a key informant approach. *J Nutr Educ.* 2001;33(5):266-277.

75. Thornton A, Lower Mississippi Delta Nutrition Intervention Research Consortium. Demographic, social, and economic characteristics. In: Harrison G, ed. *Nutrition and Health Status in the Lower Mississippi Delta of Arkansas, Louisiana, and Mississippi: A Review of Existing Data*: Rockville, MD: Westat; 1997:9-23.

76. Smith J, Lensing S, Horton JA, et al. Prevalence of self-reported nutrition-related health problems in the Lower Mississippi Delta. *Am J Public Health.* 1999;89:1418-1421.

77. National Research Council. *Food and Nutrition Board Diet and Health Implications for Reducing Chronic Disease Risk.* Washington, DC: National Academy Press; 1989.

78. MacIntyre U. A culture-sensitive quantitative food frequency questionnaire used in an African population: Relative validation by 7-day weighted records and biomarkers. *Public Health Nutr.* 2001;4(1 pt 2):63-71.

79. US Dept of Agriculture, Economic Research Service. Food security assessment. http://www.ers.usda.gov/. Accessed February 16, 2016.

80. Pekkarinen M. Methodology in the collection of food consumption data. *World Rev Nutr Diet.* 1970;12:145-171.

81. Klaver W, Knuiman JT, Van Staveren WA. Proposed definitions for use in the methodology of food consumption studies. In: Hautvast JG, Klaver W, eds. *The Diet Factor in Epidemiological Research: Euronut Report 1.* Wageningen, The Netherlands: Ponsen and Loogen; 1982:77-85.

82. Frank-Spohrer G. *Community Nutrition: Applying Epidemiology to Contemporary Practice.* 2nd ed. Sudbury, MA: Jones and Bartlet; 2008.

83. Iris S, Bernard AR, Danit RS. Dietary evaluation and attenuation of relative risk: Multiple comparisons between blood and urinary biomarkers, food frequency, and 24-hour recall questionnaires the DEARR study. *J Nutr.* 2005;135(3):573-579.

84. US Dept of Agriculture, Economic Research Service. The Community Nutrition Mapping Project (CNMap). http://www.ars.usda.gov/Serviccs/. Accessed March 9, 2016.

85. Persky VVP. The effect of dietary sucrose of blood pressure in spontaneously hypertensive rats. *Nutr Res.* 1986;6(9):1111-1115.

86. Bliss RM. Putting community nutrition on the map. https://agresearchmag.ars.usda.gov/ar/archive/2003/apr/map0403.pdf. Accessed February 19, 2017.

87. Center for Disease Control and Prevention. Behavioral risk factor surveillance system. https://www.cdc.gov/brfss/about/about_brfss.htm. Accessed February 19, 2017.

88. Ghirardelli A, Quinn V, Foerster SB. Environmental approaches to obesity prevention: Using geographic information systems and local food store data in California's low-income neighborhoods to inform community initiatives and resources. *Am J Public Health.* 2010;100(11):2156-2162.

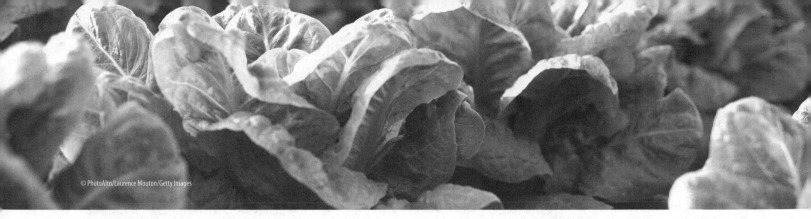

# CHAPTER 3

# Nutritional Epidemiology and Research Methods

## CHAPTER OUTLINE

- Introduction
- Epidemiology in Community Health
- Nutritional Epidemiology
- Interpretation of Cause and Effect in Nutritional Epidemiology
- Types of Public Health Nutritional Epidemiology Research
- Descriptive Measures of Community Health
- The Epidemiological Methods
- Quantitative and Qualitative Methods
- Types of Sampling
- Concepts of Collaborative Research
- Reporting Research Results
- Epidemiological Approaches to Community Health Assessment

## LEARNING OBJECTIVES

- Define nutritional epidemiology.
- Discuss the different types of epidemiological research.
- Discuss the difference between quantitative and qualitative research methods.

# ▶ Introduction

Community and public health nutrition research has increased over the years, but nutritionists must continue to increase the scientific knowledge base that is unique to their practice to provide high-quality, scientifically oriented, evidence-based services and solutions to today's nutrition-related health conditions. **Community nutrition research** is defined as the "organized study of a trend at both the basic and more applied levels that focuses on social, structural, and physical environmental inequities through active involvement of community members, organizational representatives, and researchers in all aspects of the research process with the specific topics varying between investigators and the public."[1] Learning to conduct successful research and epidemiological studies is crucial to community nutrition.

**Epidemiology** is the study of the determinants, occurrence, and distribution of health and disease in a defined population.[2,3] It studies scientifically the factors that affect the health of individuals in the community. It also serves as the foundation for intervention programs that use evidence-based information to address the prevention of health conditions.[2-4] Today, epidemiologists employ a range of study designs, from observational to experimental, with the purpose of revealing unbiased relationships between **exposures** (e.g., nutrition, biological agents, stress, or chemicals) and outcomes (e.g., diseases, wellness, and health indicators). Epidemiological studies are usually categorized as follows[3,5]:

- Descriptive (organizing data by time, place, and person)
- Analytic (aiming to examine associations or commonly hypothesized causal relationships, and incorporating a case-control or cohort study)
- Experimental (clinical or community trials of treatments and other interventions)

This chapter discusses the basic research process and epidemiological studies in dietetic practice. A more advanced research process is presented in Appendix F.

# ▶ Epidemiology in Community Health

Epidemiological and demographic measures and research methods are used to study health-related conditions. For example, they are used to investigate outbreaks of food poisoning, chickenpox, measles, and acquired immunodeficiency syndrome (AIDS). They are also used to investigate environmental conditions, lifestyles, health-promotion strategies, and other factors that affect

health.[6] The science of epidemiology is important to community and public health nutritionists because it can be utilized to assess and understand health, diseases, and injury in a community or target population. Epidemiology is a population-focused applied science that uses research and a statistical data collection methodology to determine the following[7]:

- The population that is affected by a disease or disorder
- The incidence or prevalence of a health problem in the community
- The likelihood the causes and risk factors contributing to the health problem may or may not be determined

One example of epidemiological research in the community is that of the Racial and Ethnic Approaches to Community Health Across the United States (REACH U.S.) Program. The Centers for Disease Control and Prevention (CDC) created REACH U.S. to address the problem of health disparities among different racial and ethnic groups and to show that the health status of groups most affected by health inequities can be improved. REACH U.S. supports strategies that address health disparities throughout the life span.[8] One of the success stories of the REACH U.S. program was conducted at the Genesee County (Michigan) Health Department. The department coordinated a multifaceted community effort to reduce the high death rates among African American infants born in and around Flint, Michigan. The program's activities included the following[8]:

- Case-management services designed to reach pregnant women and new mothers in high-risk areas of the county
- Community dialogue sessions designed to educate residents about infant death rates and available resources
- Workshops conducted to help participants understand the connections between racism and health care

Social marketing efforts were used to communicate important health messages about how to reduce infant deaths, and a medical services committee was formed to identify and promote best clinical practices.

Results showed that the death rate for African American infants in Genesee County dropped from a high of 23.5 deaths per 1,000 live births in 1999 to a low of 15.2 in 2005. In comparison, the rate among Caucasian American infants in 2005 was 6.3 deaths per 1,000 live births. The disparity ratio between African Americans and Caucasian Americans also dropped from a high of 3.6 African American infant deaths for every 1 Caucasian American infant death in 2001 to 2.4:1 in 2005.[8]

# ▶ Nutritional Epidemiology

**Nutritional epidemiology** is the study of dietary intake and the occurrence of disease in human populations.[9] In nutritional epidemiology, accurate quantification of nutritional exposure is critical. Exposure is the characteristics or agents (e.g., food, medications, time in the sun) that a person comes in contact with that may be related to disease risk (see **TABLE 3-1**).[10] It is complicated and challenging to evaluate and associate dietary intake with disease risk. For instance, cigarette smoking can be accurately assessed as an activity with a simple yes or no question. It has been reported that cigarette smoking is addictive, and smokers seem to be consistent in their habits, instead of stopping and starting. Most smokers seem to smoke about the same number of cigarettes per day, and, because of the expense, most people know how many cigarettes they smoke per day.[11,12]

In comparison, it is difficult for clients to report accurately the food consumed for more than 1 week because they may consume hundreds, even thousands of different foods during that period. In addition, the difficulty may be due to the following[9]:

■ Other people preparing the meals (e.g., restaurant, friends, spouse, prepackaged foods) so that the client does not know what, or how much, he or she has consumed
■ Seasonal variations in food intake
■ Life events (e.g., weekends, holidays, vacations, birthdays)

Indeed, the daily variability in food intake makes it difficult to identify any critically consistent pattern.[13] This means that researchers must depend on food composition databases to calculate the exposure variable. These issues have made it difficult to obtain consistent and strong evidence about how diet affects disease risk.

In the past 20 years, nutritional epidemiological research has focused on nutrient-based analyses to help guide the search for underlying causes of disease risk.

**TABLE 3-1** Examples of Exposures Relevant to Nutritional Epidemiological Studies

| Exposure | Diet-Related Example | Other Example |
|---|---|---|
| Agent that may cause or protect from disease | Fruit and vegetable consumption may provide protection against colon cancer, heart disease, and stroke. | Physical activity may provide protection against colon cancer, obesity, and heart disease. |
| Constitutional host factors | Persons can have a genetic predisposition to nutrition-related diseases (e.g., diabetes, heart disease, cancer). | Older adults and low-income individuals are more predisposed to chronic disease. |
| Other host factors | Food preferences learned during childhood can determine food choices. | More educated adults may have better disease screening. |
| Agents that may confound the association between another agent and disease | Correlation between dietary constituents (e.g., a diet high in fruits and vegetables is usually low in calories and fat and high in antioxidants). | Alcohol and substance abusers and smokers are less likely to engage in physical activity. |
| Agents that may modify the effects of other agents | Fruits and vegetables may protect against lung cancer among smokers. | Smoking causes an increased risk for lung cancer. |
| Agents that may determine the outcome of disease | Malnutrition. | Medical treatment and medical nutrition therapy. |

Reprinted from *Nutrition in the Prevention and Treatment of Disease*, Coulston A, Rock C, Monsen E. (Eds), Copyright Academic Press (2001), with permission from Elsevier.

However, food-based hypotheses and analyses have been shown to complement this philosophy and can be an effective method to link food intake to a health condition. For example, Ness and Powles [14] conducted a systematic review of the reported associations between the consumption of fruits and vegetables and the risk for cardiovascular diseases. Results showed that 9 of 10 ecological studies, 2 of 3 case-control studies, and 6 of 16 cohort studies found a significant protective association between the consumption of fruits and vegetables and coronary heart disease. For stroke, 3 of 5 ecological studies and 6 of 8 cohort studies found a significant protective association with consumption of fruits and vegetables. For total circulatory disease, one of two cohort studies reported a significant protective association. [15] Hence, the tools and methods of nutritional epidemiology can be developed to deal with scientific issues unique to the biology of chronic diseases. Specifically, epidemiological methods were designed to address the following [9]:

- The length of time for disease development
- The multifactorial nature of chronic diseases
- The fact that research using human beings prevents direct observations of cause and effect

## ▶ Interpretation of Cause and Effect in Nutritional Epidemiology

Epidemiology is the study of associations, and statistical methods are used to test the strength of these associations. However, it is important to note that the existence of a statistically significant association does not indicate that the observed relationship is one of cause and effect. For any observed association, the following should be considered [16,9]:

- The observed association may be due to chance.
- The association may be due to improper study design or implementation or inappropriate analysis of data.
- The association may be weak or strong.
- A credible biological mechanism may exist.
- There could be an association between exposure and the outcome.
- The significance of the results depends on the context of all the available evidence. Causality is supported when studies that are conducted at different times, using different methods, and performed among different populations show similar results.

- The result correlates with other criteria of causality (given in Appendix G).

It is not uncommon in the field of nutritional epidemiology for a cause-and-effect relationship to be beyond doubt. However, research information should not be ignored or discarded. [17] One must exercise caution and use thoughtful consideration before acting on epidemiological evidence. This chapter's Successful Community Strategies feature presents a successful cohort research study that verified the association between plant-based diets and the rate of mortality.

## ▶ Types of Public Health Nutritional Epidemiology Research

Public health nutritional epidemiology research and research design can be divided into observational and experimental/clinical categories. The difference between an experimental and an observational study is the control the researcher may have over participants, the methods and procedures, and the exposures (see **FIGURE 3-1**). In an experimental/clinical study, the researchers can control some of the clients' entire dietary intake. In an observational study, the researcher does not intervene in or manipulate the clients' dietary intake. [9,18,19] We will first discuss observational studies. The types of observational studies for individuals include *cross-sectional, case-control*, and *cohort/ prospective* studies; observational studies of groups are referred to as *ecological studies*. After that, we will discuss experimental studies. Figure 3-1 presents types of epidemiological research design.

### Observational Studies of Individuals

In a **cross-sectional study**, sometimes described as prevalence or descriptive survey, nutrient intake and outcome are both measured at the same point in time.

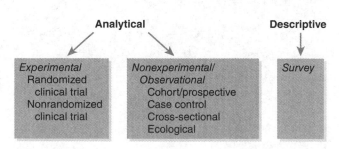

**FIGURE 3-1** Types of epidemiological research design.

The aim of the study is to describe the relationship between diseases and dietary intake in a specified community at a particular time. It can provide a snapshot of the frequency and characteristics of a disease in a population at a particular point in time.[20] An example of a cross-sectional study question would be: What is the association between nutrient intake and disease outcome? For example, the National Health and Nutrition Examination Survey (NHANES) and the International Study on Macronutrients and Blood Pressure (INTERMAP) are cross-sectional studies. INTERMAP is a cross-sectional study of associations between macronutrients and blood pressure. In this study, participants had their blood pressure measured twice on each of four occasions and completed a 24-hour recall on each day that their blood pressure was measured.[18,11,21] Similarly, the National Center for Health Statistics conducts the NHANES survey biannually to measure the health and nutritional condition of adults and children living in the United States. The survey utilizes both questionnaire and examination techniques. In this study, a sample of 1,890 12- to 16-year-olds with measured height and weight were obtained from the NHANES III survey to identify factors to potentially combat obesity in 12- to 16-year-olds with one or two obese parents and those with no obese parents. NHANES III surveys were conducted in two stages: 1) an initial interview was conducted in the respondents' homes, where health histories and sociodemographic characteristics were obtained, and 2) 3 weeks later, dietary intake assessments and physical examinations were conducted on the participants in a mobile examination center.

Results show that eating breakfast every day or some days was significantly protective against obesity in adolescents with obese parent(s), and this proved to be the strongest protective factor in this group of children. Findings from the NHANES studies have been used to create public health education and intervention programs.[22,15,23]

In nutritional **case-control studies**, also referred to as retrospective and case-referent studies, persons recently diagnosed with a diet-related disease and a group of persons without the disease (the control) from the same population are interviewed concerning their dietary habits. The differences between both groups' findings are compared. Case-control studies are a commonly used method of observational epidemiological studies. The aim of this type of study is to identify the cause of a disease among a group of people, or the cause-and-effect relationships of the health condition.[24] Typical study questions could be: Do people with the disease or health condition have a different lifestyle than persons who

have not been diagnosed with the health condition? Or, do people diagnosed with hypertension smoke cigarettes and consume foods higher in sodium than persons without hypertension?[18] For example, in 2004, Lubin et al.[25] conducted a case-control study in Israel. The aim of the study was to determine the association between body size and the risk for breast cancer. The study used a population of 1,065 breast cancer patients, 964 surgical controls, and 981 neighborhood controls. Heights and weights at three periods throughout the participants' lives (at age 18, for "most of adult life," and most recent) were ascertained. The authors analyzed these parameters and the body mass index (BMI) for each period, as well as BMI changes throughout life, controlling for age, menstrual status, and ethnic origin. Results showed an increase in risk for breast cancer with greater recent BMI among postmenopausal women ages 60 years and older.[25]

In another retrospective study, the Alaska Native Medical Center diabetes program analyzed diabetes care and outcomes audit data from 1994 to 2004 to evaluate the impact of the Special Diabetes Program for Indians (SDPI) funding on process and intermediate outcomes.[26] Congress established the SDPI grant program in 1997 to respond to the diabetes epidemic among American Indians and Alaska Natives. The SDPI program provides funding for diabetes treatment and prevention services at 399 Indian Health Service (IHS) and Tribal and Urban Indian Health Programs in all 12 IHS areas across the United States. The IHS Division of Diabetes administers the program with guidance from the Tribal Leaders Diabetes Committee.[27] The researchers conducted a retrospective analysis of data[28,29] from randomly selected standardized medical records for trends from regional sites in Alaska. Results show that hemoglobin A1c, total and low-density lipoprotein (LDL) cholesterol, triglycerides, and blood pressure significantly improved from the pre-SDPI to the SDPI period.

In **cohort studies**, sometimes called prospective, follow-up, and longitudinal studies, baseline risk factors are evaluated and participants are followed over time to monitor disease occurrence. It is the analytic method of epidemiological studies. Participants are typically free of disease. A typical study question would be: Do people with a higher intake of a nutrient develop or die from a particular disease more frequently or sooner than persons with a lower intake? Cohort studies are usually very large, exceeding 50,000 participants; may take many years to be conducted; and are expensive.[28] An example of a cohort study is the Women's Health Initiative (WHI), a 15-year study investigating the degree to which diet, hormone replacement therapy, calcium,

**TABLE 3-2** Dietary Assessment in Different Study Sessions

| Study Situation | Methods Commonly Used |
|---|---|
| Cross-sectional | 24-Hour recall; food frequency questionnaire (FFQ); brief methods |
| Case-control (retrospective) | FFQ; diet history |
| Cohort | FFQ; diet history; 24-hour recall |
| Intervention | FFQ; brief methods; 24-hour recall |
| Clinical screening | 24-Hour recall; brief methods; diet history |
| Surveillance | 24-Hour recall; brief methods |

Reprinted from *Nutrition in the Prevention and Treatment of Disease*, Coulston A, Rock C, Monsen E. (Eds), Copyright Academic Press (2001), with permission from Elsevier.

and vitamin D might prevent heart disease, breast and colorectal cancer, and osteoporosis in postmenopausal women. The main advantage of cohort studies is that exposure to potential risk factors is assessed before the development of the disease. **TABLE 3-2** shows examples of cohort studies.

**TABLE 3-3** presents examples of cohort studies utilizing nutrition assessments.

## Observational Studies of Groups

**Ecological studies** compare collective data that represent entire populations. An ecological study focuses on the comparison of groups, not individuals. The purpose of an ecological analysis may be to make biological implications about the association between exposure (e.g., water contaminant) and disease outcome in various communities within a population or to make ecological inferences about effects on group rates.[4] Ecological studies may be very useful for monitoring national trends in health, social, cultural, economic, and environmental factors that influence health that cannot be measured at an individual level. For example, migration studies, a type of ecological study, show a significant increase in the risk for several chronic diseases, such as breast cancer, when people move from an Eastern to a Western country.[24,25,34]

## Experimental Studies

Experimental studies involve intentional alteration of or intervention in the course of a disease. Nutritional intervention studies include metabolic studies and randomized clinical trials.[9,18] In metabolic or feeding studies, the researcher develops nutritionally adequate diets that vary on one or more components, to investigate the effect of this diet on internal physiological reactions (e.g., carbohydrate, lipid, and energy utilization and storage in relation to obesity and diabetes), metabolic processes (e.g., absorption, transport, and utilization of minerals, vitamins, and protein), and specific enzyme systems in experimental animals and humans.[14] An example of an experimental study is a metabolic ward study that reported changes in total cholesterol from changes in intakes of saturated and polyunsaturated fatty acids and dietary cholesterol.[18,35-37] Crossover research design is common in metabolic/feeding studies. In this design, each volunteer participant serves as his or her own control.

Another type of experimental study is the randomized clinical trial, which is a prospective study in which participants are randomly assigned to intervention and control groups. The participants are followed over time to assess the effectiveness and safety of the intervention after randomization.[34] An example of a randomized study is the Fracture Intervention Trial, which was designed to test the hypothesis that hormone replacement therapy would reduce the rate of fracture in postmenopausal women.[38]

## Genetic Epidemiological Studies

Genetic epidemiological studies use genetic epidemiology and molecular epidemiology. The investigation could be a cross-sectional and/or an intervention study. In genetic epidemiology, a question could be: Do genes determine eating behaviors, such as how much one eats, preferences for certain types of foods, and frequency or patterns of eating?[18,39] Research implies that there is a resemblance among family members for these behaviors, but it is not clear whether genes, shared environments, or both are the cause.[40,41] In molecular epidemiology, questions relate to the physical and hormonal mechanisms leading to taste preferences, hunger, and satiety. For example, taste receptors are clearly genetically determined, although the gene(s) may not all be identified yet.[35,42] For example, genes encoding hormones and proteins that regulate hunger and satiety have just been identified recently.[36,43,44] It has been known for some time that certain enzyme deficiencies, which have a genetic cause, give rise to specific nutritional problems; examples of these are phenylketonuria and galactosemia.[36,43]

**TABLE 3-3** Examples of Cohort Studies Utilizing Nutrition Assessments[30-33]

| Cohort Study | Years Conducted | Sample Studied | Purpose | Nutritional Intake Assessment | Results |
|---|---|---|---|---|---|
| Early risk factors for increased adiposity: A cohort study of African American subjects followed from birth to young adulthood | Baseline: Between 1959 and 1965 | 447 African American pregnant women | The aim of this study was to identify risk factors, present at birth, for increased adiposity in adulthood in an African American population | Baseline: Anthropometric measurements and socioeconomic factors | Three variables measured at birth were independently associated with adiposity in young adulthood. |
| Framingham Study: Heart and Vascular Disease Program Dietary patterns, smoking, and subclinical heart disease in women: opportunities for primary prevention from the Framingham nutrition studies | 1947–1972 | 1,423 women in the population-based Framingham Offspring/Spouse group | To investigate the relationship between a heart-healthy dietary pattern and subclinical heart disease in women, and to identify potential opportunities for primary prevention | Ultrasound at 12-year follow-up Food Frequency Questionnaire and 24-hour recall | Women who ate a heart-healthy diet at baseline had less cardiovascular disease risk factor profiles. Women who had heart-healthy eating pattern, plus avoidance of smoking, had lower chances of subclinical heart disease. |
| Family Structure and Childhood Obesity, Early Childhood Longitudinal Study—Kindergarten Cohort | 1998–1999 | Kindergarten (n = 14,493), third grade (n = 11,855), and fifth grade (n = 10,036) | This study examines the effect of number of parents and number of siblings on children's body mass index and risk of obesity | Face-to-face assessments or interviews, telephone interviews, and questionnaires, height and weight, body mass index (BMI) | Children living with single mothers had more tendency to obesity by fifth grade than were children living with two parents. Children with siblings had lower BMI and were less likely to be obese than children without siblings. Also, living with a single mother or no sibling was associated with increases in BMI from kindergarten through fifth grade. |
| Nurses' Health Study: Waist circumference, waist-to-hip ratio, and risk for breast cancer in the Nurses' Health Study. | 1986 through May 1994 | 47,382 U.S. registered nurses | The associations of waist circumference and waist-to-hip circumference ratio with risk for breast cancer | Waist circumference, hip circumference, and waist-to-hip ratio. Questionnaire | Higher waist circumference is associated with the risk for breast cancer, especially among postmenopausal women. |

Sources:

Chen AY, José JE. Family structure and childhood obesity: early childhood longitudinal study—kindergarten cohort. *Prev Chronic Dis.* 2010;7(3):A50-A60.

Huang Z, Willett WC, Colditz GA, Hunter DJ, et al. Waist circumference, waist:hip ratio, and risk of breast cancer in the Nurses' Health Study. *Am J Epidemiol.* 1999;150(12):1316-1324.

Millen BE, Quatromoni PA, Nam BH, O'Horo CE, et al. Dietary patterns, smoking, and subclinical heart disease in women: opportunities for primary prevention from the Framingham Nutrition Studies. *J Am Diet Assoc.* 2004;104(2):208-214.

Stettler N, Tershakovec T, Zemel B, Leonard MB, et al. Early risk factors for increased adiposity: A cohort study of African American subjects followed from birth to young adulthood. *Am J Clin Nutr.* 2000;72:378-383.

# ▶ Descriptive Measures of Community Health

Descriptive epidemiological studies explain the occurrence of disease and are collected using various methods. The data are then assembled based on time (e.g., changes of eating habits over a long period), place (geographic areas), and person (e.g., age, gender, ethnicity, lifestyle).[5,45] These data can be used to quantify the extent and location of nutrition problems within a population and to suggest associations between diet and disease that can be evaluated in analytic research.[39,46]

## Demographic Measures

**Demography** is an analytic tool used to measure a population by recording births, deaths, age distribution, and other vital statistics.[6,7] Some human characteristics, or demographics, may be associated with wellness or illness. Age, race, gender, ethnicity, income, and educational level are important demographics that may affect health outcomes. For example, men are more likely than women to develop certain heart diseases, and African Americans are more likely than Caucasian Americans to experience hypertension.[23,29,47] Community nutritionists must be familiar with the demographic characteristics of the community they serve and with the health problems associated with that community before developing a health promotion program.

## Morbidity and Mortality

Epidemiology studies both wellness and illness. Wellness is hard to measure; therefore, the measures of health are expressed in terms of morbidity (illness) and mortality (death).[6] The CDC's website (http://www.cdc.gov) is an excellent source of morbidity and mortality data organized by states and for select cities.[48]

## Incidence and Prevalence

Two types of disease frequency measures are used to determine the morbidity rate in a defined population—incidence and prevalence. Incidence is the rate of acquisition of a new health condition or the number of persons in a defined population who *developed* the condition during a specified period.[6] The calculation of incidence, therefore, requires that a population be followed over a period in a prospective or cohort (forward-looking) study.[38,45]

On the other hand, prevalence is the total number of persons in the defined population who *are affected by* a certain disease or condition at a specified time. This includes both new and existing cases.[39,38] Therefore, prevalence

may be calculated in a "one-shot" cross-sectional ("slice of time") or retrospective (backward-looking) study.[6]

**Interpretation of Incidence and Prevalence.** In both incidence and prevalence, it is important to clearly define the condition being studied; otherwise, scientists may make a mistake in differentiating between incidence (new cases) and prevalence.[49,50] Scientists must allow enough time to identify new cases to determine incidence and prevalence. This period must be long enough to adequately detect the condition, especially in the case of rare diseases or diseases with a low rate of diagnosis. However, the period cannot be so long that it will be affected by mortality and other follow-up losses.[51]

Measures of incidence and prevalence provide different information and have different implications. For example, an increase in the prevalence of diabetes or endometrial cancer means that there are more persons with these health conditions in the population. This may be due to more new cases (in other words, increased incidence) or because individuals with these health conditions are living longer. In either case, the community may need to direct resources toward treating the problem. However, if knowledge of incidence is lacking, it will be difficult to decide whether to target the resources toward primary prevention or toward secondary and tertiary treatment services.

Here is a specific example of differentiating incidence from prevalence. In a community health center, 120 infants free from measles are followed for 3 weeks. In this period of time, 45 developed measles. Remember, incidence gives an approximation of the likelihood (or risk) that a client will develop a particular health condition during a specified period. Therefore, there is an incidence rate of 45 per 120 (or 37.5 percent) during the 3-week period. However, prevalence computes the proportion of a given population with the problem. So at the same community health center, 150 infants were screened for the presence of measles and 30 infants were affected. This results in a prevalence of measles of 20 percent (30 ÷ 150). In this case, prevalence means the proportion of infants with the problem (e.g., measles) at the specified period.[52] The formulas for calculating both are in **BOX 3-1**.

## Rates

The mathematical measures used to articulate incidence and prevalence are known as rates. Epidemiological studies must relate the occurrence of a health condition to the population base. Rates express a mathematical relationship in which the numerator is the number of persons experiencing the condition, and the denominator is the population at risk, or the total number of persons who have the possibility of experiencing the condition.

---

**BOX 3-1** The Formulas for Both Prevalence and Incidence

Incidence rate (IR) = Number of new cases (people who developed the disease) during a specified period

$$IR \frac{}{\text{Total number of a defined population at risk at the time of getting the disease}}$$

Prevalence = Number of both existing and new cases during a specified period

$$P \frac{}{\text{Total number of a defined population at risk}}$$

---

The formula for calculating rate is shown in the following section.[6] Epidemiologists use rates to examine the experiences of particular groups of people at specified times, in different cities or countries. Another important use of rates is in calculating the risks to individuals and groups of experiencing an event such as a heart attack or an occurrence such as cancer or obesity.

**Example of a Rate.** In the United States, an acceptable definition for infant mortality rate is the number of deaths during the first year of life (i.e., the number of both neonatal and postneonatal deaths) per 1,000 live births. To calculate infant mortality rate, add the number of neonatal (the first 28 days of life) and postneonatal (between the 28th and 365th days of life) deaths and divide by the number of live births; then, multiply the result by 1,000. The numerator represents the number of infants experiencing the "condition" of dying in the first year of life, and the denominator represents the population of infants at risk of dying in that year.[3,53]

If 500,000 live births and 10,000 infant deaths were reported in the United States for a given year, the rate can be calculated as follows[6]:

1.  Infant mortality rate =
    $$\frac{\text{Number of infant deaths (age} < 1 \text{ year during time interval)}}{\text{Total live births during time arrival}} \times 1,000$$

2.  Divide 10,000 by 500,000 = 0.020 of the infants died during the first year of life.

3.  Because it is difficult to relate to 0.020 infants, multiply 0.020 by a constant, in this case 1,000, resulting in 20 infants who died during the first year of life per 1,000 live births. This means that the infant mortality rate was 20 infant deaths per 1,000 live births for that year.

**Interpretation of Rates.** International comparisons and rankings of infant mortality should be interpreted with caution. For example, a study investigated how infant mortality rates are reported in the United States, Norway, and Israel. Results showed that the United States reported live births less than 750 g, whereas other countries did not report live births less than 750 g. Disparities among countries resulted from differences in birth and death registration practices.[48]

Also, to determine if the population in a specific community is at greater or lesser risk for a condition, the research must compare the rates for the community with rates from similar communities, the state, or the country. Most often, rates are based on data from a calendar year, which may create some problems. When calculating an infant mortality rate, it is important to recognize that some of the infants who die during a given calendar year may not be a part of the demographics, such as those who died in 2005 but who were actually born in 2004 and thus were not part of the 2005 population at risk. Also, some of the infants who were born in 2005 might die in 2006 and not be reflected in the 2005 infant mortality rate.[6] A cohort research study (discussed earlier) can help overcome the limitations of the conventionally calculated calendar year rate.[48]

---

### ✎ Think About It

What type of research methodology did Peter use for his case-control study?

Peter, a nutrition professor, received funding from the Special Diabetes Program for Indians to conduct further analysis on the data he collected from diabetes care and nutrition education program. The information he collected included the participants' dietary preferences, knowledge, and awareness of diabetes care, attitude about nutrition education, and management of diabetes.

---

## ▶ The Epidemiological Methods

Epidemiological research methods can be descriptive, analytic, or experimental. Although all can be used in studying the occurrence of disease, the method used most often is descriptive epidemiology. Once the basic epidemiology of disease has been described, analytic methods can be used to study the disease further, and an experimental approach can be developed to test a hypothesis.[3]

In epidemiological studies, the investigator attempts to identify risk factors for particular diseases, conditions, behaviors, or risks that result from particular causes, such as environmental or industrial agents.[50,54] Epidemiology uses different methods—such as statistical, pathological, clinical, demographic, microbiological, and sociological—to study disease processes. These are not exclusive to epidemiology; however, the ways in which they are used distinctively define the epidemiological method.[39] The following examples use the investigation of the diet–disease hypothesis to show the scientific approach of epidemiologists.

## Observation

There are many instances of disease control based on epidemiological observations. In an observational study (descriptive method), the investigators observe the behaviors of participants without interfering. For example, epidemiological researchers observed consistently that vegetarian groups in the United States and overseas have lower blood pressure than nonvegetarians in most studies. The term *vegetarian* includes several heterogeneous groups, but in general, vegetarian diets are usually high in whole grains, beans, fruits, and vegetables, and sometimes fish, dairy products, and eggs. The aspects of the vegetarian diet that have been observed to be protective against hypertension include low intake of animal products and high intake of potassium, magnesium, fiber, and (sometimes) calcium.[52]

## Counting Cases or Events

Counting cases is a descriptive epidemiological method sometimes useful for health policy. It can be used to know the number of people with a particular characteristic or number of events that occurred in a given region or community. For example, the migration studies of indigenous populations showed that the prevalence of hypertension increased because of urbanization. With urbanization, people consumed more processed foods and less fresh foods (that were previously available). In addition, researchers observed lifestyle changes (e.g., lack of physical activity, overeating) that caused increases in body weight, sodium intake, and dietary fat during the process of acculturation.[55]

## Relating Cases or Events to Population at Risk

Inherent in the epidemiological method is the need for measuring the number of disease cases or events in a population and relating the number of cases to a population base. Cases that fit the case description are identified, counted, and correlated to time, place, and individuals. In reviewing 53 observational studies of calcium and hypertension, 5 studies were prospective and 48 were cross-sectional, of which 4 also contained a longitudinal component. Various dietary methodologies were used; the most common was the 24-hour dietary recall. Most studies controlled for age, sex, and BMI, with variable control for other confounding variables.[56] Together, these studies showed only modest associations between calcium and blood pressure. But in the beginning, the higher calcium and magnesium content of "hard" water, and its relation to cardiovascular mortality, triggered epidemiological inquiry into the relationship of both minerals to blood pressure.[57]

## Making Comparisons

Another scientific approach epidemiologists use is making comparisons. The Dietary Approaches to Stop Hypertension (DASH) sodium multicenter trial, for example, was created to resolve the controversy surrounding sodium intake and blood pressure.[58] The effect of dietary composition on blood pressure is an important public health topic. The National Heart Lung and Blood Institute funded the DASH study, which compared the effects of three sodium levels on blood pressure versus a control. The subjects were asked to eat either a control diet typical of intake in the United States or the DASH diet, a diet rich in fruits, vegetables, and low-fat dairy foods; low in saturated fat, total fat, and cholesterol; high in dietary fiber, potassium, calcium, and magnesium; and moderately high in protein. Within each diet (control and DASH), subjects ate foods with high, intermediate, and low levels of sodium. The investigators found that reducing the sodium intake from the high to the intermediate level reduced systolic blood pressure by 2.1 mm Hg.[58,59] Reducing the sodium intake from the intermediate to the low level caused additional reductions of 4.6 mm Hg on the control diet and 1.7 mm Hg on the DASH diet. The effects of sodium intake were observed in those subjects with and without hypertension, all races, and both women and men. Compared to the control diet with the highest sodium level, the DASH diet with the lowest sodium level reduced systolic blood pressure by 8.9 mm Hg in subjects with hypertension and 7.1 mm Hg in those without hypertension.[56]

In another comparative study, the Caucasian Prospective Investigation into Cancer and Nutrition (EPIC) study recruited 20,343 participants for a cohort study. The participants had no hypertension. The investigators examined whether the Mediterranean diet (see the Successful Community Strategies feature in this chapter), and olive oil in particular, can reduce blood pressure. Results showed that intakes of olive oil, vegetables, and fruit were associated with a reduction in blood pressure whereas intakes of cereals, meat and meat products, and alcohol were associated with higher blood pressure.[60]

In addition, another study conducted a 1-year randomized controlled trial to determine the degree to which dietary change is influenced by providing seven home-delivered therapeutic meals weekly to adults age 60 years or older with hyperlipidemia or hypertension. Fifty percent of participants received seven therapeutic meals per week for 12 months. The nutrients that make up the DASH diet were measured using 24-hour food recalls at baseline, 6 months, and 12 months. Results showed that delivery of seven DASH meals per week increased compliance with dietary recommendations among noncompliant older adults with cardiovascular disease.[61]

## Developing the Hypothesis

The hypothesis or research question is an assumption written in a clear, concise manner about what the investigator thinks will happen in the research project. For example, after reviewing the results of the migration studies and the vegetarian group's studies in the United States, researchers developed the hypothesis that diets low in sodium and high in fruits, vegetables, and fiber can reduce blood pressure.

## Testing the Hypothesis

In testing the hypothesis, research observations have shown a direct relationship between higher sodium intake and higher blood pressure across population groups.[9,13] The INTERSALT study (International Study of Salt) measured the relationship between 24-hour urinary sodium excretion and blood pressure in 10,079 men and women from 52 centers around the world.[13] Results showed a positive relationship between mean urinary sodium excretion and blood pressure; that is, the participants' blood pressure increased with an increase in sodium excretion. A slight positive relationship also was observed when the researchers adjusted for alcohol and BMI. The researchers also reported a strong positive relationship between sodium intake and the slope of blood pressure increase with age across populations, indicating a role for sodium in age-related blood pressure increase.

In a recent reanalysis of the original INTERSALT data, corrected for measurement error due to the use of single 24-hour urine collections, results were stronger: a 100 mmol/day (2,300 mg sodium) increase in urinary sodium was associated with an increase of 3 to 6 mm Hg in systolic blood pressure and of 0 to 3 mm Hg diastolic blood pressure.[62,63] In a meta-analysis of observational studies, Law et al.[64] reported stronger results than INTERSALT, especially in the elderly and those with higher baseline blood pressures, but diet and other variables were not assessed in a standard manner across studies.[9]

## Drawing Scientific Inferences

The data showing that diet modification can prevent and lower blood pressure are significant. The intervention approaches and methods involved in some data collection are still being clarified. Because of a variety of research design limitations, inadequate statistical power, and measurement issues, studies of single nutrients (except for potassium) have mainly been inconsistent.[65] However, when several nutrients, lifestyle, or dietary factors are combined in the same intervention studies, as in the DASH study, blood pressure was effectively reduced.[66] It has been shown that nutrients have interactive effects when they are consumed together in a diet.[62] In addition to the DASH dietary pattern, other factors such as reduced sodium intake, weight loss, and moderate alcohol intake have been shown to reduce blood pressure. Simultaneous observance of several recommendations (as with the DASH diet) is likely to be the best strategy for preventing and lowering blood pressure. Future research should center on methods to motivate and maintain dietary changes for controlling blood pressure, plus address the unanswered nutritional hypotheses.

The implication of these findings is that the success of dietary intervention depends on support from clinicians, government agencies, private institutes, and industries at both the population and individual levels. In particular, industries can improve the nutritional value of the food supply, such as reducing the sodium and fat content of processed foods; this is a very critical role in implementing dietary changes. Dietetic and other healthcare professionals must also play a significant role in educating the public and promoting adherence to nutritional guidelines for the prevention of hypertension and other health conditions.[16,67]

## Conducting Experimental Studies

Another scientific approach that epidemiologists use is conducting experimental studies. One such study examined the effects of garden-based nutrition education on adolescent fruit and vegetable consumption. Sixth-grade students at three different elementary schools were used as a control group and two treatment groups. Students in the treatment groups participated in a 12-week nutrition education program, and one treatment group also participated in garden-based activities. Students in all three groups were required to complete three 24-hour food-recall workbooks before and after the intervention. Results showed that adolescents who participated in the garden-based nutrition intervention increased their servings of fruits and vegetables more than students in the control groups. Also, the experimental group's vitamin A, vitamin C, and fiber intake increased significantly.[68]

In an analytical research design, the aim is to evaluate hypotheses based on existing knowledge or findings. The DASH trial, discussed earlier, was a randomized, multicenter, controlled feeding study to compare the effects of three dietary patterns on blood pressure. The control group consumed fruits and vegetables and a combination diet (having less total fat, less saturated fat, and less cholesterol than the fruit and vegetable diet or the control diet). The dietary patterns differed in selected nutrients hypothesized to alter blood pressure. This study examined the food-group structure and nutrient composition of the study diets and participant nutrient consumption during the intervention. Participants consumed the control dietary pattern during a 3-week start-up period. They were then randomized either to continue on the control diet or to change to the fruits and vegetables or the combination diet for 8 weeks. Sodium intake and body weight were constant during the entire feeding period. Analysis of variance models compared the nutrient content of the three diets.

Targeting a few nutrients thought to influence blood pressure resulted in diets that were very different in their food-group and nutrient composition. The control and fruits and vegetables diets contained more oils, table fats, salad dressings, and red meats and were higher in saturated fat, total fat, and cholesterol than was the combination diet. The fruits and vegetables and combination diets contained relatively more servings of fruits, juices, vegetables, and nuts/seeds, and were higher in magnesium, potassium, and fiber than was the control diet. Both the fruits and vegetables and combination diets were low in sweets and sugar-containing drinks. The combination diet contained a greater variety of fruits, and its high calcium content was obtained by increasing low-fat dairy products. In addition, the distinct food grouping pattern across the three diets resulted in substantial differences in the levels of vitamins A, $B_6$, C, and E; folate; and zinc.[69]

**FIGURE 3-2** presents examples of the scientific method used by epidemiologists.

## ▶ Quantitative and Qualitative Methods

The methodologies appropriate for answering the research question need to be considered. Quantitative methods have been the standard methodology used in

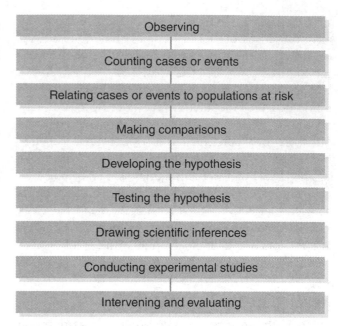

**FIGURE 3-2** Examples of the scientific method of epidemiologists.

nutrition research because they depend on isolation of one or more variables that can be measured and analyzed statistically. In quantitative (objective) research, random sample surveys and structured interviews are used to collect mostly quantifiable data that are analyzed using statistical techniques. This method promotes gathering data that can be verified by another researcher and generalized to other populations. Deductive reasoning, objectivity, quasi-experiments, statistical techniques, and control characterize these methods.[70]

Although many nutrition research questions are open to traditional methodologies, others require a different approach. There is a growing acceptance of nutrition science as a composite of different viewpoints and varied research methodologies.[70,71] Although recognition of qualitative (subjective) methods for scientific study is relatively recent in nutrition literature, they began to be used in the United States during the late 1800s.[5] Qualitative strategies were used to reveal the rapidly developing social problems in cities at that time caused by industrialization, urbanization, and mass immigration. Munhall and Boyd[72] stated that qualitative descriptions encouraged social change by making urban problems visible to the public.

Qualitative methods may be more beneficial for a particular incident being studied. For example, qualitative approaches are rarely appropriate in genetic engineering but may be appropriate when analyzing a social behavior, such as food choice and dieting. They use semi-structured or interactive interviews to collect data relating to people's judgments, attitudes, preferences, priorities, and/or perceptions about a nutrition issue; the data are then analyzed through sociological or anthropological research techniques. Inductive reasoning, subjectivity, discovery, description, and the meaning of an experience to an individual or groups typify qualitative methods.[73]

Both quantitative and qualitative data collection methods can be combined in a single research study. This is known as a mixed method study. For example, adding subjective and open-ended questions to a standard household survey could provide a better approach to defining and measuring poverty.[74] The use of mixed methods will increase as the ability to acquire and analyze large amounts of quantitative data improves along with improvements in electronic technologies. For example, it is now possible to measure and record in an accessible database every step and movement made by an individual, as well as every word he or she speaks and hears.[74]

An example of research that utilized both quantitative and qualitative methods was a study that examined the awareness and acceptability of brown rice in Chinese adults, and the possibility of introducing brown rice into their diet. This was part of a large, long-term randomized clinical trial to lower the risk for acquiring type 2 diabetes. The authors used questionnaires (quantitative) and focus-group discussions (qualitative) to collect data from participants, who resided in Shanghai. The focus group discussion was about their dietary preferences, purchasing practices for specific varieties of rice, and their knowledge and awareness of brown rice. Ninety-four percent of the participants consumed white rice daily; only 8 percent of the participants had previously consumed brown rice. Before tasting, most participants considered brown rice inferior to white rice in terms of taste and quality. However, after tasting brown rice and learning about its nutritional value, the majority indicated greater willingness to consume brown rice. The main barriers to acceptance were the perception of rough texture and unpalatable taste, as well as higher price. All participants suggested that large-scale promotion was needed to change societal attitudes toward brown rice. In addition, most of the participants articulated their willingness to participate in a future long-term brown rice intervention study. These results provided valuable information for the design of the future brown rice intervention trial and highlighted the importance of increasing awareness about the nutritional value of brown rice.[75]

Another example is a community audit qualitative and quantitative research method in which researchers drive through a community to observe its physical and social attributes, mainly through windshield tours and **ground truthing**. Ground truthing is a verification process that uses data gathered by direct observation to validate data gathered from secondary sources.[76] This method was used to conduct research in 10 communities in a rural eastern North Carolina county. The purpose of the study was to describe an approach to conducting a community audit (consisting of windshield tours and ground truthing) to compute resources, to assess community characteristics, and to inform revisions to a community guide on nutrition and physical activity resources. Community audits have been used for epidemiological studies and in program planning for health-promotion interventions.[77] In this study, the researchers used Google Earth mapping software to examine commercial and residential districts for the presence of sidewalks using both aerial and street-level views. They also determined the number of fast-food restaurants through the Reference USA business database. The researchers compared their observations on community characteristics with available secondary data sources to examine the level of agreement. The initial resource guide included 42 resources; the community audits identified 38 additional resources. Results showed that there was moderate to high agreement between windshield tour observations and secondary data sources for several community characteristics, such as number of fast-food restaurants (67 percent agreement) and existence of sidewalks (100 percent agreement). Moreover, the audit resulted in an enhanced understanding of the related barriers and facilitators to lifestyle change. The techniques presented in this article may serve as a model for health-promotion professionals in other rural communities.[76]

# ▶ Types of Sampling

Regardless of the type of research methodology, the research questions and methodologies chosen must guide the plan for data analysis. It is helpful to identify the computer software that will assist with data analysis and decide how results will be presented. For example, the researcher may want to prepare tables for the data once they are collected. These tables will help ensure all the data necessary for answering the research questions have been collected.

The research questions and plan for data analysis will guide sample selection and size. There are many methods of sample selection, but two will be considered here: random and deliberate sampling. **Random sampling** means that every case or participant has an equal opportunity to be included in the study.[5] For example, first the target group or community is informed about the research study's purpose/aim, as well as its risks, and is asked to participate. Then, individuals consenting to participate in the study are assigned randomly to one, two, or more treatment or intervention groups. The individuals randomized to receive the standard intervention treatment serve as the control group. The main

| **TABLE 3-4** The Nine Steps for the Development of a Questionnaire | |
|---|---|
| **Steps** | **Examples** |
| Decide the information required. | Dietary behavior, cultural influence, physical activity, food insecurity |
| Describe the target participants. | Pregnant women, teenagers, children, older adults, households, college students |
| Select the research methodology appropriate for the target participants. | Food frequency questionnaire, 24-hour questionnaire, and others |
| Decide on question content. | Nutrient intake, physical activity levels, food availability, demographics |
| Develop the question wording. | Avoid technical terms and jargon, be clear and concise, measure one thing per question, avoid leading questions |
| Put questions into a meaningful order and format. | Administer by telephone, in-person, online, mail. |
| Check the length of the questionnaire. | Keep the questionnaire short |
| Pretest the questionnaire. | Administer the questionnaire to a few participants for feedback and modification |
| Develop the final survey form. | Getting the permission from participants. If it is online, how it looks, consider the readability |

factor is random assignment; that is, chance determines the intervention assignment. **Deliberate sampling** means that specific target groups or communities are invited to participate in the study.[5] The choice of research methodologies will determine the characteristics of the sample population.

After consultation with a statistician, the researcher determines the factors, such as the sample size, gender, and age range. The researcher may use power analysis software to help determine sample size. Most of the time, it is impossible to know the exact number of people living in the community being studied, so the nutritionist may estimate the total population based on census data.

### General Rules for Writing Survey Questions

In addition, the nutritionist may need to write or modify an existing questionnaire for collecting data from the targeted community. The general rules for writing a survey questionnaire include, but are not limited to, the following[78]:

- Measuring the fundamental concept it is intended to obtain
- Must not measure other concepts

- Must mean the same thing to all respondents
- Must determine the hypotheses around which the questionnaire is to be designed

**TABLE 3-4** presents nine steps involved in the development of a questionnaire.[79,78]

## ▶ Concepts of Collaborative Research

**Collaboration** is very important in research and sometime is required for community types of grants. Collaboration involves mutual participation in decision making and working with others toward a common goal. It is a process of joint decision making in an atmosphere of shared respect and cooperation.[73] Collaboration should always involve interaction among community nutritionists, clients, and other healthcare practitioners. Nutrition professionals work as members of a team in all healthcare settings. In community nutrition settings, the nutritionist is part of a multidisciplinary team that includes other healthcare workers, as well as community organizations, social service agencies, and the judicial system. The multidisciplinary team can conduct research studies that can benefit the public. The need for collaborative research is especially strong now due to the prevalence of health disparities in the United States. In addition, there is a belief that partnerships between researchers and community members can contribute not only to the ability of communities to effectively address local issues, but also to the development of new knowledge.[80,81]

Successful collaboration requires that the multidisciplinary team develop a common purpose, communicate to coordinate efforts, and recognize the unique and complementary skills possessed by each team member. Each team member brings special abilities and expertise to the collaborative process. Collaboration does not work when one team member designs a research project or nutrition program and then "coordinates" by informing others of the plan. For a nutrition program or research to be successful, collaboration must be a joint effort on the part of the clients and all team members to identify mutual goals and acceptable means for meeting those goals.[82]

Although they do share some similarities, collaboration and coordination are different. **Coordination** is the act of managing interdependencies among activities. It is the ability to manage services without gaps or overlaps.[80] The nutritionist, as coordinator, may or may not consult others when carrying out a management function. Collaboration, on the other hand, involves joint decision making between two or more people.

Collaboration also can enhance the opportunity for obtaining grant money. Many granting agencies encourage collaborative efforts. A community nutritionist can collaborate with statisticians, epidemiologists, nurses, social workers, physicians, and colleagues to complement his or her nutrition expertise.[39] Collaboration is especially helpful for a new university faculty member, first-time grant seeker, or nutritionist who wants to change his or her focus area of research. Community nutritionists can find collaborators by networking with colleagues and community members and communicating with other professionals or experts in the area of interest.

Amuwo and Jenkins[81] outlined four distinct phases necessary for successful partnership building in community-based research, based on their experiences with collaborative work: networking, cooperation, collaboration, and partnership. Within these four phases, they identified 12 concrete, systematic steps that a partnership-building effort must complete in a rather sequential order, as follows[81]:

1. Involve the community early so they can see the importance of the program.
2. Be aware that partnership building is a nonlinear procedure.
3. Recruit and empower important community-based personnel.
4. Conduct a community needs assessment (both human and capital resources).
5. Recognize that other grassroots community organizations are potential partners.
6. Recruit community-based staff.
7. Engage in strategic planning.
8. Meet training needs.
9. Involve other relevant community members, public institutions, and organizations.
10. Communicate and pursue research and service agendas at the community level.
11. Facilitate the transfer of knowledge.
12. Maintain trusting and collaborative relationships.

# ▶ Reporting Research Results

Reporting research findings is an essential aspect of conducting research activities. Reporting the results of research outcomes in professional journals and at professional meetings facilitates the growth and use of nutrition knowledge. By applying research results, nutritionists can institute social change. Policy makers, other professionals, and the community can then learn that the research findings are relevant and applicable. The results of a study involving the community could support expansion of community or public health nutrition services. The nutrition profession is in urgent need of research documenting the cost effectiveness of nutrition care. Effectiveness, however, can be measured in many ways beyond cost, including quality of care, client satisfaction, and the ability for a person to maintain independence.[83]

# ▶ Epidemiological Approaches to Community Health Assessment

The changing disease patterns throughout the world are linked to changing lifestyles. One of the functions of epidemiological approaches is to determine the etiology or cause of the disease or risk factors for the disease. One way that epidemiologists study the cause and effect of disease is through a three-sided conceptual model known as the epidemiological triangle.[5] This model explains how changes in one element can influence the occurrence of a disease by increasing or decreasing an individual's risk for the health condition.

## The Epidemiological Triangle

The epidemiological triangle explores health and disease using three elements: an agent, a host, and an environment (each of which is discussed in this section).

All three of the components of this model are of equal strength. **FIGURE 3-3** shows the model in its normal state of equilibrium. Equilibrium does not mean optimal health, but it does signal the usual patterns of illness and health in a population. Any change in one of the components (agent, host, or environment) will result in disequilibrium (i.e., a change in the usual patterns).[6]

The nutritionist using the epidemiological triangle in a situation such as teenage obesity might focus on diet as the agent causing teenage obesity. However, behavior also could be a factor. An example of a behavioral factor is a sedentary lifestyle that promotes weight gain. The nutritionist would strive to determine whether there has been a change in any of the possible agents.

The host factors are personal characteristics of the teenage population who are at risk for obesity and other health-related conditions, such as diabetes. The personal characteristics include age, ethnicity, gender, socioeconomic status, eating patterns, exercise behavior, and lifestyle. Some personal characteristics, such as gender, age, and ethnicity, are not modifiable, but others are. Characteristics that can be changed include nutritional status, physical activity, and income level. By evaluating these factors, it may be possible to identify groups of teenagers who are at an increased risk for dying from obesity-related health conditions.

Finally, the environment must be assessed. Environmental factors are external factors that encompass an agent and a host. They may be exclusively physical, such as climate or surroundings (e.g., an urban housing area in the Midwestern United States). An environmental factor also may have multiple levels, such as low, middle, and high socioeconomic status. Low socioeconomic status is associated with the reduced availability of health and social services.[84] High socioeconomic status is associated with excessive behaviors, such as heavy drinking, overeating, and risk taking.[85,86]

The analysis of these three areas—agent, host, and environment—should provide information regarding groups at risk for increased rates of obesity and may provide direction toward a program aimed at reducing the risks. Therefore, the epidemiological triangle can provide a useful guide for investigating different health problems of teenage obesity, as well as other health problems.

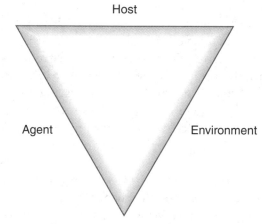

**FIGURE 3-3** Epidemiological triangle model.

Modified from: Stanhope M, Lancaster J. *Community and Public Health Nursing*. 5th ed. St. Louis, MO: Mosby; 2000.

# Successful Community Strategies

## EPIC Elderly Cohort Research Study[87-97]

The Mediterranean diet has been reviewed in many studies because several of its components have been related to decreases in common chronic diseases. Ecological evidence suggests that such a diet may be beneficial to health, and variants of this diet have improved the prognosis of patients with coronary heart disease. The Mediterranean diet is characterized by a high intake of vegetables, legumes, fruits, and cereals; a moderate to high intake of fish; a low intake of saturated lipids but a high intake of unsaturated lipids, particularly olive oil; a low to moderate intake of dairy products, mostly cheese and yogurt; a low intake of meat; and a modest intake of ethanol, mostly as wine. Several studies have reported that a diet that adheres to the principles of the traditional Mediterranean diet is associated with longer survival. Trichopoulou and Vasilopoulou[87] used a 10-unit dietary score to determine whether adherence to a Mediterranean diet was associated with a longer life expectancy among elderly Caucasians. However, several studies have used variations of this score and reported opposite associations with overall mortality. These studies, however, relied on small samples of mostly elderly participants or only on the Greek population.

The Caucasian Prospective Investigation into Cancer and Nutrition (EPIC) study used a multicenter, prospective cohort study to investigate the role of biological, dietary, lifestyle, and environmental factors in cancer and other chronic diseases and to examine whether adherence to the modified Mediterranean diet, in which unsaturated fats were substituted for monounsaturated fats, is associated with longer life expectancy among elderly persons.

Between 1992 and 2000, 519,978 healthy volunteers were recruited in 23 centers from 10 European countries (Denmark, France, Germany, Greece, Italy, the Netherlands, Norway, Spain, Sweden, and the United Kingdom). After initial

*(continues)*

## Successful Community Strategies (continued)

screening, only 74,607 individuals were included in the study. Data were collected from participants ages 60 or over. Information on the vital status of participants was obtained from mortality registries and by active follow-up. The earliest and latest years of follow-up were 1999 (some participants in the Netherlands) and December 2003 (most of the centers). Participants were classified as alive at last follow-up, dead, emigrated, refused to participate further, or unknown.

Dietary intakes were assessed through compatible instruments (food frequency questionnaires and, in some centers, records of intake over 7 or 14 days) that had been developed and validated within each center. In addition, a computerized instrument for recall of dietary intake over 24 hours was developed to collect information from a standardized random sample of the aggregate cohort. The aim was to calibrate the measurements across countries.

Nutrient intakes were calculated using food composition tables specific to the country. Fourteen food groups and nutrients were considered: potatoes, vegetables, legumes, fruits, dairy products, cereals, meat and meat products, fish and seafood, eggs, monounsaturated lipids, polyunsaturated lipids, saturated lipids, sugar and confectionery (candy, pastry, etc.), and nonalcoholic beverages.

Results showed that an increase in the modified Mediterranean diet score was associated with lower overall mortality. When dietary exposures were calibrated across countries, the reduction in mortality was 7 percent (ranging from 1 to 12 percent). The study concluded that the Mediterranean diet, modified so as to apply across Europe, was associated with increased survival among older people.

### Children and Adolescents, National Health and Nutrition Examination Survey[98]

The National Health and Nutrition Examination Survey (NHANES) is designed to assess the health and nutritional status of adults and children in the United States. The survey is a combination of interviews and physical examinations. The objective of this NHANES study was to describe perceptions of child weight status among U.S. children, adolescents, and their parents and to examine the degree in which personal and parental perception of weight status is associated with self-reported attempted weight loss.

The sample included 2,613 participants aged 8–15 years in the NHANES from the two most recent consecutive cycles (2007–2008 and 2009–2010). Classifications of weight perception were developed by comparing measured to perceived weight status. Multivariable logistic regression analyses were used to examine the association between weight misperception and self-reported attempted weight loss.

Results showed that among children and adolescents, 27.3 percent underestimated and 2.8 percent overestimated their weight status. Among parents, 25.2 percent underestimated and 1.1 percent overestimated their child's weight status. Logistic regression analyses showed that the odds of self-reported attempted weight loss was 9.5 times as high among healthy-weight children and adolescents who overestimated their weight status as among those who perceived their weight status accurately; the odds of self-reported attempted weight loss were 3.9 and 2.9 times as high among overweight and obese children and adolescents, respectively, who accurately perceived their weight status than among those who underestimated their weight status. Parental misperception of weight was not significantly associated with self-reported attempted weight loss among children and adolescents who were overweight or obese.

The authors recommended that to prevent childhood obesity both children and parents should be included in the education regarding the appropriate identification and interpretation of actual weight status. Interventions for appropriate weight loss can target children directly because of the child's perception of his or her weight status.

# Learning Portfolio

## Chapter Summary

- A community nutritionist is a member of a multidisciplinary team and can conduct research studies that can benefit the public.
- Epidemiological and demographic measures and research methods are used to study nutrition and health-related conditions.
- Measures of incidence and prevalence provide different information and have different implications. For instance, an increase in the prevalence of diabetes or breast cancer means that there are more persons with these health conditions in the population.
- Successful collaboration requires that the multidisciplinary team develop a common purpose, communicate to coordinate efforts, and recognize the unique and complementary skills possessed by each team member.
- The three components of the epidemiological triangle model are agent, host, and environment, and they are used to explore health and disease.

- In experimental studies, the investigator has control over participants, procedures, and exposures.
- Epidemiology is the study of associations, and statistical methods are used to test the associations. The existence of a statistically significant association does not indicate that the observed relationship is one of cause and effect. Causality is supported when a number of studies that are conducted at different times, using different methods, and performed among different populations show similar results.
- In quantitative research, random sample surveys and structured interviews are used to collect quantifiable data; qualitative research analyzes social behavior such as food choice and dieting.

## Critical Thinking Activities

- Identify a research study in the literature relevant to community and public health nutrition. Then identify the strengths and limitations of the research.
- Communicate/present the research findings in class.
- Meet with the librarian as a class/group and learn how to use the Medline database; ERIC database; CINAHL database; Ingenta: The Global Research Gateway (http://www.ingenta.com), a portal to online information around the world; and other search engines for finding grant sources.

## 🔍 CASE STUDY 3-1: Collaboration Efforts Between Nutrition Students and Business

Damian and Monica, two senior baccalaureate nutrition students in a community nutrition course, had their community outreach experience at a rural community clinic. They were involved with the owner of a local candy factory in planning for disease prevention and health promotion activities for the employees. After consulting with the faculty member responsible for the course and the director of the community clinic, they designed a survey to distribute to employees to assess their needs for health education programming. The students submitted the survey, which included blood pressure screening, to the nutrition professor for approval before distributing it to the employees. The students also reviewed the medical records of the participants, with their consent.

Some of the employee priorities identified from the survey data that need to be addressed were the following problems:

- High blood pressure (160/90 on average)
- Smoking cessation (2 packs a day on average)
- Weight loss (average body fat percentage of 49 percent)
- High stress level

The students met with the factory owner, the faculty member, and a representative of the local chapter of the American Lung Association to plan for implementation of this initiative. A timeline was established to notify employees of an opportunity to participate in the weight loss, stress reduction, and smoking cessation program. This included notices distributed in employee paychecks and signs posted in prominent locations throughout the factory. The students discussed plans for conducting a research study related to implementation and evaluation of the weight loss, stress reduction, and smoking cessation program with the faculty member. The students collected a 3-day dietary record and observed that the participants consumed high-fat, high-sodium snacks and plenty of candy, mostly from the vending machine located in their break rooms. After reviewing their medical records with permission, data showed a fasting blood glucose level of 150/100 mg/dl.

### Questions

1. What is community nutrition research?
2. What is the definition of epidemiology? Describe the methods of epidemiological studies. What kind of epidemiological study could Damian and Monica use for their proposed research study?
3. Describe each of the stages of the research process that Damian and Monica must understand.
4. What are the differences between collaboration and coordination? Who could Damian and Monica collaborate with (other than their current collaborators) on their new research study?
5. What is the epidemiological triangle? Describe a situation in which Damian and Monica could utilize the epidemiological triangle.
6. What is the difference between the quantitative and qualitative methods that Damian and Monica must know before they can carry out the project?
7. What are some of the negative implications of cigarette smoking?

*(continues)*

*(continued)*

# 🔍 CASE STUDY 3-1: Collaboration Efforts Between Nutrition Students and Business

8. What types of dietary assessments could be used in a cross-sectional research study? What type of dietary assessment would be useful for Damian and Monica's research study?
9. Describe the difference between incidence and prevalence that Damian and Monica must know before carrying out the project.
10. Work in small groups or individually to discuss the case study and practice using the Nutrition Care Process chart provided on the companion website. You can also add other nutrition and health-related conditions or assessments to the case study to make it more challenging and interesting.

## Think About It

**Answer:** Qualitative research method

## Key Terms

**case-control study:** Exposure and other characteristics of cases of the disease under investigation are compared with a control group of persons unaffected by the disease. The results are analyzed to acquire effect estimates.

**cohort study:** Groups of individuals, defined in terms of their exposures, are followed over time to see if there are differences in the development of new cases of the disease of interest (or other health outcome) between the groups with and without exposure.

**collaboration:** Working with others toward a common goal.

**community nutrition research:** Organized study of a trend at both the basic and more applied levels that focuses on social, structural, and physical environmental inequities through active involvement of community members.

**coordination:** Efficient management of services without gaps or overlaps.

**cross-sectional study:** Measures the prevalence of disease and measures exposure and effect at the same time.

**deliberate sampling:** Inviting specific people to participate in a study.

**demography:** An analytic tool used to measure a population by recording births, deaths, age distribution, and other vital statistics.

**ecological study:** Involves the investigation of a group of people, such as those living within a geographic area such as a region or state.

**epidemiology:** The study of the determinants, occurrence, and distribution of health and disease in a defined population. It studies scientifically the factors that affect the health of individuals in the community.

**exposure:** Characteristics or agents (e.g., food, medications, sunlight) that the participant comes in contact with that may be related to disease risk.

**nutritional epidemiology:** Study of dietary intake and the occurrence of disease in human populations.

**random sampling:** When every case or participant has an equal opportunity to be included in a study.

**ground truthing:** A verification process that uses data gathered by direct observation to corroborate data gathered from secondary sources.

## References

1. Israel BA, Schulz AJ, Parker EA, Becker AB. Review of community-based research: assessing partnership approaches to improve public health. *Annu Rev Public Health.* 1998;19:173-202.
2. Frank-Spohrer G. *Community Nutrition: Applying Epidemiology to Contemporary Practice.* Rockville, MD: Aspen; 2007.
3. Brachman PS. *Epidemiology General Concepts.* 4 ed. Galveston, TX: The University of Texas Medical Branch; 1996.
4. Morgan R, Jain M, Miller A. A comparison of dietary methods in epidemiologic studies. *Am J Epidemiol.* 2006;107(6):488-498.
5. Stanhope M, Lancaster J. *Community and Public Health Nursing: Population-Centered Health Care in the Community.* 9th ed. New York, NY: Elsevier; 2015.
6. Anderson E, McFarlane, J. *Community as Partner: Theory and Practice in Nursing.* 3rd ed. Philadelphia PA: Lippincott; 2010.
7. Hitchcock J, Schubert, PE, Thomas, SA. *Community Health Nursing.* 2nd ed. United States: Thomson Delmar Learning; 2003.
8. Center for Disease Control and Prevention. REACH U.S. finding solutions to health disparities: at a glance 2010. www.cdc.gov. Accessed March 12, 2016.
9. Berdanier CD. *Handbook of Nutrition and Food.* New York NY: CRC Press; 2013.
10. Abramson JH, Abramson ZH. *Survey Methods in Community Medicine.* 5th ed: Edinburgh & London: Livingstone; 2000.

11. Stamler J, Elliott P, Dennis B. INTERMAP: background aims, design methods and descriptive statistics (nondietary). *J Hum Hypertens*. 2003;17:591–608.

12. Zimlichman E, Kochba I, Mimouni FB, Shochat T, et al. Smoking habits and obesity in young adults. *Addiction*. 2005;100(7):1021-1025.

13. Tande DDL. The associations between blood lipids and the Food Guide Pyramid: findings from the Third National Health and Nutrition Examination Survey. *Prev Med*. 2004;38(4):452-457.

14. Ness AR, Powles JW. Fruit and vegetables and cardiovascular disease: a review. *Int J Epidemiol*. 1997;26:1-13.

15. Fiore H, Travis S, Whalen A, Auinger P, et al. Potentially protective factors associated with healthful body mass index in adolescents with obese and nonobese parents: a secondary data analysis of the Third National Health and Nutrition Examination Survey 1988–1994. *J Am Diet Assoc*. 2006;106(1):55-64.

16. Coulston A, Rock C, Monsen E. *Nutrition in the Prevention and Treatment of Disease*. New York NY: Academic Press; 2001.

17. Eugene W, Kaplan H, James S. The epidemiologic evidence for a relationship between social support and health. *Am J Epidemiol*. 2005;17(5):521-537.

18. Lubin F, Ruder M, Wax Y, Modan B. Overweight and changes in weight throughout adult life in breast cancer etiology. *Am J Epidemiol*. 2004;122(4):579-588.

19. Berdanier CD, Feldman EB, Flatt WP, St. Jeor ST. *Handbook of Nutrition and Food*. New York, NY: CRC Press LLC; 2007.

20. Ramesh M, Schraer C, Mayer AM, Asay E, et al. Effect of special diabetes program for Indians' funding on system changes in diabetes care and outcomes among American Indian/Alaska Native people 1994-2004. *Int J Circumpolar Health*. 2008;67:203–212.

21. Indian Health Service. Special Diabetes Program for Indians. http://www.ihs.gov/. Accessed March 12, 2016.

22. Cade JE. The UK Women's Cohort Study: comparison of vegetarians, fish-eaters and meat-eaters. *Public Health Nutr*. 2004;7(7):871-878.

23. Franco O. Blood pressure in adulthood and life expectancy with cardiovascular disease in men and women: life course analysis. *Hypertension*. 2005;46(2):280-286.

24. Kant A, Block G, Schatzkin A, Ziegler RG, et al. Dietary diversity in the U.S. population NHANES II 1976-1980. *J Am Diet Assoc*. 1991;91:34-38.

25. Grant W. A multicountry ecologic study of risk and risk reduction factors for prostate cancer mortality. *Eur Urol*. 2004;45(3):271-279.

26. Dreon DM, Fernstrom HA, Campos H, et. al. Change in dietary saturated fat intake is correlated with change in mass of large low-density-lipoprotein particles in men. *Am J Clin Nutr*. 1998;67:828-836.

27. Sukhinder KC, Luis BA. Metabolism of cholesterol is altered in the liver of C3H mice fed fats enriched with different C-18 fatty acids. *J Nutr*. 1999;129:1718-1724.

28. Greenspan SL, Resnick NM, Parker RA. Combination therapy with hormone replacement and alendronate for prevention of bone loss in elderly women a randomized controlled trial. *JAMA*. 2003;289:2525-2533.

29. Perusse LB, Bouchard CE. The genetics of obesity. In: Bouchard CE, ed. *Family Studies*. Boca Raton, FL: CRC Press; 1994:125.

30. Stettler N, Tershakovec T, Zemel B, Leonard M, et al. Early risk factors for increased adiposity: a cohort study of African American subjects followed from birth to young adulthood. *Am J Clin Nutr*. 2000;72:378–383.

31. Chen AY, José JE. Family structure and childhood obesity, early childhood longitudinal study—kindergarten cohort. *Prev Chronic Dis* 2010;7(3):A50-A60.

32. Huang Z, Willett WC, Colditz GA, Hunter DJ, et al. Waist circumference, waist:hip ratio, and risk of breast cancer in the Nurses' Health Study. *Am J Epidemiol*. 1999;150(12):1316-1324.

33. Millen BE, Quatromoni PA, Nam BH, O'Horo CE, et al. Dietary patterns, smoking, and subclinical heart disease in women: opportunities for primary prevention from the Framingham Nutrition Studies. *J Am Diet Assoc*. 2004;104(2):208-214.

34. Winitz M, Seedman DA, Graff J. Studies in metabolic nutrition employing chemically defined diets. I. Extended feeding of normal human adult males. *Am J Clin Nutr*. 1970;23(5):525-545.

35. Cummings DE, Schwartz MW. Genetics and pathophysiology of human obesity. *Annu Rev Med*. 2003;54:453-471.

36. Behrens MM. The human taste receptor hTAS2R14 responds to a variety of different bitter compounds. *Biochem Biophys Res Commun*. 2004;319(2):479-485.

37. Smith J, Lensing S, Horton JA, Lovejoy J, et al. Prevalence of self-reported nutrition-related health problems in the Lower Mississippi Delta. *Am J Public Health*. 1999;89:1418-1421.

38. Schneider MJ. *Introduction to Public Health*. Boston MA: Jone and Bartlett; 2006.

39. Monsen ER. *Research: Successful Approaches.* 2nd ed. Chicago, IL: American Dietetic Association; 2003.

40. Sheats NN, Sheats NN. Prevalence, treatment, and control of hypertension among African Americans and Caucasians at primary care sites for medically under-served patients. *Ethn Dis.* 2005;15(1):25-32.

41. Prutkin J, Fisher EM, Etter L, et al. Genetic variation and inferences about perceived taste intensity in mice and men *Physiol Behav.* 2000;69:161-173.

42. Arnold A, Arnold AM. Incidence of cardiovascular disease in older Americans: the cardiovascular health study. *J Am Geriatr Soc.* 2005;53(2):211-218.

43. National Center for Health Statistics. National vital statistics reports. http://www.cdc.gov/nchs/. Accessed March 12, 2016.

44. Freeman J, Hutchison, G. Prevalence, incidence and duration. *Am J Epidemiol.* 2005;112(5):707–723.

45. Flanders WD, O'Brien TR. Inappropriate comparisons of incidence and prevalence in epidemiologic research. *Am J Public Health.* 1989;79(9):1301-1303.

46. Robinson K. Family care giving: who provides the care, and at what cost? *Nurs Econ.* 1997;15(2):243.

47. Paulette GB. Populations at risk across the lifespan reducing infant mortality rates using the perinatal periods of risk model. *Public Health Nurs.* 22(1):2-7.

48. Kramer MS, Platt RW, Yang H, Haglund B, et al. Registration artifacts in international comparisons of infant mortality. *Paediatr Perinat Epidemiol.* 2002;16(1):16-22.

49. Silva AA, Barbieri MA, Gomes UA. Trends in low birth weight: a comparison of two birth cohorts separated by a 15-year interval in Ribeirao Preto, Brazil. *Bull World Health Organ.* 1998;76(1):73-84.

50. Wakeford R, McElvenny, D. From epidemiological association to causation. *Occup Med.* 2007;57(7):464-465.

51. McDonald JC, McDonald AD, Hughes JM, Rando RJ, et al. Mortality from lung and kidney disease in a cohort of North American industrial sand workers: an update. *Ann Occup Hyg.* 2005;49(5):367-373.

52. Alexander GL. Dietary sodium intake and its relation to human health: a summary of the evidence. *J Am Coll Nutr.* 2006;25(3):165-169.

53. Barry MP. Urbanization lifestyle changes and the nutrition transition. *World Dev.* 1999;27:1905-1916.

54. Pryer J, Cappuccio FP, Elliott P. Dietary calcium and blood pressure: a review of the observational studies. *J Hum Hypertens.* 1995;9(8):597-604.

55. Troyer JL, Racine EF, Ngugi GW, McAuley WJ. The effect of home-delivered Dietary Approach to Stop Hypertension (DASH) meals on the diets of older adults with cardiovascular disease. *Am J Clin Nutr.* 2010;91(5):1204-1212.

56. INTERSALT Cooperative Research Group. Sodium, potassium, body mass, alcohol, and blood pressure: the INTERSALT study. *J Hypertens.* 1988;6(4):S584-S586.

57. Crawford MD, Gardner MJ, Morris JN. Mortality and hardness of local water supplies. *Lancet.* 1968:827-831.

58. Sacks FFM. Effects on blood pressure of reduced dietary sodium and the Dietary Approaches to Stop Hypertension (DASH) diet. DASH-Sodium Collaborative Research Group. *N Engl ed.* 2001;344(1):3-10.

59. Sacks FM, Appel LJ, Moore TJ, Obarzanek E. A dietary approach to prevent hypertension: a review of the Dietary Approaches to Stop Hypertension (DASH) Study. *Clin Cardiol.* 1999;22 (7 Suppl):1116-1110.

60. Trichopoulou A, Orfanos P, Norat T, Bueno-de-Mesquita B, et al. Modified Mediterranean diet and survival: EPIC elderly prospective cohort study. *BMJ.* 2005;330:7498.

61. Alpert JE, Fava, M. Nutrition and depression: the role of folate. *Nutr Rev.* 1997;55:145.

62. Sacks FM, Willett WC, Smith A, Brown LE, et al. Effect on blood pressure of potassium, calcium, and magnesium in women with low habitual intake. *Hypertension.* 1998;31:131.

63. Beevers DG. The epidemiology of salt and hypertension. *Clin Auton Res.* 2002;12(5):353-357.

64. Law MR, Frost CD, Wald NJ. Analysis of data from trials of salt reduction. *Br Med J.* 1991;302:819-824.

65. Haddy FJ, Vanhoutte PM, Feletou M. Role of potassium in regulating blood flow and blood pressure. *Am J Physiol Regul Integr Comp Physiol.* 2006;290:R548-R552.

66. Lawrence J. Lifestyle modification as a means to prevent and treat high blood pressure. *J Am Soc Nephrol.* 2003;14:S99-S102.

67. Persky VP. The effect of dietary sucrose of blood pressure in spontaneously hypertensive rats. *Nutr Res.* 1986;6(9):1111-1115.

68. McAleese JD, Rankin LL. Garden-based nutrition education affects fruit and vegetable consumption in sixth-grade adolescents. *J Am Diet Assoc.* 2007;107(4):662–665.

69. Karanja N. Descriptive characteristics of the dietary patterns used in the Dietary Approaches to Stop Hypertension Trial. DASH Collaborative Research Group. *J Am Diet Assoc.* 1999;99(8):S19-27.

70. Robinson JR, Young TK, Roos LL, Gelskey DE. Estimating the burden of disease. *Med Care.* 1997;35:932-947.

71. Geng Z, Vasanti SM, Shuba K. Substituting brown rice for white rice to lower diabetes risk:

a focus-group study in Chinese adults. *J Am Diet Assoc.* 2010;110(8):1216-1221.

72. Munhall PL, Boyd, CO. *Nursing Research: A Qualitative Perspective.* New York, NY: National League for Nursing; 1993.

73. Sullivan MB, Camer L. Benefits, barriers and enablers of university-community research: input from health and social service agencies. *Soc Mark Q.* 2000;4:9-25.

74. National Institute of Medicine. *The Future of Public Health.* Washington, DC: National Academy Press; 1998.

75. Vega WA. Theoretical and pragmatic implications of cultural diversity for community research. *Am J Community Psychol.* 1992;20:375-391.

76. McGuirt JT, Jilcott SB, Keyserlingm TC. Conducting community audits to evaluate community resources for healthful lifestyle behaviors: an illustration from rural eastern north carolina. *Prev Chronic Dis.* 2011;8(6):A149-A160.

77. Valdés Hernández MC, Morris Z, Dickie DA, Royle NA, et al. Close correlation between quantitative and qualitative assessments of white matter lesions. *Neuroepidemiology.* 2013;40:13-22.

78. Research HUPS. Questionnaire design tip sheet. http://psr.iq.harvard.edu/files/psr/files/PSRQuestionnaireTipSheet_0.pdf?m=1357530492. Accessed March 10, 2016.

79. Agriculture and Consumer Protection. The steps preceding questionnaire design. http://www.fao.org/docrep/w3241e/w3241e05.htm. Accessed March 10, 2016.

80. Malone TW, Crowston K. *Toward an Interdisciplinary Study of Coordination.* Cambridge, MA: Center for Coordination Science, MIT; 1991.

81. Amuwo S, Jenkins E. True partnership evolves over time. In: Sullivan M, James K, eds. *Collaborative Research: University and Community Partnership.* Washington, DC: American Public Health Association; 2001:25-43.

82. Clark MJ. *Nursing in the Community.* 3rd ed. Stamford, CT: Appleton & Lange; 1999.

83. Hinke M, Maurits W, Seidell C, Thijs A, et al. Effectiveness and cost-effectiveness of early screening and treatment of malnourished patients. *Am J Clin Nutr.* 2005;82:1082-1089.

84. Mellora JM. Exploring the relationships between income inequality, socioeconomic status and health: a self-guided tour? *Int J Epidemiol.* 2002;31:685-687.

85. Frank-Spohrer G. *Community Nutrition: Applying Epidemiology to Contemporary Practice.* 2nd ed. Sudbury, MA: Jones and Bartlet; 2008.

86. Hill AB. The environment and disease: association or causation? *Proc Roy Soc Med.* 1965;65(58):295–300.

87. Trichopoulou A, Vasilopoulou E. Mediterranean diet and longevity. *Br J Nutr.* 2000;84(2):S205-209.

88. De Groot LC, Staveren WA, Burema J. Survival beyond age 70 in relation to diet. *Nutr Rev.* 1996;54:211-212.

89. Keys A. *Seven Countries. A Multivariate Analysis of Death and Coronary Heart Disease.* Cambridge, MA: Harvard University Press; 1980.

90. De Lorgeril M, Renaud S, Mamelle N, Salen P, et al. Mediterranean alpha-linolenic acid-rich diet in secondary prevention of coronary heart disease. *Lancet.* 1994;343:1454-1459.

91. Singh RB, Dubnov G, Niaz MA. Effect of an Indo-Mediterranean diet on progression of coronary artery disease in high risk patients (Indo-Mediterranean diet heart study): a randomized single-blind trial. *Lancet.* 2002;360:1455-1461.

92. Osler M, Schroll M. Diet and mortality in a cohort of elderly people in a north European community. *Int J Epidemiol.* 1997;26:155-159.

93. Lasheras C, Fernandez S, Patterson AM. Mediterranean diet and age with respect to overall survival in institutionalised, nonsmoking elderly people. *Am J Clin Nutr.* 2000;71(4):987-992.

94. Knoops KT, de Groot LC, Kromhout D. Mediterranean diet, lifestyle factors, and 10-year mortality in elderly European men and women: the HALE project. *JAMA.* 2004;292:1433-1439.

95. Slimani N, Kaaks R, Ferrari P. European prospective investigation into cancer and nutrition (EPIC) calibration study: rationale, design and population characteristics. *Public Health Nutr.* 2002;5:1125-1145.

96. Deharveng G, Charrondiere UR. Comparison of nutrients in the food composition tables available in the nine European countries participating in EPIC. European prospective investigation into cancer and nutrition. *Eur J Clin Nutr.* 1999;53:60-79.

97. Kaaks R, Riboli E. Validation and calibration of dietary intake measurements in the EPIC project: methodological considerations. European prospective investigation into cancer and nutrition. *Int J Epidemiol.* 1997;26(Suppl 1):S15-25.

98. Chen HL, Pagoto SL, Barton BA, Lapane KL, et al. Personal and parental weight misperception and self-reported attempted weight loss in US children and adolescents, National Health and Nutrition Examination Survey, 2007–2008 and 2009–2010. *Prev Chronic Dis.* 2014;11:140123-1401143.

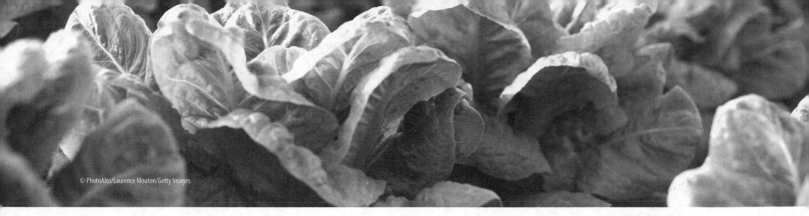

© PhotoAlto/Laurence Mouton/Getty Images

# CHAPTER 4

# U.S. Nutrition Monitoring and Food Assistance Programs

## CHAPTER OUTLINE

- Introduction
- The History of Food Assistance Programs in the United States
- Monitoring Nutrition in the United States
- Food Insecurity
- The Current Status of Food Insecurity in the United States
- Welfare Reform
- The Importance of Food Assistance Programs
- Food Distribution Programs
- Child Nutrition and Related Programs
- Programs for Women and Young Children
- Programs for Older Adults

## LEARNING OBJECTIVES

- Describe the purpose of U.S. food assistance programs.
- Identify entitlement and nonentitlement programs.
- Define nutrition monitoring in the United States.
- Outline and describe the adult and child nutrition programs in the United States.
- Discuss the status of food insecurity in the United States.
- Discuss the impact of welfare reform.
- Identify the federal domestic nutrition assistance programs.

## ▶ Introduction

Providing guidelines or food selection information to someone does not guarantee optimal nutrition if that person does not have access to adequate food or the money to buy it. A variety of food and nutrition programs have become available to assist low-income families in obtaining a safe and wholesome food supply in adequate amounts. Among some of the U.S. landmark programs are the **National School Lunch Program**, the **WIC** program (Special Supplemental Nutrition Program for Women, Infants, and Children), the **Supplemental Nutrition Assistance Program (SNAP)** (formerly the Food Stamp Program), food distribution programs, and senior adult meals.

The nutrition assistance programs are a uniquely American invention, with nearly all the resources provided by the federal government but with most of the operational responsibility located as close as possible to the communities they serve. The success of U.S. nutrition assistance programs means that extreme forms of hunger and malnutrition, common in developing countries, have been practically eliminated. However, less severe forms of food insecurity and hunger are still found within the United States and remain a reason for concern.[1] This chapter discusses nutrition monitoring in the United States, food insecurity, and food assistance programs.

## ▶ The History of Food Assistance Programs in the United States

W.O. Atwater discovered the link among food composition, dietary intake, and health in 1890. The predominant nutritional problems then were low caloric intake and inadequate intakes of certain vitamins and minerals.[2,3] Because of food restrictions and shortages during World War I, scientific discoveries in nutrition were translated quickly into public health policy. In 1917, the U.S. Department of Agriculture (USDA) issued the first dietary recommendations based on five food groups.[4]

In 1921, the Maternal and Infancy Act, formerly known as the Sheppard-Towner Act, was adopted by Congress and remained in effect until 1929. The passage of the act resulted in federal grant-in-aid to states for child and adult health programs. Another major result of the act was the development of full-time units of maternal and child health services in state health departments. The act also enabled state health departments to employ nutritionists. During the 1930s, the federal government developed food relief and food commodity distribution programs, including school feeding, nutrition education programs, and national food consumption surveys.[5]

The growth of publicly funded nutrition programs accelerated during the early 1940s because of reports that 25 percent of military draftees showed evidence of past or present malnutrition. A frequent cause of rejection from military service was tooth decay or loss caused by conditions that might have been prevented or corrected by adequate nutrition in early childhood.[5,6]

## U.S. Department of Agriculture Food Plans

In the 1930s, the USDA began developing family food plans at four separate cost levels: Economical, Low-Cost, Moderate-Cost, and Liberal. In 1974, the USDA replaced the Economical Plan with the Thrifty Plan. These plans are still the official food plans maintained by the USDA Center for Nutrition Policy and Promotion (CNPP).[7]

Each plan represents a set of market baskets applicable to one of 12 age/gender groups. Each market basket contains a selection of foods in quantities that reflect dietary recommendations, food consumption patterns, food composition data, and food prices. The four plans have various policy uses, including the following[7,8]:

- Bankruptcy courts often use the value of the Low-Cost Plan to determine the portion of a bankruptee's income to allocate for necessary food expenses.
- The Department of Defense uses the values of the Moderate-Cost and Liberal Food Plans to set the Basic Allowance for Subsistence rate for all enlistees.
- Many divorce courts use the value of the food plans to set alimony payments, and all four plans are used in the USDA's Expenditures on Children by Families Report, which is used to set state child support guidelines and foster care payments.
- Policy makers and others use the food plans as national standards in educational programs and as references for policies that are designed to help families budget their food dollars effectively and improve their diets.

In 1955, the USDA National Food Consumption Study found that the average U.S. family spent about one third of its net income on food.[9] Therefore, the poverty line was established at three times the cost of the USDA's Low-Cost Food Plan for a family of four. After the USDA established the Thrifty Plan in 1974—using more frugal food choices than the Low-Cost Food Plan—they switched to that plan. The Thrifty Plan is now multiplied by three and adjusted for the size of the family and the current consumer price index to determine the official poverty income guidelines each year. The Thrifty Plan is also used to calculate SNAP allowances. These guidelines are used by federal agencies as criteria for eligibility for different federal assistance programs and as a basis for compiling data on poverty. **TABLE 4-1** lists an example of estimated different costs of the four USDA food plans for the month of January 2016.[10,11]

**TABLE 4-1** Official USDA Food Plans: Cost of Food at Home at Four Levels, U.S. Average, February 2016*

| Age/Gender Groups | Weekly Cost[†] | | | | Monthly Cost[†] | | |
|---|---|---|---|---|---|---|---|
| | Thrifty Plan (USD) | Low-Cost Plan (USD) | Moderate-Cost Plan (USD) | Liberal Plan (USD) | Thrifty Plan (USD) | Low-Cost Plan (USD) | Moderate-Cost Plan (USD) |
| **Individuals[‡]** | | | | | | | |
| **Child** | | | | | | | |
| 1 year | 22.00 | 29.80 | 33.70 | 41.10 | 95.30 | 129.10 | 146.10 |
| 2–3 years | 23.90 | 30.60 | 36.90 | 45.00 | 103.70 | 132.40 | 159.90 |
| 4–5 years | 25.20 | 31.70 | 39.40 | 48.10 | 109.10 | 137.50 | 170.90 |
| 6–8 years | 32.40 | 44.90 | 53.70 | 63.60 | 140.20 | 194.60 | 232.80 |
| 9–11 years | 36.70 | 48.10 | 62.50 | 73.00 | 159.20 | 208.40 | 270.90 |
| **Male** | | | | | | | |
| 12–13 years | 39.20 | 55.40 | 69.50 | 81.60 | 169.70 | 239.90 | 301.20 |
| 14–18 years | 40.40 | 56.60 | 71.90 | 82.70 | 175.20 | 245.30 | 311.50 |
| 19–50 years | 43.60 | 56.30 | 70.50 | 86.80 | 189.00 | 244.10 | 305.70 |
| 51–70 years | 39.80 | 53.00 | 65.70 | 79.60 | 172.30 | 229.80 | 284.80 |
| 71+ years | 39.90 | 52.30 | 65.20 | 81.00 | 173.10 | 226.80 | 282.60 |
| **Female** | | | | | | | |
| 12–13 years | 39.20 | 47.80 | 57.80 | 70.60 | 169.80 | 207.30 | 250.30 |
| 14–18 years | 38.60 | 48.20 | 58.30 | 71.90 | 167.10 | 208.80 | 252.50 |
| 19–50 years | 38.50 | 48.90 | 60.30 | 76.90 | 166.80 | 211.70 | 261.50 |
| 51–70 years | 38.20 | 47.40 | 59.10 | 71.00 | 165.50 | 205.40 | 255.90 |
| 71+ years | 37.50 | 46.90 | 58.50 | 70.60 | 162.30 | 203.20 | 253.60 |
| **Families** | | | | | | | |
| **Family (male and female) of 2[§]** | | | | | | | |
| 19–50 years | 90.30 | 115.70 | 144.00 | 180.10 | 391.30 | 501.40 | 623.80 |
| 51–70 years | 85.70 | 110.50 | 137.30 | 165.70 | 371.50 | 478.70 | 594.80 |

*(continues)*

**TABLE 4-1** Official USDA Food Plans: Cost of Food at Home at Four Levels, U.S. Average, February 2016* (*continued*)

| Age/Gender Groups | Weekly Cost[†] | | | | Monthly Cost[†] | | |
|---|---|---|---|---|---|---|---|
| | Thrifty Plan (USD) | Low-Cost Plan (USD) | Moderate-Cost Plan (USD) | Liberal Plan (USD) | Thrifty Plan (USD) | Low-Cost Plan (USD) | Moderate-Cost Plan (USD) |
| **Family of 4** | | | | | | | |
| **Couple (male and female) 19–50 years and children** | | | | | | | |
| 2–3 and 4–5 years | 131.20 | 167.50 | 207.20 | 256.90 | 568.50 | 725.70 | 897.90 |
| 6–8 and 9–11 years | 151.20 | 198.20 | 247.10 | 300.40 | 655.20 | 858.80 | 1070.80 |

* The Food Plans represent a nutritious diet at four different cost levels. The nutritional bases of the Food Plans are the 1997 to 2005 Dietary Reference Intakes, 2005 Dietary Guidelines for Americans, and 2005 MyPyramid food intake recommendations. In addition to cost, differences among plans are in specific foods and quantities of foods. Another basis of the Food Plans is that all meals and snacks are prepared at home. For specific foods and quantities of foods in the Food Plans, see Thrifty Food Plan, 2006 (2007) and The Low-Cost, Moderate-Cost, and Liberal Food Plans, 2007 (2007). All four Food Plans are based on 2001 to 2002 data and updated to current dollars by using the Consumer Price Index for specific food items.

[†] All costs are rounded to nearest 10 cents.

[‡] The costs given are for individuals in 4-person families. For individuals in other size families, the following adjustments are suggested: 1-person—add 20 percent; 2-person—add 10 percent; 3-person—add 5 percent; 4-person—no adjustment; 5- or 6-person—subtract 5 percent; 7- (or more) person—subtract 10 percent. To calculate overall household food costs, (1) adjust food costs for each person in household and then (2) sum these adjusted food costs.

[§] Ten percent added for family size adjustment.

Source: Center for Nutrition Policy and Promotion. 2011. Available at: http://www.cnpp.usda.gov. Accessed March 31, 2016.

# Monitoring Nutrition in the United States

**Nutrition monitoring** provides an ongoing description of nutrition conditions in the population, paying particular attention to subgroups defined in socioeconomic terms. It is used to plan, analyze the effects of policies and programs on nutrition problems, and predict future trends.[11]

Nutrition programs rely on data from nutrition monitoring surveys to identify the needs of those they serve. Data from national surveys are used to monitor the dietary status of the population, assess the nutritional adequacy of the food supply, measure the economics of food consumption, make public policies related to nutrition education programs, evaluate the effects of food assistance and regulatory programs, and provide the public with guidelines for food selection.[12-14] The data also are used to direct program development and determine national, state, and local funding.

The United States is recognized as having one of the most comprehensive nutrition monitoring programs in the world. The United States and some other developed countries, such as the United Kingdom, France, Japan, Norway, and Canada, have integrated a data collection and reporting system into a national nutrition monitoring program to provide comprehensive nutrition and diet and health information. Programs in the United States such as the SNAP, National School Lunch Program, and WIC support myriad nutrition and health policy needs, regulatory reviews, and research studies.

The food and nutrient intakes reported from national food consumption surveys reflect either daily or usual consumption patterns; information is obtained on the types of foods consumed, commercially prepared or home-prepared foods, quantities of food consumed per meal or per day, and food preparation methods and recipe ingredients. Nutrition monitoring programs provide broad management capability to ensure that surveillance surveys exist to detect and report changes so that appropriate actions can be taken.[15,16]

In 1990, the National Nutrition Monitoring System (NNMS) was renamed the National Nutrition Monitoring and Related Research Program (NNMRRP).[17-19] The aim of this nutrition monitoring program is to strengthen nutrition monitoring efforts in the United States and have a coordinated, comprehensive system that provides information about the dietary and nutritional status of the U.S. population, the conditions that affect the dietary and nutritional status of individuals, and the relationships between diet and health.[20,21]

## National Center for Health Statistics and Centers for Disease Control and Prevention Growth Charts

The National Center for Health Statistics (NCHS) and Centers for Disease Control and Prevention (CDC) growth charts are an example of how nutrition monitoring data have been used for the development of population reference standards.[22] In 2000, data from the third National Health and Nutrition Examination Survey (NHANES III) were used to develop the revised NCHS and CDC growth charts.[23] The revised charts represent racial and ethnic diversity in the United States and contain a mixture of growth data from infants who were breastfed and formula-fed that is more accurate than the 1977 NCHS reference growth charts.[24,25] They also include information for children from infancy up through 20 years of age, as well as a new chart for body mass index (BMI) by age.[23,26] Visit the CDC website at http://www.cdc.gov/growthcharts to view or download the charts.

The USDA conducted the Continuing Survey of Food Intakes by Individuals (CSFII) in 1977 to 1978, 1985 to 1986, 1989 to 1991, and 1994 to 1996 before it was combined with the NHANES in 2000 and referred to as What We Eat in America (WWEIA)-NHANES. The two surveys were integrated to improve the coordination of nutrition monitoring across agencies. WWEIA-NHANES is the dietary component of NHANES that includes data collection about food intake, dietary supplement intake, food program participation, and other diet-related data from 5,000 respondents. WWEIA is conducted as a partnership between the USDA and the U.S. Department of Health and Human Services (DHHS). The DHHS is responsible for the sample design and data collection, and the USDA is responsible for the survey's dietary data collection methodology and maintenance of the databases.

## Programmatic Uses

National nutrition monitoring programs provide information for developing and promoting nutrition education activities and programs such as the *Dietary Guidelines for Americans*[13] and Fruits and Veggies—More Matters program,[27] public health programs such as the National Cholesterol Education Program,[28] the National High Blood Pressure Education Program,[29] and federally supported food assistance programs such as SNAP and WIC.[30,31]

## Regulatory Uses

Nutrition monitoring data have been used by regulatory agencies to develop and examine U.S. food fortification,[32,33] food safety, and food labeling policies to enlighten and educate consumers.[34] The data have been used to provide dietary estimates for nutrient and nonnutrient food components. For instance, national nutrition monitoring data collected in NHANES III were used to evaluate folate status and the relationship among serum determinations, diet, and other nutrition and health variables before the U.S. Food and Drug Administration (FDA) ruled on the need for folate food fortification.[34-35,36]

## Scientific Uses

Nutrition monitoring data are used by scientists to revise the standards of human nutrient requirements and study the relationships among diet, nutrition, and health.[37,38] National data on the population's dietary intake and serum nutrient levels have been used to investigate nutrient requirements throughout the life cycle, to identify areas of nutrition research needed to increase the knowledge base, and for the development of the Dietary Reference Intakes by the National Academy of Sciences.[37,38,39] Current research, such as the Human Genome Project, is being used to develop nutrition status indicators, which will be important for future monitoring efforts.

Nutrition monitoring data are also used to evaluate progress toward the 2010 Healthy People Objectives, discussed in Chapter 1, and determine and prioritize the food and nutrition research needs of the community.[39-43] For example, national nutrition monitoring data have been used in the Surgeon General's *Report on Nutrition and Health* to provide important information about the link between diet and chronic health conditions[44] and the National Academy of Sciences report *Diet and Health: Implications for Reducing Chronic Disease Risk*.[39] The link for the directory of federal and state nutrition monitoring and related research activities is https://www.cdc.gov/nchs/data/misc/direc-99.pdf and for food and nutrition surveys is https://www.nal.usda.gov/fnic/food-and-nutrition-surveys.

## ▶ Food Insecurity

Nutrition monitoring data are also used to estimate food insecurity. In the United States, food security is defined as access to enough food for an active, healthy life and includes at a minimum the ready availability of nutritionally adequate and safe foods and the ensured ability to acquire acceptable foods in socially acceptable ways (i.e., without resorting to emergency food supplies or other coping strategies).[45]

**Food insecurity** exists whenever the availability of nutritionally adequate and safe foods or the ability to acquire acceptable foods in socially acceptable ways is limited or uncertain.[46,47] Four main conceptual elements define this phenomenon[48]:

- Food insecurity is experienced at the household and individual levels in different ways. Individual-level experience relates to issues of food consumption and allocation and includes the physiological sensation of hunger. Food supply management and acquisition issues define the household situation.[49]
- The experience of food insecurity is not static but dynamic, defined by a sequence of events and experiences that can be considered in terms of frequency, duration, and periodicity.
- The sequence of stages that define the experience reflects graded levels of severity, ranging from qualitative compromises in food selection and consumption to quantitative compromises in intake and the physical sensation of hunger, as resources become depleted. At its most severe stage, food insecurity is experienced as absolute food deprivation (i.e., individuals not eating at all).
- Within households, individuals' experiences of food insecurity differ. Mainly, adults seem to compromise their own intakes first, in an effort to minimize the extent and nature of compromise experienced by children in the household. This suggests that food insecurity is a managed process in which the sequence of events and severity of experience for different household members is, to some extent, controlled and predictable.[50-53]

## Assessing Food Insecurity

Since 1995, the U.S. Census Bureau has conducted an annual survey of food security among a nationally representative sample of people living in the United States using the food security module in the Current Population Survey (CPS). The questions asked were about the following[54,55]:

- Anxiety or the perception that the household budget is inadequate to buy enough food
- A perception of inadequacy in the quantity or quality of food eaten by adults and children in the household
- Instances of reduced food intake or consequences of reduced food intake for adults and children
- Periods of a decrease in food intake, hunger, and/or weight loss by household members

The CPS questionnaire contains 18 items. Households without children were asked to respond to 10 questions, and households with children were asked to respond to all 18 questions. Questions 1, 1a, and 1b are not used to calculate the food security or hunger scale and may be used, in conjunction with income, as a preliminary screener to reduce respondent burden for high-income households. Therefore, question 1 was not included in **TABLE 4-2**. The CPS can be administered in approximately 2 minutes.[54] The questions reflect the different classifications of households' food insecurity levels. For example, the least severe item is an adult-referenced item that asks whether the household members worried that food would run out before they got money to buy more. See **BOX 4-1** for a method of measuring the severity of household food insecurity and hunger.

A CPS food security form is available in Spanish that has been validated.

Households are classified into one of four categories of food security[54]:

- *Food Secure:* Households with no or minimal evidence of food insecurity.
- *Food Insecure Without Hunger:* Food insecurity is evident in the household's concerns and in adjustments to household food management, including reduced quality of diets. Little or no reduction in household members' food intake is reported.
- *Food Insecure with Moderate Hunger:* Food intake for adults in the household has been reduced to an extent that it implies the adults have repeatedly experienced the physical sensation of hunger. Such reductions are not observed at this stage for children in the household.
- *Food Insecure with Severe Hunger:* Households with children that have reduced the children's food intake to an extent that it implies the children have experienced the physical sensation of hunger. Adults in households with and without children have repeatedly experienced more extensive reductions in food intake at this stage.

The food security scale measures the respondents' levels of food security or insecurity in terms of a numeric value that ranges between 0 and 18. A respondent who has not experienced any of the food insecurity situations would have a scale value of zero. A respondent who has experienced all of the situations covered in the questions would have a scale value of 10 or 18, depending on which version of the survey they took. For categorizing or assigning respondents to levels of food insecurity, the maximum raw score for being classified as food insecure based on the standard value is level 3 in households with or without children. Respondents with a score of zero are classified as food secure. At the other extreme, respondents who reported experiencing all or nearly all of the conditions receive high scale values of level 3 and are classified as food insecure with severe hunger.

| **TABLE 4-2** | Questions Included in the Core Food Security Scale[51,52] |
|---|---|
| | **Stage 1 (Screen 1 asked of all households)** |
| | Now I'm going to read you several statements that people have made about their food situation. Please tell me whether the statement was *often, sometimes,* or *never true* in the last 12 months. |
| **Q2** | "I worried whether our food would run out before we got money to buy more." Was that often, sometimes, or never true for you in the last 12 months? |
| **Q3** | "The food that we bought just didn't last, and we didn't have money to get more." Was that often, sometimes, or never true for you in the last 12 months? |
| **Q4** | "We couldn't afford to eat balanced meals." Was that often, sometimes, or never true for you in the last 12 months? |
| **Q5** | "We relied on only a few kinds of low-cost food to feed the children because we were running out of money to buy food." Was that often, sometimes, or never true for you in the last 12 months? |
| **Q6** | "We couldn't feed the children a balanced meal because we couldn't afford that." Was that often, sometimes, or never true for you in the last 12 months? |
| | **Stage 2 (asked of households after passing of the first screen)** |
| **Q7** | "The children were not eating enough because we just couldn't afford enough food." Was that often, sometimes, or never true for you in the last 12 months? |
| **Q8** | In the last 12 months, did you or other adults in your household ever cut the size of your meals or skip meals because there wasn't enough money for food? |
| **Q9** | In the last 12 months, did you ever eat less than you felt you should because there wasn't enough money to buy food? |
| **Q10** | In the last 12 months, were you ever hungry, but didn't eat because you couldn't afford enough food? |
| **Q11** | Sometimes people lose weight because they don't have enough to eat. In the last 12 months, did you lose weight because there wasn't enough food? |
| **Q12** | In the last 12 months, did you or other adults in your household ever not eat for a whole day because there wasn't enough money for food? How often did this happen—almost every month, some months but not every month, or in only 1 or 2 months? |
| **Q13** | In the last 12 months, did you ever cut the size of any of the children's meals because there wasn't enough money for food? |
| **Q14** | In the last 12 months, did any of the children ever skip meals because there wasn't enough money for food? How often did this happen—almost every month, some months but not every month, or in only 1 or 2 months? |
| **Q15** | In the last 12 months, were the children ever hungry, but you just couldn't afford more food? |
| **Q16** | In the last 12 months, did any of the children ever not eat for a whole day because there wasn't enough money for food? |

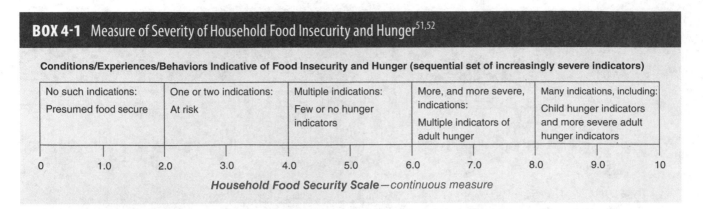

**BOX 4-1** Measure of Severity of Household Food Insecurity and Hunger[51,52]

**Conditions/Experiences/Behaviors Indicative of Food Insecurity and Hunger (sequential set of increasingly severe indicators)**

| No such indications: Presumed food secure | One or two indications: At risk | Multiple indications: Few or no hunger indicators | More, and more severe, indications: Multiple indicators of adult hunger | Many indications, including: Child hunger indicators and more severe adult hunger indicators |

0     1.0     2.0     3.0     4.0     5.0     6.0     7.0     8.0     9.0     10

*Household Food Security Scale—continuous measure*

**TABLE 4-3** USDA's New Labels Describing the Ranges of Food Security

| General Categories | Detailed Categories | | |
|---|---|---|---|
| | **Old Label** | **New Label** | **Description of Conditions in the Household** |
| Food security | Food security | High food security<br>Marginal food security | No reported indications of food-access problems or limitations<br>One or two reported indications—typically of anxiety over food sufficiency or shortage of food in the house<br>Little or no indication of changes in diets or food intake |
| Food insecurity | Food insecurity without hunger<br>Food insecurity with hunger | Low food security<br>Very low food security | Reports of reduced quality, variety, or desirability of diet<br>Little or no indication of reduced food intake<br>Reports of multiple indications of disrupted eating patterns and reduced food intake |

Reproduced from: USDA/ERS. Recommendation by the Committee on National Statistics (CNSTAT) of the National Academies. Available at: http://www.ers.usda.gov/Briefing/FoodSecurity/labels.htm. Accessed April 5, 2016.

See **TABLE 4-3** for measures of severity of household food insecurity and hunger.[56] The CPS questionnaire and instructions can be downloaded in PDF format from http://www.ers.usda.gov. The Spanish version has been validated and is also available.

## ▶ The Current Status of Food Insecurity in the United States

In 2014, 48.1 million people in the United States lived in households experiencing food insecurity, up significantly from 35 million in 2005, 38.2 million in 2004, and 36.3 million in 2003.[55,56] In 2010, 86.0 percent of U.S. households were food secure throughout the entire year, implying that they had access, at all times, to enough food for an active, healthy life for all household members.[7,57,58] The remaining 14.5 percent of households were food insecure at least some time during that year. (See **FIGURE 4-1**.) The prevalence of food insecurity increased from 10.7 percent in 2001 to

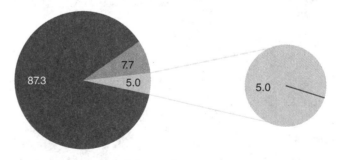

■ Food-secure households

▩ Households with low food security

▨ Households with very low food security

**FIGURE 4-1** U.S. households by food security status, 2015 pie chart.

Reproduced from Economic Research Services/USDA. Household Food Security in the United States, 2014. Available at www.ers.usda.gov/. Accessed March 31, 2016.

11.9 percent in 2004, but decreased slightly to 11 percent in 2005 before increasing to 14.5 percent in 2010. The prevalence of low food security increased from 3.7 percent in 2004 to 7.1 percent in 2005, and then increased again to 9.1 percent in 2010. Nearly 6 percent of households experienced very low food security (food security with hunger) in 2010. In 2014, 5.6 percent of U.S. households had very low food security. The rates of food insecurity for all households with children was 19.2 percent and households with children headed by a single woman was 35.3 percent or a single man 21.7 percent.[59] See Table 4-3 for a description of the ranges of food security.[54, 58, 60] **TABLE 4-4** shows a summary of the trends in U.S. food insecurity and hunger from 1995 to 2009. The rates of the prevalence of food insecurity and food insecurity with hunger were not statistically significant from 2002 to 2003 and stayed below the levels of the 1995 prevalence rate, when it was first measured.

| **TABLE 4-4** | Trends in Prevalence of Food Insecurity and Food Insecurity with Hunger in U.S. Households, 1995–2014 | | | |
|---|---|---|---|---|
| **Years** | **All Households Percentage** | **Food Secure Percentage** | **Low Food Security Percentage** | **Very Low Food Security Percentage** |
| 1995 | 10.3 | 89.6 | 6.4 | 3.9 |
| 1996 | 10.4 | 89.6 | 6.3 | 4.4 |
| 1997 | 8.7 | 91.3 | 5.6 | 3.1 |
| 1998 | 10.2 | 88.2 | 6.6 | 3.6 |
| 1999 | 10.1 | 89.9 | 7.1 | 3.1 |
| 2000 | 10.5 | 89.5 | 7.3 | 3.1 |
| 2001 | 10.7 | 89.3 | 7.4 | 3.3 |
| 2002 | 11.1 | 88.9 | 7.6 | 3.5 |
| 2003 | 11.2 | 88.8 | 7.7 | 3.5 |
| 2004 | 11.9 | 88.1 | 8.0 | 3.9 |
| 2005 | 11.0 | 89.0 | 7.1 | 3.9 |
| 2006 | 10.94 | 89.0 | NA | 3.99 |
| 2007 | 11.10 | 89.0 | NA | 4.10 |
| 2008 | 14.60 | 85.0 | NA | 5.7 |
| 2009 | 14.70 | 85.3 | NA | 5.7 |
| 2010 | 14.5 | 85.5 | 9.1 | 5.4 |
| 2011 | 14.9 | 85.1 | 8.8 | 5.7 |
| 2012 | 14.5 | 85.5 | 8.8 | 5.7 |
| 2013 | 14.3 | 85.7 | 8.7 | 5.6 |
| 2014 | 14.0 | 86.0 | 8.4 | 5.6 |

Modified from: Nord M, Andrews M, Carlson S. Household food security in the United States. Available at: http://www.ers.usda.gov/Briefing/FoodSecurity/. Accessed March 31, 2016.

**FIGURE 4-2** shows the prevalence of food insecurity and hunger among various socioeconomic, geographic, and demographic groups. The difference in the rates of food insecurity and hunger was not statistically significant. However, the figures show that poverty and hunger continued in households with children headed by single women, African Americans, Hispanics, and those with income below the poverty threshold.[58,61] The data also indicated that households were more likely to be hungry or food insecure if they lived in states in the Southern region of the country.[61,62] Overall, households with children reported food insecurity more than households without children. The following sections describe the groups that are experiencing the most food insecurity and hunger in the United States today.

## Low-Income People

Poverty is one of the contributing factors to food insecurity and hunger. For example, in 2014, food insecurity was significantly higher in households with annual incomes below 130 to 185 percent of the poverty line than in households with incomes above that range. However, many factors that might affect a household's food security (such as job loss, divorce, or other unexpected events)

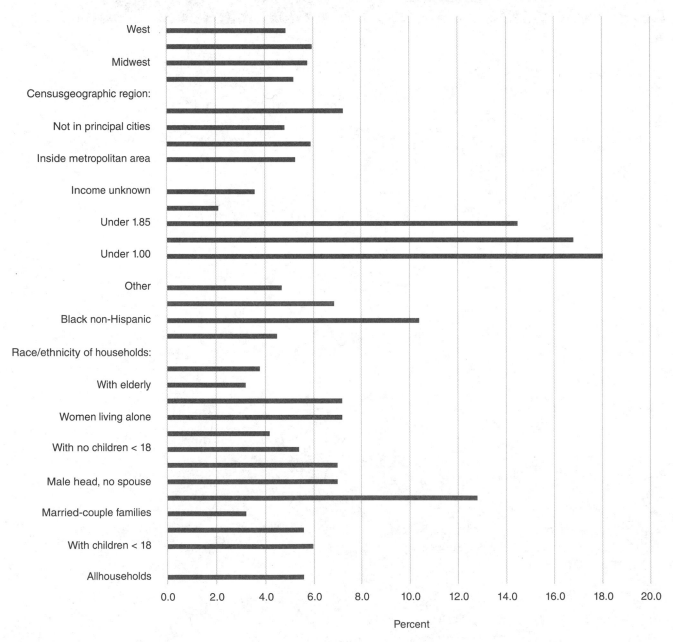

**FIGURE 4-2** Prevalence of food insecurity by selected households.

[1]Households with children in complex living arrangements, such as children of other relatives or unrelated roommate or boarder.
[2]Hispanics may be of any race.
[3]Metropolitan area residence is based on 2013 Office of Management and Budget delineation. Prevalence rates by area of residence are not precisely comparable with those of previous years.
[4]Households within incorporated areas of the largest cities in each metropolitan area. Residence inside or outside of principal cities is not identified for approximately 17 percent of households in metropolitan statistical areas.
Reproduced from USDA. Calculated by ERS using data from the December 2014 Current Population Survey Food Security Supplement.

are not recognized by any annual income measure.[63,64] Reports show that low-income households with children were more affected by food insecurity than low-income households without children (19.2 vs. 9.7 percent). Low-income single mothers with children were more vulnerable to both food insecurity and hunger; 35.3 percent of these households were food insecure.[65,66] Households with income below 130 percent of the poverty line can receive assistance from the SNAP, and children in these households are eligible for free meals in the National School Lunch and School Breakfast Programs.

## The Working Poor

In 2013, 45.3 million people (14.5 percent of the population) lived at or below the official poverty threshold; in 2004, 37 million (12.7 percent) were at or below the threshold. Although the nation's poor were mainly children and adults who were not in the labor force, 10.5 million individuals were classified as working poor. The **working poor** are those who spent at least 27 weeks of the year in the labor force (working or looking for work), but whose incomes are below the official poverty threshold. (See **TABLE 4-5**.) In 2014, 46.7 million people (14.8 percent of the population) include the following[65][67]:

■  Of those employed full time, 4.1 percent were classified as working poor, compared with 13.5 percent of part-time workers.

■  The likelihood of being classified as working poor greatly diminishes as workers achieve higher levels of education. Only 2.0 percent of college graduates were counted among the working poor, compared with 18.3 percent of people with less than a high school diploma. Women who maintain families are twice as likely as their male counterparts to be among the working poor.

Of all individuals in the labor force for at least half of the year, more women than men heads of households were poor (7.2 percent vs.5.5 percent). Although approximately 6.1 percent of the working poor were Caucasian Americans workers, African American and Hispanic workers were more than twice as likely as their Caucasian American counterparts to be among the working poor. The poverty rate for both African Americans and Hispanics was 11.7 percent.[66,68]

Reports show that younger workers were more vulnerable to being poor than older workers. The poverty rate for children 16 to 19 was 10.4 percent. In 2013, government-sponsored survey showed that the majority of families who go to food pantries for emergency help work or have children. The use of food pantries varied considerably by household structure and by race and ethnicity.[67] In 2014, approximately 54 percent of households used food pantries.[69]

In 2014, of those who used food pantries, 10.5 were African American, 8.2 percent were Hispanic, and 4.2 percent were Caucasian Americans. Caucasian Americans comprise a majority of food pantry users because of their larger share in the general population. Approximately 69.1 percent of households with incomes below the poverty line received food from food pantries, compared with 16.0 percent of households with incomes above 185 percent of the poverty line.[69] The use of food pantries in suburban and rural areas was 8.0 percent.[69]

## Ethnic Groups

Low-income and minority persons are more likely to experience food insecurity than those in the majority group. The prevalence of food insecurity with hunger for African American households in 2014 was 32.4 percent; for Hispanic households it was 26.9 percent. Food insecurity represents lack of enough food and lack of nutritious food. Both socioeconomic status and race have been shown to affect household diets.[62]

## The Elderly

In 2014, the poverty rate for the elderly increased to 10.0 percent. In 2005, 2.6 percent of the elderly population lived in severe poverty (below 50 percent of the poverty threshold), and 16.7 percent were classified as near poor (incomes between 100 percent and 125 percent of poverty).[68] A significant number of the elderly encounter poverty at some time during their lifetime. After age 65, the probability of a person experiencing a year below the poverty line at some point is 40 percent.[68]

Rates of food insecurity and hunger among elderly households depended on household composition, household income, race and ethnicity, and area of residence. The rates of food insecurity were higher among those living alone (9.3 percent). The rates of food insecurity among elderly households with incomes below the federal poverty line were higher compared to those of elderly households with incomes above 185 percent of the poverty line.[70]

## State-by-State Variations

The rates of food insecurity and food insecurity with hunger vary from state to state. Data compiled from 2013 to 2015 showed that the rate of food insecurity increased above national average by statistically significant percentages in 12 states. The prevalence of food insecurity during the 3 years ranged from 8.4 percent in North Dakota to 22.0 percent in Mississippi. During the same period, the prevalence of very low food security ranged from 2.9 percent in North Dakota to 8.1 percent in Arkansas[70,71]

**TABLE 4-5** Poverty Status of Persons and Primary Families in the Labor Force for 27 Weeks or More, 2001 to 2013 (Numbers in Thousands)

| Characteristics | 2001 | 2002* | 2003† | 2004 | 2005 | 2006 | 2007 | 2008 | 2009 | 2010 | 2011 | 2012 | 2013 |
|---|---|---|---|---|---|---|---|---|---|---|---|---|---|
| Total Persons‡ | 138,143 | 139,728 | 140,007 | 140,876 | 142,824 | 145,229 | 146,567 | 147,838 | 147,902 | 146,859 | 147,475 | 148,735 | 149,483 |
| In poverty | 6,802 | 7,359 | 7,429 | 7,837 | 7,744 | 7,427 | 7,521 | 8,883 | 10,391 | 10,512 | 10,382 | 10,612 | 10,450 |
| Poverty rate (percentage) | 4.9 | 5.3 | 5.3 | 5.6 | 5.4 | 5.1 | 5.1 | 6.0 | 7.0 | 7.2 | 7.0 | 7.1 | 7.0 |
| Unrelated individuals | 29,387 | 29,847 | 29,898 | 30,373 | 31,422 | 31,887 | 33,226 | 32,785 | 33,798 | 34,099 | 33,731 | 34,810 | 35,061 |
| In poverty | 2,388 | 2,584 | 2,472 | 2,720 | 2,846 | 2,741 | 2,558 | 3,275 | 3,947 | 3,947 | 3,621 | 3,851 | 4,141 |
| Poverty rate | 8.1 | 8.7 | 8.3 | 9.0 | 9.1 | 8.6 | 7.7 | 10.0 | 11.7 | 11.6 | 10.7 | 11.1 | 11.8 |
| Primary families§ | 62,251 | 63,352 | 63,567 | 64,063 | 64,360 | 65,388 | 65,158 | 65,907 | 65,467 | 64,931 | 66,225 | 66,541 | 66,462 |
| In poverty | 3,697 | 3,973 | 4,167 | 4,279 | 4,094 | 3,960 | 4,169 | 4,538 | 5,193 | 5,269 | 5,469 | 5,478 | 5,137 |
| Poverty rate (percentage) | 5.9 | 6.3 | 6.6 | 6.7 | 6.4 | 6.1 | 6.4 | 6.9 | 7.9 | 8.1 | 8.3 | 8.2 | 7.7 |

* Data, beginning in 2002 with the collection of the 2003 Annual Social and Economics Supplement to the Current Population Survey, are not strictly comparable with data for earlier years because of the introduction in the January 2003 survey of revised population controls.
† Data, beginning in 2003 with the collection of the 2004 Annual Social and Economic Supplement to the Current Population Survey, are not strictly comparable with data for earlier years because of the introduction in the January 2004 survey of revised population controls.
‡ Includes persons in families, not shown separately.
§ Refers to primary families with at least one member in the labor force for more than half the year. A primary family includes the reference person (householder) and all people living in the household who are related to the reference person.
Source: U.S. Department of Labor, U.S. Bureau of Labor Statistics. A profile of working poor. March 2010. Available at: http://www.bls.gov/. Accessed March 30, 2016.

## The Homeless

**Homeless people** are individuals who do not have a fixed, regular, and adequate nighttime residence. They may be sleeping on the streets, with friends or family, in cars, in abandoned buildings, or in shelters.[72] In 2014, a survey by the U.S. Conference of Mayors found that of the population surveyed, 41 percent of the homeless households with children had a male head of household and 84 percent had a female head of household. However, 63 percent of the single homeless population was male, and they made up 76 percent of the homeless populations surveyed.[73]

Homelessness affects the health and well-being of individuals throughout the life span. Consider the effect of homelessness on children, pregnant women, adolescents, or older persons. Each group has different nutritional needs, and dietitians need to be aware of their unique needs. For example, homeless pregnant women have less access to prenatal care, poorer nutritional status, and a higher incidence of poor birth outcomes (lower-birth-weight infants) than those who are not homeless.[74] Homeless children are at greater risk for inadequate nutrient intake that can contribute to failure to thrive, obesity, and poor growth.[75] In addition, homeless older persons experience untreated nutrition-related conditions such as obesity, heart disease, hypertension, and malnutrition.[76] Similar to other homeless people, older persons must focus their energy on survival.

It is not easy to know the number of homeless people and who they are. The high cost of housing, mental illness, low-paying jobs, substance abuse, domestic violence, and unemployment limits the food budget and creates the problems of hunger and homelessness. Becoming homeless is a gradual process. Once the home is lost, the individual or family may live with family or friends and only go to the shelter or seek refuge on the streets when all other options are depleted.[77] Several factors can contribute to homelessness and hunger, including poverty, unemployment, and emergency demands on income. However, the two factors that contribute most to homelessness and hunger are unaffordable housing units and low or lack of income. The national **housing wage** is the amount a person working full time must earn to pay for a two-bedroom rental unit at fair market rent without paying more than 30 percent of his or her income in rent.[77] In 2016, the housing wage increased to $18.92 an hour. This is almost three times the federal minimum wage of $7.25 an hour. The housing wage has increased significantly since 1999, when a person had to earn $11.08 an hour to pay for fair market rent.[77] Consequently, minimum-wage workers in Illinois must work about 90 hours per week to afford a two-bedroom unit. Additional contributing factors to homelessness are presented in **BOX 4-2**.

**BOX 4-2**  Contributing Factors to Homelessness and Hunger[78]

- Low-paying job
- High housing costs
- Medical or health costs
- Substance abuse
- Mental illness
- Reduced public benefits
- Childcare costs
- Limited life skills (lack of education)
- Weakening of the economy
- Transportation expenses or lack of transportation
- Lack of information about the Supplemental Nutrition Assistance Program
- Lack of nutrition education and income in older population
- Divorce
- Jail or prison (prison release)
- Domestic violence
- Reluctance to participate in food assistance programs, especially among older persons, due to the stigma associated with being on welfare

Homeless people are at high risk for food insecurity because they lack both money and cooking facilities.[79] They regularly depend on soup kitchens and shelters to obtain adequate food. The consequences of inadequate food intake are poor nutritional status (due to lack of folate, vitamin A, vitamin C, magnesium, zinc, vitamin $B_{12}$, iron, etc.) and nutrition-related health conditions such as anemia, dental caries, stunted growth, failure to thrive, low-birth-weight infants, infant mortality, and obesity.[78,80] In some states, homeless individuals may be required to provide an identification card or home address to participate in WIC or SNAP.

Homeless individuals have minimal (on an emergency basis only) or no access to health care and in most cases have problems following a prescribed diet. For example, it is impossible for a homeless diabetic woman who lives on the street or in a shelter to eat regular meals, get adequate rest and exercise, and administer insulin on schedule. Also, crowded living conditions put homeless people at risk for exposure to viruses and bacteria that cause pneumonia, food poisoning (e.g., *Escherichia coli*), and tuberculosis.[81] The number of homeless individuals with AIDS has increased because of high housing and medical costs. HIV infection in the homeless is estimated to be at least double that found in the general population.[67,82]

Community nutritionists have an important role to play in providing nutrition services to the poor or homeless. They can advocate for accessible nutrition services and coordinate a network of services and providers to help prevent malnutrition. Some homeless individuals are eligible for programs such as WIC and SNAP. (See examples of food programs later in the chapter in Table 4-10.) Even with federal assistance programs, many poor people depend on churches and charitable emergency food services to provide for their nutritional needs. For example, Second Harvest, the nation's largest charitable hunger relief organization, provides foods to approximately 23 million people each year.[83] See the Successful Community Strategies feature for exemplary programs for responding to hunger.

## Successful Community Strategies

### Responding to Problems of Hunger

#### Chicago[78]

The Greater Chicago Food Depository (GCFD) reduced the problems of hunger by developing a food program that picked up foods from supermarket delis, restaurants, hotels, and other institutional kitchens in refrigerated trucks and delivered the foods to Chicago Community Kitchens. Chicago Community Kitchens trains underemployed and unemployed individuals for careers in food service. The students were challenged by the variety of foods GCFD delivered to the kitchen to create nutritious and appealing meals for children. The food was then frozen and delivered again in Food Depository refrigerated vehicles to Kids Cafés across the city. The meals released the Kids Café volunteers and staff from preparing the meals, which made them more available to spend time with the children, often latchkey kids living in dangerous neighborhoods.

#### San Antonio[78]

Another exemplary program can be found in the city of San Antonio. The San Antonio Food Bank started a program called Project HOPE. This program served hungry senior citizens by acting as a direct partner with the city's Senior Nutrition Centers. These centers are safe nurturing places where neighborhood seniors go to receive a hot lunch. In addition, the San Antonio Food Bank provided the seniors with two bags of groceries each month. Most of the Project HOPE participants were single and low-income individuals. Some of the achievements of the joint project were that it strengthened the communities and families and created the opportunity to form friendships. Also, participants shared meals together and restocked their pantries. In October 2003, the city invested an additional $270,000 in the program. The San Antonio Food Bank plans to expand the program by including a Supplemental Nutrition Assistance Program education program and nutrition classes.

U.S. Conference of Mayors, Sodexho USA. Hunger and Homelessness Survey. Available at: http://www.usmayors.org/uscm/hungersurvey/2004/onlinereport/HungerAndHomelessnessReport2004.pdf. Accessed April 03, 2016.

## ▶ Welfare Reform

On August 22, 1996, the Personal Responsibility and Work Opportunity Reconciliation Act of 1996, P.L. 104-193 (PRWORA), became law. This comprehensive, bipartisan legislation changed the U.S. welfare system to one that requires work in exchange for time-limited cash assistance. It created the **Temporary Assistance for Needy Families (TANF)** program, which replaced the Aid to Families with Dependent Children (AFDC), Emergency Assistance (EA), and Job Opportunities and Basic Skills Training (JOBS) programs under Title IV of the Social Security Act. The law marked the end of federal entitlement to assistance that began in 1935 when the AFDC was established to provide monetary public assistance to poor single mothers and their children.[84] TANF was reauthorized in February 2006 under the Deficit Reduction Act of 2005. States and territories operate programs, and Native American tribes have the option to carry out their own programs in TANF. States, territories, and tribes each receive a block grant allocation, and states, territories, and tribes must maintain a historical level of spending known as maintenance of effort. The basic block grant includes cash benefits, administrative expenses, and services targeted to needy families.

PRWORA significantly changed the structure of income support for poor single parent families in the United States by the following[84]:

- Eliminating the entitlement to cash assistance
- Imposing a time limit on federal aid
- Granting broad discretion to states in designing a "work-based safety net" for poor families with children

The provisions in federal law often identified as the key elements of TANF's "work-based safety net" include the elimination of the entitlement to cash assistance, block grant funding, mandatory work requirements, sanctions, and a 5-year time limit on cash assistance (see **TABLE 4-6**).

## The Impacts of Welfare Reform

The impacts of welfare reform on families may be positive due to greater self-esteem associated with joining the workforce. However, this advantage may not result in increased financial security. Studies show that welfare reform causes a higher incidence of depression, poorer child health status, household food insecurity, and loss of federal financial support and assistance from the SNAP.[85] Symptoms of depression were also observed in inner-city pediatric clinical populations[78,86] and children participating in a **Head Start program**.[87] The incidence of depression was associated with changes in federal financial assistance and SNAP support. In addition, families were more likely to face a decrease in income from direct loss of benefits and related barriers to employment, such as poor physical and mental health, inadequate past employment experience, discrimination, and low education.[78] Mothers' emotional state has been

---

**TABLE 4-6**   Key Provisions: The Personal Responsibility and Work Opportunity Reconciliation Act

**Establishes Temporary Assistance for Needy Families (TANF)**

- Replaces former entitlement programs with federal block grants
- Transfers authority and responsibility for welfare programs from federal to state government
- Emphasizes moving from welfare to work through time limits and work requirement

**Changes eligibility standards for Supplemental Security Income (SSI) child disability benefits**

- Restricts certain formerly eligible children from receiving benefits
- Changes eligibility rules for new applicants and eligibility predetermination

**Requires states to enforce a strong child support program for collection of child support payments**

**Restricts aliens' eligibility for welfare and other public benefits**

- Denies illegal aliens most public benefits, except emergency medical services
- Restricts most legal aliens from receiving food stamps and SSI benefits until they become citizens or work for at least 10 years
- Allows states the option of providing federal cash assistance to legal aliens already in the country
- Restricts most new legal aliens from receiving federal cash assistance for 5 years
- Allows states the option of using state funds to provide cash assistance to nonqualifying aliens

**Provides resources for foster care data systems and a national child welfare study**

**Establishes a block grant to states to provide childcare for working parents**

**Alters eligibility criteria and benefits for child nutrition programs**

- Modifies reimbursement rates
- Makes families (including aliens) who are eligible for free public education also eligible for school meal benefits

**Tightens national standards for food stamps and commodity distribution**

- Institutes an across-the-board reduction in benefits
- Caps standard deduction at fiscal year 1995 level
- Limits receipt of benefits to 3 months in every 3 years by childless able-bodied adults ages 18 to 50 unless working or in training

Reproduced from: Economic Research Service. United States Department of Agriculture. Food and Nutrition Assistance Programs: Welfare Reform and Food Assistance Briefing Room.
Available at: www.ers.usda.gov/briefing/foodnutritionassistance/gallery/keyprovisions.htm. Accessed February 20, 2008.

shown to be associated with material circumstances. Worry about debt was the strongest independent socioeconomic predictor of maternal depression.

The most quoted impact of welfare reform is the decrease in the number of families receiving cash public assistance. The national welfare caseload reached its peak in 1994, with 5 million families receiving cash public assistance. Before the passage of welfare reform in 1996, the caseload had decreased to 4.4 million families. After welfare reform, it decreased further to 2.5 million in 1999.[88]

Another often-quoted impact of welfare reform is the increase in the employment rates of various groups of single mothers. National labor force data show that the number of all mothers participating in paid work was 74.8 percent in 2013. The participation rate for single mothers (widowed, divorced, separated, or never married) was 64.7 percent in 2013.[87,89,90] State and national studies consistently show that approximately 60 percent of those who have left the TANF program were employed shortly after leaving the program.[87,91,92]

Studies have also shown that although the rate of employment has increased, these mothers' earnings, income, and poverty did not improve. For example, those leaving welfare for employment usually take jobs that pay below poverty-level wages and have no employer-provided benefits, such as health insurance and paid sick or vacation leave. In addition, many of these families do not receive important public income supports, including Medicaid, childcare assistance, and SNAP aid, although their incomes are low enough to meet eligibility requirements.[87,93,94]

In addition, "dire" or "deep" poverty (i.e., family income below 50 percent of the poverty level) has increased among some families headed by single mothers. This means that some groups of poor single mothers and children remained poor after welfare reform.[94-99]

## The Importance of Food Assistance Programs

The goal of food assistance programs is to achieve food security for all Americans.[100,101] The USDA and DHHS conduct a variety of health-related programs that significantly affect the nutritional status of the population, from newborn infants to the elderly. Some of these programs are known as **nonentitlement programs**. Nonentitlement programs[5] compete for funds through the congressional appropriation process and establish eligibility requirements for recipients. The National School Lunch Program and WIC program are examples of nonentitlement programs. The SNAP, in contrast, is an **entitlement program**.[6]

U.S. food assistance programs are designed to improve the nutrition and health status of target recipients and beneficiaries by improving their access to food. The other aims of these programs are to support agriculture and ultimately reduce food insecurity in many U.S. households.[101,102] All the assistance programs, including those administered by the DHHS and the Department of Homeland Security (DHS), are often referred to as a food or nutrition "safety net."[99]

## Federal Domestic Nutrition Assistance Programs

In the United States, the major food assistance programs designed to make sure that all people have access to an adequate diet are the Supplemental Nutrition Assistance Program (SNAP); Special Supplemental Nutrition Program for Women, Infants, and Children (WIC); Child Nutrition Program; and The Emergency Food Assistance Program (TEFAP). Under TEFAP, the USDA distributes commodities to states, which then provide the food to local agencies they have selected, usually food banks, which in turn distribute the food to soup kitchens and food pantries that serve the public. The commodities vary depending on market conditions. Products that are typically available include canned and dried fruits, canned vegetables, canned meats, cheese, peanut butter, butter, and pasta products.[103] Programs that target specifically women, infants, children, and the elderly will be discussed in detail in Chapters 8, 9, and 11, respectively. A brief description of some of the food assistance programs is presented in this section.

## Supplemental Nutrition Assistance Program and Related Programs

The SNAP, formerly known as Food Stamp Program, provides a basic safety net to millions of people. The program provided monthly coupons to eligible low-income families that could be used to purchase food. However, the **electronic benefit transfer (EBT) system** replaced paper coupons with a benefits card, similar to a bankcard. The USDA reports that all 50 states, Washington, D.C., and Puerto Rico are now using EBT systems.

SNAP is designed to supplement the food-buying power of eligible low-income people. In April 2003, all legal immigrants who had worked in the United States continuously for 5 years became eligible to apply for SNAP. In October 2003, all legal immigrants' children, regardless of date of entry to the United States, became eligible to apply. SNAP is the largest of the food assistance programs in the United States, and one of its strengths is the ability to respond to local, state, and national economic changes and emergencies.[102] For example, participation in SNAP increased to 27.5 million in September 2005, mainly due to the Disaster Supplemental Nutrition Assistance Program for victims of Hurricane Katrina.

Changes from PRWORA affected the SNAP. Its expenditures declined by 33 percent from 1996 to 2000, and average monthly participation rates also decreased from 25.5 million to 17.2 million recipients.[104] It is estimated that 65 percent of the decrease in SNAP participation was due to welfare reform and 35 percent to an improved economy.[101]

As part of an effort to more fully understand the factors that influence SNAP participation, the Economic Research Service (ERS) funded the Supplemental Nutrition Assistance Program Access Study, which examined the extent to which policies implemented at the local level, as well as local office practices, affect households' decision to apply for SNAP and their decision to continue participating once they are approved for benefits. Although most nonparticipant households (69 percent) said that they would apply for SNAP benefits if they were sure they were eligible, 27 percent would not apply even in those circumstances. Factors that would prevent some households from participating in SNAP include the following[101]:

1. Stigma (41 percent)
2. Previous bad experience (24 percent)
3. **Costs of application or participation** (61 percent)
4. Personal independence (91 percent)
5. Did not know how to apply (12 percent)

## How Much Could a Household Receive?

The amount of benefit that each household could receive is called an allotment, which varies according to family size and income. The net monthly income of the household is multiplied by 30 percent, and the result is subtracted from the maximum allotment for the household size (see **TABLE 4-7**).[105] This is because SNAP households are expected to spend about 30 percent of their resources on food. For example,

The 2017 allotment for a family of 5 is $771.00.

The family's net monthly income is $455.00.

30 percent of net monthly income = $455.00 × 0.3 = $136.50

To determine the maximum monthly allotment for a family of 5: $771.00 – $136.50 = $634.50.

In this situation, the maximum SNAP allotment for a household is $656.50.

**TABLE 4-7** Maximum Monthly Allotment If Household Has No Income

| People in Household | Maximum Monthly Allotment (USD) |
|---|---|
| 1 | 194 |
| 2 | 357 |
| 3 | 511 |
| 4 | 649 |
| 5 | 771 |
| 6 | 925 |
| 7 | 1,022 |
| 8 | 1,169 |
| Each additional person | 146 |

Modified from: U.S. Department of Agriculture, Food and Nutrition Service. Available at: http://www.fns.usda.gov/2011. Accessed September 30, 2016.

Net income is the household's total cash income from earnings, welfare, and other sources, minus certain allowable items that count in determining SNAP benefits. Most households may have up to $2,000 in countable resources, such as bank accounts, stocks/bonds, cash, and others. Items not included in the assets limit are vehicles, houses, and property lot values. In addition, households may have $3,000 if at least one person is 60 years or older or is disabled. Any household with a net income of zero receives the maximum benefit level, which is based on the Thrifty Food Plan and varies according to household size (see Table 4-1). For low-income households that receive the maximum benefit amount from SNAP, the cost of a nutritious diet modeled on the Thrifty Food Plan is affordable because the maximum benefit amount is equal to the cost of that food plan.[106] However, the maximum SNAP benefit amount may not cover the full costs of the Thrifty Food Plan in periods of high food price inflation. During FY 2008, the loss in purchasing power for a family of four increased from $12 at the beginning of the year to $56 by July.

The Supplemental Nutrition Assistance Program Map Machine is a very important interactive web-based mapping utility that shows program participation and benefit levels up to the county level. The Map Machine can show per capita participation, per capita benefits, changes from year to year, and more. For example, an individual can select any state or region of the United States and display a map showing how program participation changed in each county between 1994 and 2017To access the Map Machine, visit http://maps.ers .usda.gov.

## Supplemental Nutrition Assistance Program Nutrition Education

In the 1990s, the USDA's Food and Nutrition Service (FNS) began to provide funds for **Supplemental Nutrition Assistance Program Nutrition Education (SNAP-Ed)** by matching the dollars a state spends on SNAP-Ed activities. This provided links to state-level maps and data to assist in assessing the impact of SNAP-Ed. The goal of the SNAP-Ed program is to provide educational programs that increase, within a limited budget, the possibility that all SNAP recipients will make healthy food and lifestyle choices consistent with the most recent dietary advice (the *Dietary Guidelines for Americans* and MyPlate).[103] The goals of SNAP-Ed include the following[107]:

- Assisting SNAP households to implement healthy eating and active lifestyles that are consistent with the *Dietary Guidelines for Americans* and MyPlate
- Increasing practices related to economical shopping and preparation of nutritious foods
- Increasing food security of SNAP households and making certain that people eligible for SNAP but not participating are aware of its benefits and how to apply for them as part of nutrition education activities
- Increasing SNAP households' safe handling, preparation, and storage of food

Studies show that SNAP and WIC clients enrolled in SNAP-Ed increased their vegetable, fruit, dairy product, and grain intake to an amount consistent with the *Dietary Guidelines for Americans* and MyPlate. In addition, the participants engaged in behaviors that reflected improvements in safe food handling practices.[108-110]

## ▶ Food Distribution Programs

Several commodity distribution programs assist in preventing food insecurity and hunger. The purpose of food distribution programs is to strengthen the food and nutrition safety net through commodity distribution and other nutrition assistance to low-income individuals and families.[111] Some of the food distribution programs include the Commodity Supplemental Food Program (CSFP), Food Distribution Program on Indian Reservations (FDPIR), The Emergency Food Assistance Program (TEFAP), Nutrition Services Incentive Program, and Schools/Child Nutrition Commodity Programs.

## Commodity Supplemental Food Program

The aim of the **Commodity Supplemental Food Program (CSFP)** is to improve the health of low-income pregnant and breastfeeding women, infants, children up to age 6, and elderly people at least 60 years of age by supplementing their diets with nutritious USDA commodity foods. CSFP provides food and administrative funds to states to supplement the diets of these groups. The CSFP state agencies are responsible for determining the income eligibility for participants. Some states may need the participants to be at nutritional risk before they can participate. The assessments that can be used to determine whether individuals are at nutritional risk include blood tests and height and weight measurements. Examples of nutritional risk conditions are anemia and underweight.[112]

The commodities available each year vary depending on the market conditions. Food packages include a variety of foods, such as infant formula and cereal; nonfat dry and evaporated milk; juice; farina; oats; ready-to-eat cereal; rice; pasta; egg mix; peanut butter; dry beans or peas; canned meat, poultry, or tuna; and canned fruits and vegetables. The packages are designed to address the nutritional needs of the clients. In fiscal year 2016, approximately 619,000 people participated in the program from January 1 to December 31 (Clients may not participate in WIC and CSFP at the same time.)

## Food Distribution Program on Indian Reservations

The purpose of the **Food Distribution Program on Indian Reservations (FDPIR)** is to help low-income American Indian and non-Indian households living on a reservation to maintain a nutritionally balanced diet. Those who do not have access to SNAP offices or authorized food stores can participate in the FDPIR. The Indian Tribal Organizations (ITOs) or an agency of the state government administers FDPIR locally. About 243 tribes receive benefits under the FDPIR through 98 ITOs and 5 state agencies. The USDA purchases the commodities, based on a list of available foods, and ships them to the ITOs and state agencies. However, some commodities offered through FDPIR may be donated to the program from agricultural surpluses. These administering agencies store and distribute the food, determine applicant eligibility, and provide nutrition education to recipients. The USDA also provides the administering agencies with funds for program

---

**BOX 4-3** Examples of Commodity Foods[111]

- Frozen ground beef
- Canned meats
- Poultry and fish
- Canned fruits and vegetables
- Canned soups
- Spaghetti sauce
- Macaroni and cheese
- Pastas
- Cereals
- Rice
- Grains
- Cheese
- Egg mix
- Nonfat dry evaporated milk
- Flour
- Chicken
- Reduced-sodium crackers
- Dried beans
- Low-fat refried beans
- Dehydrated potatoes
- Vegetable oil
- Juices
- Dried fruit
- Peanuts
- Peanut butter
- Corn syrup
- Shortening
- Canned juices
- Bakery mix
- Cornmeal

---

administrative costs.[113] Participants may select from over 70 products (see **BOX 4-3**).

Participants on most reservations can choose fresh produce instead of canned fruits and vegetables and may decide from month to month whether to participate in SNAP or the Food Distribution Program. Administering agencies are responsible for providing nutrition education to participants, which can include individual nutrition counseling, cooking demonstrations, proper storage of commodities, nutrition classes, and information on how to use commodities to make a nutritious diet. A collection of test recipes submitted by program participants can be found at http://www.fns.usda.gov.

## Emergency Food Assistance Program

The purpose of **The Emergency Food Assistance Program (TEFAP)**, formerly known as the Temporary Emergency Food Assistance Program, is to reduce federal food inventories and storage costs and help poor people, including the elderly, at the same time.

The amount that each state receives from the USDA depends on its low-income and unemployed population. TEFAP distributes the commodities to state agencies (food banks), which distribute the foods to the public, including homeless people via soup kitchens and food pantries. The state is responsible for setting the eligibility criteria. The foods TEFAP distributes vary depending on the preferences of states and agricultural market conditions. More than 60 products were made available for fiscal year 2011, including canned and dried fruits, canned vegetables, fruit juice, dried egg mix, meat, poultry, fish, nonfat dry milk, pasta, peanut butter, rice, grits, cereal, and soups.

## Nutrition Services Incentive Program

The purpose of the **Nutrition Services Incentive Program (NSIP)** is to provide incentives to states and tribes for the effective delivery of nutritious meals to older adults. The program originally was administered by the USDA, which provided cash and/or commodities to supplement meals provided under the authority of the Older Americans Act (OAA). The OAA was amended in 2003 to transfer the NSIP from the USDA to the Administration on Aging (AOA) within the DHHS.[114] The only eligibility criterion is age. People 60 years of age or older and their spouses, regardless of age, are eligible for NSIP benefits. ITOs may choose an age below 60 for defining an older person for their tribes. Additionally, the following individuals also may receive meals through NSIP[114]:

1. Disabled people under age 60 who live in elderly housing facilities where congregate meals are served
2. Disabled persons who reside at home and accompany elderly participants to meals
3. Volunteers who assist in the meal service

## Food Distribution Disaster Assistance

**Food distribution disaster assistance programs** distribute commodity foods directly to households that are in need as a result of an emergency. Such direct distribution takes place when normal commercial food supply channels such as grocery stores have been disrupted, damaged, or destroyed, or cannot function (e.g., lack of electricity). The FNS of the USDA is the agency in charge of food during a period of disaster. The Federal Emergency Management Agency (FEMA) in the DHS coordinates overall disaster relief efforts.[114] In an emergency situation, the USDA can authorize states to release food stocks to disaster relief agencies (e.g., Salvation Army, Red Cross) to feed people at shelters and mass feeding sites. If the president declares a disaster, states, with USDA approval, also can distribute commodity foods directly to households that are in need as a result of an emergency.[115] FNS uses the term *situation of distress* when a natural catastrophe or other event has not been declared by the president to be a disaster, but in the judgment of the state distributing agency or FNS warrants the use of USDA-donated foods for congregate feeding or household distribution or the issuance of emergency SNAP assistance. A situation of distress could be caused by a hurricane, tornado, storm, flood, tidal wave, tsunami, earthquake, volcanic eruption, landslide, mudslide, snowstorm, drought, fire, or other natural catastrophe. There are also situations other than natural catastrophes, such as strikes or explosions that, in the judgment of FNS, may warrant the use of donated foods. It is recommended that state distributing agencies use commodities provided through the National School Lunch Program whenever possible. These commodities are easy for disaster feeding organizations to use in preparing congregate meals, and they are easy for FNS to replace or reimburse.

## ▶ Child Nutrition and Related Programs

There are several nutrition programs that target children. This section discusses some of these programs. Chapter 9 and Table 4-9 (later in this chapter) provide more information on child nutrition programs, including the Head Start Program.

### The National School Lunch Program and School Breakfast Program

Both the National School Lunch Program and the School Breakfast Program were designed to improve children's diet, nutrient intake, and well-being. These meals make a very important contribution to children's mental and physical development. Both meals must meet the nutritional requirements outlined in the *Dietary Guidelines for Americans*, published jointly by the USDA and the DHHS, which recommends that no more than 30 percent of an individual's calories come from fat and less than 10 percent from saturated fat. In addition, breakfasts must provide one fourth of the Recommended Dietary Allowance for protein, calcium, iron, vitamin A, vitamin C, and calories. The **School Breakfast Program (SBP)** provides children with nutritious foods before their school day begins; this helps improve their diets and encourages the learning process. An example of a good breakfast consists of a serving of orange juice, toast with jelly, and oatmeal with milk and raisins. This breakfast provides about

450 calories plus protein; B vitamins; vitamins C, A, and D; and the minerals calcium and iron.[116] The School Lunch Program must provide one third of the children's nutritional requirements for the day.

Most of the support the USDA provides to schools in the School Breakfast and Lunch Programs comes in the form of a cash reimbursement for each meal served. In addition to cash reimbursements, schools are entitled by law to receive commodity foods, called entitlement programs foods, at a value of 17.25 cents for each meal served. Schools also can receive "bonus" commodities as they are available from surplus agricultural stocks.

These school programs help children from families with income at or below 130 percent of the federal poverty level obtain free meals. Those with income between 130 percent and 185 percent of the poverty level are eligible for reduced-price meals (see **TABLE 4-8**). Children from families over 185 percent of poverty level pay full price. Children from families that qualify for

**TABLE 4-8** 2016 DHHS Poverty Guidelines

| Size of Family Unit | 48 Contiguous States and Washington, D.C. (USD) | Alaska | Hawaii |
|---|---|---|---|
| 1 | 11,880 | 14,840 | 13,670 |
| 2 | 16,020 | 20,020 | 18,430 |
| 3 | 20,160 | 25,200 | 23,190 |
| 4 | 24,300 | 30,380 | 27,950 |
| 5 | 28,440 | 35,560 | 32,710 |
| 6 | 32,580 | 40,740 | 37,470 |
| 7 | 36,730 | 45,920 | 42,230 |
| 8 | 40,80 | 51,120 | 47,010 |
| For each additional person, add: | 4,160 | 5,200 | 4,780 |

Tables containing various percentage multiples (e.g., 100 percent, 120 percent, 133 percent, etc.) of the 2006 poverty guidelines commonly used in federal and state programs are available online.

Modified from: Federal Register, 2016;76(13):3637–3638.

SNAP automatically qualify for free school breakfasts and lunches.[117] Visit http://www.ns.usda.gov for more information about these programs.

## After-School Snack Program

An after-school snack gives children a nutritional enhancement and encourages them to participate in supervised activities that are safe and filled with learning opportunities. All programs that meet the eligibility requirements can participate in the National School Lunch Program and receive USDA reimbursement for after-school snacks. **After-school snack programs** are designed to promote the health and well-being of children and youth through the age of 18. In order for schools to qualify for the program they must provide children with regularly scheduled activities in an organized, structured, and supervised environment. The activities must be educational or enrichment-based (e.g., mentoring or tutoring programs). Competitive interscholastic sports teams are not eligible for the after-school program. The programs must meet state or local licensing requirements, if available, or state or local health and safety standards.[118] The USDA reimburses the schools for the snacks.[119]

## Special Milk Program

The FNS of the USDA administers the Special Milk Program at the federal level. The **Special Milk Program** provides milk to children in schools, childcare institutions, and eligible camps that do not participate in other federal child nutrition meal service programs. The program reimburses schools and institutions for the milk they serve to the children.[117]

## Summer Food Service Program for Children

Millions of low-income children lose access to the school breakfasts, lunches, and after-school snacks when school is no longer in session. The **Summer Food Service Program (SFSP)** fills this gap. Many of the children served may be at nutritional risk if they do not have access to school meals. SFSP provides free meals to all eligible participants and children up to the age of 18 years from households with incomes at or below 185 percent of the poverty guidelines. Most SFSP sites can provide up to two meals (breakfast and lunch or breakfast and dinner) or one meal and a snack a day.

Sites that serve migrant children and certain types of summer camps are "open sites," which means that they are open to all children who go to the site during meal service times. These sites are especially important for migrant workers' children, who may not have the opportunity to officially enroll in the program. An open site is eligible for federal SFSP funds for all the children if it is located in a geographic area in which at least 50 percent of the children are from low-income families. Some sites are called "enrolled sites"; these sites serve only children who are officially enrolled in the program. An enrolled site is eligible for federal funds to serve all the children enrolled in the program if at least 50 percent of the children enrolled can qualify for free or reduced price school meals (documented).

Many SFSP sites provide not just meals, but educational enrichment and recreational activities that help children continue to learn and stay safe when school is not in session. Accordingly, the NYSP provides youth from low-income communities the opportunity to receive benefits from structured sports and education programs and at least one USDA-approved meal daily. Local universities, colleges, schools, parks and recreation departments, summer camps, community action agencies, and other nonprofit organizations manage NYSP.[120]

## Child and Adult Care Food Program

The purpose of the **Child and Adult Care Food Program (CACFP)** is to serve nutritious meals and snacks to eligible children and adults who are enrolled for care at participating childcare centers, daycare homes, and adult daycare centers. CACFP also provides meals to children residing in homeless shelters and snacks to youths participating in after-school care programs. The USDA's FNS administers CACFP through grants to states. The program is administered within most states by the state educational agency.

Childcare centers and daycare homes may be approved to claim up to two reimbursable meals (breakfast, lunch, or dinner) and one snack, or two snacks and one meal, to each eligible participant, each day. Shelters may serve each child up to three reimbursable meals (breakfast, lunch, and dinner) each day. After school care programs may claim reimbursement for serving each child one snack each day. In childcare centers, participants from households with incomes at or below 130 percent of poverty level are eligible for free meals. Participants with household incomes between 130 percent and 185 percent of poverty level are eligible for meals at a reduced price. Institutions must determine each enrolled participant's eligibility for free and reduced-price meals served in centers. Children whose families receive benefits from SNAP, FDPIR, or state programs funded through TANF are categorically eligible for free meals. Children who were eligible to participate in the Head Start program are automatically eligible for free meals.[120,121]

## ▶ Programs for Women and Young Children

Among many nutrition programs designed to serve vulnerable people are programs to assist low-income women and their children obtain nutritious foods. (See Chapters 8 and 9 and later in this chapter for more information.) This section provides a brief discussion of women and young children's programs.

### Special Supplemental Nutrition Program for Women, Infants, and Children

WIC is a federally funded program that provides healthy supplemental foods and nutrition counseling for pregnant women, new mothers, infants, and children up to age 5. The program has an extraordinary record of over 30 years of preventing children's health problems and improving their long-term health, growth, and development. WIC is not an entitlement program; that is, Congress does not set aside funds to allow every eligible individual to participate in the program. Instead, WIC is a federal grant program for which Congress authorizes a specific amount of funding each year for program operations. The FNS, which administers the program at the federal level, provides these funds to WIC state agencies (state health departments or comparable agencies) to pay for WIC foods, nutrition counseling and education, and administrative costs. A few WIC state agencies distribute the WIC foods through warehouses or deliver the foods to participants' homes. The foods provided are high in one or more of the following nutrients: protein, calcium, iron, and vitamins A and C.

In most WIC state agencies, WIC participants receive the following[122]:

1. Checks or vouchers to purchase specific foods each month that are designed to supplement their diets. Different food packages are provided for different categories of participants.
2. Special therapeutic infant formulas and medical foods are provided when prescribed by a physician for a specified medical condition.
3. Nutrition education and counseling are provided.
4. Referrals to other healthcare services are offered.

On December 6, 2007, WIC created new food packages that were linked with the 2005 *Dietary Guidelines for Americans* and the infant feeding practice guidelines of the American Academy of Pediatrics. These food packages are a more efficient method of promoting and supporting the establishment of successful, long-term breastfeeding; providing WIC participants with a wider variety of foods, including fruits, vegetables, and whole grains, and providing WIC state agencies greater flexibility in prescribing food packages to accommodate the cultural food preferences of WIC participants. Visit http://www.fns.usda.gov for more information on the food packages.

An individual whose income is at or below 185 percent of the U.S. Poverty Income Guidelines is eligible to participate in WIC. A person who participates or has family members who participate in certain other benefit programs, such as SNAP, Medicaid, or TANF, automatically satisfies the income eligibility requirement.[122]

### WIC Farmers' Market Nutrition Program

The **WIC Farmers' Market Nutrition Program (FMNP)** was established in 1992 to provide fresh, unprepared, locally grown fruits and vegetables to WIC participants and expand the awareness, sales, and use of farmers' markets. FMNP participants receive vouchers in addition to their regular WIC food provisions. The vouchers issued to the participants may not be less than $10 and not more than $30 per year.[123] However, state agencies may supplement the benefit level. These are used to buy fresh, unprepared locally grown fruits, vegetables, and herbs from farmers' markets or roadside stands that have been approved by the state agency to accept FMNP coupons. Participants also receive nutrition education through an arrangement with the local WIC agency. The nutrition education is designed to encourage FMNP participants to improve and expand their diets by adding fresh fruits and vegetables, as well as to educate them on how to select, store, and prepare the fresh fruits and vegetables.[124]

### Expanded Food and Nutrition Education Program

The Expanded Food and Nutrition Education Program (EFNEP) is a unique program that currently operates in all 50 states and in American Samoa, Guam, Micronesia, Northern Marianas, Puerto Rico, and the Virgin Islands. It provides community-based nutrition education programs designed to help individuals, families, and communities acquire knowledge, skills, attitudes, and changed behavior needed to support health, economic, and social well-being. EFNEP is offered to families who are eligible for WIC and SNAP.

County Extension professionals provide on-the-job training and supervise paraprofessionals and volunteers who teach EFNEP. The paraprofessionals usually live in the communities where they work. They recruit families and receive referrals from neighborhood contacts and community agencies (e.g., SNAP and WIC). EFNEP activities may include the following[125]:

1. Direct teaching in group or one-on-one situations
2. Mailings and telephone teaching
3. Mass media efforts to promote the educational program
4. Development and training of volunteers to assist with direct teaching of adults and youth
5. Assist limited-resources individuals and families to improve their physical activity

The Cooperative State Research Education Extension Service (CSREES) provides funds for the EFNEP programs. The goal of CSREES is to advance knowledge of agriculture, the environment, human health and well-being, and communities by supporting research, education, and Extension programs in the land-grant university system and other partner organizations (e.g., Economics and Commerce; Families, Youth, and Communities; Food, Nutrition, and Health; and Natural Resources and Environment).

Research shows that EFNEP has made a significant impact in improving low-income families' nutrient intake. For example, dietary intake of six important nutrients that are frequently limited in the diets of low-income people (protein, iron, calcium, vitamin A, vitamin C, and vitamin $B_6$) increased considerably due to participation in EFNEP.[123]

## Successful Community Strategies

### New York State WIC and FMNP[126]

Three New York State (NYS) agencies embarked on a statewide initiative to enhance the effectiveness of the WIC Farmers' Market Nutrition Program (FMNP) for both families and farmers. The agencies involved in the FMNP initiative were the NYS Department of Agriculture and Markets (DAM), the NYS Department of Health (DOH), and the Division of Nutritional Sciences/Cornell Cooperative Extension (CCE) at Cornell University. The program enhancements included four components intended to influence market and consumer behavior:

1. A statewide CCE staff member, who was hired to initiate and coordinate FMNP promotion efforts
2. Increased collaboration among state-level agencies
3. Increased local-level community capacity-building
4. Dissemination of newly developed nutrition education resources

Thirty-eight local Extension associations committed to organizing capacity-building efforts in their communities, including hosting of pre- and post-FMNP season meetings among stakeholders, identification of community goals and means for accomplishing them, and identification of parties responsible for taking certain actions toward accomplishing those goals. Several new FMNP nutrition education resources were made available and promoted for the FMNP season to both WIC and CCE in the communities. The resources used for the program, called *Get Fresh!* included a set of videos, recipe cards, ideas for using the videos and recipe cards, and an activity booklet for children (CCE only). *Get Fresh!* was promoted through CCE in-service and WIC training events. Videos were mailed to all local WIC agencies and to the 38 participating local CCE associations. In addition, the resources were incorporated into local educational activities at WIC sites, CCE activities, and farmers' markets.

Among the local 89 WIC agencies and 38 local CCE associations, 90 percent utilized the resources.

The aim of the nutrition education using these resources was to increase program participation by decreasing barriers to purchasing and preparing fresh produce.

At the end of the intervention, the redemption rate was significantly higher than the earlier trend. Also, results showed that FMNP goals were advanced through a coordinated, collaborative initiative with activities at state and local levels, resulting in increased utilization of FMNP benefits by WIC participants and increased income to local farmers. In addition, evaluation showed that efforts resulted in increased delivery of FMNP nutrition education at farmers' markets and WIC agencies, as well as changes in market operation times and locations to suit community needs.

# ▶ Programs for Older Adults

There are many federal, local, and private programs designed to promote the nutritional health of older persons in the United States. Chapter 11 and Table 4-9 (later) provide more information about the programs. This section provides a brief discussion of some of the programs.

## Elderly Nutrition Program

The DHHS AOA provides funding for the **Elderly Nutrition Program (ENP)**. All seniors 60 years of age or older and their spouse of any age, regardless of income, are eligible to participate in the ENP. Some tribal organizations set the age eligibility limit lower than 60 years of age because Native Americans are likely to have lower life expectancies and higher rates of illness at younger ages. Although the program does not set particular income limits to participate, outreach efforts are focused on low-income older persons and low-income minority older persons.

The purpose of the ENP is to[127]:

1. Improve the dietary intakes of older persons
2. Create informal support networks
3. Provide positive social contacts with other seniors at the group meal sites
4. Make community-based services available to older adults who may be at risk for losing their independence
5. Educate them on how to shop, plan, and prepare nutritious meals that are economical
6. Enhance their health and well-being

The ENP provides a congregate meal program at locations such as churches and senior community centers. Sometimes called Meals on Wheels, home-delivered meals are delivered to homebound seniors who are unable to travel to a congregate meal site.

The program must provide at least one third of the recommended dietary allowances established by the Food and Nutrition Board of the Institute of Medicine of the National Academy of Sciences, as well as the *Dietary Guidelines for Americans*. In practice, the ENP's 3.1 million elderly participants are receiving an estimated 40 to 50 percent of most required nutrients.[126]

## Senior Farmers' Market Nutrition Program

In fiscal year 2001, the **Senior Farmers' Market Nutrition Program (SFMNP)** was established. The purpose of the program is to provide low-income older persons coupons that can be used to purchase locally grown fresh, unprepared fruits, vegetables, and herbs at farmers' markets, roadside stands, and community-supported agriculture programs. The eligibility criteria are income not more than 185 percent of poverty level and age 60 years or older (with some exceptions). In fiscal year 2007, $15 million was used to operate SFMNP in 46 states; federally recognized Indian tribal governments also are supposed to operate the SFMNP.[123]

**TABLE 4-9** presents federally funded food and nutrition programs. **TABLE 4-10** presents the limitations and advantages of federal food assistance programs.

| **TABLE 4-9** Federally Funded Food and Nutrition Programs | | | | | |
|---|---|---|---|---|---|
| **Food Assistance and Nutrition Program** | **Service Provider** | **Who Qualifies** | **Service/Benefits** | **Funding** | **Administrative Agency** |
| **National School Lunch Program** | | | | | |
| Provides nutritious low-cost lunches to children enrolled in school | All public schools; voluntary in private schools | All children attending school may participate; reduced-price meals to children from families with incomes between 130 percent and 185 percent of poverty level; free meals to children from families with income at or below 130 percent of poverty level | Nutritious low-cost lunch at full or reduced prices or free | USDA | State departments of education; local school districts |

| Food Assistance and Nutrition Program | Service Provider | Who Qualifies | Service/Benefits | Funding | Administrative Agency |
|---|---|---|---|---|---|
| **School Breakfast Program** | | | | | |
| Provides nutritious breakfast to children in participating schools or institutions | Voluntarily by public and private schools | All children attending schools where the breakfast program operates may participate; reduced-price breakfast available to children from families with income between 130 percent and 185 percent of poverty level; free breakfast to children from families with incomes at or below 130 pecent of poverty level | Nutritious low-cost breakfast at full or reduced prices or free | USDA | State departments of education; local school districts |
| **Special Milk Program** | | | | | |
| Provides milk to school-age children in childcare centers and in schools or institutions where there is no school lunch program | Schools, camps, and childcare institutions not participating in other school nutrition programs | All children attending schools or institutions with this program | Milk at reasonable price or free | USDA | State departments of education; local school districts |
| **Summer Food Service Program for Children** | | | | | |
| Provides one nutritious meal to children as a substitute for the National School Lunch and School Breakfast Programs during summer vacation | Public and nonprofit private schools; public or nonprofit private residential facilities of local, municipal, or county government | Children under 18 years and persons over 18 years who are handicapped and participate in a sponsored program of county government; no income requirements; eligibility is determined by location and sponsor | Nutritious meals (breakfast, lunch, and/or snacks) | USDA | State departments of education; local sponsors |

*(continues)*

**TABLE 4-9**  Federally Funded Food and Nutrition Programs (*continued*)

| Food Assistance and Nutrition Program | Service Provider | Who Qualifies | Service/Benefits | Funding | Administrative Agency |
|---|---|---|---|---|---|
| **Childcare Food Program** | | | | | |
| Provides financial assistance for nutritious food in childcare settings . | Licensed childcare centers or family daycare homes; Head Start programs | Children 12 years or younger; children of migrant workers 15 years or younger; physically/mentally handicapped individuals provided care in a center where majority are age 18 or younger | Free or reduced-price meals to eligible children in centers and free meals to all children in family daycare homes; reimbursements for up to two meals and one snack daily | USDA | State departments of education; local providers |
| **Head Start** | | | | | |
| Provides comprehensive health, educational, nutrition, social, and other services to low-income preschool children and their families | Local Head Start program | Children ages 3–5 years from low-income families receiving public assistance or total annual income not more than 100 percent of poverty level; at least 10 percent total enrollment available for handicapped children | Education; comprehensive medical, dental, nutrition, and social services through assessment, early intervention, and prevention; nutritious meals and snacks (through Child Care Food Program); nutrition education; family counseling and referrals for social services | DHHS | DHHS regional offices; local providers |
| **Special Supplemental Food Program for Women, Infants, and Children (WIC)** | | | | | |
| Provides supplemental food and nutrition education as an adjunct to health care to low-income pregnant, postpartum, and breastfeeding women, infants, and children at nutritional risk | Health agencies, social services, community action agencies | Pregnant women, postpartum women (6 months), breastfeeding women (up to 1 year); infants and children (up to 5 years); must be certified to be at nutritional risk; household income determined to be at or below 185 percent of poverty level | Monthly foods or coupons for milk, cheese, eggs, fruit juice, cereal, peanut butter or legumes, infant formula, and infant cereal; nutrition education | USDA | State health agencies; local agencies |

| Food Assistance and Nutrition Program | Service Provider | Who Qualifies | Service/Benefits | Funding | Administrative Agency |
|---|---|---|---|---|---|
| **Commodity Supplemental Food Program (CSFP)** | | | | | |
| Provides commodity foods to low-income women (pregnant, breastfeeding, or postpartum), infants, children up to 6 years of age, and the elderly in certain cases | Public and private nonprofit agencies (community health or social service agencies) | Pregnant women, postpartum women, breastfeeding women, infants, and children (up to 6 years); household income determined to be at or below 185 percent of poverty level; low-income elderly may be served if it does not reduce the benefits to eligible women, infants, and children | Monthly commodity canned or packaged food, including fruits, vegetables, meats, infant formula, farina, beans, and others as available | USDA | State health agencies |
| **\*Supplemental Nutrition Assistance Program (SNAP)** | | | | | |
| Provides low-income households with voucher to increase food purchasing power | Local public assistance or social services offices | U.S. citizen; recognized refugee with visa status or legal alien; households with low income and with resources (aside from income) of $2,000 or less/$3,000 or less with at least one elderly person (age 60 or older); eligibility determined after formal application to local public assistance or social services | Food voucher to purchase foods at participating food markets | USDA | State welfare, social service, or human service agencies |
| **The Emergency Food Assistance Program (TEFAP)** | | | | | |
| Provides commodity foods to low-income households through local public or private nonprofit agencies; quarterly distributions by emergency providers | Public and private nonprofit agencies (community action agencies, councils on aging, or local health/local school districts) | Households with incomes at or below 150 percent of poverty level | Quarterly distribution of cheese, butter, rice, and occasionally flour, cornmeal, and dry milk; emergency food available once per month; dairy products, rice, flour, cornmeal | USDA | State and local agencies |

*(continues)*

**TABLE 4-9**  Federally Funded Food and Nutrition Programs *(continued)*

| Food Assistance and Nutrition Program | Service Provider | Who Qualifies | Service/Benefits | Funding | Administrative Agency |
|---|---|---|---|---|---|
| **Nutrition Assistance Program (NAP) for Puerto Rico** | | | | | |
| Block grant program in which Puerto Rico receives the cost of food assistance benefits (provided to recipients and half of the Commonwealth) and administrative costs, up to a legislatively set total | Commonwealth of Puerto Rico | Program operates under eligibility rules similar to SNAP | Cash to be used by recipients to supplement their food budget | USDA | Puerto Rico Commonwealth Government |
| **Food Distribution Program on Indian Reservations (FDPIR)** | | | | | |
| Operates as a substitute for SNAP for eligible needy families living on or near Indian reservations | Local agency | Indian families living on or near reservations | Offers USDA commodities monthly | USDA | Indian tribal Councils |
| **Meal Program for the Elderly** | | | | | |
| Provides older Americans with meals and nutrition education in congregate setting or delivered to their homes | Area agency on aging or other aging services provider | People age 60 or older with social or economic needs; spouses of eligible people; handicapped or disabled people under 60 who reside in housing occupied primarily by the elderly | Nutritious meals; nutrition education; access to social and rehabilitative services; transportation | DHHS; Administration on Aging; state; individual donations | State agencies on aging; area agencies on aging |
| **Cooperative Extension—Expanded Food and Nutrition Education Program (EFNEP)** | | | | | |
| Provides nutrition education to low-income families and individuals | Local Cooperative Extension office where program is available | Families with children under 19 years; income at or below 125 percent of federal poverty level; at nutritional risk | Education and training on food and nutrition for homemakers and youth | USDA | State land grant universities; Cooperative Extension |

*Indicates entitlement programs.

Modified from: Kaufman M. *Nutrition in Public Health: A Handbook for Developing Programs and Services.* Rockville, MD: Aspen; 1990.

**TABLE 4-10** The Limitations and Advantages of Federal Food Assistance Programs

| Limitations | Advantages |
|---|---|
| The federal poverty level is an inappropriate index of hunger. | Reduce food insecurity in many U.S. households |
| The U.S. social welfare system does not insulate individuals and families from repetitive economic difficulties. | Increase household food expenditures |
| Voluntary activities and private charity cannot cure the hunger problem. | Reduce child poverty |
| Hunger, poverty, unemployment, and the costs of housing and basic needs are interrelated. | Reduce the incidence of anemia in children |
| The SNAP benefit formula does not account for geographic differences in food prices (except in Alaska and Hawaii, where food prices and benefits are higher). | Increase lunchtime intakes of riboflavin, vitamin $B_{12}$, calcium, phosphorus, magnesium, and zinc in children |
| The maximum SNAP benefit amount may not cover the full costs of the Thrifty Food Plan in periods of high food price inflation | |

Reproduced from: United States Department of Agriculture Food and Nutrition Service. Available at http://www.fns.usda.gov. Accessed September 19, 2011.

## ✍ Think About It

Janet, a community nutritionist, works in a retirement community composed of both men and women who are experiencing food insecurity. What food assistance programs would Janet recommend to her clients, and what benefits would each program provide?

# Learning Portfolio

## Chapter Summary

1. In the 1930s, the USDA began developing family food plans at four separate cost levels. The Thrifty Food Plan continues to be used as the nutritional basis for the benefits of the Supplemental Nutrition Assistance Program.

2. National nutrition monitoring programs provide data to assess food and nutrient inadequacies as well as malnutrition and chronic diseases related to overconsumption. Scientific research utilizes nutrition monitoring data to revise the standards of human nutrient requirements and study the relationship among diet, nutrition, and health.

3. During the 1930s, the federal government developed food relief and food commodity distribution programs, including school food programs, nutrition education programs, and the national food consumption survey.

4. The U.S. Department of Health and Human Services (DHHS) administers the majority of public health and nutrition programs. It is the second largest federal agency in terms of dollars received from the federal budget for its programs.

5. The National School Lunch Program, established in 1946, provides nutritious lunches and the opportunity to practice skills learned in nutrition education classrooms.

6. Federal cash reimbursements and donated foods from the Commodity Food Program are provided to schools that serve a lunch meeting the specified nutritional requirements under the School Lunch Program.

7. The Special Milk Program, established in 1955 by the USDA, provides reimbursement for milk served to children.

8. The Special Supplemental Nutrition Program for Women, Infants, and Children (WIC) and the National School Lunch Program (NSLP) are nonentitlement programs.

9. WIC was established as a pilot program in 1972 and was made permanent in 1974. The Food and Nutrition Service administers WIC at the federal level.

10. The Supplemental Nutrition Assistance Program (SNAP) is an entitlement program; eligible individuals are entitled to receive benefits. To qualify for SNAP, households must have gross incomes below 130 percent of the official poverty level.

11. The National Youth Sports Program (NYSP) is a federal program designed to assist low-income children ages 10 to 16 in a summer program. It provides a comprehensive developmental and instructional sports program to low-income children as well as one USDA-approved meal per day.

12. School nutrition services integrate nutritious, affordable, and appealing meals; nutrition education; and an environment that promotes healthful eating behaviors.

13. The Emergency Food Assistance Program (TEFAP) provides commodity foods to emergency kitchens (often referred to as soup kitchens), homeless shelters, and similar organizations that serve meals to low-income individuals. An eligibility criterion is set between 130 and 150 percent of the poverty line for some states.

14. Federally funded food and nutrition programs are the safety net through which families are provided a reasonable supply of nutritious food, knowledge, and the skills required to make healthy food choices.

## Critical Thinking Activities

1. Help a community nutritionist provide nutrition education on how to plan and prepare low-cost meals using MyPlate and other educational tools.

2. Observe a community nutritionist for 2 days and write a reflective journal/log about the experiences/observations.

3. Interview an individual or a household who has participated in a food assistance program. Ask them to describe their experiences with food assistance programs.

4. Plan a 1-day meal for a family of five within SNAP allotments.

5. Carry out a discussion on whether SNAP should or should not be more restricted and/or exclude certain foods.

6. Obtain and critique a research article about working-poor issues that are related to nutrition.

7. Collect data on population groups that are new to the community, such as migrant workers, Asian groups, or refugees, to determine the availability of food and their eligibility for any of the federal programs.

8. Create a list for individuals participating in a food pantry, showing where and how to shop for the most economical and nutritious foods in the community.

9. Survey two participants in food pantries, a homeless shelter, the WIC program, or the like about the effectiveness of food assistance programs.

10. Contact different businesses (such as restaurants, grocery stores, churches, and senior citizen clubs) to donate time, food items, and other products to organizations such as homeless shelters, the Salvation Army, Catholic Charity sites, and so on.

11. Work with a classmate on a service-learning activity. Each pair should observe and participate/work in a community-based food assistance program for 1 to 3 days. It is more rewarding to vary the experiences by working at two different sites. Examples of assistance programs include homeless shelters, WIC, Peace Meal/Congregate Meal Programs, food banks/pantries, and Catholic meal programs in the community. You can help serve meals and/or engage in conversation with the clients. (Older clients in the Congregate Meal Program are especially receptive to students.)

12. Keep a reflective journal/log about how you felt after accomplishing these activities. Describe the quality of your interactions with the clients at the site and what you learned during these interactions. How will these experiences be useful to you as a community nutritionist in the future?

   Ask the supervisors/coordinators of the sites some of the following questions:

   - Who does the program serve?
   - What are the eligibility requirements?
   - Who helps carry out the duties of the program?

## ⌕ CASE STUDY 4-1: Nutrition Students Involved in Service Learning Activities to Reduce Hunger and Malnutrition

Population characteristics have an impact on the health of individuals, families, and aggregates. However, community nutritionists can address nutritional needs and minimize health risks by creating interventions for those populations at risk, such as those who are homeless, the elderly, and hungry children.

A city with a population of 200,000 was experiencing an increase in homeless people; infant mortality; underweight elderly individuals; and hungry children with tooth decay, dull sparse hair, and protein-energy malnutrition (PEM). Students enrolled in a community nutrition course in that city were assigned to help reduce these nutrition-related conditions by providing services as needed at various community sites. They served meals to the homeless and the elderly and provided nutrition education to the parents of the children and low-income families receiving help at food pantries. The students also included information about the different food assistance programs available to them as part of the nutrition education. At the end of the school year, the students decided to establish a community-based emergency food delivery network by involving different student organizations and local businesses in the community.

### Questions

1. What is the definition of nutrition monitoring? What are the different subcategories of the federal nutrition monitoring surveys and surveillance activities since 1990 that the students must understand?
2. The students learned about food insecurity before working in the community. How are households classified in terms of food security or insecurity? What are the USDA's labels to describe the ranges of food security?
3. What is the goal/purpose of the U.S. food assistance programs?
4. What is the difference between entitlement and nonentitlement programs?
5. What are the major food assistance programs in the United States?
6. What is Supplemental Nutrition Assistance Program Nutrition Education? What are the goals of this food assistance program?
7. The city in the case study was experiencing an increase in homeless people, infant mortality, and the underweight elderly population. What are some food assistance programs to which the students could have referred these at-risk families and populations?
8. What are the food assistance programs that target health and nutrition in school-age children? In what programs would children be eligible to participate if they are 8 years of age and their family's income is at 145 percent of the national poverty level?
9. What is the impact of welfare reform?
10. Who are considered the working poor?
11. Work in small groups or individually to discuss the case study and practice using the Nutrition Care Process chart provided on the companion website. You also can add other nutrition and health-related conditions or assessments to the case study to make the case study more challenging and interesting.

- How many people (staff) work for the program, and what are the skills required?
- What is the purpose of the program?
- Who funds the program, and what are the eligibility criteria for funding?
- What challenges/difficulties does the program encounter?

Use this information for an in-class discussion.

## Think About It

**Answer:** *Elderly Nutrition Program:* Provides nutritious meals (lunch), nutrition education, access to social and rehabilitative services, and transportation.

*Commodity Supplemental Food Program (CSFP):* Provides monthly commodity canned or packaged food, including fruits, vegetables, meats, farina, beans, and others as available.

*SNAP:* Provides food voucher to purchase foods at participating food markets.

*Senior Farmers' Market Nutrition Program:* Provides low-income older persons coupons that can be used to purchase locally grown fresh, unprepared fruits, vegetables, and herbs at farmers' markets, roadside stands, and community-supported agriculture programs.

## Key Terms

**after-school snack program:** Gives children a nutritional enhancement and encourages them to participate in supervised activities that are safe and filled with learning opportunities.

**Child and Adult Care Food Program (CACFP):** Serves nutritious meals and snacks to eligible children and adults who are enrolled for care at participating child-care centers, daycare homes, and adult daycare centers.

**Commodity Supplemental Food Program (CSFP):** Provides food and administrative funds to states to supplement the diets of low-income pregnant and breastfeeding women, infants, children up to age 6 and elderly people at least 60 years of age.

**Elderly Nutrition Program (ENP):** Provides grants to support nutrition services to older people throughout the country. It provides for congregate and home-delivered meals programs.

**electronic benefit transfer (EBT) system:** An electronic system that allows a recipient to authorize transfer of their government benefits from a federal account to a retailer.

**entitlement programs:** Programs funded by Congress for any person who qualifies due to level of income or other eligibility requirements; SNAP is an entitlement program.

**food distribution disaster assistance programs:** Distribute commodity foods directly to households in need as a result of an emergency. Such direct distribution takes place when normal commercial food supply channels, such as grocery stores, have been disrupted, damaged, or destroyed or cannot function (e.g., lack of electricity).

**Food Distribution Program on Indian Reservations (FDPIR):** The USDA purchases commodities and ships them to Indian Tribal Organizations (ITOs) to help low-income American Indian and non-Indian households living on a reservation to maintain a nutritionally balanced diet.

**food insecurity:** The inability to obtain sufficient food for any reason.

**Head Start program:** A comprehensive child development program for low-income preschool children and their families.

**homeless people:** Individuals who do not have a fixed, regular, and adequate nighttime residence.

**housing wage:** The amount a person working full time must earn to pay for a two-bedroom rental unit at fair market rent.

**National School Lunch Program:** Child nutrition program started in 1946 that provides cash reimbursement to schools so they can provide a free or reduced price lunch that meets specified nutritional requirements.

**nonentitlement programs:** Programs that compete for funds through the congressional appropriation process and establish eligibility requirements for recipients.

**nutrition monitoring:** An ongoing description of nutrition conditions in the population with particular attention to subgroups defined in socioeconomic terms, for purposes of planning, analyzing the effects of policies and programs on nutrition problems, and predicting future trends.

**Nutrition Services Incentive Program (NSIP):** Provides incentives to states and tribes for the effective delivery of nutritious meals to older adults. The USDA provides cash and/or commodities to supplement meals provided under the authority of the Older Americans Act (OAA).

**School Breakfast Program:** Provides a nutritious breakfast to children in participating schools or institutions.

**Senior Farmers' Market Nutrition Program (SFMNP):** Provides low-income older persons coupons that can be used to purchase locally grown fresh, unprepared fruits, vegetables, and herbs at farmers' markets, roadside stands, and community-supported agriculture programs.

**Special Milk Program:** Provides milk to school-age children in childcare centers and in schools or institutions where there is no School Lunch Program.

**Summer Food Service Program:** Provides nutritious meals to children during summer as a substitute for the National School Lunch and School Breakfast Programs.

**Supplemental Nutrition Assistance Program (SNAP):** A federal entitlement program established in 1964 as the Food Stamp Program and administered by the USDA to give more food-buying power to low-income persons or families through monthly allotments of stamps.

**Supplemental Nutrition Assistance Program Nutrition Education (SNAP-Ed):** Provides educational programs that help all SNAP recipients make healthy food choices consistent with the most recent dietary advice as reflected in the *Dietary Guidelines for Americans* and MyPlate.

**Temporary Assistance for Needy Families (TANF):** A program created by 1996 welfare reform to replace Aid to Families with Dependent Children (AFDC). It is the major source of funding for cash welfare for needy families with children. There are federal requirements about work and time limits for families receiving assistance.

**The Emergency Food Assistance Program (TEFAP):** Distributes commodities to state agencies (food banks), which distribute the foods to the public, including homeless people via soup kitchens and food pantries.

**WIC:** The Special Supplemental Nutrition Program for Women, Infants, and Children was established in 1972 to improve the nutritional status of medically high-risk pregnant and lactating women as well as children up to 5 years of age from low-income families. WIC is funded through the USDA.

**WIC Farmers' Market Nutrition Program:** Provides fresh, unprepared, locally grown fruits and vegetables to WIC participants; also expands the awareness, sales, and use of farmers' markets.

**working poor:** Those who spent at least 27 weeks in the labor force (working or looking for work), but whose income is below the official poverty threshold.

# References

1. Jung Sun L, and Frongillo, E.A. Understanding needs is important for assessing the impact of food assistance program participation on nutritional and health status in U.S. elderly persons. *J Nutr.* 2001;131:765-773.

2. Hess AF. Newer aspects of some nutritional disorders. *JAMA.* 1921;76:693-700.

3. Atwater WO. *Food: Nutritive Value and Cost.* Washington, DC: USDA;1894. No. 23.

4. Langer PL. *History of Goitre: In Endemic Goitre.* Geneva, Switzerland: World Health Organization;1960.

5. Center Disease Control and Prevention. Achievements in public health, 1900-1999: Safer and healthier foods. 1999. www.cdc.gov/epo/mmwr/preview. Accessed April 15, 2005.

6. Kaufman M. *Nutrition in Promoting the Public's Health: Strategies, Principles, and Practice.* Burlington, MA: Jones and Bartlett; 2009.

7. Economic Research Service/USDA. Household food security in United States. *USDA's Thrifty Food Plan.* 2016; https://www.cnpp.usda.gov/sites/default/files/CostofFoodDec2016.pdf. Accessed February 20, 2017.

8. Andrew M, Scott L, Lino M. Using USDA's Thrifty Food Plan to assess food availability and affordability - United States Department of Agriculture. 2001. http://www.findarticles.com/p/articles/mi_m3765/is_2_24/ai_80517266. Accessed April 1, 2016.

9. Kaufman M. *Nutrition in Public Health A Handbook for Developing Programs and Services.* Rockville, MD: Aspen; 2007.

10. US Department of Agriculture and US Department of Health Human Services. *Dietary Guidelines for Americans.* Washington, DC: U.S. Printing Office;2000:232.

11. US Department of Agriculture. Income eligibility guidelines. 2005. http://www.fns.usda.gov/cnd/Governance/notices/iegs/IEGs.htm. Accessed April 14, 2005.

12. Nutrition and Your Health. *Dietary Guidelines for Americans.* Washington, DC: Departments of Agriculture and Health and Human Services; Home and Garden Bulletin No. 32.;2000.

13. US Department of Agriculture, US Department of Health Human Services. *Nutrition and Your Health: Dietary Guidelines for Americans.* 8th ed: Home and Garden Bulletin; 2015.

14. Sims LS. Research aspects of public policy in nutrition generating research questions to determine the impact of nutritional, agricultural, and healthcare policy and regulations on the health and nutritional status of the public. The research agenda for Dietetics Conference. In: American Dietetic Association, ed. Chicago, IL: Proceedings; 1993:25-38.

15. Caballero B, Allen L. *Encyclopedia of Human Nutrition.* 1st ed. St. Louis, MO: Elsevier Academic Press; 1999.

16. St-Onge MP, Keller KL, Heymsfield SB. Changes in childhood food consumption patterns: a cause for concern in light of increasing body weights. *Am J Clin Nutr.* 2003;78(6):1068-1073.

17. Mitchell CO, Chernoff R, eds. *Geriatric Nutrition: The Health Professional's Handbook.* 2nd ed. Gaithersburg, MD: Aspen Publishers; 1999.

18. Congress. US. *P.L. 101-445. National Nutrition Monitoring and Related Research Act of 1990.* Washington, DC: 1st Congress; October 22, 1990.

19. U.S. Department of Health and Human Services. *Ten-year comprehensive plan for the national nutrition monitoring and related research program.* and U.S. Department of Agriculture; June 11, 1993. 58:32752-32806.

20. Briefel RR. Assessment of the US diet in national nutrition surveys: national collaborative efforts and NHANES. *Am J Clin Nutr.* 1994;59:164S-167S.

21. Berdanier CD, Feldman EB, Flatt WP, St. Jeor ST. *Handbook of Nutrition and Food.* New York, NY: CRC Press LLC; 2007.

22. Centers for Disease Control and Prevention National Center for Health Statistics. *National Center for Health Statistics-at-a-Glance.* Hyattsville, MD: CDC; 2002.

23. Kuczmarski RJ, Ogden CL, Grummer-Strawn LM, Flegal KM, et al. CDC growth charts: United States. *Adv Data.* 2000;8(314):1-27.

24. Cole TJ, Bellizzi MC, Flegal KM, Dietz WH. Establishing a standard definition for child overweight and obesity worldwide: international survey. *Br Med J.* 2000;320:1240-1243.

25. Beker L. Principles of growth assessment. *Pediatr Rev.* 2006;27:196–198.

26. Ogden CL, Kuczmarski RJ, Flegal KM, Mei Z, et al. Centers for Disease Control and Prevention 2000 growth charts for the United States: improvements to the 1977 National Center for Health Statistics version. *Pediatrics.* 2002;109(1):45-60.

27. Centers for Disease Control and Prevention. How many fruits and vegetables do you need? [Fruits and Veggies More Matters]. http://www.fruitsandveggiesmorematters.org/cdc-resources/. Accessed February 20, 2017.

28. National Cholesterol Education Program (NCEP). Summary of the second expert panel of the National Cholesterol Education Program (NCEP) Expert

Panel on Detection, Evaluation, and Treatment of High Blood Cholesterol in Adults (Adult Treatment Panel II). *JAMA.* 1993;269:3015-3023.

29. National Heart L, and Blood Institute. *Sixth report of the Joint National Committee on Detection, Evaluation, and Treatment of High Blood Pressure.* Washington, DC: U.S.: DHHS Publ. No. 98-4080. Department of Health and Human Services; November, 1997.

30. Koplan J, Liverman CT, Kraak VI. *Preventing Childhood Obesity: Health in the Balance.* Washington, DC: National Academies Press; 2005.

31. Prevention CfDCa. Nutritional status of children participating in the Special Supplemental Nutrition Program for Women, Infants, and Children—United States. *1988–91. MMWR Morb Mortal Wkly Rep.* 1995;45(3):65-69.

32. Crane NT, Wilson DB, Lewis CJ, Cook DA, et al. Evaluating food fortification options: general principles revisited with folic acid. *Am J Public Health.* 1995;85:660-666.

33. Lewis C, Crane NT, Wilson DB, Yetley EA. Estimated folate intakes: data updated to reflect food fortification, increased bioavailability, and dietary supplement use. *Am J Clinical Nutr.* 1999;70:198-207.

34. Wright J, Bialostosky K, Gunter EW, Najjar MF, et al. Blood folate and vitamin B12: United States, 1988–1994. *Vital Health Stat.* 1998;11(243):1-13.

35. Institute of Medicine. *Dietary Reference Intakes for Calcium, Phosphorus, Magnesium, Vitamin D, and Flouride.* Washington, DC: National Academy Press; 1997.

36. Institute of Medicine. *Dietary Reference Intake: Folate, Other B Vitamins and Choline.* Washington, DC: National Academy Press;1998.

37. Council NR. *Diet and Health Implications for Reducing Chronic Disease Risk.* Washington, DC: National Academy Press;1989:12.

38. U.S. Department of Health and Human Services Public Health Service. Healthy People 2000 National Health Promotion and Disease Prevention Objectives. Vol PHS Publication 91-50212. Washington, DC: U.S. Government Printing Office; 1991.

39. U.S. Department of Health and Human Services. *Healthy People 2010 Understanding and Improving Health.* 2nd ed. Washington, DC: Department of Health and Human Services; 2000.

40. Sims LS. Public policy in nutrition: a framework for action. *Nutr Today.* 1993;28(2):10-20.

41. Office of Science and Technology Policy (OSTP). Meeting the Challenge: A Research Agenda for America's Health Safety and Food. Washington, DC: U.S. Government Printing Office; 1996.

42. U.S. Department of Health and Human Services. *The Surgeon General's Report on Nutrition and Health. PHS Publication No. 88-50210.* Washington, DC: U.S. Department of Health and Human Services;1988.

43. Anderson SA. The 1990 Life Sciences Research Office (LSRO) Report on Nutritional Assessment defined terms associated with food access. Core indicators of nutrtional state for difficult to sample populations. *J Nutr.* 1990;102:1559-1660.

44. Radimer K. Measurement of household food security in the USA and other industrialized countries. *Public Health Nutr.* 2002;5:859–864.

45. Life Sciences Research Office. Federation of American Societies for Experimental Biology. *J Nutr.* 1990;120S:1559-1600.

46. Canada H. What is Food Insecurity? 2016. http://proof.utoronto.ca/food-insecurity/. Accessed February 20, 2017.

47. Campbell CC, Desjardins E. A model and research approach for studying the management of limited food resources by low income families. *J Nutr Educ.* 1989;21(4):162-171.

48. Radimer KL, Olson CM, Greene JC, Campbell CC, et al. Understanding hunger and developing indicators to assess it in women and children. *J Nutr Educ.* 1992;24(1):36S-45S.

49. Radimer KL, Olson CM, Campbell CC. Development of indicators to assess hunger. *J Nutr.* 1990;120:1544-1548.

50. Nord M, Andrews M, Winicki J. Frequency and duration of food insecurity and hunger in US households. *J Nutr Educ Behav.* 2002;34(4): 194-200.

51. Furness BW, Simon PA, Wold CM, Asarian-Anderson J. Prevalence and predictors of food insecurity among low-income households in Los Angeles County. *Public Health Nutr.* 2004;7(6):791-794.

52. U.S. Department of Agriculture. Food security. www.ers.usda.gov. Accessed April 05, 2016.

53. Hamilton WL, Cook JT, Thompson WW, Buron LF, et al. *Household Food Security in the United States in 1995-Summary Report of the Food Security Measurement Project.* Washington, DC: Office of Analysis and Evaluation, Food and Consumer Service;1997.

54. Nord M, Andrew M, Carlson S. Household Food Security in the United States in 2011; https://www.ers.usda.gov/webdocs/publications/err141/30967_err141.pdf. Accessed February 20, 2017.

55. Andrews M, Nord M, Bickel G, Carlson S. *Household Food Security in the United States 1999. Food Assistance and Nutrition Research,* (FANRR-8). USDA;2000.

56. Service UER. Food Security in the United States: Conditions and Trends. https://www.ers.usda.gov/publications/pub-details/?pubid=79760. Accessed February 20, 2017.

57. Nord M, Andrews M, Carlson S. *Household Food Security in the United States, 2003*. USDA;2004. (FANRR42) 69.

58. Bogle M. Lower Mississippi Delta Nutrition Intervention Research Initiative. *Annual report* 2007. https://portal.nifa.usda.gov/web/crisproject pages/0407913-lower-mississippi-delta-nutrition-intervention-research-initiative--earline-strickland.html. Accessed February 20, 2017.

59. Coleman-Jensen A, Rabbitt MP, Gregory C, Sing A. Household Food Security in the United States in 2014. 2015. https://www.ers.usda.gov/webdocs/publications/err215/err215_summary.pdf. Accessed February 20, 2017.

60. Nord M, Brent P. Food Insecurity in Higher Income Households. 2002. https://www.ers.usda.gov/topics/food-nutrition-assistance/food-security-in-the-us/key-statistics-graphics.aspx#trends. Accessed February 20, 2017.

61. Gundersen C, Gruber J. The dynamic determinants of food insecurity. In: Andrews M, Prell M, eds. *Second Food Security Measurement and Research Conference.* Vol II: USDA, Economic Research Service; 2001.

62. Nord M, AndrewsM, Carlson S. *Household Food Security in the United States, 2002.* USDA;2003.

63. Nord M, Andrews M, Carlson S. Household Food Security in the United States, 2015. https://www.ers.usda.gov/topics/food-nutrition-assistance/food-security-in-the-us/key-statistics-graphics.aspx#trends. Accessed February 20, 2017.

64. DeNavas-Walt C, Bernadette DP, Hill L. *Current Population Reports, P60-231, Income, Poverty, and Health Insurance Coverage in the United States: 2005.* Washington, DC: U.S. Census Bureau; 2006.

65. U.S. Department of Labor U.S. Bureau of Labor Statistics. A Profile of the Working Poor, 2016. https://www.bls.gov/opub/mlr/2016/home.htm. Accessed February 20, 2017.

66. Harvest AsS. Hunger Study. 2007; http://www.hungerinamerica.org/key_findings. Accessed January 1, 2016.

67. Nord M, Coleman-Jensen A, Andrews M, Carlson S. Measuring Food Security in the United States Household Food Security in the United States, 2009. http://www.ers.usda.gov/. Accessed April 1, 2016.

68. Feeding America. Hunger in America 2010 Natio National Report Prepared for Feeding America. 2010. http://feedingamerica.issuelab.org/. Accessed April 1, 2011.

69. Project HOME. Facts on homelessness. 2002. http://www.projecthome.org/Advocacy/facts.html. Accessed August 6, 2016.

70. Beal AC, Redlener I. Enhancing perinatal outcome in homeless women: the challenge of providing comprehensive health care. *Semin Perinatol.* 1995;19(4):307-313.

71. Homeless NC. How Many People Experience Homelessness? http://www.nationalhomeless.org/. Accessed April 1, 2011.

72. Johnson LJ, McCool AC. Dietary intake and nutritional status of older adult homeless women: a pilot study. *J Nutr Elder.* 2003;23(1):1-21.

73. National Low Income Housing Coalition. Housing Remains "Out of Reach" for Millions of Americans. 2006. http://www.nlihc.org/oor2004_new/press release.htm. Accessed August 6, 2005.

74. Tarasuk VT, Dachner N, Li J. Homeless youth in toronto are nutritionally vulnerable. *J Nutr.* 2005;135(8):1926-1933.

75. Luder E, Ceysens-Okada E, Koren-Roth A, Martinez-Weber C. Health and nutrition survey in a group of urban homeless adults. *J Am Diet Assoc.* 1990;90(10):1387-1392.

76. Drake MM. The nutritional status and dietary adequacy of single homeless women and their children in shelters. *Public Health Rep.* 1992;107(3):312-319.

77. Whit MC, Tulsky JP, Dawson C, Zolopa AR. Association between time homeless and perceived health status among the homeless in San Francisco. *J Community Health.* 1997;22(4):271.

78. United States Conference of Mayors-Sodexho-USA. Hunger and homelessness survey. http://www.usmayors.org/. Accessed February 20, 2017.

79. Nord M. Food security in the United States. https://www.ers.usda.gov/topics/food-nutrition-assistance/food-security-in-the-us/. Accessed February 20, 2017.

80. Miller CL, Spittal PM, Frankish JC, Li K, et al. HIV and hepatitis C outbreaks among high-risk youth in Vancouver demands a public health response. *Can J Public Health.* 2005;96(2):107-108.

81. Jones-DeWeever A, Peterson J, Xue S. Before and After Welfare Reform: The Work and Well-Being of Low-Income Single Parent Families. 2003. http://www.iwpr.org/publications/pubs/before-and-after-welfare-reform-the-work-and-well-being-of-low-income-single-parent-families. Accessed February 20, 2017.

82. Casey PP. Maternal depression, changing public assistance, food security, and child health status. *Pediatrics.* 2004;113(2):298-304.

83. Bartlett SJ, Kolodner K, Butz AM, Eggleston P, et al. Maternal depressive symptoms and emergency department use among inner-city children with asthma. *Arch Pediatr Adolesc Med.* 2001;155: 347-353.

84. Heneghan AM, Silver EJ, Bauman LJ, Stein REK. Do pediatricians recognize mothers with depressive symptoms? *Pediatrics.* 2000;106: 1367-1373.

85. Lanzi RG, Pascoe JM, Keltner B, Ramey SL. Correlates of maternal depressive symptoms in a national Head Start Program sample. *Arch Pediatr Adolesc Med.* 1999;153:801-807.

86. Smith LA, Wise PH, Chavkin W, Romero D, et al. Implications of welfare reform for child health: emerging challenges for clinical practice and policy. *Pediatrics.* 2000;106:1117-1125.

87. United States Department of Labor Statistics. Employment Characteristics of Families Summary. 2007. http://www.bls.gov/news.release/famee.nr0 .htm. Accessed January 2, 2016.

88. Kaestner R, Tarlov E. Changes in the welfare caseload and the health of low-educated mothers. *J Policy Analysis Manage.* 2006;25(3):623–643.

89. Haskins R. Effects of welfare reform on family income and poverty. In: Bland R, Haskins R, eds. *The New World of Welfare* . Washington, DC: Brookings Institute Press; 2001.

90. Soss J, Sanford, FA. Public transformed: Welfare reform as policy feedback. *Am Polit Sci Rev.* 2007;101:111–127.

91. Nnakwe N. Dietary pattern and prevalence of food insecurity among low-income families participating in food assistance programs in midwest. *Fam Consum Sci Res J.* 2008;36:229-242.

92. Pati S, Romero D, Chavkin W. Changes in use of health insurance and food assistance programs in medically underserved communities in the era of welfare reform: an urban study. *Am J Public Health.* 2002;92(9):1441–1445.

93. Porter K, Dupree A. *Poverty Trends for Families Headed by Working Single Mothers, 1993-1999.* Washington, DC: Center on Budget and Policy Priorities; 2001.

94. Pavetti L. Welfare Policy in Transition: Redefining the Social Contract for Poor Citizen Families with Children. *Focus.* 2000;21(2):44-50.

95. Lyter D. *Education and Job Training Build Strong Families.* Washington, DC: Institute for Women's Policy Research; 2002.

96. O'Neill MK, Primus W. Recent data trends show welfare reform to be a mixed success: significant policy changes should accompany reauthorization. *Rev Policy Res.* 2005;22(3):301–324.

97. Kendall A, Olson CM, Frongillo EA. Relationship of hunger and food insecurity to food availability and consumption. *J Am Diet Assoc.* 1996;96:1019-1024.

98. Wilde P. Strong economy and welfare reforms contribute to drop in food stamp rolls. *Food Rev.* 2001;24:2-7.

99. Sonya J, Jahns L, Laraia BA, Haughton B. Lower risk of overweight in school-aged food insecure girls who participate in food assistance: results from the panel study of income dynamics child development supplement. *Arch Pediatr Adolesc Med.* 2003;157:780-784.

100. Frank GC. *Community Nutrition: Applying Epidemiology to Contemporary Practice.* Rockville, MD: Aspen; 2007.

101. Economic Research Service USDA. Supplemental Nutrition Assistance Program. http://www.fns .usda.gov/snap/. Accessed April 5, 2016.

102. Rowe G. *Assessing the New Federalism: Welfare Rules Databook.* Washington, DC: State TANF policies as of July 1999: Urban Institute;2000.

103. Zedlewski SR. Family economic resources in the post-reform era. *Future Child.* 2002;12:120-145.

104. Bartlett S, Burstein N, Andrews M. Supplemental Nutrition Assistance Program access study: eligible nonparticipants. http://www.fns.usda.gov/snap/. Accessed April 3, 2016.

105. Drewnowski A, Eichelsdoerfer P. Can low-income Americans afford a healthy diet? *Nutr Today.* 2009;44(6):246–249.

106. Cason K. About Food Stamp Nutrition Education. http://www.clemson.edu/fsne/about_fsne.php. Accessed July 26, 2016.

107. Anding J, Fletcher RD, Van Laanen P, Supak C. The food stamp nutrition education program's impact on selected food and nutrition behaviors among Texans. *J Extension.* 2001;39(6):1-10.

108. Perez-Escamilla R, Rerris AM, Haldeman L. Food stamps are associated with food security and dietary intake of inner-city preschoolers form hartford, Connecticut. *J Nutr.* 2000;130:2711-2717.

109. Campbell MK, Farrell D, Carbone E, Brasure M. Effects of a tailored multimedia nutrition education program for low income women receiving food assistance. *Health Educ Res.* 1999;14:246-256.

110. Food and Nutrition Service. Food Distribution Programs. 2005. http://www.fns.usda.gov/fdd/. Accessed August 9, 2016.

111. Food and Nutrition Service. Commodity Supplemental Food Program. 2005. http://www.fns.usda .gov/fdd/programs/csfp/pfs-csfp.pdf. Accessed August 9, 2016.

112. Service FN. Food Distribution Program on Indian Reservations. 2005. http://www.fns.usda

.gov/fdd/programs/fdpir/pfs-fdpir.pdf. Accessed August 9, 2016.

113. U.S. Department of Agriculture Food and Nutrition Service. Nutrition Services Incentive Program. 2007; http://www.fns.usda.gov/fdd/programs/nsip/. Accessed February 9, 2016.

114. Food Nutrition Service. FNS Commodity Disaster Program. http://www.fns.usda.gov/fdd/programs/fd-disasters/CommodityDisasterManual.pdf. Accessed April 3, 2016.

115. Grosvenor MB, Smolin LA. *Nutrition form Science to life*. New York, NY: Harcourt College; 2002.

116. Food and Nutrition Service. 2016. http://schoolmeals.nal.usda.gov. Accessed April 18, 2016.

117. Food and Nutrition Service. National School Nutrition Programs. http://www.fns.usda.gov/cnd/. Accessed February 20, 2017.

118. U.S Department Department of Agriculture Food and Nutrition Service. National School Lunch Program. https://www.fns.usda.gov/nslp/national-school-lunch-program-nslp. Accessed February 20, 2017.

119. Program NYS. 2016. http://www.nyscorp.org/nysp/home.html. Accessed August 10, 2016.

120. USDA. Child and Adult Care Food Program. http://www.fns.usda.gov/pd/ccsummar.htm. Accessed April 3, 2016.

121. USDA FN. Women, Infants, and Children. 2016. https://www.fns.usda.gov/wic/about-wic-wic-glance. Accessed February 20, 2017.

122. Food Nutrition Service. Senior Farmers' Market Nutrition Program. 2016. http://www.fns.usda.gov/wic/SeniorFMNP/SeniorFMNPoverview.htm. Accessed August 10, 2016.

123. U.S Department of Agriculture. Expanded Food and Nutrition Education Program. 2016. http://www.csrees.usda.gov/nea/food/efnep/about.html. Accessed February 20, 2017.

124. Cooperative State Research E, and Extension Service,. Expanded Food and Nutrition Education Program Success Stories - Collaboration. http://www.csrees.usda.gov/nea/food/efnep/success-collaboration.html. Accessed February 20, 2017.

125. Administration on Aging Department of Health and Human Services. The Elderly Nutrition Program. http://www.aoa.gov/. Accessed March 21, 2016.

126. Conrey EJ. Integrated program enhancements increased utilization of Farmers' Market Nutrition Program. *J Nutr.* 2003;133(6):1841-1844.

127. National Library of Medicine and the National Institutes of Health. Nutrition for Senior. https://www.nih.gov/health-information. Accessed February 20, 2017.

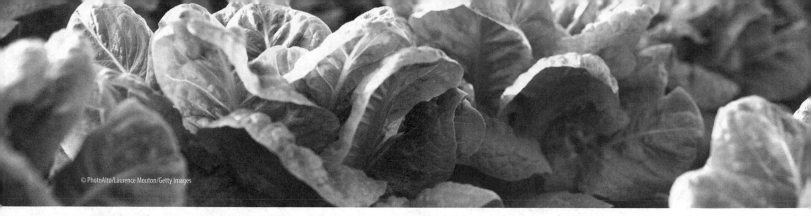

# CHAPTER 5

# Cultural Influences and Public Health Nutrition

## CHAPTER OUTLINE

- Introduction
- U.S. Cultural Demographics
- Health Disparities in the United States
- Culture, Race, and Ethnicity
- Developing Cultural Competence in Community Nutrition
- Dietary Acculturation
- Barriers to Multicultural Health Promotion and Disease Prevention
- The Importance of Communication
- Designing Health Promotion Programs for Multicultural Groups
- Strengthening Organizational Cultural Competence
- Dietary Patterns of Different Cultural Groups in the United States

## LEARNING OBJECTIVES

- Discuss different determinants of health.
- List different acculturation scales for developing health promotion programs for multicultural groups.
- Discuss different components of cultural competency.
- Identify different ways of acquiring cultural competency.
- Identify barriers to multicultural health promotion and disease prevention.
- Explain the historical food habits of different ethnic groups and their influence on current dietary practices.
- Discuss the dietary patterns of different cultural groups in the United States.

# ▶ Introduction

In the past few decades, an influx of refugees has come into the United States due to political, social, cultural, religious, and economic oppression in Central America, South America, the Caribbean Islands, Eastern Europe, Africa, and Southeast Asia.[1,2] The life of immigrants is laden with difficulties, such as going from an old to a new way of life, learning a new language, and adapting to a new climate, new attire, new foods, and new culture. In addition, they have to choose new foods from large supermarkets, and traditional foods may be expensive, if available. They also have to use new high-tech kitchen equipment to prepare foods. Hence, they need support and culturally appropriate nutrition education to improve their diets, break the cultural barriers, and experience healthy, productive lives. However, there are not enough ethnically and linguistically diverse community nutritionists and other healthcare professionals to help reduce the cultural barriers these immigrants experience.[3]

Community and public health nutritionists are in a position to work with a variety of different cultures and are faced with the challenge of providing services to different cultural groups they may have never previously met. The challenge of serving multicultural groups in a rapidly changing population accentuates the importance of cultural competence skills. As people become acculturated in the United States, their dietary habits begin to change from whole-grain to high fat intake, and, consequently, chronic health conditions begin, such as obesity and heart disease. Community nutritionists need to have strategies that can bridge the cultural gaps and prevent malnutrition and other nutrition-related health conditions. This chapter discusses health disparities, cultural competence, and the dietary patterns of different cultural groups in the United States.

# ▶ U.S. Cultural Demographics

The world is now smaller, and the United States is an ethnically diverse country. People from around the world have joined Native Americans and Mexican indigenes in the United States. According to the 2010 census, the United States' total population was approximately 308.7 million people, an overall increase of 9.7 percent from the 281.4 million in 2000. The fastest growing population group is Hispanics. The total number of Hispanics was estimated to be 50.5 million in the 2010 census, an increase of 43 percent from their total of 35.3 million in the 2000 census. African Americans, including those who declared mixed backgrounds, totaled 38.9 million persons, an increase of 12.3 percent since the 2000 census.[4] People of Asian backgrounds are also a fast-growing group. The numbers of other racial groups, including Native Americans, Alaskan natives, and Pacific Islanders, are increasing as well.[4] In 2000, the U.S. Census Bureau provided data on the U.S. foreign-born population by region of birth. These data are presented in **FIGURE 5-1**.

Due to the demographic diversity in the United States, community nutritionists should build nutrition education programs based on their clients' cultural food preferences and customs and use culturally appropriate nutrition education materials to improve the quality of their clients' diets. The use of pictorial graphics such as MyPlate and illustrations of traditional foods to communicate nutrition messages has been effective. Pictures and educational material should be field tested with the target audience to determine whether the educational materials are acceptable and easy to comprehend. Also, nutritionists should not assume that all clients are able to read, either in English or in their native language, or that they understand basic nutrition and health information, including food labels, food preparation education (e.g., meal and/or infant formula preparation, etc.), and dietary plans. Community nutritionists should consider these barriers when providing educational interventions and materials. Simple, informal methods are available that can identify individuals with low English proficiency without causing embarrassment to the client. Methods include asking open-ended questions about the materials received, listening to the individual's comments, and asking the clients if they need an interpreter. The following are ideas that can serve as a starting point for providing effective nutrition education programs to culturally diverse groups[1]:

- Assess common cultural food patterns.
- Complete an individual assessment to determine the main foods that the clients eat regularly.
- Determine the nutrient content of these foods.
- Determine the main food preparation methods of these foods.

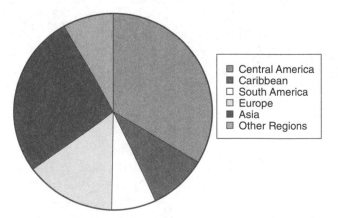

**FIGURE 5-1** U.S. foreign born population by region of birth.

Legend:
- Central America
- Caribbean
- South America
- Europe
- Asia
- Other Regions

- Before introducing new foods, emphasize familiar or comparable foods.
- Know about program eligibility criteria for federal or state assistance programs and make referrals as needed.

# ▶ Health Disparities in the United States

Health is defined as the status of an individual's condition (i.e., the presence or absence of a health condition or illness, such as high blood pressure, asthma, obesity, drug use, etc.) and the individual's state of complete physical, mental, and social well-being. Health care refers to the process of treating an illness or injury.[5] Health disparities are the differences in the incidence, prevalence, mortality, and burden of diseases and other adverse health conditions that exist among specific population groups in the United States.[6,7] Disagreements exist about the definition and use of the terms *health disparity, inequality*, and *inequity*.[8] The definition of these terms can have important practical consequences; it determines the measurements that are monitored by governments and international agencies and the activities that will be supported by resources allocated to address health disparities.[9] It also reflects different political ideas. The definition of disparities can be reviewed at https://www.healthypeople.gov/2020/about /foundation-health-measures/Disparities.

Healthy People 2010 is a comprehensive national health promotion and disease prevention agenda. Two broad goals were established with the intent to affect the health of U.S. citizens—to increase quality and years of life and eliminate health disparities.[10] The current attention to health disparities is in response to significant evidence that many minority populations are being disproportionately affected by major health problems. According to a comprehensive study by the Institute of Medicine (IOM), evidence of racial and ethnic disparities in health care were consistent and remained even after adjustments were made for socioeconomic differences and healthcare access–related factors.[11] The study further reported that health disparities were associated with poor outcomes for minority populations.[12] The IOM report also stated that "racial and ethnic disparities occurred in the context of broader historic and contemporary social and economic inequality and evidence of persistent racial and ethnic discrimination in many sectors of American life."[11]

The causes for the disparity and the determinants of health are many and have been broadly categorized by some as either avoidable or unavoidable or biological or socioeconomic/sociocultural.[12] The specific effects of these determinants, how they should be measured, and the magnitude of their effects are not well known.[13-15] In addition, recent discoveries in the area of the human genome have added to the complexity of the discussion and raised questions related to race as a specific determinant.[16,17] It has been theorized that an understanding of the molecular basis for chronic diseases and what genetic variants exist may help show what predisposes some groups to health disparities.[17] However, research indicates that there is no genetic basis for the concept of race, suggesting that race may not be a useful category.[13,18] In addition, the few genes responsible for factors such as skin color cannot be linked to genetically complex diseases such as diabetes mellitus.[13,16,17,19]

Topics covered by the objectives in Healthy People 2010 reflect the variety of critical influences that determine the health of individuals and communities. For example, individual behaviors and environmental factors are responsible for approximately 70 percent of all premature deaths in the United States.[20] Developing and implementing policies and preventive interventions that effectively address these determinants of health can reduce the burden of illness, enhance quality of life, and increase longevity.

## Race and Ethnicity

It is reported that the biological and genetic characteristics of African Americans, Hispanics, American Indians, Alaska Natives, Asians, Native Hawaiians, and Pacific Islanders do not offer any explanation about the health disparities these groups experience compared with the European American, non-Hispanic population in the United States.[21] It is believed that these disparities are due to the complex interactions among genetic variations, environmental factors, and specific health behaviors.[10,22]

Although the U.S. infant mortality rate has lowered, the infant mortality rate among African Americans is still significantly higher than that of Caucasians. In addition, heart disease death rates are over 40 percent higher for African Americans than for Caucasians.[23-25] The death rate for all cancers is 30 percent higher for African Americans than for Caucasians; for prostate cancer, it is significantly higher than for Caucasians.[26] African American women have a higher death rate from breast cancer despite mammography screening. The death rate from HIV/AIDS for African Americans is seven times higher than that of Caucasians, and the rate of homicide is six times higher than that of Caucasians.[6,23,27,28]

Hispanic Americans are two times more likely to die from diabetes compared to non-Hispanic Caucasians. In the United States, in Hispanics and other minority populations, rates of tuberculosis increased significantly in 2007.

It is also reported that Hispanics have higher rates of high blood pressure and obesity than non-Hispanic Caucasians. Research studies also show that there are differences among Hispanic populations. For example, the rate of low-birth-weight infants is lower for the total Hispanic population compared with that of Caucasians, but Puerto Ricans have a low-birth-weight rate that is up to 50 percent higher than the rate for Caucasians.[23,27,29,30]

It has been reported that American Indians and Alaska Natives have a significantly higher infant mortality rate than Caucasians. They also have two times the rate of diabetes as Caucasians.[31] The Pima tribe of Arizona has one of the highest rates of diabetes in the world. Additionally, American Indians and Alaska Natives also have significantly higher unintentional injuries and suicide death rates.[32]

It is reported that Asians and Pacific Islanders, on average, are the healthiest population groups in the United States. However, results from a national survey found that the same proportions of Asian and non-Hispanic Americans have diabetes, but after accounting for the lower body mass index (BMI) of Asians, the adjusted prevalence of diabetes was 60 percent higher in Asian Americans.[33] New cases of hepatitis and tuberculosis also are higher in Asians and Pacific Islanders in the United States than for Caucasians.[32] A great diversity exists within the Asian population group, and there are differences in health disparities for some specific segments of the group. For instance, women of Vietnamese origin have cervical cancer at about five times the rate for European American women.[23,34]

## Socioeconomic Factors

Socioeconomic factors may contribute to health and illness among minority groups. For instance, Gordon-Larsen et al.[35] reported that minority groups with lower socioeconomic status had reduced access to facilities, which in turn was associated with decreased physical activity and increased overweight and subsequently chronic health conditions such as diabetes and heart disease. Also, individuals with lower socioeconomic status do not have similar opportunities for education, occupation, and income as do those with higher socioeconomic status. According to the U.S. Census Bureau, there are more European American families (accounts for 72 percent of the population) than minorities who are below poverty level; however, the concentration of poor minority families is greater. For example, European American families represent 8.5 percent of those in poverty, whereas African Americans represent 26.4 percent and Hispanics represent 27.0 percent. The negative impact of poverty and nutritional status is well documented.[36,37]

One research study measured the difference between dietary intake and eating habits across socioeconomic

groups. For the study, 116 participants from a high socioeconomic group and 206 from a low socioeconomic group were recruited. Results showed that participants in the low socioeconomic status group were less educated and less physically active. Dietary intake among the participants in the low socioeconomic group was significantly lower in protein, monounsaturated fat, and most vitamins and minerals (thiamine, riboflavin, niacin, vitamin C, calcium, magnesium, and iron). In the low socioeconomic group, the main contributors to energy intake were breads, oils, and sugars. The participants in the low socioeconomic group consumed more oils, fats, and citrus fruits, whereas participants in the high socioeconomic group consumed more dairy products, grains, and legumes.[38] Overall, the study found that the participants in the low socioeconomic group consumed a poorer quality diet.

Another effect of the socioeconomic factor is the obesity–hunger paradox. Both obesity and hunger (and, more broadly, food insecurity) are serious public health problems, sometimes coexisting in the same person within the same household.[39] This phenomenon is called the *hunger–obesity paradox*.[40,41] This trend is supported by published scientific literature and research studies, including a study by Drewnowski and Darmon[42] that showed the highest rates of obesity and diabetes in the United States were among the lower income groups. The observed links between obesity and socioeconomic position may be related to dietary energy density and energy cost. Refined grains, added sugars, and fats are among the lowest cost sources of dietary energy. They are inexpensive, taste good, and are convenient. In contrast, the more nutrient-dense lean meats, fish, fresh vegetables, and fruit are more expensive.[42] Another study using the nationally representative 1994 to 1996 Continuing Survey of Food Intakes by Individuals (CSFII) sample of 4,537 women and 5,004 men showed that the prevalence of overweight among women increased as food insecurity increased from 34 percent for those who were food secure to 41 percent for those who were mildly food insecure, to 52 percent for those who were moderately food insecure.[41]

The coexistence of obesity and hunger seems contradictory, but individuals lacking the resources to purchase adequate and high-quality foods can still be overweight, for various reasons that researchers now are beginning to understand. The possible explanation for this phenomenon is that, among the mix of coping strategies, food quality is affected before the quantity of food intake. It is possible that households would spend less by purchasing lower quality or less of a variety of foods instead of reducing the quantity of food eaten. Consequently, although families get enough food to avoid feeling hungry, they also are poorly nourished because they cannot afford consistently adequate diets that promote health and prevent obesity. In the short term, the stomach registers that it is full, not whether a meal was nutritious.[43] In addition, obesity can be an adaptive response to periods when people are unable to get enough to eat. A research study showed that chronic lack of food caused people to eat more when food is available.[44] When money or Supplemental Nutrition Assistance Program (SNAP) are not available for food purchases during part of the month, people may overeat during the days when food is available. Over time, this cycle can result in weight gain and subsequent obesity.[42]

## Income and Education

Inequalities in income and education contribute significantly to health disparities in the United States. They are fundamentally linked and serve as alternative measures for each other.[45] Generally, the segment of the population that experiences the worst health status also has the highest poverty rates and is the least educated. Chronic health conditions such as heart disease, diabetes, obesity, elevated blood lead levels, and low birth weight are linked to low income and education status and to illness and death.[23,46] Higher incomes provide the opportunity for individuals to have access to medical care, quality housing, and safer neighborhoods and the ability to participate in health-promoting behaviors.[23,28,31,45]

## Rural Versus Urban

Rural areas are places with fewer than 2,500 residents. Approximately 25 percent of Americans live in rural areas. A metropolitan (or urban) area is made up of many different cities. For example, the Paris metropolitan area includes 1,300 cities, the New York metropolitan area includes more than 700 cities, and the St. Louis metropolitan area includes about 400 cities. It is reported that heart disease, cancer, and diabetes rates are significantly higher in rural areas than urban areas. The reason for high rates of chronic diseases and subsequent death is irregular use of preventive screening services and lack of exercise. Timely access to emergency services and the availability of specialty care are other health-related issues for the rural segment of the population. In addition, rural residents have fewer physicians and nurses and more transportation barriers than urban residents; they visit physicians less often and later in the course of an illness than urban residents.[10,23]

## Biology and Behaviors

The interaction between an individual's biology and behaviors influences health, as does the interaction with the individual's social and physical environments. Also, the quality of health can be improved by providing

**Determinants of Health**

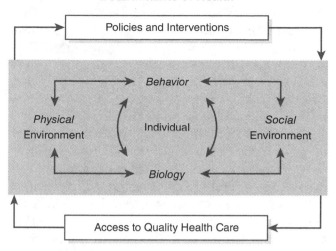

**FIGURE 5-2** The different determinants of health.

Data from: Office of Disease Prevention and Health Promotion, U.S. Department of Health and Human Services. www.healthy people.gov/document/html/uih/uih_2.htm#goals. Accessed October 25, 2007.

access to quality health care, making policies, and providing intervention programs that target factors related to individuals and their environments. **FIGURE 5-2** presents the interactions among different determinants of health.[10,23,28] Biology in the context of Figure 5-2 means the individual's genetic makeup, family history (which may suggest risk for disease), and the physical and mental health problems attained during life. However, it is reported that such factors as aging, diet, physical activity, smoking, stress, alcohol or illicit drug abuse, injury or violence, or an infectious or toxic agent may cause illness or disability and can produce a "new" biology.[11,23]

*Behaviors* are the way individuals respond or react to internal stimuli and external conditions. There may be a link between behaviors and biology (each can react to the other). For instance, smoking (behavior) can alter the cells in the lungs and result in shortness of breath, emphysema, or cancer (biology), which may cause an individual to quit smoking (behavior). Equally, a family history of cancer or heart disease (biology) may induce an individual to develop good eating habits, avoid the use of tobacco or drugs, and maintain an active lifestyle (behaviors) that may subsequently prevent the development of heart disease or cancer (biology).[23]

Other factors also can shape an individual's behavior, including social and physical environments. The social and physical environments are factors that influence the life of individuals, positively or negatively, over which they do not have immediate or direct control.[10,23] The social environment provides a sense of well-being when an individual interacts with family, friends, coworkers, and others in the community. It includes social institutions such as law enforcement, the workplace, places of worship, and schools. Other components of the social environment include housing, culture, public transportation, and the presence or absence of violence in the community.[23] Studies show that social environment is linked with morbidity, mortality, and chronic disease (e.g., heart disease, cancer). At the same time, individuals and their behaviors contribute to the quality of the social environment. Individual contributions include lack of physical activity, the use of tobacco, excessive consumption of alcohol, and poor dietary habits.[23,47]

The physical environment refers to that which can be seen, touched, heard, smelled, and tasted. It provides an opportunity for individuals and the community to be exposed to harmful situations such as toxic substances, irritants, infectious agents, and physical hazards in homes, schools, and worksites. The physical environment also can promote good health, for instance, by providing clean and safe places for people to work, exercise, and play.[23,48] The presence of a playground might promote active behavior, whereas a busy street might discourage active behavior and consequently lead to obesity.[48]

*Policies and interventions* can influence the health of individuals and the community. Examples of these policies and intervention efforts are health promotion campaigns to increase the intake of fruits and vegetables, quit smoking, and prevent cancer; policies mandating child restraints and safety belt use in automobiles; infectious disease prevention services, such as the immunization of children, adolescents, and adults; healthy school lunch and breakfast programs to prevent malnutrition; physical activity programs; and clinical services, such as better mental health care. All of these have positive effects on health. Policies and interventions are implemented by a variety of state and federal agencies—such as the state public health department and the U.S. Department of Health and Human Services—that promote individual and community health. These activities can be conducted using churches, community-based organizations, civic groups, and businesses.[49]

The community and individuals' health also depends on the availability of quality health care. High-quality health care is essential in the effort to eliminate health disparities and increase the quality and years of healthy life for all Americans. Health care includes the services received through healthcare providers, as well as health information and services received through other sources in the community.

In the determinants of health, individual biology and behavior, physical and social environments, policies and interventions, and access to high-quality health care have a significant effect on the health of individuals, communities, and the nation.[49]

## The Role of Dietetics Professionals

Whether the causes of these disparities are biological or environmental, the role of the dietetics professional in

lessening them is essential. According to Harris-Davis and Haughton, 50.4 percent of the registered dietitians they surveyed provided services to individuals who were "culturally different from themselves" or from other racial and/or ethnic groups.[50] This percentage is likely to increase. This makes it vital that dietitians in acute care settings and in primary prevention efforts acquire cultural competence and awareness in order to make a significant impact on minorities' health and life.[12]

General health status, birth outcomes, and diseases such as diabetes, obesity, hypertension, and coronary heart disease are related to diet and lifestyle, and dietitians have the nutritional science expertise to provide the appropriate care. However, it can be difficult to acquire the awareness and skills needed to work effectively with diverse populations.[12]

## ▶ Culture, Race, and Ethnicity

The concepts of culture, race, and ethnicity play a significant part in understanding human behavior, and these three concepts are frequently used inaccurately. Nutritionists are expected to understand the meaning of each when providing nutritional care to clients of diverse cultures.

**Culture** is defined in different ways, such as the customary beliefs, social norms, and material traits of a racial, religious, or social group.[51,52] Culture is an element of ethnicity that includes shared ideals, values, and assumptions about life that characterize a particular group of people. It includes technology, art, symbols, beliefs, and science, as well as moral systems and characteristic behaviors and habits.[51,52] It is a continuous, slow process that develops and changes over time. Culture provides guidance to solving life's problems in response to the needs of a cultural group's members and environment.[51]

Every culture has an organizational arrangement that differentiates it from others and provides the structure for what members of the cultural group determine to be proper or improper behavior. Culture provides strength and stability, but is not static. The organizational rudiments include, but are not limited to, child-rearing practices, dietary habits, religious practices, family structure and values, and attitudes. People learn about their culture from parents, teachers, religious and political leaders, and respected peers.[52,53]

**Race** is a social classification that relies on physical markers, such as skin color, to identify group membership.[52] There is the possibility that individuals may be of the same race, but have different cultures. Although they are a mixed group, they are often seen as culturally and racially identical. Commonly, many cultural differences of individuals from different countries are overlooked because of their similar racial characteristics.[52]

**Ethnicity** implies one or more of the following: shared origins or social background; shared, distinctive culture and traditions that are maintained between generations; and shared culture that contributes to a sense of identity and group. Most policy makers emphasize some sort of cultural distinctiveness as the mark of an **ethnic** group.[52,54]

# ▶ Developing Cultural Competence in Community Nutrition

Food is a source of nutrients needed for life. However, if food is considered only as this basic concept, the important subtleties that influence what people eat will be missed.[55,56] It would be convenient if achieving adequate nutrition for people meant defining the requirements for each person according to age and sex and then providing the nutrients in the correct amounts via supplements. Unfortunately, this approach would deprive people of the pleasures that food adds to their lives. Favorite flavors, textures, and aromas (especially when provided in familiar and preferred recipes) give immediate pleasure and stir up happy memories of people and places associated with these foods.[57] Every individual in a community has a history, and most of the time this translates to eating habits influenced by culture.[58,59] Religion is a particularly strong factor in cultural identity. Sharing common beliefs and practices that are central to a particular religion creates common threads that bind people together into a culture.[57,58]

Cultural food practices affect tastes, preferences, shopping habits, manners, communication, and personal interactions. As people from varying backgrounds become acculturated into U.S. society, dietary habits tend to change from a pattern based on whole grains and vegetables to foods that are higher in fats and sugars.[56,58] Dietetic professionals need to be sensitive to what might be considered acceptable or unacceptable by persons from different cultures by providing advice to each individual within a cultural perspective. For instance, a dietitian's advice to reduce using lard or pork may be perceived as unrealistic by many Mexican Americans because they are widely used in traditional recipes.[56,60] Community nutritionists in the United States need to be able to work with people and their total humanness, not just what they eat.

**Cultural competence** is defined as understanding the importance of social and cultural influences on individuals' health beliefs and behaviors, considering how these factors interact at multiple levels of the healthcare delivery system, and devising interventions that take these issues into account to ensure high-quality care.[61,62]

It is also the ability to work effectively with individuals from different cultural and ethnic backgrounds. Cultural competence requires a continuous developmental process that involves a long-term commitment and significant efforts in acquiring the skills, practices, and attitudes toward becoming culturally competent. However, it is important to acknowledge that a nutritionist must undergo many steps to achieve cultural competency. The integration of this knowledge into day-to-day practice takes effort and time. Practitioners in the healthcare system in locations where cultural competency was not necessary until recently may resist adopting new ideas. In addition, cultural competency is complex and multifaceted, and many facets change over time, such as demography, immigration history, poverty status, and policies.

An example of how to design a culturally competent program is a study conducted by the University of Michigan called Healthy Eating and Physical Activity for Arab-American Women. It was the nutrition part of the University of Michigan's Program for Multicultural Health. The aim of this program was to provide a culturally appropriate nutrition education to Arab-American women and reduce their risk for chronic diseases. The researchers carried out a needs assessment to determine culturally preferred foods and any challenges to modifying the participants' diet for optimal health. The main finding of the assessment was that most of the participants were not drinking enough water daily. Resources and tips on how to increase daily water consumption were provided to the participants. In addition, the participants were given a tour of a Middle Eastern grocery store to help them modify their diets. The project also included a cooking demonstration with the chef using culturally appropriate foods. For more information visit the website http://www.med.umich.edu/multicultural/projects/past.htm.

Another approach community nutritionists can use to work with a diverse population is to use professional interpreters who are fluent in the language and are familiar with the culture of the participants. It is not advisable to use nonprofessional interpreters such as the participant's child, friend, housekeeping staff, husband or wife, or other relatives because confidentiality may be compromised and/or the participant may be uncomfortable discussing personal issues. If an interpreter is not available, the nutritionist can use the AT&T Language line through the operator, which gives 24-hour service in 140 languages.

Developing cultural competence is an ongoing life process.[63] There are four steps to acquiring cultural competence, as follows[52,64,65]:

- Cultural awareness
- Cultural knowledge
- Cultural skill
- Cultural encounter

Cultural awareness is developing an understanding and sensitivity to another ethnic group's values, beliefs, practices, lifestyles, and problem-solving strategies. The process of acquiring cultural awareness includes an examination of one's own culture, beliefs, values, attitudes, and prejudices and how they are expressed in one's own life, and reviewing assumptions about individuals who are different.[52,66,67]

Cultural knowledge is another component that is essential for caring for a multicultural society. It involves acclimatizing to selected cultural characteristics such as history, values, belief systems, and behaviors of the members of another ethnic group.[52] It means that the nutritionist understands how cultures are similar and how they are different. It provides the nutritionist with organizational elements of cultures and current information on what is necessary to provide effective health promotion.[68] Nutritionists can gain cultural knowledge by reading about the language, customs, and health beliefs of participants in the program and by keeping in mind that cultural lifestyles are constantly influenced by contemporary events, including media and interaction with other cultures. It is important to observe the health beliefs and lifestyles of the participants through conversation and participation in the community's daily life. Cultural knowledge can be acquired by knowing and maintaining relationships with culturally diverse people through traveling, books, movies, attending events held by local ethnic or cultural organizations (e.g., attending weddings, birthday parties, international fairs at universities, and religious celebrations), and maintaining an open mind.[68,69] Participating in these different events will increase trust in the nutritionist and increase his or her ability to influence health-directed behaviors.[54]

The third component in developing cultural competence is acquiring cultural skill. Cultural skill reproduces effective integration of cultural awareness and cultural knowledge to meet the participants' needs. It is also the ability of people of one culture to understand and feel comfortable with the cultures of other people. During interaction with culturally diverse people, a culturally skillful nutritionist uses appropriate gestures during conversation, is receptive to the cultural differences and responses of individuals, avoids stereotyping, and interacts respectfully with people of all cultures in a way that recognizes their worth and supports their dignity.[52,69] The culturally skillful nutritionist refrains from making judgments about cultural behaviors and practices that seem strange to him or her.

A cultural encounter is the fourth step in becoming culturally competent. It involves integrating all the cultural competency components in nutrition, health promotion, and intervention in ways that accomplish the following[52,68,69]:

- Preserve the participants' cultural values, health beliefs, and health-related practices that promote and maintain their well-being
- Place the nutritionist in situations where his or her understanding of self and the world is severely challenged, as well as how he or she thinks things "are" or "should be"
- Accommodate health-related practices that are not harmful to their health
- Repattern the participants' lifestyles for new, different, and beneficial health-directed behaviors while respecting their cultural values and health beliefs

## The Importance of Cultural Knowledge in Community Nutrition

Cultural knowledge is needed for adequate nutritional practice. In nutrition assessment, it is important to collect basic information about your community's cultures, most frequently used foods, and food preparation methods. Information needed to provide adequate nutritional guidance includes the following[70]:

- Types of food available
- Accepted and preferred foods
- Safety of the food supply and related health problems
- Energy and nutrient quality of major foods chosen
- Most commonly used foods, who selects them, and how and where they are obtained
- Food preparation methods and how they are divided among family/community
- Foods eaten, how much, when, with whom, and where
- Food storage, facilities, and methods; food safety; and garbage disposal

Other strategies that may help in the assessment include observing the neighborhood and homes where clients live and where they shop for foods, as well as the types of food available. Learn more about the group by interviewing individuals from or closely associated with the client group.[71] Ask relevant questions about food and health behaviors, or ask other healthcare professionals who serve the cultural group, community leaders among the group, and any other members of the group.

Nutrition practices are an integral part of the assessment process for all families because they contribute significantly in the development of health problems. Knowing the participants' cultural nutrition practices makes it possible to develop health promotion programs that do not conflict with cultural food practices. The cultural background of a client may affect nutritional status in many ways other than disease risk and nutrient needs. Traditional food habits are related to ethnic and religious identity and have little adverse impact on diet.[50] For example, calcium deficiency may be of concern, but sensible food habits often compensate for the noticeable lack of the nutrient. For instance, some segments of the Asian population prepare their daily soups by soaking bones in an acidified broth.[72] Latinos often prepare their tortillas with lime-slaked corn.[73] Ironically, milk-drinking Caucasians are one of the groups most often affected by osteoporosis.

However, traditional food habits also may conflict with nutritional needs. A Nigerian immigrant may consider weight gain desirable and a sign of beauty, and many cultures may consider overweight an indication of well-being.[56] Also, a Chinese American mother who still observes the precepts of yin and yang in her diet may feed her baby "neutral" foods, omitting most fruits and vegetables.[74,75] Nutritionists can use the existing organizational structure within each cultural group to plan, design, develop, and implement appropriate programs that address the needs of diverse and multicultural populations.

## ▶ Dietary Acculturation

**Acculturation** is a process by which a cultural group adapts or learns the cultural norms of another group. The process is related to age, education, frequency of interaction, and income, and it occurs on a continuum.[76] **Dietary acculturation** refers to the process that occurs when immigrants adopt the dietary practices, eating patterns, and food choices of the host country.[77] For instance, dietary acculturation for a Nigerian or Mexican immigrant to the United States may be characterized by increased meat consumption and decreased consumption of whole grains, fruits and vegetables, and legumes.[78] The host country, the United States, in turn often adopts some of the foods and dietary practices of the immigrants, as evidenced by the different ethnic supermarkets and restaurants throughout most of the United States.[79]

Dietary acculturation can result in both healthful and unhealthful dietary changes. For example, among Hispanic immigrants, drinking soda instead of traditional fruit-based beverages can be considered an unhealthful change, whereas consumption of fewer highly saturated fats (e.g., lard) is a healthful change.[80,81] Adverse nutritional consequences can result from changes made in the diet through acculturation; for example, Japanese immigrants to the United States may have an increased risk for cardiovascular disease due to a diet higher in saturated fats and cholesterol.[82] In another example, the vegetable intake of Hispanic immigrants decreased with acculturation, whereas the consumption of snacks and processed foods increased.[83,84]

Most commonly used acculturation scales and indexes have been developed and validated in social science and psychological research, and some have been applied to studies examining dietary behavior. **TABLE 5-1** shows major approaches to measuring dietary acculturation. The major limitation of the single-item measures is that they are quite general, focusing on items such as length of residence in the host country, language proficiency, and generation level.[79,85] However, these items may yield general assessment information needed for designing health promotion programs, such as dietary interventions and education programs.

Acculturation scales are considerably more comprehensive and measure several facets of exposure to the host country; therefore, they are less likely to misclassify a person's level of acculturation.[86] They do not typically include diet-specific acculturation indicators, however. In addition, most of these scales were validated against single-item measures and demographic characteristics rather than any type of gold standard.[87,88]

The food-based measures (food lists and dietary acculturation scales) assess dietary acculturation by measuring eating patterns. Therefore, they directly assess the outcome of dietary acculturation that includes adoption of the eating patterns of the host country, maintenance of traditional diets, or both. However, these food-based measures do not assess other steps or factors (e.g., psychosocial factors) in the process of acculturation, which are necessary for the design of effective dietary interventions.[75]

## Ethnocentrism and Stereotyping

Public and community dietitians need to avoid an ethnocentric perspective when working with ethnic groups. **Ethnocentrism** is a way of looking at the world through a personal lens that has been influenced by personality, genetics, family and relationships, and media. It is an important concept that keeps culture viable.[93,94] In its mildest form, ethnocentrism is a subconscious disregard for cultural differences; in its most severe form, it is an authoritarian dominance over groups different from one's own.[94] This can serve as a major obstacle in establishing and maintaining good working relationships with clients of different ethnic groups. Cross-cultural counseling skills are essential for the dietitian working with clients from different ethnic or religious backgrounds. Ethnocentricity, including personal biases and background pertaining to eating certain foods as well as assumptions about what foods are eaten and when or how many meals are eaten each day, should be considered when working with individuals from different ethnic backgrounds. Respect for cultural values and personal preference is a precondition for successful health promotion in a heterogeneous society.[95]

**TABLE 5-1** Scales and Indexes That Have Been Used to Study Dietary Acculturation Among U.S. Immigrants[76,88-92]

| Single-Item Measures of General Acculturation | Examples of Questions | Comments |
|---|---|---|
| **Residency**<br>- Length of residency in host country<br>- Length of residency in country of origin<br>- Place of birth | - How long have you lived in the United States?<br>- How long did you live in Korea?<br>- Where were you born? | - Commonly and successfully used for assessing general acculturation in many studies<br>- Provides a global measure of exposure to host culture<br>- Has the advantage of using short, factual questions that do not require interpretation by respondents<br>- Is very nonspecific and may misclassify a respondent's level of acculturation |
| **Language**<br>- Proficiency<br>- Preference | - What language do you usually speak?<br>- What language do you prefer to speak?<br>Does anyone speak a different language in your home? | - Commonly used questions that are short, simple, and nonspecific<br>- Provides valuable information for many public health and intervention settings regarding the need for interpreters and translated materials |
| **Generation Level**<br>N/A | - Where was your mother/father born? | - Simple, factual question; only indirectly measures exposure to host culture |
| **Friendship Preferences**<br>N/A | - Who do you associate with in the outside community: mostly people of your same background, U.S. citizens, or both? | - Intended to assess respondent's degree of ethnic identification with host or original culture |
| **Self-Identification**<br>N/A | - How do you identify yourself (Chinese, American, or bicultural)? | - Has the advantage of allowing participant to assess own degree of acculturation<br>- Very open to interpretation by respondents<br>- Social desirability may influence responses |
| **Acculturation Scales** | **Scale Description and Characteristics** | **Comments for All Scales** |
| Acculturation Rating Scale for Mexican Americans[91] | 20 items with 4 subscales: language, familiarity, usage, and preference; ethnic identification and generation; reading, writing, and cultural exposure; ethnic interaction | - Have widespread use in studies of acculturation and have been validated in comparison with single-item questions<br>- Assess many domains related to acculturation; they are less likely to misclassify respondents than single-item questions<br>- May be too long to be practical for some research or programmatic applications<br>- Except for the scale developed by Anderson et al.,[91] do not specifically address issues related to dietary acculturation |
| Asian Self-Identity Acculturation Scale[96] | 21 items with 6 dimensions: language, identity, friendship choices, behaviors, geographic history, and attitudes | |
| Acculturation Scale for Southeast Asians[91] | 13 items with 2 subscales: language proficiency and language, social, and food preferences | |
| Short Acculturation Scale for Hispanics[91] | 12 items with 3 subscales: language use, media preferences, and social interactions | |

| Food-Based Assessments | Scale Description and Characteristics | Comments for Both Assessments |
|---|---|---|
| **Food Lists**<br>Participants identify from a food list the foods they usually eat now versus when they were in their country of origin | Yang and Fox[89] compiled a list of 47 food items common in Chinese and U.S. cuisine. Respondents indicated (yes/no) whether they ate the foods in the past month. Scores were derived by summing the responses. | ■ Both measures assess dietary acculturation by directly measuring the outcome of dietary acculturation (i.e., traditional vs. Western eating patterns or both).<br>■ Neither assesses other steps or factors in the process of dietary acculturation.<br>■ The assessments need to be supplemented with other instruments when the objective is to design effective dietary interventions. |
| **Dietary Acculturation Scales**<br>Instruments specifically designed to measure changes in dietary patterns | Satia et al.[97] developed a list of 15 food items and dietary behaviors reflective of traditional Chinese behavior and of westernization of eating patterns and identified two subscales, Chinese and Western. Scores were derived by obtaining the mean of no missing responses for each scale. | |

Data from: Satia J, Patterson RE, Kristal AR, Hislop TG, Yasui Y, Taylor VM. Development of scales to measure dietary acculturation among Chinese-Americans and Chinese-Canadians. J Am Diet Assoc. 2001;101:548;101:548–553. Copyright Elsevier (2001).

# ▶ Barriers to Multicultural Health Promotion and Disease Prevention

Many factors can be barriers or obstructions to successful health and nutrition or disease prevention programs. For the purposes of this discussion, a barrier is any obstacle that might hinder the ability of the community nutritionist, healthcare professional, or their culturally diverse clients to achieve the intended intervention program objectives.[98] Because many potential barriers cannot easily be categorized, an attempt will be made to group some of these variables.

Different demographic factors can obstruct multicultural health-promoting activities. It is important for the nutritionist to first assess the level of acculturation and assimilation of his or her clients before implementing the intervention program because many of the identified barriers may not apply to all clients. Many of these barriers are easy to understand; a brief discussion of a few of them may help emphasize the importance of demographics when working with or planning health promotion programs for a culturally diverse group. For example, gender may become an issue when providing health promotion services such as mammography or cervical screening. Holroyd et al.[99] reported that Chinese cultural values associated with modesty and sexuality coupled with medical interpersonal and interprofessional skills of the practitioners, lack of

educational materials written in Chinese, and lack of female physicians were barriers preventing Chinese women from enrolling in health promotion screening services. The authors recommended that healthcare practitioners prepare themselves with relevant social and cultural knowledge of the population groups they serve. Information on barriers to health promotion and disease prevention in rural areas can be found at https://www.ruralhealthinfo.org/community-health/health-promotion/1/barriers.

The main language spoken also can be a barrier for health promotion programs. One study showed that despite following standard diabetes self-management recommendations to a comparable degree and receiving health care in a culturally competent setting, individuals who spoke Chinese as their preferred language, even with the use of translation services, had less baseline diabetes knowledge and showed a trend toward higher glycosylated hemoglobin (HbA1c) levels than those who spoke English as their preferred language. (Glycosylated hemoglobin level determines how well a person's diabetes is being controlled over time.) Another reason for the results was the shortage of diabetes information in the Chinese language in the United States.[99]

Geographic factors, including a lack of hospital or private physician offices in the minority group communities, as well as difficulties in accessing public transportation or getting a drivers' license; social isolation; and financial constraints also can create barriers to multicultural health promotion efforts.[100]

# ▶ The Importance of Communication

Human **communication** is defined as a social interaction of giving and receiving information for facilitating understanding and creating social connection with a common set of rules.[101] These rules indicate how the communication will be carried out, the channels in which it will be carried out, when it will happen, and how feedback may or may not be provided between the sender or encoder and a receiver or decoder. For example, in Japanese cultural beliefs, indirect communication is perceived to be more ethical than direct communication when dealing with disclosure of a serious health condition (e.g., cancer, heart disease). This is based on their motivation of not extinguishing the individual's hope to live. U.S. physicians attempting to give hope to individuals may actively engage in open communication with them about their health condition. In contrast, many Japanese believe that the concealment itself can convey concern and hope. Typically, the head of the household is the primary individual communicating with the healthcare practitioner when a family member needs medical care. Also, the head of the household is the one who makes decisions about treatment options and what the family member should be told about his or her medical condition.[102]

Many factors can affect communication in general and specifically cross-cultural encounters. These factors include the communication skills, attitudes, knowledge, social system, and culture of both the sender and receiver of communication transactions and differences in cultural values, backgrounds, biases, linguistic barriers, and dietary and healthcare beliefs and practices.[101] To communicate effectively, it is essential that nutritionists avoid stereotyping by responding to the clients as individuals within their own cultural perspective. Nutritionists must also recognize the influence of their own cultural backgrounds and attitudes. Communication is sometimes challenging with those who do not share the same cultural perspective. To communicate successfully, nutritionists need to be willing to accept the discomfort of unfamiliarity and insecurity. Overcoming this challenge requires sensitivity to cultural diversity, stereotyping, and prejudice; general skills of good communication; and skills to overcome communication barriers. In addition, human interaction factors, including dominance–submission or love–hate relationships, communication transactions, and the circumstances in which they occur, have been identified as important to understanding and improving the communication process.[103-105]

The basis for achieving health promotion and disease prevention is to understand the variations in patterns of verbal and nonverbal communication.[52] The differences of communication style among cultures are reflected in the pronunciation, word meaning, voice quality, and humor and in nonverbal styles, such as eye contact, gestures, touch, interjection during conversation, body posture, facial expression, and silence.[52] For example, when gathering data from a Hispanic woman, the community nutritionist needs to be aware that her style of communication may be low-key and the woman may avoid eye contact and be hesitant to respond to questions. This behavior should not be taken as lack of interest or inability to relate to others.[106] Also, generally Latinos sit and stand much closer to one another than most Caucasians. Therefore, stepping away from a client who seems too close may be considered offensive, especially in a counseling situation.[106,107]

Dietitians who are members of the host country's main ethnic group may have goodwill, but may be ineffective when they attempt to engage a person of a different cultural group in a relationship without questioning how culture influences interactions, interpretations of events, information, beliefs, and values concerning health and healthcare practices. Preconceived ideas such as racial or ethnic identity, religion, country of origin, gender, or sexual orientation can interfere with the dietitian's ability to relate to people as individuals. At the same time, a lack of knowledge of other cultural groups can deter dietitian's understanding of the individual's point of view. Guidelines for recognizing the multicultural context of communication include the following[108,109]:

- Make an ethnocultural assessment; this is a critical component of every evaluation.
- Allow other people to define themselves.
- Respect the language of others, and do not assume superiority in language.
- Collaborate with trained translators and health promoters (persons with the same ethnic or racial background as the individuals/groups).
- Avoid the use of racist, sexist, ageist, and other forms of condescending language.
- Do not perpetuate stereotypes in communication.
- Adapt communication to the uniqueness of the individual.
- Reject humor that degrades members based on gender, race, ethnicity, religion, sexual orientation, country of origin, and so forth.
- Do not allow injustice to continue through silence.

An integral part of any culture or geographical setting is language.[108,110] It is important to give attention to the language patterns of different ethnic groups in the community. It is equally essential to accept existing dialects as a vital part of the culture and not give the impression that the dialect is incorrect or bad. Dietitians may need to use an interpreter or members of the group to explain or clarify terms when working in areas with large numbers of non–English-speaking groups; this will prevent incorrect assumptions.[107] They also need to avoid the use of jargon, technical terms, and slang and keep information simple. Any effort shown to communicate effectively conveys to people a genuine interest in their health.[110] Whether in Charleston, South Carolina, or Brooklyn, New York, learning to listen to a dialect allows the dietitian to experience the richness of people's lives. When communicating in an ethnically diverse area, the dietitian's communication approach must project trust and genuineness so that people will be receptive to the nutrition education activity.[111]

Interviewing a key informant is another effective approach dietitians can use in gathering information from the minority group. Key informant interviews are with individuals who live or work in the community and who possess a special insight into its needs and resources. **BOX 5-1** identifies interview tips and guidelines that community nutritionists can use in obtaining information from individuals.

All cultures are not the same, but they have the same basic organizational factors. These factors must be explored in a cultural assessment because of the differences among groups. The differences include communication, background, touch, family organization, time perception, self-care practice, alternative healers, and biological variations.[112] Some of these differences among cultural groups are presented in **TABLE 5-2**.

## ▶ Designing Health Promotion Programs for Multicultural Groups

As contemporary societal and demographic environments for health care continue to change, public health leaders nationwide recognize that all health practitioners need cultural sensitivity knowledge and skills to effectively serve a multicultural population.[85] Cultural sensitivity skills enable culturally relevant programs and services to be developed and implemented. Bilingual practitioners are very important in providing nutrition programs.[52]

**Cultural sensitivity** involves a heightened knowledge of the needs of the client. Culturally sensitive nutritionists respond to and accurately interpret nonverbal or other cultural cues, as evidenced in the way they provide information to culturally diverse clients.[113] This means that nutritionists and healthcare professionals must make efforts to be aware of the possible and actual cultural factors that affect their interactions with clients. It also means that they need to be willing to design programs and materials, to implement programs, and to make recommendations that are culturally relevant

**BOX 5-1** Assessment of Dietary Practices and Food Consumption Patterns[113]

- Determine the social significance of food in the family. Do they eat alone or as a family?
- Determine the foods that are purchased often.
- Determine who is responsible for buying and preparing the foods and how the foods are prepared.
- Determine the foods considered taboo or prohibited.
- Determine the influence religion has in their food selection. Any restrictions?
- Determine the amount of food that is eaten, how often, and with whom.
- Determine the living conditions and types of restaurants they use.
- Determine whether the clients have adopted foods of other cultural groups.
- Determine the types of foods they like most.
- Determine the availability of their favorite foods and the cost.

**Interview Tips**

- Listen attentively.
- Be attentive to nonverbal cues. Display pictures, books, brochures, and posters that reflect the cultures and ethnic backgrounds of clients who are being served.
- Explain why you need the information and the benefit to the client.
- Use an interpreter. (The age of the interpreter may be of concern; for example, older clients may want a more mature interpreter.) Children tend to have limited language skills, and when spoken to may have difficulty interpreting information.
- Clarify roles with the interpreter, and explain to the client what the interpreter will be doing.
- Be patient and consider periods of silence as opportunities for reflection on what has been said.
- Remember that customs regarding touching, gestures, eye contact, and relationships vary among cultures.
- Review the situation and information to be translated before and after the interview.

Modified from: Stanhope M, Lancaster J. *Community and Public Health Nursing*. 5th ed. St. Louis, MO: Mosby; 2000.

and culturally specific, and to plan interventions that are relevant and acceptable within the cultural framework.[113,114] Although the role of culture has long been acknowledged, culture has not been a central focus of nutritional care. The nutritionist developing a culturally sensitive program must move outside the paradigm of the dominant culture.[100] He or she needs to make efforts to understand the dietary patterns of clients and not rely on the dominant group's culture.

**TABLE 5-2** Variations Among Selected Cultural Groups

| | African Americans | Asians | Hispanics | Native Americans |
|---|---|---|---|---|
| Verbal communication | Asking personal questions of someone you have just met for the first time is seen as improper and intrusive. | High levels of respect for others, especially those in positions of authority. | The expression of negative feelings is considered impolite. | Speak in a low tone of voice and expect the listener to be attentive. |
| Nonverbal communication | Direct eye contact in conversation is often considered rude. | Direct eye contact with superiors may be considered disrespectful. | Avoidance of eye contact is usually a sign of attentiveness and respect. | Direct eye contact is often considered disrespectful. |
| Touch | Touching someone else's hair is often considered offensive. | It is not customary to shake hands with persons of the opposite sex. | Touching is often observed between two persons in conversation. | A light touch of the person's hand instead of a firm handshake is often used when greeting a person. |
| Family organization | Usually have close extended family networks; women play key roles in healthcare decisions. | Usually have close extended family ties. Emphasis may be on family needs rather than individual needs. | Usually have close extended family ties; all members of the family may be involved in healthcare decisions. | Usually have close extended family; emphasis tends to be on family rather than on individual needs. |
| Time perception | Often present-oriented. Believe in harmony of mind, health, body, and spirit with nature. | Often present-oriented. Enjoy balance between the "yin" and "yang" energy forces. | Often present-oriented. Enjoy balance and harmony among mind, body, spirit, and nature. | Often past-oriented. Rely on harmony of mind, body, spirit, and emotions with nature. |
| Alternative healers | "Granny," "root doctor," voodoo priest, spiritualist. | Acupuncturist, acupressurist, herbalist. | Curandero, spiritualista, yerbo. | Medicine man, shaman. |
| Self-care practices | Poultices, herbs, oils, roots. | Hot and cold foods, herbs, teas, soups, burning, rubbing, pinching. | Hot and cold foods, herbs. | Herbs, cornmeal, medicine bundle. |
| Biological variations | Sickle cell anemia, lactose intolerance, Mongolian spots, keloid formation, inverted T waves. | Thalassemia, lactose intolerance, Mongolian spots. | Lactose intolerance, Mongolian spots. | Lactose intolerance, cleft uvula (the small piece of soft tissue that can be seen dangling down from the soft palate over the back of the tongue). |

Reproduced from Stanhope M, Lancaster J. *Community and Public Health Nursing*. 5th ed. New York: Mosby, 2000. Reprinted with permission from Elsevier.

## Planning Health Promotion and Disease Prevention Programs in Multicultural Populations

Planning health promotion and disease prevention programs in multicultural populations is a challenging process. It requires efficient identification and selection of a particular course of action. Developing and implementing a health promotion program requires the dietitian and participants to work together to accomplish a wide range of activities, including the following[100,115]:

- Assessing the needs, problems, and resources of the target population
- Developing appropriate goals and objectives
- Formulating strategies and interventions that consider the peculiarities of the clients' nutrition and health-related conditions and settings
- Implementing and monitoring the interventions
- Evaluating the outcomes
- Refining approaches for greater program effectiveness and efficiency

Given these guidelines, the community nutritionist may provide a successful intervention program using the following strategies[101,116]:

- Define the level of change wanted as a result of the program (i.e., the health education level or the health promotion level).
- Make contact attempts on varied days, evenings, and weekends.
- Identify specific health-related factors that affect the health of the target group in the community, the action strategy to be used (e.g., strengthen community action, create a supportive environment, develop personal skills), and the level of action to be taken (e.g., society, a specific sector or system, community, family, individual, etc.).
- Link cultural competence to the health promotion program.
- Identify and address sociocultural barriers (language, organizational barriers such as availability and acceptability of health care, lack of interpreter services or culturally and linguistically appropriate health education materials for members of a minority group).
- Be culturally competent when interacting and working with participants in the overall health promotion and disease prevention planning process by attending continuing multicultural education seminars and workshops.
- Know your own beliefs, values, patterns, and styles of interaction with other cultures, because they could reflect biases or prejudices that could disrupt the planning process.

## Intervention Considerations

The design of well-planned and culturally appropriate interventions is critical to the success of any health promotion and disease prevention program or service offered in a community setting. Designing intervention strategies, methods, and materials so they relate to the specific cultural characteristics of the target group needs to be an integral part of the design process.[100,115] With these ideas in mind, the community nutritionist also may consider the following additional strategies and suggestions as he or she begins the intervention phase[68,101,115-117]:

- Tailor the program to the intended target group using MyPlate, flipcharts, and brochures. If possible, print materials in the target group's language.
- Utilize the community's strengths, resources, and assets, all of which promote community ownership and involvement with the health promotion and disease prevention program.
- Involve the target group whose members will be the recipients of the program.
- Consider other factors such as issues related to being a new immigrant and linguistic, literacy, gender, and cultural factors in the design of the intervention program for the community.
- Consider using churches or places of worship as sites for conducting health promotion and disease prevention programs. However, it is not easy to involve some sites in health promotion and disease prevention efforts because many of them have their own causes, which may or may not have a health or nutrition focus.
- Take the intervention program to the community instead of asking the community to come to the intervention site.
- Use peer educators from the community. This is a very effective method for delivering health promotion and disease prevention programs or services to the community.
- Develop educational materials that reflect relevant cultural values, themes, and literacy levels of the target group.
- Develop partnerships with local media. This can be an effective way to disseminate information about the health promotion and disease prevention program or service being planned and offered to the community.

The Successful Community Strategies feature presents the University of California's Cooperative Extension culturally relevant nutrition education success story.

## Successful Community Strategies

### University of California Cooperative Extension Culturally Appropriate Nutrition Education[34,118,119]

Immigrants come to the United States seeking religious and political freedom and economic opportunities. The Vietnamese population is the fastest growing segment of the Asian/Pacific Islander population in the United States. Currently, approximately 46 percent of the Vietnamese population resides in California. From 1993 to 1996, the University of California Cooperative Extension (UCCE) received a U.S. Department of Agriculture grant to evaluate the diets of Vietnamese-speaking women who were eligible for the Special Supplemental Nutrition Program for Women, Infants, and Children (WIC) and to provide culturally appropriate nutrition education to improve their dietary quality. A secondary goal of the program was to increase interagency cooperation between the UCCE and WIC.

At the beginning of the project, 1-day joint in-service training meetings were held in each county for staff from UCCE's Expanded Food and Nutrition Education Program (EFNEP) and WIC to facilitate communication and cooperation.

A total of 112 professional and paraprofessional staff members attended the meetings. The purpose of these meetings was to educate project staff about Vietnamese foodways and culture and to introduce this joint project. At the meetings, a bicultural, bilingual Vietnamese American registered nurse spoke about traditional Vietnamese health beliefs and food practices related to pregnancy and the postpartum period, including lactation. A total of 152 homemakers were recruited to participate in a nutrition education program, with 76 receiving the intervention and 76 serving as the control group. Non–English-speaking Vietnamese American women eligible for WIC with incomes below 185 percent of the poverty level living in five California counties participated in the program.

### Intervention

For this project, five California EFNEP curriculum modules were revised and rewritten in Vietnamese by two bicultural, bilingual Vietnamese American nutritionists, one of whom was a registered dietitian. These were then translated into English so that nutrition professionals who were not literate in Vietnamese could use them with Vietnamese clients. The five modules were Nutrition for a Healthy Mother and Baby, Calcium-Rich Foods, Protein and Iron-Rich Foods, Grains, and Fruits and Vegetables. The modules emphasized the health benefits of the traditional Vietnamese diet that is rich in fruits, vegetables, and complex carbohydrates and low in fat. The modules were made culturally appropriate for the audience by integrating drawings of traditional nutrient-rich Vietnamese foods into flipchart and handout illustrations and by addressing traditional Vietnamese food practices. Information on how to purchase, store, and prepare "new" American foods from each food group was also included. Bicultural, bilingual Vietnamese American nutrition education assistants taught five to seven lessons using nutrition education materials written in the Vietnamese language. Twenty-four-hour food recalls were obtained before and after the 8-week interval on the treatment and control groups to examine if changes occurred over time in nutrient intake and nutrient density within groups.

Analysis of covariance techniques determined differences between groups. Results showed that over time the number of intervention group participants who had the recommended number of servings from each food group increased significantly in comparison to the control group. The dietary nutrient density of calcium, riboflavin, and vitamin $B_6$, as well as potassium, of the intervention group significantly improved in comparison to the control group. As a result, officials in all five counties acknowledged the importance of having bicultural, bilingual Vietnamese nutrition education assistants on staff to work with the increasing number of Vietnamese clients. The teaching modules developed for the program were distributed to WIC agencies and other Cooperative Extension county offices throughout the state and nation, as well as to other agencies working with Vietnamese clients.

Practitioners involved in nutrition education for immigrant populations whose native language is not English are encouraged to hire bilingual, bicultural professionals and paraprofessionals to reach these populations. In this project, Vietnamese American nutrition professionals designed culturally appropriate educational materials for the project and were involved in the training of paraprofessionals working at the local level. The paraprofessionals were invaluable in recruiting and working with women from their communities. They were able to relate to the difficulties new immigrants had in shopping at Western supermarkets; learning about new food products; discovering new methods of food handling, preparation, and storage; and dealing with language barriers in communicating with health professionals who did not speak Vietnamese.

# ▶ Strengthening Organizational Cultural Competence

Cultural training for dietetics students usually consists of a background course in anthropology or a related social or behavioral science combined with dietetics education about traditional food preferences and associated health problems of certain racial and ethnic groups. This educational step is valuable for introducing students to basic information, but does not prepare them to incorporate cultural concepts into dietetics practice. Accordingly, nutrition and other healthcare providers can benefit from a conceptual model of cultural competence.[120]

The current incentive to address the needs of cultural sensitivity includes Healthy People 2010 and 2020 goals set by the federal government to eliminate health disparities. In addition, an agency's policy and mission statements can provide the organization and staff the drive toward higher levels of culturally competent care and programming.[121] Every organization needs to ensure that cultural competence philosophies are incorporated into its policy and mission statements and that all are followed. If these features already exist in policy and mission statements, an assessment of how well they are being followed is important. Examples of the variables that can be monitored and observed include the following[100,113,121,122]:

- The interaction between staff and management and among themselves
- How management and personnel value diversity
- How the management and staff adapt to the diversity and cultural contexts of individuals and communities served (accepting the differences within the community)
- The interactions in the clinic, waiting area, educational area, and other areas where the target group and facility staff interact
- The environment in which services are provided, including location, hours of operation, physical resources, and information systems
- Service models that are adapted to the culture-specific needs of the population
- The materials given to the target group: Are they well received, perceived, and read? Are they written in a language the target group can read and understand at the appropriate grade or reading levels?

The agency also should assess whether signs of the agency's policy about culture are placed within and around the facility and other locales where services, including health promotion programming, may be offered. Additional strategies for strengthening organizational cultural competence include the following[100,113]:

- Explain the Western concepts of health, disease, prevention, and treatment in culturally understandable terms that are relevant to the target group.
- Design and employ educational materials that are relevant and culturally appropriate to the target group.
- Use well-trained bilingual/bicultural staff.
- Provide adequate fiscal resources to support translation and interpretation of services, hire qualified staff, and purchase teaching materials (videotapes, pens, papers, etc.) and equipment (computers, tables, chairs, etc.).
- Employ indigenous health workers/dietitians when working in and with diverse multicultural communities.
- Seek ways to improve access to services for multicultural populations.
- Include strategic goals, plans, policies, and procedures as part of a comprehensive management strategy.
- Create a cultural competence plan that includes defined steps for its integration at every level of organizational planning and the related policy or procedural changes needed.

## The U.S. Department of Health and Human Services' National Standards for Culturally and Linguistically Appropriate Services

Until the late 1990s, many healthcare providers did not have clear guidance on how to prepare for or respond to culturally sensitive situations. No comprehensive nationally recognized standards of cultural or linguistic competence in healthcare service delivery had been developed. Instead, federal health agencies, state policy makers, and national organizations independently developed their own standards and practices. Some developed definitions of cultural competence, whereas others mandated providing language services to speakers with limited English. Some specified the collection of language, race, and ethnicity data. Many approaches attempted to be comprehensive, whereas others targeted only a specific issue, geographic area, or subfield of health care, such as mental health. The result was a wide spectrum of ideas about what constitutes culturally competent health services, including significant differences with respect to target population, scope, and quality of services.[122]

In 1997, the U.S. Department of Health and Human Services (DHHS), Office of Minority Health (OMH) undertook the development of national standards for culturally and linguistically appropriate services (CLAS) to help guide providers, policy makers, accreditation and credentialing agencies, purchasers, patients, advocates, educators, and the general healthcare community.[119] These guidelines were developed with input from a national project advisory committee of policy makers, providers, and researchers. The full report is available online at http://www.omhrc.gov. Each standard is accompanied by commentary that addresses its relationship to existing laws and standards and offers recommendations for implementation and oversight to providers, policy makers, and advocates. These 14 standards must be met by most healthcare-related agencies. The standards are based on an analytical review of key laws, regulations, contracts, and standards currently in use by federal and state agencies and other national organizations.

Culture and language have a considerable impact on how individuals access and respond to healthcare services. To ensure equal access to quality health care by diverse populations, healthcare organizations and providers need to follow these standards[113]:

- *Standard 1:* Promote and support the attitudes, behaviors, knowledge, and skills necessary for staff to work respectfully and effectively with patients and each other in a culturally diverse work environment.
- *Standard 2:* Have a comprehensive management strategy to address culturally and linguistically appropriate services, including strategic goals, plans, policies, procedures, and designated staff responsible for implementation.
- *Standard 3:* Utilize formal mechanisms for community and consumer involvement in the design and execution of service delivery, including planning, policy making, operations, evaluation, training, and, as appropriate, treatment planning.
- *Standard 4:* Develop and implement a strategy to recruit, retain, and promote qualified diverse and culturally competent administrative, clinical, and support staff that are trained to address the needs of the racial and ethnic communities being served.
- *Standard 5:* Require and arrange for ongoing education and training for administrative, clinical, and support staff in culturally and linguistically competent service delivery.
- *Standard 6:* Provide all clients who have limited English proficiency access to bilingual staff or interpretation services.
- *Standard 7:* Provide oral and written notices, including translated signage at key points of contact, to clients in their primary language informing them of their right to receive interpreter services free of charge.
- *Standard 8:* Translate and make available signage and commonly used written patient educational materials as well as other materials for members of the predominant language groups in service areas.
- *Standard 9:* Ensure that interpreters and bilingual staff can demonstrate bilingual proficiency and receive training that includes the skills and ethics of interpreting and knowledge of the terms and concepts relevant to clinical or nonclinical encounters. Family or friends are not considered adequate substitutes because they usually lack these abilities.
- *Standard 10:* Ensure that the client's primary spoken language and self-identified race/ethnicity are included in the healthcare organization's management information system as well as any patient records used by provider staff.
- *Standard 11:* Use a variety of methods to collect and utilize accurate demographic, cultural, epidemiological, and clinical outcome data for racial and ethnic groups in the service area, and become informed about the ethnic/cultural needs, resources, and assets of the surrounding community.
- *Standard 12:* Undertake ongoing organizational self-assessments of cultural and linguistic competence, and integrate measures of access, satisfaction, quality, and outcomes for CLAS into other organizational internal audits and performance improvement programs.
- *Standard 13:* Develop structures and procedures to address cross-cultural ethical and legal conflicts in healthcare delivery and complaints or grievances by patients and staff about unfair, culturally insensitive discriminatory treatment, or difficulty in accessing services, or denial of services.
- *Standard 14:* Prepare an annual progress report documenting the organization's progress with implementing CLAS standards, including information on programs, staffing, and resources.

# ▶ Dietary Patterns of Different Cultural Groups in the United States

The migration of different ethnic groups into the United States has created a blend of cultures often addressed in metaphors. Originally, it was the melting pot, then a set of tributaries, a tapestry, and then a garden salad. Community nutritionists in the United States need to be able to consider all aspects of their clients, not just what they eat. This section of the chapter creates cultural awareness for nutritionists working with different cultural groups. It is important to note that variations exist in each cultural group (e.g., socioeconomic status, religion, age, education, social class, location, length of time in the United States, country of origin, and variation within country of origin). Therefore, nutritionists must be cautious and not generalize or imply that the characteristics discussed in this section apply to all individuals of a cultural group. This section discusses the historical perspective, current nutrition practices, and health-related issues of the major ethnic groups in the United States.

## Working with African American Food Patterns

### Historical Perspective

African Americans are descendants of African ancestry whose lineal relatives, such as parents, grandparents, or great-grandparents, have resided in the United States for several generations or are recent immigrants. "Soul food," a metaphor of group identity, emphasizes both the content and preparation styles of food. African Americans adopted soul food in the 1960s as a way of identifying their ethnicity.[3] Blank et al.[21] found that older African Americans in the South added wild animals, such as squirrels, rabbits, opossums, and deer, to their soul food diet. Flour-based gravies are a favorite with meats and rice. Many African Americans still eat Hoppin' John, or rice and black-eyed peas, on New Year's Day for good luck in the upcoming year.[21]

Soul food is high in fat, salt, and sugar. Most of the time, meats and other foods are fried, and most vegetables are stewed with pork fat. Soul food is also spiced with red pepper (cayenne) and malagueta peppers. Hot pepper sauces, mace, allspice, cinnamon, cloves, sesame seeds (benne), Cajun from sassafras leaves, thyme, and vinegar are also used to prepare soul foods. Drinks and desserts are usually very sweet. Heavily sweetened iced tea is the traditional drink, but unsweetened tea, lemonade, and Kool-Aid made with 1 cup of sugar to 7 cups of water are favorite summer drinks. Fat (butter) and sugar are also used liberally in the preparation of favorite side dishes such as candied "yams," a sweet potato dish, and desserts such as apple or peach cobblers or pies; sweet potato pie and pudding; banana pudding; and chocolate, pineapple, coconut, lemon, and pound cakes.[56]

There is similarity between African and Caucasian' food preferences in comparable socioeconomic groups living in the same region of the United States. However, African Americans often include black-eyed peas, okra, peas, and green leafy vegetables (e.g., chard, collard greens, kale, mustard greens, spinach, and turnip greens) in their diets.[56]

### Current Nutrition Practices and Health-Related Issues

It is difficult to characterize the most current nutritional status of African Americans because a limited number of studies have investigated this population. Research has shown that African American nutritional intake is associated with socioeconomic status because poor families of any ethnic group often depend on subsidies such as SNAP, school breakfast and lunch programs, and emergency food programs.[56,65] In the United States, a large number of African Americans experience nutrient deficiencies at or near poverty levels.[123] Haytowitz et al.[124] studied the variety of foods consumed daily and found that the percentage of African Americans reporting lower servings of dairy, meat, grains, fruits, or vegetables and higher salty food intakes was higher than that of Caucasians.[125] High levels of income and education increased the variety of foods they consumed. Also, African Americans consumed more calories from animal proteins than did Caucasians.[125]

Obesity is a major health problem for African American adolescents and adults because it contributes to most chronic health conditions, such as diabetes and heart disease. It is estimated that 29.1 percent of African American women and 35.9 percent of African American men are overweight compared to 24.8 percent of European American women and 40.7 percent of European American men.[126,127] The high incidence of weight gain may be due to several factors, such as socioeconomic status, poor eating habits, genetic predisposition, and a more permissive attitude about obesity.[42]

Obesity is a contributing factor to non–insulin-dependent diabetes mellitus, prevalent in African American communities, which affects approximately 20 percent of the African American population. The incidence of non–insulin-dependent diabetes mellitus is three to four times higher for African Americans than for the total U.S. population.[56] Non–insulin-dependent diabetes mellitus is credited to be one of the contributing factors to the high mortality rate among African Americans. Also, there is a direct link between diabetes and heart disease, which has increased the rate of death, especially among African American women.[56,128]

The incidence of hypertension is very high for African Americans—almost twice that of the European American population. Although data comparing normotensives and hypertensives by ethnic groups is limited, reports show that African Americans have the highest proportion of hypertension of any group.[56] Furthermore, African Americans experiencing hypertension are five times more likely to have chronic heart failure and 10 times more likely to develop kidney failure.[56,129]

The reason for the prevalence of hypertension among African Americans is not clear in approximately 95 percent of all cases. Studies show that sub-Saharan Africans have the lowest prevalence of hypertension, although hypertension increases with urbanization of sub-Saharan Africans.[130,131] It is reported that the rate of hypertension among Caribbean Africans is moderately high.[132] Several studies have reported that there is a link between negative stressors and low socioeconomic status, including low education levels and hypertension.[133,134] Research also found that chronic discrimination and the struggle for social acceptance can lead to continuous stress and an increased prevalence of high blood pressure.[23,135]

It is reported that low calcium, magnesium, and potassium intakes are associated with hypertension.[133] It is estimated that a higher percentage of African Americans are lactose-intolerant, which may be a contributing factors to the low calcium intake. It is also believed that salt retention is associated with calcium retention, which may account for why many African American women have high bone mineral densities and low rates of osteoporosis despite low calcium intake.[56,136-138] One of the recommendations for reducing blood pressure is to lower salt intake and increase calcium, magnesium, and potassium intakes. Another effective method for reducing blood pressure is a diet that is low in total fat, saturated fat, and cholesterol and high in fruits, vegetables, and low-fat dairy foods, especially in African Americans, even with no reduction in salt intake or weight loss.[56,139-141]

Although differences in cultural beliefs, attitudes, and practices exist between rural and urban African Americans, they have some basic cultural beliefs. The core of African American culture is family and religion. The family is the strongest institution for them, and it provides strong extended kinship bonds with grandparents, aunts, uncles, and cousins. The family is the main source of support, especially during crisis and illness. Religion and religious behavior are essential parts of the African American community.[56,142,143] Their perception is that health is a feeling of well-being and the ability to fulfill role expectations. Spiritual balance is also a major component of their culture.[54]

An African American client may not consider himself or herself as active during interaction with community or public health nutritionists and, therefore, may not communicate his or her needs or ask questions. On the other hand, his or her participation in conversational types of communication is engaging and expressive, but prolonged eye contact is viewed as rude.[54] When planning nutrition education for African American clients, consider using action- or task-oriented activities. An in-depth interview is important with African American participants.

It is important to consider the variability in diet related to region, socioeconomic conditions, and degree of ethnic identity when planning health promotion programs. In the United States, Caribbean or Central American participants are more likely to identify with the foods and food habits of Latinos than with those of African Americans.[54] Some African Americans have Islamic or Eastern Orthodox religious affiliations, and community nutritionists must consider the influence of religion on dietary practices.

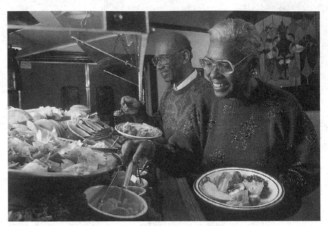

Interpretation of messages is based on one's cultural framework, and interpretation of visual elements varies considerably by ethnic group.
Courtesy of Bill Branson/National Center Institute.

## Working with Hispanic/Latino American Food Patterns

### Historical Perspective

Hispanics comprise approximately 16 percent of the U.S. population and are the fastest growing ethnic group in the country.[4] Hispanic immigrants come to the United States from Central America, South America, and the Caribbean, but the greatest number come from Mexico. The cultural foods and food preparation methods of Hispanic populations vary significantly, depicting indigenous, African, and European influences.[56] For example, Mexican cuisine is influenced by indigenous, Spanish, and French cultures. Chilies, cocoa, and tomatoes are among the flavors used in preparing traditional Mexican dishes.[56]

The Aztec Indians contributed corn, tomatoes, roast turkey, quail, duck, fish, lobster, frogs, green plums, cocoa, beans, peas, and squash to Mexican cuisine. The Spanish contributed cinnamon, garlic, onions, rice, wheat, sugarcane, and pork. Mexican clients also consume meats such as goat, poultry, and beef. Mexicans experience high incidences of lactose intolerance, which causes a reduction in the diet of dairy foods.[56,144] They often use traditional foods and ingredients to prepare Mexican dishes such as tacos, enchiladas, tamales, quesadillas, burritos, stews, tortillas, chili rellenos, flan, guacamole, and salsas.[56]

Some Hispanics think illness is due to 1) excessive emotion, 2) dislocation of internal organs, 3) magic, or

4) an imbalance in hot or cold; they also may consider health conditions such as pneumonia and appendicitis to be European diseases.[56,145] In addition, some Hispanic Americans believe that the origins of disease and illness are due to spiritual or natural punishments, natural diseases, and mental issues.[56,146]

They base their treatment of an illness on the cause of the health condition. Some Mexican Indians practice a hot–cold system of diet and health; the rural poor also have similar practices. This is derived from the Arab system of humoral medicine brought to Mexico by the Spanish, combined with the native Indian practice.[56,145,147]

Hispanic Americans believe in prayer and depend on spiritual strength to help them in illness and death. They trust God and believe that living life in accord with God's intention is essential in maintaining health. Hence, offending God necessitates punishment.[56,144]

## Current Nutrition Practices and Health-Related Issues

In the United States, Hispanic immigrants adhere strongly to their food traditions. Nevertheless, it has been reported that as Hispanic immigrants become assimilated into the host country's culture, traditional foods are consumed less often than when they lived in their country.[56] The dietary acculturation of Hispanics is often characterized by an increased consumption of high-fat, high-sugar, highly processed foods associated with mainstream culture.[148] It is also reported that with the alteration in the traditional diet, Hispanic immigrants show a significant increase in diet-related chronic conditions such as obesity, hypertension, cardiovascular disease, and diabetes.[149-151] These observations are supported by clinical data documenting a high incidence of these conditions among Hispanic immigrants in the United States.

The birth rate for Mexican women between the ages of 15 and 44 years is 114 births per 1,000 women. This is about half the figure for Caucasian women. The pregnancy rate for unmarried teenage girls is twice that of Caucasians.[56] It was reported that half of teenage Hispanic mothers do not obtain prenatal care during the first trimester. However, infant mortality is lower for Mexican American infants than for European American infants, despite the risk factors associated with the delay in enrolling in prenatal care. Breastfed infants are usually weaned from the breast to the bottle.[56] Prolonged use of a feeding bottle, containing both milk and/or sweetened liquids (i.e., Kool-Aid, fruit juice, tea), is a problem because it causes iron-deficiency anemia, obesity, and extensive tooth decay among toddlers.[152,153]

Many Mexican Americans like fried foods, which results in the increased intake of high-fat foods and a lesser intake of fruits and vegetables than European

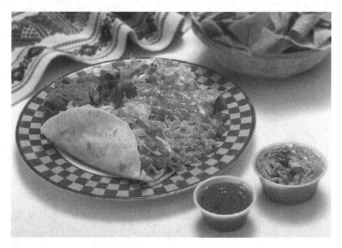

Dietary acculturation can result in both healthful and unhealthful dietary changes.
© LiquidLibrary.

Americans of similar backgrounds. Acculturation exacerbates these dietary intake differences.[56] It is reported that second-generation Mexican Americans consume more meat and cheese and less beans; eat vegetables as side dishes with added butter, dressings, or mayonnaise; and choose sweetened fruit drink mixes (Kool-Aid) over fresh, blended fruit drinks.[56,154,155]

Lack of money may cause Hispanic people to disregard healthcare services. About 27 percent of all Hispanic families in the United States live below the poverty line. In addition, Hispanics are very proud and very private when it comes to family problems.[56,156] It is not easy for a family to help a member who has alcohol abuse problems and still more difficult to recommend external help. This value influences receptivity to community nutrition programs and printed materials.[56] The following is a list of general recommendations for working with Hispanic populations[56,157-159]:

- Target prevention and intervention efforts to the entire family and their religious leaders.
- Help Hispanic/Latino fathers recognize how important their role is to their children.
- Encourage mothers to learn strategies for including their spouses in family interactions.
- Educate mothers and daughters to reduce the shame associated with asking for help.
- Emphasize the family as a unit in printed materials. Tailor separate versions for males and females.
- Emphasize participation in healthy eating and exercise programs to adjust to the American culture without abandoning their own.
- **Reach Hispanic/Latino audiences through** Spanish-speaking, community-level organizations and leaders.
- Educate community nutritionists and assistants about traditional gender roles to aid their efforts.

# Working with Native American Food Patterns

## Historical Perspective

American Indians/Native Americans (both are appropriate terms) are diverse groups of indigenous people who have lived north of Mexico and south of Canada since at least 12,000 B.C. Both hunting and gathering (foraging) contributed significantly to the diet of all American Indian groups at the time of contact with Europeans, whether or not they were horticulturalists. More than 550 sovereign Indian nations currently live within the political boundaries of the United States, so it is difficult to summarize their different foods and dietary habits.[56]

Native North Americans consume a variety of foods based on the diverse plant and animal communities found throughout the continent. They link food to spirituality and physical health, balance, and harmony. Corn has a special healing significance.[159] Fry bread (bread dough deep-fried in fat) is a popular food at Indian fairs and gatherings. The dish can actually be traced to medieval Europe.[160] Native Americans also have made a significant contribution to the current American diet. Native Americans contributed, among many other items, corn, squash, beans, cranberries, and maple syrup to European settlers.

Food has significant religious and social meaning to many Native Americans. It is an integral component of many festivities, including powwows and other ceremonies. They like to give foods to guests, and extra food is frequently given to members of the extended family. Meals are prepared and eaten communally in some Native American nations in the southwest. A large amount of one dish is prepared by every woman, and they share it with other families, who in turn share what they have prepared.[56,161]

## Current Nutrition Practices and Health-Related Issues

Native Americans believe that a state of health exists when a person lives in total harmony with nature. The earth is seen as a living entity that should be respected, and failure to do so would harm the body. Native Americans believe their healing practices and traditions function in the context of the relationship among spirituality (Creator, Mother Earth, Great Father), community (family, clan, tribe/nation), environment (daily life, nature, balance), and self (inner passions and peace, thoughts, and values).[56,161]

Native Americans experience many social problems (e.g., alcohol/drug abuse and violence) at a rate that is significantly higher than the national average. The rate of adult-onset (type 2) diabetes for American Indians is more than three times that of the entire U.S. population.[162] Research on the nutritional status

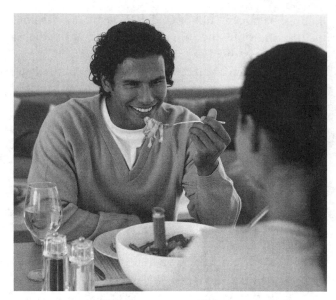

The cultural foods and food preparation methods of Hispanic populations are diverse, reflecting indigenous, African, and European influences.
© Stockdisc/age footstock

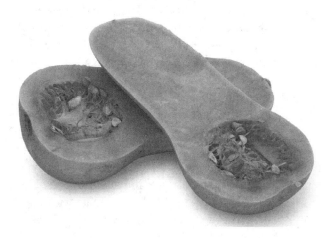

Traditional Native American foods, such as squash, are a part of today's American diet.
© Elena Schweitzer/ShutterStock, Inc.

of Native Americans is limited, but it does show that fetal malnutrition may be the cause of type 2 diabetes and, in subsequent generations, transmitted by disturbances in the intrauterine environment.[163] Many Native Americans experience low socioeconomic status and a lack of transportation, fuel, refrigeration, and running water, which contribute to inadequate diet intake. The resulting problems include dental caries, goiter, growth retardation, female obesity, and low levels of hemoglobin, vitamin A, thiamin, and riboflavin.[56,164]

One explanation for Native Americans' poor health status is the "thrifty genotype" model, which states that such a genotype gave a genetic advantage to populations who experienced periods of feast and famine. If maximizing their caloric intake of fat for storage, which could be utilized during times of famine, they would have a selective advantage over other populations.[56] A problem occurs when the feasting, especially in the form of high-fat, carbohydrate-rich foods, becomes permanent. The result has been high rates of obesity, insulin resistance, and diabetes.[162]

The high incidence of diet-related health conditions such as diabetes, coronary heart disease, hypertension, and obesity has been most pronounced in the decades following World War II. The promotion of an American diet and lifestyle was one of the many facets of attempting to assimilate Native Americans into the U.S. mainstream. It included home economics instruction for Native American women showing them how to utilize the surplus commodities being provided to poor Indian communities.[56]

Current research on Native American meal patterns is limited. It is assumed that three meals per day has become the norm. One study of Dakotas reported that there was little variety in daily menus. Current dietary intakes include cereal with milk, fried potatoes, fried eggs, chopped meat, milk, bread with butter, oatmeal or cornmeal, and high white sugar consumption.[56,165]

It is reported that the life expectancy for Native Americans has increased in recent years, but it is still lower than that of the overall U.S. population. The age-adjusted mortality rate for Native Americans is approximately 50 percent higher than that of the rest of the United States, and one third of Native Americans die before the age of 45, compared to just 11 percent of the total U.S. population.[56,165] Chronic conditions complicating diabetes, including hypertension and end-stage renal diseases, were found to be more prevalent among northern plains Indians than among the general population.[166]

Healthcare providers who counsel American Indians must recognize traditional beliefs and practices. For example, varying according to tribe or region, either all individuals speak for themselves because no other can speak for them or, in some cases, the elder can speak for others. Also, "yes" and "no" are considered complete responses, and explanations are not thought to be warranted. Also, in Native American culture, direct eye contact is not common.[56]

## Think About It

A community nutritionist was hired to work in the Native American community and conduct nutrition assessment and provide nutrition education. What basic information about the clients should he collect to provide adequate nutritional guidance?

# Working with Asian American Food Patterns
## Historical Perspective

The term *Asian American* refers to people of Asian descent who are citizens or permanent residents of the United States. The term encompasses at least 23 subgroups including persons from China, Mongolia, Pakistan, Sri Lanka, Maldives, India, Nepal, Bhutan, Bangladesh, Burma, Laos, Thailand, Vietnam, Cambodia, North Korea, South Korea, Japan, Hong Kong, Macao, Taiwan, Philippines, Malaysia, and Polynesia.[56,167] They constituted 4.8 percent of the total population of the United States in 2010. It is projected that by 2050, this figure will be 10.1 percent. High rates of tuberculosis, parasitic infection, and hepatitis B have been found in many Asian American immigrants.[56]

Asian cultural values are imbedded in their health beliefs and practices, which help them determine what is important in life. Although variations are the norm rather than the exception, Asian groups share some similarities based on their religious backgrounds and the influence of Chinese culture throughout Asia.[168]

Asians view health as a state of harmony with nature or freedom from symptoms or illness. The concept of balance is related to health promotion, and the concept of imbalance is related to disease.[56] This balance or equilibrium relates to temperature in foods, climate, and body elements, and diet, and it influences people's activities of daily living and health promotion. To achieve health and avoid illness, they believe people must adjust to the environment in a holistic manner. Traditional practitioners assist people in achieving this through energy balance.[169]

In the Chinese culture, food is viewed as more than something to eat. The decision about what to eat is carefully planned. Food plays a significant role in preventing and treating diseases as well as addressing certain health conditions. For example, foods and herbs are frequently boiled in soup or tea for treatments of various diseases and conditions. The preferred beverage is hot green tea. Older Chinese individuals rarely drink cold beverages.[56,170,171] The Japanese believe that certain foods and herbs have harmful or beneficial effects; for example, a study using the Japanese diet and herbal medicine formula Hochu-ekki-to (containing *Astragalus* root, licorice, jujube, ginseng, white *Atractylodes* rhizome, fresh ginger, and Chinese Angelica root) found it to be effective as an alternative therapy for difficult atopic dermatitis.[172]

Asian individuals eat a wide variety of foods. The traditional Asian diet is low in fat and dairy products and high in complex carbohydrates and sodium; research with elderly foreign-born Americans of Chinese descent indicates that their dietary pattern is mostly continued in the United States. However, Asians' diets become more like the diets of the majority of Americans as the length of stay and the number of generations living in the United States increases. The diet becomes higher in fat, protein, sugar, and cholesterol and lower in complex carbohydrates.[56,173]

## Current Nutritional Practices and Health-Related Issues

In general, Chinese diets are high in sodium, which may contribute to hypertension; however, hypertension rates among Chinese Americans in California are significantly lower than for Caucasians, but research is limited.[173]

Some Chinese Americans avoid fresh dairy products because of lactose intolerance, which may be found in as many as 75 percent of Asians.[56] It has been reported that their calcium intake is low.[89,174] However, a recent study shows an increase in the consumption of dairy products such as milk and cheese.[90]

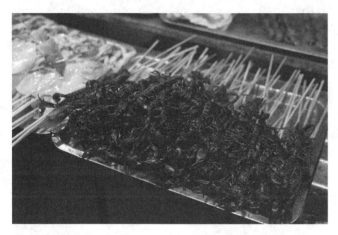

One person's favorite food is another person's dismay.

© ksbank/ Getty Images

The Asian American meal pattern includes eating three meals and several snacks a day. Some of the foods the Asian communities use include soy sauce, rice, pickled dishes, raw fish, and tea.[56] A study of acculturation and diet in Chinese American women found that Chinese-language newspapers and friends were the primary sources of nutrition information.[97]

Koreans relate health to happiness, to the ability to live life fully, to function without impairment, and to not be a burden on one's children.[56] There are limited research studies on the health of Korean Americans. One comparison of the nutritional status of elderly Korean Americans indicated that native Koreans had the poorest diet.[175,176] Nearly half consumed inadequate amounts of energy, vitamin A, and riboflavin. Almost one fourth consumed less than two thirds of the recommended daily allowance (RDA) of protein, phosphorus, and vitamin

C.[176] Of the total, 25 percent of both the men and women had inadequate protein intakes. Korean Americans also reported low calcium consumption.[56,176,177]

The variations in the health status of Asian Americans are due to subcultures within the larger group. Asian Americans have health problems similar to those of the European American population. Cardiovascular problems are common, and they have a high incidence of strokes. The prevalence of cardiovascular disease among Japanese Americans is only half that for Caucasians; however, it is expected that death rates will climb steadily as further acculturation occurs.[178] Heart disease rates are estimated to be one and one-half to four times greater among Asian Indian immigrants than among Caucasians. Researchers have reported that Asian Indians living in urban and westernized regions have a significantly higher risk for cardiovascular disease and type 2 diabetes mellitus than the native population in India or the European American population in the United States, and diabetes rates also are calculated to be at least four times higher.[56,179-181] Changes in diet also have been implicated in the high rates of type 2 diabetes found among Japanese American men. Hypertension is usually an accompanying chronic problem, resulting from a high salt intake.[181] The rate of hypertension in Asian Indians is associated with the high incidence of cardiovascular disease, which is slightly higher than that of Caucasians.[182]

Cancers are also leading health problems for Asian men and women. Breast, colorectal, and lung cancers are the leading causes of death.[56,183] The incidence of liver cancers is high among foreign-born Asians with a history of hepatitis B infection. Cancers, such as breast and rectal, have increased in Japanese Americans as their residency in the United States increases. The leading cause of death among Koreans is stomach cancer, and higher incidences of stomach, liver, and esophageal cancer have been reported among Korean Americans compared to Caucasians.[56,184] A low intake of vitamins A (including beta-carotene) and C and a high intake of sodium and chili peppers are reported to be the contributing factors to the high risk of these cancers. Aflatoxins, which have been linked to liver cancer, are also sometimes found in Korean soy sauce.[185,186]

In addition, the rate of hepatitis B (responsible for most liver cancers) is very high in Korean Americans. The prevalence of hepatitis B infection among Asian Americans ranges from 15 to 30 percent.[187] **TABLE 5-3** presents some food practices, health issues, dietary concerns, and strategies for the main minority groups in the United States. **TABLE 5-4** presents a sample menu of traditional versus contemporary food choices of multiethnic groups in the United States.

**TABLE 5-3** Some Food Practices, Health Issues, Dietary Concerns, and Strategies for the Main Minority Groups in the United States[56,58,96,187-191]

| Cultural Group | Food Practices | Diet-Related Heath Issues | Dietary Concerns | Strategies |
|---|---|---|---|---|
| African American | Traditional foods include collard greens, other leafy green and yellow vegetables, beans, legumes, rice, and potatoes. Starches and vegetables are often seasoned with fat, such as bacon, ham hocks, or salt pork. Meats are often fried or barbecued and served with sauce or gravy. Home-baked cakes and pies are popular. Religion plays some role in their diets. For example, some Christians will avoid meat on holy days such as Good Friday and Ash Wednesday (Catholics). Those practicing Islam are required to avoid all pork and pork products; all meat must be slaughtered according to ritual draining of blood. | High incidence of diabetes, hypertension, heart disease, obesity, and some types of cancer; lactose intolerance. | Overall diet may be low in fiber, calcium, and potassium and high in fat and sodium. | ▪ Encourage continued intake of leafy greens, vegetables, legumes, rice, and potatoes.<br>▪ Offer tips for modifying food preparation methods to reduce fat and sodium.<br>▪ Encourage increased intake of fruits.<br>▪ Suggest ways to include low-fat dairy foods. |
| Asian American | Traditional diets vary widely by country and region of origin. Some common elements include a diet largely composed of rice, vegetables, and fruits; low intake of dairy foods except for ice cream or some yogurt; protein primarily from fish, pork, and poultry, as well as nuts, legumes, and/or tofu. Food is prepared by stir-frying, steaming, grilling, deep-frying, baking, or boiling. | Some types of cancer, osteoporosis, and stroke; lactose intolerance; risk for heart disease, diabetes, and obesity increases with dietary acculturation. | Overall diet may be low in calcium and high in carbohydrates and sodium. | ▪ Encourage continued variety.<br>▪ Evaluate calcium intake and suggest other food sources of calcium if inadequate.<br>▪ Provide tips for reducing sodium intake. |
| Hispanic | Traditional diets vary by country and region of origin. Often the same foods are prepared and/or integrated into meal patterns in different ways. Common elements include beans, rice, breads, and, for some, corn and corn products. Protein sources include legumes, eggs, shellfish, fish, and a variety of meats and poultry. Minimal use of low-fat dairy foods. Foods are mainly fried or baked. With acculturation, there is an increased intake of milk, certain vegetables and fruits, fats, and sugars. | High incidence of obesity, diabetes, heart disease, hypertension, dental caries, and both overnutrition and undernutrition. | Overall diet is high in fat and low in calcium, iron, folic acid, and vitamins A and C. | ▪ Preserve healthy cultural food practices, such as continued use of complex carbohydrates.<br>▪ Suggest modifications of traditional dishes to lower intake of fat and sodium.<br>▪ Encourage intake of low-fat dairy foods, lean meats, fresh vegetables, and fruits.<br>▪ Reduce intake of soft drinks and sweetened beverages. |

*(continues)*

**TABLE 5-3** Some Food Practices, Health Issues, Dietary Concerns, and Strategies for the Main Minority Groups in the United States[56,58,96,187-191] *(continued)*

| Cultural Group | Food Practices | Diet-Related Health Issues | Dietary Concerns | Strategies |
|---|---|---|---|---|
| Navajo (American Indians) and Alaska Natives | Traditional diets vary according to culture and seasons. Most diets include meats such as sheep, goat, wild game (deer, antelope, rabbits, and prairie dogs). pigs, chickens, and cattle; vegetables, such as celery, onion, spinach, potatoes, and pigweed; and fruits such as wolfberries, juniper berries, squaw berries or wax currants, prickly pear fruit, wild bananas, and yucca fruit. Other items added to food include gray clay and culinary ash from burned cedar and juniper boughs, tumbleweed, and greasewood. Gray clay decreases the bitterness of foods such as wolfberries and wild potatoes. The added clay also increases the mineral content of foods. Ash helps soften foods such as hominy and helps maintain the blue color in blue corn products. Other items in the diet include cantaloupe, watermelon, beans, squash, and fish. | Diabetes, obesity, coronary heart disease, hypertension, and end-stage renal diseases. | Overall diet may be high in fat, sugar, and alcoholic intake with a low potassium intake. | ▪ Encourage continued intake of leafy greens, vegetables, legumes, and potatoes.<br>▪ Promote modifying food preparation methods to reduce fat and sodium.<br>▪ Encourage low-fat foods.<br>▪ Encourage regular physical activities. |
| Jewish | Dietary practices vary because Jews originate from many different countries. Also, religious belief plays a significant role in dietary practice. Most commonly used foods include bagels with cream cheese, rye bread, corned beef, pastrami, and matzo (popular in the United States). Some Jewish people observe strict dietary laws (kosher) that require restriction of all pork and pork products and all fish without scales and fins. Dairy products are not eaten at the same meal that contains meat and meat products. All kosher meat must be slaughtered and prepared according to Biblical ordinances. Since blood is forbidden as food, meat must be drained thoroughly. Bakery products and prepared food mixtures must be prepared under acceptable kosher standards. All noncloven-hoofed animals such as beef and chicken that have been blessed by a rabbi are allowed. Dairy, eggs, grains, legumes, vegetables, and fruits are permitted. Leavened bread and cake are forbidden during Passover; unleavened bread or flat bread is permitted. Mixing meat and dairy products is not allowed. | Type 2 diabetes, breast cancer, obesity, and coronary heart disease. | Overall diet may be high in intake of fat and sugar and low in intake of fiber, zinc, iron, and calcium. | ▪ Encourage the use of low-fat foods and complex carbohydrate (whole wheat, rice, and whole grains).<br>▪ Encourage physical activity.<br>▪ Encourage reducing foods containing high levels of simple sugars. |

**TABLE 5-4**  Sample Menu of Traditional Versus Contemporary Food Choices of Multiethnic Groups in the United States

| Ethnic Group | Traditional Meal | Contemporary Meal |
|---|---|---|
| **Hispanic Americans** | **Breakfast**<br>Corn tortillas, eggs with chorizo (sausage), salsa<br>Mexican sweet bread and fruit<br>Hot chocolate or coffee with milk<br><br>**Lunch**<br>Corn tortillas; beef, chicken<br>Fried fish tacos<br>Stew with chili and tomatoes<br>Soft drinks or coffee with milk<br><br>**Dinner**<br>Enchiladas, rice, and beans<br>Cactus with pork and onion, beans and corn tortillas<br>Rice and beans<br>Soft drinks or coffee with milk | **Breakfast**<br>Traditional foods or Americanized choices:<br>Bacon, scrambled eggs, and toast, or cold cereal with milk<br>Fruit juice or coffee with milk<br><br>**Lunch**<br>Traditional foods at home or fast food (pizza, hamburgers, burritos, and sandwiches)<br>Tortilla chips, cheese<br>School lunch for most children<br>Milk, fruit juice, or soft drinks<br><br>**Dinner**<br>Traditional food choices such as rice, beans, a meat dish, and fried tortillas<br>Typical Americanized food choices such as spaghetti or barbecued chicken, corn, salad, and bread<br>Fruit juice, soft drinks, or coffee with milk |
| **African American** | **Breakfast**<br>Eggs, country ham with red-eye gravy, biscuits, and fried potatoes or grits<br>Coffee or milk<br><br>**Dinner (the traditional lunch meal)**<br>Fried chicken or catfish, boiled cabbage or collard greens and potatoes<br>Beef-vegetable stew with cornbread<br>Rice and black-eyed peas<br>Fruit cobbler<br>Buttermilk and fruit-flavored drinks<br><br>**Supper (the traditional dinnertime meal)**<br>Boiled legumes or greens with ham hocks, coleslaw, and cornbread<br>Fried okra<br>Apple or peach cobblers<br>Buttermilk or fruit-flavored drinks | **Breakfast**<br>Much lighter than traditional<br>May include toast; eggs and bacon; and cream of wheat, oatmeal, or grits<br><br>**Lunch**<br>Typical fast-food choices: hamburgers, hot dogs, sandwiches, pizza<br>School lunches for most children<br>Milk, fruit juice, or coffee<br>Barbeque sandwich<br>Corn bread<br><br>**Dinner**<br>Baked chicken with bread stuffing, green beans, green salad, bread and butter<br>Macaroni and cheese<br>Apple cobblers<br>Coffee, tea, fruit-flavored drinks, or milk |
| **Asian American/ Chinese** | **Breakfast**<br>Rice porridge seasoned with small amounts of meat or fish<br>Bowl of noodles with vegetables and meat<br><br>**Lunch**<br>Rice or fried noodles, Chinese greens, and a seasoned meat dish with clear soup<br>Chicken and vegetable stir fry<br>Tea | **Breakfast**<br>Similar to traditional choices but may include westernized selections of cold cereal with milk, or eggs with toast<br><br>**Lunch**<br>Traditional choices including rice with leftovers<br>Sandwiches and other take-out foods<br>School lunch for most children<br>Tea, fruit juice, or milk |

*(continues)*

**TABLE 5-4** Sample Menu of Traditional Versus Contemporary Food Choices of Multiethnic Groups *(continued)* in the United States

| Ethnic Group | Traditional Meal | Contemporary Meal |
|---|---|---|
| | ***Dinner (a larger version of lunch)*** <br> Rice, tofu with sausage, several vegetable dishes, and clear soup <br> Tea or soup (In northern China, soup is usually the beverage at meals; in southern China, the beverage is usually tea) | ***Dinner*** <br> Most similar to traditional pattern including rice, meat or fish dishes, sautéed vegetables with soy sauce or oyster sauce, and clear soup <br> Tea, fruit juice, or milk |
| Navajo (American Indians) and Alaska Natives | ***Breakfast*** <br> Fruited millet cereal <br> Yogurt <br> Wolfberries <br> Melons (or wild banana) <br> Juice (apple, orange, grapefruit) <br> Herbal tea, nonfat milk, decaffeinated coffee <br><br> ***Lunch*** <br> Corn chowder soup <br> Baked halibut <br> Pear, fruit <br> Mixed vegetables and mushrooms <br> Herbal tea, evaporated milk, water <br><br> ***Dinner*** <br> Roast mutton or dried salmon <br> Baked deer meat with rice <br> Seaweed <br> Blue corn <br> Juniper berries <br> Fried bread <br> Regular soda, herbal tea, coffee with evaporated milk | ***Breakfast*** <br> Traditional foods at home such as sourdough pancakes with salmonberry syrup <br> Oatmeal <br> Bacon, eggs, and white bread <br> Cold cereal with milk <br> Pancake with margarine <br> Soda, fruit juice, coffee <br><br> ***Lunch*** <br> Traditional foods at home or fast food: pizza, hamburgers <br> Soda, coffee with sugar <br><br><br><br> ***Dinner*** <br> Traditional foods at home such as duck soup, rice, carrots, and wild berries <br> Pizza <br> Fried bread <br> Fried potatoes <br> Soda, coffee with sugar |
| Jewish | ***Breakfast*** <br> Bagel with cream cheese <br> Orange juice, milk <br><br> ***Lunch*** <br> Soup (beet) <br> Smoked salmon <br> Unleavened bread <br> Grapes <br> Sweet potatoes <br> Soda, coffee with milk and sugar <br><br> ***Dinner*** <br> Corned beef or baked kasha and goat meat <br> Babka (spongy yeast cake) or unleavened bread <br> Vegetables (spinach, carrots) <br> Fruit (blintz) <br> Rye bread <br> Tea or coffee | ***Breakfast*** <br> Wheat toast with jam or jelly <br> Fried eggs, bacon, or potato pancakes (latkes) <br> Milk <br><br> ***Lunch*** <br> Traditional foods at home or fast food: pizza, hamburgers <br> Turkey sandwich <br> Hot dog <br> Soda, coffee with milk and sugar <br><br><br> ***Dinner*** <br> Baked fish, fried chicken and rice <br> Green beans, fried mushrooms <br> Prunes <br> Tea or coffee, milk |

## Working with Caucasian American Food Patterns

### Historical Perspective

In the United States, Southern and Northern Europeans make up Caucasian/White Americans. The terms *Caucasian American* and *White American* are used interchangeably. Caucasian Americans are not recognized as a group by the U.S. Census Bureau on their own, but are included in the category of "White." The U.S. Census Bureau defines "White" as a person having origins in any of the original peoples of Europe, the Middle East, or North Africa.[192] *Non-Hispanic white* is the term used as a substitute for European Americans that also includes a small fraction of peoples of Middle Eastern descent, and excludes Hispanics directly from Spain.

Caucasian Americans seem to value individualism and independence. They believe in responsibility for self, and their destinies are not controlled by fate, but rather by individuals. Caucasian Americans generally have a logical, problem solving learning style. For example, if a healthcare system is not working, they typically analyze the issue and takes steps to solve the problem. They are not reluctant to challenge authority to overcome problem. Caucasian Americans tend to be disproportionately represented in powerful positions and control almost all political, economic, and cultural institutions.[193,194]

Caucasian Americans typically prepare traditional ancestral dishes on holidays and special occasions. Example of the dishes are:

- Stollen (German)
- Lutefisk and lefse (Scandinavian)
- Corned beef and cabbage or soda bread (Irish)

New Englanders were the origin of dishes typically consumed by Americans today, especially during special occasions, such as apple pie and the oven-roasted Thanksgiving turkey.[56,194]

### Current Nutrition Practices and Health-Related Issues

Caucasian Americans usually consume the Western Pattern Diet (or Standard American Diet), characterized by red meat, high-fat salty foods, processed foods, sugary desserts, and often alcohol. One-third of an American's daily calories are from fast foods and other junk foods. This diet is low in dietary fiber, complex carbohydrates, plant-based foods, vitamins, and minerals. The incidence of chronic health conditions, such as heart disease, obesity and hypertension have increased due to inadequate consumption of fresh fruits, vegetables, whole-grain foods, and fish.[195,196]

Compared to prudent dietary consumption, the Western dietary habits are linked to obesity, heart disease, and cancer.[197,198]

In working with this group, Community Nutritionists need to include community involvement, schools, neighborhoods, and worksites to increase access to and consumption of affordable healthy foods.[199]

# Learning Portfolio

## Chapter Summary

- Culture is a learned set of ideals, values, and assumptions about life that are widely shared among a group of people.
- Nutritionists can gain cultural competence by reading about the language and customs of other cultures and by attending events held by local ethnic or cultural organizations, such as weddings, birthday parties, international fairs, and religious celebrations.
- Cultural knowledge is a needed base for adequate nutritional practice. When working with multicultural groups in nutrition assessment, it is important to collect basic information about the culture, the foods most frequently used, and food preparation methods.
- The current information about the biological and genetic characteristics of African Americans, Hispanics,

American Indians, Alaska Natives, Asians, Native Hawaiians, and Pacific Islanders does not explain the health disparities experienced by these groups.
- The U.S. infant mortality rate has lowered, but the infant death rate among African Americans is still more than double that of Caucasians. In addition, heart disease death rates are more than 40 percent higher for African Americans than for Caucasians.
- Some of the factors that may affect communication when working with a multicultural group include the communication skills, attitudes, knowledge, social system, and culture of both the sender and receiver of communication transactions.
- It is important to understand the variations in patterns of verbal and nonverbal communication that are the basis for achieving health promotion and disease prevention goals. Variations among cultures are reflected in verbal styles, such as pronunciation,

word meaning, voice quality, and humor, and in nonverbal styles, such as eye contact, gestures, touch, interjection during conversation, body posture, facial expression, and silence.

- Nutrient deficiencies are prevalent among the large number of African American families at or near poverty levels in the United States.
- Dietitians may need to use an interpreter or members of the cultural group to explain or clarify terms to prevent incorrect assumptions.

## Critical Thinking Activities

A community nutritionist, Angelina Okoro, and a community nurse, Lucy Tsai, conducted diabetes and dietary screenings at a free clinic to a culturally diverse population in the community. Analysis revealed that a high percentage of participation was due to print media advertising in the participants' native language. However, the families of

5 percent of the Asian group who were diabetic (children) were unwilling to provide their children the prescribed diet.

- Determine the factors that may have caused this group to refuse the prescribed diet.
- Determine the different ways to socialize with different ethnic groups in your community to determine the best way to assess their nutritional needs.
- Identify major values of the dominant American group. Determine how these values differ from the values of minority cultural groups.
- Determine the strategies you can use when caring for clients who do not speak your language and for whom no translator is readily available.
- Taste different cultural foods by attending international fairs, restaurants, and the like.
- Identify foods that are taboo or prohibited for Asian Indians, Hispanics, Filipinos, Native Americans, and African Americans.

## ⌕ CASE STUDY 5-1: Nutrition and Health Promotion in a Small City

A small city is the focus of a health promotion activity to prevent heart disease, obesity with BMI of 40 on average, hypertension, and diabetes. Report showed evidence of high-fat, high-sugar (candy), low-fruit, and low-vegetable intakes. Community nutritionist Omari was hired to implement the activities, which will include exercise and nutrition education. Sample diets were constructed, and a videotape was purchased for exercise demonstration. However, the videotape and the educational materials were only in English and did not depict people of different ethnic backgrounds. Omari noted that of the 60 participants who enrolled in the program, 15 were Hispanic with limited English-speaking abilities, 10 were African American, 10 were new Asian immigrants, and the others were European American.

### Questions

1. What are some ideas for Omari that can serve as starting points for providing effective nutrition education programs to culturally diverse groups?
2. Omari's learning more about health disparities will help his program. What is the definition of health disparities? What are some health disparity issues in the United States?
3. The concepts of culture, race, and ethnicity play an important role in the success of Omari's program. What are the differences between culture, race, and ethnicity that Omari must know before starting the health promotion program?
4. Omari needs to develop cultural competence. What are the four steps for acquiring cultural competence? What does a cultural encounter involve?
5. Omari needs to know if the different ethnic groups need help adjusting to their new diets. What is acculturation? Dietary acculturation?
6. What are the cultural barriers to health promotion and disease prevention that Omari may encounter?
7. A lack of knowledge of other cultural groups can prevent Omari's understanding of the individual's point of view. Therefore, Omari reviewed the guidelines for recognizing the multicultural context of communication. What are the guidelines for recognizing the multicultural context of communication?
8. Culturally, Omari must be knowledgeable of the needs of his clients. What is cultural sensitivity?
9. What are some of the strategies for strengthening Omari's organizational cultural competence?
10. Briefly describe the dietary concerns and strategies for African Americans, Asian Americans, and Hispanic Americans outlined in Table 5-3.
11. The organizational factors of all cultures must be explored in a cultural assessment because of the differences among cultures, including communication and background. Describe at least three variations among African Americans, Asian Americans, and Hispanic Americans.
12. Work in small groups or individually to examine the case study and practice using the Nutrition Care Process chart provided on the companion website. You can add other nutrition and health-related conditions or assessments to the case study to make the case study more challenging and interesting.

## Think About It

**Answer:** Information needed to provide adequate nutritional guidance includes the following[75]:

- Types of food available
- Accepted and/or preferred foods
- Safety of the food supply and related health problems
- Energy and nutrient quality of major foods chosen
- Most commonly used foods, who selects them, and how and where they are obtained
- Food preparation methods and how they are divided among family/community
- Foods eaten, how much, when, with whom, and where
- Food storage, facilities, and methods; food safety; and garbage disposal

Other strategies that may help in the assessment include observing the neighborhood and homes where clients live, where they shop for foods, and the types of food available. He could learn more about the group by interviewing individuals from or closely associated with the client group.[75] He could ask relevant questions about food and health behaviors, or ask other healthcare professionals who serve the cultural group, community leaders among the group, and any other members of the group.

## Key Terms

**acculturation:** Repeated exposure to influences from a different culture. The process is related to age, education, frequency of interaction, and income and occurs on a continuum.

**communication:** A process of information sharing in which those involved in the communication share a common set of rules.

**cultural competence:** Understanding the importance of social and cultural influences on individuals' health beliefs and behaviors, considering how these factors interact at multiple levels of the healthcare delivery system, and devising interventions that take these issues into account ensure quality of care.

**cultural sensitivity:** Planning interventions that are relevant and acceptable within the cultural framework of the population to be reached.

**culture:** The customary beliefs, social forms, and material traits of a racial, religious, or social group.

**dietary acculturation:** The process that occurs when members of a minority group adopt the eating patterns or food choices of the majority group.

**ethnic:** The commonality of a group expressed by its nationality, language, or race.

**ethnicity:** Implies one or more of the following: shared origins or social background; shared, distinctive culture and traditions that are maintained between generations; and shared culture that contributes to a sense of identity and group.

**ethnocentrism:** The belief that one's own group view of the world is superior to that of others.

**race:** A social classification that relies on physical markers, such as skin color, to identify group membership.

## References

1. Edelstein S. *Nutrition in Public Health: A Handbook for Developing Programs and Services.* 2nd ed. Boston, MA: Jones and Bartlett; 2006.
2. US Dept of Homeland Security. *2002 Yearbook of Immigration Statistics: Immigration Information.* Washington, DC: Dept of Homeland Security; 2002.
3. Katz SH, Weaver WW. *Encyclopedia of Food and Culture.* New York, NY: Scribner; 2003.
4. US Bureau of the Census. *Projections of the Population of the United States, by Age, Sex, and Race: 1983-2008.* Washington, DC: US Bureau of the Census.
5. World Health Organization. Constitution of the World Health Organization. 2007. htt://www.who.int/governance/eb/who_constitution_en.pdf. Accessed March 12, 2016.
6. National Institutes of Health. NIH strategic research plan to reduce and ultimately eliminate health disparities. 2005. http://www.minority.unc.edu/reports/strategic.html. Accessed February 22, 2017.
7. National Institute of Health, National Cancer Institute. What are health disparities? https://www.nlm.nih.gov/hsrinfo/disparities.html. Accessed February 22, 2017.
8. Braveman P. Health disparities and health equity: concepts and measurement. *Annu Rev Public Health.* 2006;27:167-194.
9. Braveman P, Starfield B, Geiger HJ. World health report 2000: how it removes equity from the agenda for public health monitoring and policy. *BMJ.* 2001;323:678-681.
10. US Dept of Health and Human Services. *Healthy People 2010* (conference edition). Washington, DC: US Dept of Health and Human Services; 2000.
11. Smedley BD, Stith AY, Nelson AR. *Unequal Treatment Confronting Racial and Ethnic Disparities in Healthcare.* Washington, DC: National Academies Press; 2002.
12. Gordon-Larsen L. Facing racial and ethnic health disparities. *J Am Diet Assoc.* 2004;104(12):1779-1780.
13. Garte S. The racial genetics paradox in biomedical research and public health. *Public Health Rep.* 2002;17:421-425.
14. Carter-Pokras O, Baquet C. What is a health disparity? *Public Health Rep.* 2002;117(5):426-434.

15. Thomas SB. The color line: race matters in the elimination of health disparities. *Am J Public Health*. 2001;91(7):1046-1048.

16. Venter JC, Adams MD, Myers EW, et al. The sequence of the human genome. *Science*. 2001;291:1304-1351.

17. Cooper RS, Kaufman JS, Ward R. Race and genomics. *N Engl J Med*. 2003;348(12):1166-1170.

18. Oppenheimer GM. Paradigm lost: race, ethnicity, and the search for a new population taxonomy. *Am J Public Health*. 2001;91(7):1049-1055.

19. Schwartz RS. Racial profiling in medical research. *N Engl J Med*. 2001;344(18):1392-1393.

20. Arah OA, Westert GP, Delnoij DM, Klazinga NS. Health system outcomes and determinants amenable to public health in industrialized countries: a pooled cross-sectional time series analysis. [electronic resource]. *(BMC Public Health)*. 2005;5:81.

21. Blank RM, Dabady M, Citro CF. *Measuring Racial Discrimination*. Panel on methods for assessing discrimination, Committee on National Statitistics, Division of Behavioral and Social Sciences and Education. Washington, DC: Nation Research Council; 2004.

22. Quanhe Y, Muin JK, Friedman J, Flanders DW. How many genes underlie the occurrence of common complex diseases in the population? *Int J Epidemiol*. 2005:1-9.

23. Heathy People 2010. A systematic approach to health improvement. 2005. https://www.healthy people.gov/2020/topics-objectives. Accessed February 22, 2017.

24. Glover MJ, Greenlund KJ, Ayala C, Croft JB. Racial/ ethnic disparities in prevalence, treatment, and control of hypertension: United States, 1999–2002. *MMWR Morb Mortal Wkly Rep*. 2005;54(1);7-9.

25. Centers for Disease Control and Prevention. Heart disease facts. 2016. http://www.cdc.gov /heartdisease/facts.htm. Accessed April 24, 2016.

26. Howe HL, Wingo PA, Thun MJ, et al. Annual report to the nation on the status of cancer (1973 through 1998), featuring cancers with recent increasing trends. *J Natl Cancer Inst*. 2001;93(8):24-42.

27. Gargiullo P, Wingo PA, Coates RJ, Thompson TD. Recent trends in mortality rates for four major cancers, by sex and race/ethnicity: United States, 1990–1998. *MMWR Morb Mortal Wkly Rep*. 2002;51(3);49-53.

28. Ploeg M, Perrin E. *Eliminating Health Disparities Measurement and Data Needs*. Washington, DC: National Academies Press, National Research Council; 2004.

29. Office of Minority Health. 2007. https://minority health.hhs.gov/. Accessed Ferbruary 22, 2017.

30. Office of Minority Health. Health disparities experienced by black or African Americans: United States. *MMWR Morb Mortal Wkly Rep*. 2005;54(1):1-3.

31. Centers for Disease Control and Prevention, National Center on Health Statistics. National Center or Health Statistics. CDC growth charts: United States. http://www.cdc.gov/. Accessed February 22, 2017.

32. Liao Y, Tucker P, Okoro CA, Giles WH, et al. REACH 2010 surveillance for health status in minority communities: United States, 2001-2002. 2004. http://www.cdc.gov/mmwr/preview/mmwrhtml /ss5306a1.htm. Accessed February 8, 2016.

33. McNeely MJ, Boyko EJ. Type 2 diabetes prevalence in Asian Americans: results of a national health survey. *Diabetes Care*. 2004;27(1):66-69.

34. Ikeda JP, Pham L, Nguyen KP, Mitchell RA. Culturally relevant nutrition education improves dietary quality among WIC-eligible Vietnamese immigrants. *J Nutr Educ Behav*. 2002;34(3): 151-158.

35. Gordon-Larsen P, Nelson MC, Page P, Popkin BM. Inequality in the built environment underlies key health disparities in physical activity and obesity. *Pediatrics*. 2006;117:417-424.

36. Mishra GG. Socio-demographic inequalities in the diets of mid-aged Australian women. *Eur J Clin Nutrition*. 2005;59(2):185-195.

37. Park SSY. Dietary patterns using the Food Guide Pyramid groups are associated with socio-demographic and lifestyle factors: the multiethnic cohort study. *J Nutr*. 2005;135(4):843-849.

38. Shahar D, Shai I, Vardi H, Shahar A, et al. Diet and eating habits in high and low socioeconomic groups. *Nutrition*. 2005;21(5):559-566.

39. Benjamin D. *Food Insecurity and Hunger: A Preventable Public Health Problem*. Minneapolis, MN: Maternal and Child Health Program School of Public Health Division of Epidemiology and Community Health, University of Minnesota; 2006.

40. Scheier LM. What is the hunger-obesity paradox? *J Am Diet Assoc*. 2005;105:883-886.

41. Townsend MS, Peerson J, Love B, Achterberg C, et al. Food insecurity is positively related to overweight in women. *J Nutr*. 2001;131:1738-1745.

42. Drewnowski A, Darmon N. The economics of obesity: dietary energy density and energy cost. *Am J Clin Nutr*. 2005;82(1):265S-273S.

43. Blaak EE. Prevention and treatment of obesity and related complications: a role for protein? *Int J Obesity* 2006;30:S24–S27.

44. Casey PH. The association of child and household food insecurity with childhood overweight status. *Pediatrics.* 2006;118:e1406-e1413.

45. National Center for Health Statistics. *Health, United States 2003 with Chartbook on Trends in the Health of Americans.* Hyattsville, MD: Centers for Disease Control and Prevention; 2006.

46. Phares TM, Morrow B, Lansky A. Surveillance for disparities in maternal health-related behaviors—selected states. Pregnancy Risk Assessment Monitoring System (PRAMS). 2000–2001. *MMWR Morb Mortal Wkly Rep.* 2004;53(S04):1-13.

47. Louik C, Hernandez-Diaz S, Mitchell A. Nausea and vomiting in pregnancy: maternal characteristics and risk factors. *Paediatr Perinat Epidemiol.* 2006;20:270-278.

48. Foster C, Hillsdon M. Changing the environment to promote health-enhancing physical activity. *J Sports Sci.* 2004;22(8):755-769.

49. Chappel M, Funk L, Carson A, MacKenzie P, et al. Multilevel community health promotion: how can we make it work. *Community Dev J.* 2006;41(3):352-366.

50. Harris-Davis E, Haughton B. Model for multicultural nutrition counseling competencies. *J Am Diet Assoc.* 2000;100:1178-1185.

51. Marshall MI, Johnson A, Fulton J. Writing a successful grant proposal. Purdue Extension, EC-737. 1990. http://www.ces.purdue.edu/extmedia/EC/EC-737.pdf. Accessed February 22, 2017.

52. Stanhope M, Lancaster J. *Community and Public Health Nursing: Population-Centered Health Care in the Community.* 9th ed. New York, NY: Elsevier; 2015.

53. Brach C, Fraserirector I. Can cultural competency reduce racial and ethnic health disparities? A review and conceptual model. *Med Care Res Rev.* 2000;57(suppl 1):181-217.

54. Senior P, Bhopal, R. Ethnicity as a variable in epidemiological research. *Brit Med J.* 1994;30:327-328.

55. McWilliams M, Heller, H. *Food Around the World: Cultural Perspective.* Upper Saddle River, NJ: Prentice Hall; 2003.

56. Kittler PG, Sucher K, Nahikian-Nelms M. *Food and Culture.* 7th ed. Belmont CA: Wadsworth Thomson Learning; 2017.

57. Harrison GG, Kagawa-Singer M, Foerster SB. Seizing the moment: California's opportunity to prevent nutrition-related health disparities in low-income Asian American population. *Cancer.* 2005;104(12):2962-2968.

58. Lutz C, Przytulski K. *Nutrition and Diet Therapy.* 5th ed. Philadelphia, PA: F.A. Davis; 2010.

59. Dein S. Race, culture and ethnicity in minority research: a critical discussion. *J Cult Divers.* 2006; 13(2):68-75.

60. Dunham DD, Czysczon A, Chavez N, Piorkowski J, et al. Dietary differences among women of Polish descent by country of birth and duration of residency in the United States. *Ethn Dis.* 2004;14(2):219-226.

61. Arredondo EM, Elder JP, Ayala GX, Slymen D, et al. Association of a traditional vs shared meal decision-making and preparation style with eating behavior of Hispanic women in San Diego County. *J Am Diet Assoc.* 2006;106(1):38-45.

62. Betancourt JR, Green AR, Carrillo JE, Ananeh-Firempong 2nd O. Defining cultural competence: a practical framework for addressing racial ethnic disparities in health and health care. *Public Health Rep.* 2003;118(4):293-302.

63. Boyle MA, Holben D. *Community Nutrition in Action: An Entrepreneurial Approach.* 4th ed. Belmont, CA: Thomson Wadsworth; 2013.

64. White K. *Excutive Summary: Building Cultural Competence.* Tumwater, WA: Community and Family Health Multicultural Work Group. Washington State Department of Health; 2003.

65. Wittig DR. Knowledge, skills, and attitudes of nursing students regarding culturally congruent care of Native Americans. *J Transcult Nurs.* 2004;5(1):54-61.

66. Campinha-Bacote JT. *The Process of Cultural Competence in the Delivery of Healthcare Services: A Culturally Competent Model of Care.* Cincinnati, OH: Transcultural C.A.R.E. Associates; 2002.

67. Griswold KK, Zayas L, Kernan JB, Wagner CM. Cultural awareness through medical student and refugee patient encounters. *J Immigr Minor Health.* 2007;9(1):55-60.

68. Alfonso M. Cross-cultural encounter as an opportunity for personal growth. *J Humanist Psychol.* 2004;44(2):243-265.

69. Van Dyne L. Cultural Intelligence: an essential capability for individuals in contemporary organizations. 2005. http://globalEDGE.msu.edu. Accessed February 22, 2017.

70. Williams SR, Schlenker ED. *Essentials of Nutrition and Diet Therapy.* 10th ed. Davis CA: Mosby; 2010.

71. Tripp-Reimer TF, Skemp LK, Enslein JC. Cultural barriers to care: inverting the problem. *Diabetes Spectr.* 2001;14:13-22.

72. Perlas LA, Gibson R. Household dietary strategies to enhance the content and bioavailability of iron, zinc and calcium of selected rice- and maize-based Philippine complementary foods. *Matern Child Nutr.* 2005;1(4):263-273.

73. Jorge L, Margarita DR, Rosas A, Ian G, et al. Calcium absorption from corn tortilla is relatively high and is dependent upon calcium content and liming in Mexican women. *J Nutr.* 2005;135:135(11):2578-2581.

74. Yu-chih C. Chinese values, health and nursing. *J Advan Nurs.* 2001;36(2):270-273.

75. Satia-Abouta J, Patterson RE, Neuhouser ML, Elder J. Dietary acculturaiton: applications to nutrition research and dietetics. *J Am Diet Assoc.* 2002;102(8):1105-1118.

76. Satia-Abouta JJ. Psychosocial predictors of diet and acculturation in Chinese American and Chinese Canadian women. *Ethn Health.* 2002;7(1):21-39.

77. Aldrich L, Variyam JN. Acculturation erodes the diet quality of U.S. Hispanics. *Food Rev.* 2000; 23(1):51-55.

78. Sujata L. Acculturation and dietary intake. *J Am Diet Assoc.* 2005;105(3):411-412.

79. Bermúdez OI, Falcón LM, Tucker KL. Intake and food sources of macronutrients among older Hispanic adults: association with ethnicity, acculturation, and length of residence in the United States. *J Am Diet Assoc.* 2000;100:665-673.

80. Gray VB, Cossman JS, Dodson WL, Byrd SL. Dietary acculturation of Hispanic immigrants in Mississippi. *Salud Publica Mex.* 2005;47(5): 351-360.

81. Wiking E, Sven-Erik J, Sundquist J. Ethnicity, acculturation, and self reported health: a population based study among immigrants from Poland, Turkey, and Iran in Sweden. *J Epidemiol Community Health.* 2004;58:574-582.

82. Saskia J, Wind M, Lenthe FJ, Knut-Inge K, et al. Differences in fruit and vegetable intake and determinants of intakes between children of Dutch origin and non-Western ethnic minority children in the Netherlands: a cross sectional study. *Int J Behav Nutr Phys Act.* 2006;3(31).

83. Colby SE, Morrison S, Morales S, Budd L, et al. *Dietary Acculturation of Mexican American Immigrants: A Case Study.* Philadelphia, PA: US Dept of Agricultural Research; 2005.

84. Cabassa LJ. Measuring acculturation: where we are and where we need to go. *Hisp J Behav Sci.* 2003;25(2):127-146.

85. Satia-Abouta JJ. Dietary acculturation: applications to nutrition research and dietetics. *J Am Diet Assoc.* 2002;102(8):1105-1118.

86. Satia J, Patterson RE, Neuhouser M, Elder J. Dietary acculturation: applications to nutrition research and dietetics. *J Am Diet Assoc.* 2002;102(8):1105-1118.

87. Gim Chung RH, Bryan SK, Aabreu J. Asian American multidimensional acculturation scale: development, factor analysis, reliability, and validity. *Cult Divers Ethnic Minor Psychol.* 2004; 10(1):66-80.

88. Cuellar I, Harris LC, Jasso R. An acculturation scale for Mexican Americans: normal and clinical populations. *Hispanic J Behav Sci.* 1980;2:199-217.

89. Yang GP, Fox HM. Food habit changes of Chinese persons living in Lincoln, Nebraska. *J Am Diet Assoc.* 1979;75:420-424.

90. Satia J, Patterson RE, Kristal AR, Hislop TG, et al. Development of scales to measure dietary acculturation among Chinese-Americans and Chinese-Canadians. *J Am Diet Assoc.* 2001;101:548-553.

91. Anderson J, Moeschberger M, Chen MS, Kunn P, et al. An acculturation scale for Southeast Asians. *Soc Psychiatr Psychiatr Epidemiol.* 1993;289: 134–141.

92. Garner EM, Olmstead MP, Polivy J. Development and validation of a multidimentional eating disorder inventory of anorexia nervosa and bulimia. *Int J Eat Disord.* 1983;2:15-34.

93. Hammond K. Assessment: dietary and clinical data. In: Mahan L, Escott-Stump S, eds. *Krause's Food, Nutrition and Diet Therapy.* 12th ed. Philadelphia, PA: Saunders; 2004:383-410.

94. Sutherland LL. Ethnocentrism in a pluralistic society: a concept analysis. *J Transcult Nurs.* 2002;13(4):274-281.

95. Seyed-Mahmoud A. Managing workforce diversity as an essential resource for improving organizational performance. *Int J Prod Perf Manag.* 2004;53(6):521-531.

96. American School Health Association, Association for the Advancement of Health Education, Society for Public Health Education. *The National Adolescents Student Health Survey: A Report on the Health of America's Youth.* Oakland, CA: American School Health Association, Association for the Advancement of Health Education, Society for Public Health Education; 1988.

97. Satia J, Patterson RE, Taylor VM, Cheney CL, et al. Use of qualitative methods to study diet, acculturation, and health in Chinese-American women. *J Am Diet Assoc.* 2000;100:934-940.

98. Huff RM, Kline MV. *Promoting Health in Multicultural Populations: A Handbook for Practioners.* New Delhi, India: Sage Publication; 1999.

99. Holroyd E, Twinn S, Adab P. Socio-cultural influences on Chinese women's attendance for cervical screening. *J Adv Nurs.* 2004;46(1):42-52.

100. Hsu WC, Cheung S, Ong E. Identification of linguistic barriers to diabetes knowledge and glycemic control in Chinese Americans with diabetes. *Diabetes Care.* 2006;29:415-416.

101. Goins T, Williams KA, Carter MW, Spencer M, et al. Perceived barriers to health care access among rural older adults: a qualitative study. *J Rural Health.* 2005;21(3):206-213.

102. Hitchcock J, Schubert PE, Thomas SA. *Community Health Nursing.* 2nd ed. Clifton Park, NY: Thomson Delmar Learning; 2003.

103. Hisako K. A double standard in bioethical reasoning for disclosure of advanced cancer diagnoses in Japan. *Health Commun.* 2002;14(3):361-376.

104. Luckmann J. *Transcultural Communication in Healthcare.* Clifton Park, NY: Delmar Thomson Learning; 2000.

105. Schouten BB, Meeuswesen LS. Cultural differences in medical communication: a review of the literature. *Patient Educ Couns.* 2006;64(1-3):21-34.

106. Haunani D, Dillard JP, Anderson JW. Episode type, attachment orientation, and frame salience: evidence for a theory of relational framing. *Human Commun Res.* 2002;28(1):136-152.

107. Delgadillo L. Guidelines for reaching out and counseling low income monolingual Latino clients. *J Extension.* 2003; 41(6):51-78.

108. Bairstow R, Berry H, Driscoll DM. Tips for teaching non-traditional audiences. *J Extension.* 2002;40(6).

109. Edelman M. *Health Promotion Throughtout the Lifespan.* St. Louis, MO: Mosby; 2002.

110. Johnson RL, Saha S, Arbelaez JJ. Racial and ethnic differences in patient perceptions of bias and cultural competence in health care. *J Gen Intern Med.* 2004;19(2):101-110.

111. Clark CC. *Health Promotion in Communities: Holistic and Wellness Approaches.* New York, NY: Springer Publishing; 2002.

112. Giger JN, Davidhizar, R. *Transcultural Nursing Assessment and Intervention.* 3rd ed. St. Louis: Mosby; 1999.

113. US Dept of Health and Human Services, Health Resources and Services Administration. Services Administration study on measuring cultural competence in health care delivery settings. 2007. http://www.hrsa.gov/culturalcompetence/measures/sectionii.htm. Accessed March 2, 2016.

114. Kumpfer K, Alvarado R, Smith P, Bellamy N. Cultural sensitivity and adaptation in family-based prevention interventions. *Prev Sci.* 2001; 3(3):241-246.

115. **Tanjasiri SP, Kagawa-Singer M, Foo MA,** Chao M, et al. Designing culturally and linguistically appropriate health interventions: the life is precious—Hmong breast cancer study. *Health Educ Behav.* 2007;34(1):140-153.

116. Erwin DO, Johnson VA, Trevino M, Duke K, et al. A comparison of African American and Latina social networks as indicators for culturally tailoring a breast and cervical cancer education. *Cancer.* 2007;109(2):368-377.

117. Goodman MJ, Ogdie A, Kanamor MJ, Cañar J, et al. Barriers and facilitators of colorectal cancer screening among Mid-Atlantic Latinos: focus group findings. *Ethn Dis.* 2006;16(1):255-261.

118. Fawcett JT, Carino BV. *The New Immigration from Asia and the Pacific Islands.* Staten Island, NY: Center for Migration Studies; 1987.

119. McPhee SJ, Jenkins CNH, Hung S, Nguyen KP, et al. Behavioral risk factor survey of Vietnamese: California, 1991. *MMWR Morb Mortal Wkly Rep.* 1992;41:69-72.

120. Purnell L. A description of the Purnell Model for Cultural Competence. *J Transcult Nurs.* 2000; 11(1):40-46.

121. National Center for Cultural Competence. Cultural competency: concepts and definitions. 2005. http://www.allianceonline.org/members/library/diversity/cc.concept. Accessed February 14, 2016.

122. US Dept of Health and Human Services, Office of Minority Health. National standards on culturally and linguistically appropriate services (CLAS). 2001. http://www.omhrc.gov/templates/browse.aspx?lvl=2&lvlID=15. Accessed February 14, 2016.

123. Cook JT, Frank DA, Berkowitz B, Black MM, et al. Food insecurity is associated with adverse health outcomes among human infants and toddlers. *J Nutr.* 2004;134(6):1432-1438.

124. Haytowitz DB, Pehrsson PR, Holden JM. Adapting methods for determining priorities for the analysis of foods in diverse population. *J Food Comp Anal.* 2000;13:425-433.

125. Byers KK. The myth of increased lactose intolerance in African-Americans. *J Am Coll Nutr.* 2005;24(6):569S-573S.

126. Flegal KM, Carroll MD, Ogden CL, Johnson CL. Prevalence and trends in obesity among US adults, 1999–2000. *JAMA.* 2002;288(14):1723-1727.

127. Centers for Disease Control and Prevention. Overweight among U.S. children and adolescents. http://www.cdc.gov. Accessed February 22, 2017.

128. Steinberger J, Daniels SR. Obesity, insulin resistance, diabetes, and cardiovascular risk in children. *Circulation.* 2003;107:1448.

129. Ayala C, Croft JB, Wattigney WA, Mensah JA. Trends in hypertension-related death in the United States: 1980-1998. *J Clin Hypertens.* 2004;6(12):675-681.

130. Opie LH, Seedat YK. Hypertension in Sub-Saharan African populations. *Circulation.* 2005; 112(23):3562-3568.

131. Jahoor FF, Badaloo A, Reid MA, Forrester M, et al. Protein kinetic differences between children with edematous and nonedematous severe childhood undernutrition in the fed and postabsorptive states. *Am J Clin Nutr.* 2005;82(4):792-800.

132. Agyemang C, Bhopal R, Bruijnzeels M. Negro, Black, Black African, African Caribbean, African American or what? Labelling African origin populations in the health arena in the 21st century. *J Epidemiol Commun Health.* 2005;59:1014-1018.

133. Fernander AF, Durán REF, Saab PG, Schneiderman N. John Henry Active Coping, education, and blood pressure among urban blacks. *J Natl Med Assoc.* 2004;96(2):246-255.

134. Petersen KK. Community socioeconomic status is associated with carotid artery atherosclerosis in untreated, hypertensive men. *Am J Hypertension.* 2006;19(6):560-566.

135. Scott RP, Heslin KC. Historical perspectives on the are of African Americans with cardiovascular disease. *Ann Thorac Surg.* 2003;76:S1348-S1355.

136. Peters RM, Flack JM. Salt sensitivity: common findings. *Prog Cardiovasc Nurs.* 2000;15(4):138-144.

137. Flack JJ, Sica DA. Therapeutic considerations in the African-American patient with hypertension: considerations with calcium channel blocker therapy. *J Clin Hypertens (Greenwich).* 2005; 7(4 suppl 1):9-14.

138. Pothiwala PP, Evans EM, Chapman-Novakofki KM. Ethnic variation in risk for osteoporosis among women: a review of biological and behavioral factors. *J Womens Health (Larchmt).* 2006;15(6):709-719.

139. Appel LJ. Lifestyle modification as a means to prevent and treat high blood pressure. *J Am Soc Nephrol.* 2003;14(7 suppl 2):S99-S102.

140. Appel LJ, Champagne CM, Harsha DW, Cooper LS, et al. Effects of comprehensive lifestyle modification on blood pressure control. *JAMA.* 2003;289:2083-2093.

141. Hermansen K. Diet, blood pressure and hypertension. *Br J Nutr.* 2000;83(suppl 1):113-119.

142. Kulkarni KD. Food, culture, and diabetes in the United States. *Clin Diabetes.* 2004;22(4):190-192.

143. Medical News Today. Positive influence of religion and spirituality on blood pressure. 2006. http://www.medicalnewstoday.com/medicalnews.php?newsid=44202. Accessed February 14, 2016.

144. Auld GG, Boushey C, Bock M. Perspectives on intake of calcium-rich foods among Asian, Hispanic, and white preadolescent and adolescent females. *J Nutr Educ Behav.* 2002;34(5):242-251.

145. Dillinger TL, Barriga P, Escárcega S, Jimenez M, et al. Food of the gods: cure for humanity? A cultural history of the medicinal and ritual use of chocolate. *J Nutr.* 2000;130(8S suppl):2057S-2072S.

146. Fleuriet KJ. Health and health care problems among the Kumiai of San Antonio Necua and their indigenous relatives in Baja California: reflections of poverty, marginality, and a history of colonization. *Californian J Health Promot.* 2003;1(1):140-157.

147. Alejandro M, Rolf P, Zea M. Use and implications of ethnomedical health care approaches among Central American immigrants. *Health Social Work.* 2003;28(1):43-51.

148. McArthur LH, Ruben P, Viramontez A, Deigo N. Maintenance and change in the diet of Hispanic immigrants in Eastern North Carolina. *Fam Consum Sci Res J.* 2001;29(4):309-335.

149. Hai L, Bermudez OI, Tucker KL. Dietary patterns of Hispanic elders are associated with acculturation and obesity. *J Nutr.* 2003;133(11): 3651-3657.

150. Mazur R, Marquis GS, Jensen HH. Diet and food insufficiency among Hispanic youths: acculturation and socioeconomic factors in the third National Health and Nutrition Examination Survey. *Am J Clin Nutr.* 2003;78(6):1120-1127.

151. Neuhouser ML, Thompson B, Coronado GD, Solomon CC. Higher fat intake and lower fruit and vegetables intakes are associated with greater acculturation among Mexicans living in Washington State. *J Am Diet Assoc.* 2004;104(1): 51-57.

152. Harris R, Nicoll AD, Adair PM, Pine CM. Risk factors for dental caries in young children: a systematic review of the literature. *Community Dent Health.* 2004;21:S71-S85.

153. Bonuck KA. Prolonged bottle use and its association with iron deficiency anemia and overweight: a preliminary study. *Clin Pediatr.* 2002;41(8): 603-607.

154. Matheson DM, Killen JD, Wang Y, Varady A, et al. Children's food consumption during television viewing. *Am J Clin Nutr.* 2004;79(6):1088-1094.

155. Artinian NT, Schim SM, Vander Wal JS, Nies MA. Eating patterns and cardiovascular disease risk in a Detroit Mexican American population. *Public Health Nurs.* 2004;21(5):425-434.

156. Duraski SA. Meeting the needs of the community: a project to prevent stroke in Hispanics. *Top Stroke Rehabil.* 2003;9(4):46-56.

157. Umana-Taylor AJ, Bámaca MY. Conducting focus groups with Latino populations: lessons from the field. *Fam Relat.* 2004;53(3):261-272.

158. Hobbs BB. Latino outreach programs: why they need to be different. *J Exension.* 2004;42(4):1-4.

159. Rundle A, Carvalho M, Robinson M. *Cultural Competence in Healthcare: A Practical Guide.* Boston, MA: Jossey-Bass; 2002.

160. Garrett JT, Garrett MT. *The Cherokee Full Circle: A Practical Guide to Ceremonies and Traditions.* Santa Fe, NM: Bear & Company; 2004.

161. Tarrell AA, Portman A, Garrett MT. Native American healing traditions: indigenous and complementary and alternative healing practices. *Int J Disabil Dev Educ.* 2006;53(4):452-469.

162. Flesher ME, Archer ME, Katharine KA, McCollom RA, et al. Assessing the metabolic and clinical consequences of early enteral feeding in the malnourished patient. *JPEN J Parenter Enteral Nutr.* 2005;29(2):108-117.

163. Benyshek DC, Martin JF, Johnston CS. A reconsideration of the origins of the type 2 diabetes epidemic among Native Americans and the implications for intervention policy. *Med Anthropol.* 2001;20(1):25-64.

164. McGanity WJ. The story of the Interdepartmental Committee on Nutrition for National Defense's North American Activities (1958-1970). *J Nutr.* 2005;135:1268-1271.

165. Jimenez MM, Receveur O, Trifinopoulos M, Kuhnlein H, et al. Comparison of the dietary intakes of two different groups of children (grades 4 to 6) before and after the Kahnawake schools diabetes prevention project. *J Am Diet Assoc.* 2003;103:1191-1194.

166. Di Noia J, Schinke SP, Contento IR. Dietary patterns of reservation and non-reservation Native American youths. *Ethn Dis.* 2005;15(4):705-712.

167. Abizadeh A. Ethnicity, race, and a possible humanity. *World Order.* 2001;33(1):23-34.

168. Obarzanek E, Kimm S, Barton B, Van Horn L, et al. Long-term safety and efficacy of cholesterol-lowering diet in children with elevated low-density lipoprotein cholesterol: seven-year results of the Dietary Intervention Study in Children (DISC). *Pediatrics.* 2001;107:256-264.

169. Luo L. A preliminary study on the concept of health among the Chinese. *Couns Psychol Q.* 2002;15(2):179-189.

170. Cabrera C, Artacho R, Giménez R. Beneficial effects of green tea: a review. *J Am Coll Nutr.* 2006;25(2):79-99.

171. Nan L, Brown J, Liu B. Factors influencing dairy product consumption of Chinese Americans in Pennsylvania: enhancing nutrition consumption in the American diet. *Top Clin Nutr.* 2007;22(3):258-271.

172. Kobayashi H, Mizuno N, Teramae H, Kutsuna H, et al. Diet and Japanese herbal medicine for recalcitrant atopic dermatitis: efficacy and safety. *Drugs Exp Clin Res.* 2004;30(5-6):197-202.

173. Lv N, Cason K. Dietary pattern change and acculturation of Chinese Americans in Pennsylvania. *J Am Diet Assoc.* 2004;104(5):771-778.

174. Kwok TT. Does low lactose milk powder improve the nutritional intake and nutritional status of frail older Chinese people living in nursing homes? *J Nutr Health Aging.* 2001;5(1):17-21.

175. Greenspan SL, Resnick NM, Parker RA. Combination therapy with hormone replacement and alendronate for prevention of bone loss in elderly women a randomized controlled trial *JAMA.* 2003;289:2525-2533.

176. Park SYS-Y, Murphy S, Sangita S, Colonel L. Dietary intakes and health-related behaviours of Korean American women born in the USA and Korea: the Multiethnic Cohort Study. *Public Health Nutr.* 2005;8(7):904-911.

177. Abate N, Chandalia M. Ethnicity and type 2 diabetes. *J Diabetes Complications.* 2001;15:320 327.

178. Oh SSY. Food insecurity is associated with dietary intake and body size of Korean children from low-income families in urban areas. *Eur J Clin Nutr.* 2003;57(12):1598-1604.

179. Katsuhiko Y, Grove JS, Chen S, Rodriguez BL, et al. Plasma fibrinogen as a predictor of total and cause-specific mortality in elderly Japanese-American men. *Arterioscler Thromb Vasc Biol.* 2001;21:1065-1070.

180. Alka M, Kanaya MD, Grady D, Barrett-Connor E. Explaining the sex difference in coronary heart disease mortality among patients with type 2 diabetes mellitus. *Arch Intern Med.* 2002;162:1737-1745

181. Barbato A, Cappuccio FP, Folkerd EJ, Strazzullo P, et al. Metabolic syndrome and renal sodium handling in three ethnic groups living in England. *Diabetologia.* 2004;47(1):40-46.

182. Kwoka TCY, Woob J. Relationship of urinary sodium/potassium excretion and calcium intake to blood pressure and prevalence of hypertension among older Chinese vegetarians. *Eur J Clin Nutr.* 2003;57:299-304.

183. Centers for Disease Control and Prevention. Cancer selected U.S. National research findings. 2007. http://www.cdc.gov/Women/natstat/cancer.htm. Accessed February 23, 2016.

184. Jee SH, Yun JE, Park EJ, Cho ER, et al. Body mass index and cancer risk in Korean men and women. *Int J Cancer.* 2008;123(8):1892-1896.

185. Oh SW, Yoon YS, Shin SA. Effects of excess weight on cancer incidences depending on cancer sites and histologic findings among men: Korea

National Health Insurance Corporation Study. *J Clin Oncol.* 2005;23(23):4742-4754.

186. Suinn RM, Rickard-Figueroa K, Lew S, Vigil P. The Suinn-Lew Asian Self-Identity Acculturation Scale: an initial report. *Educ Psychol Meas.* 1987;47:401-407.

187. Rozen GGS, Rennert GG, Rennert HHS, Diab GG, et al. Calcium intake and bone mass development among Israeli adolescent girls. *J Am Coll Nutr.* 2001;20(3):219-224.

188. Ohio State University Extension. Fact sheets: cultural diversity: eating in America: African-American, Asian, Mexican-American. 2004. http://ohioline .osu.edu/hyg-fact/5000/. Accessed February, 2017.

189. Donelle LL, Hoffman-Goetz LL, Clarke JJN. Ethnicity, genetics, and breast cancer: media portrayal of disease identities. *Ethn Health.* 2005; 10(3):185-197.

190. American Dietetic Association, American Diabetes Association. *Ethnic and Regional Food Practices: A Series (Soul and Traditional Southern, Mexican American, Chinese American, Jewish, and Navajo).* Chicago, IL: American Dietetic Association; 1989-1998.

191. Kraft Foods. Spring-summer 2005 nutrition update: providing nutrition guidance to a multicultural population—the importance of cultural competency. 2011. http://www.kraftnutrition .com. Accessed April 10, 2016.

192. Coon CS. *The Races of Europe.* New York, NY: Macmillan; 1939:400-401.

193. University of Missouri–St. Louis. Key American values. 2016. http://www.umsl.edu/~intelstu /Admitted%20Students/Visitor%20Handbook /keyvalues.html. Accessed July 6, 2016.

194. David H, Fischer AS. *Four British Folkways in America.* New York, NY: Oxford University Press; 1991:30-50.

195. Association AH. Sugar-sweetened drinks linked to increased risk of heart disease in men. 2016. http://newsroom.heart.org/news/sugar-sweetened -drinks-linked-230144. Accessed July 6, 2016.

196. Cahill LE, An Pan S, Qi Sun W, Frank BH, et al. Fried-food consumption and risk of type 2 diabetes and coronary artery disease: a prospective study in 2 cohorts of US women and men. *Am J Clin Nutr.* 2014;18:1-9.

197. Xia WY, Yingying O, Jun L. Fruit and vegetable consumption and mortality from all causes, cardiovascular disease, and cancer: systematic review and dose-response meta-analysis of prospective cohort studies. *BJM.* 2014;349:2-14.

198. Schwab U, Lauritzen L, Tholstrup T, Thorhallur, H. Effect of the amount and type of dietary fat on cardiometabolic risk factors and risk of developing type 2 diabetes, cardiovascular diseases, and cancer: a systematic review. *Food Nutr Res.* 2014;58:25-45.

199. Stratis Health. European Americans in Minnesota. 2016. http://www.culturecareconnection .org/matters/diversity/european.html. Accessed July 6, 2016.

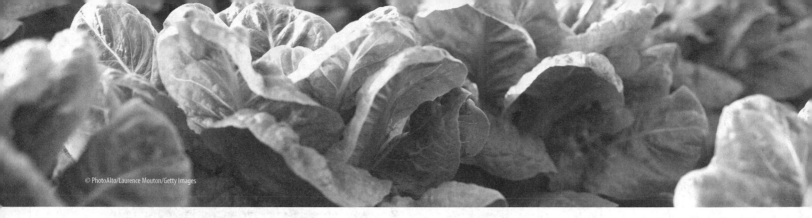

# CHAPTER 6

# Public Policy and Nutrition

## CHAPTER OUTLINE

- Introduction
- Legislation and Public Policy
- Implementing and Enforcing Nutrition Policy in the United States
- The Policymaking Process
- Policymaking Strategies
- State and Local Policy
- The Links Among Nutrition Monitoring, Nutrition Research, and Nutrition Policy
- Emerging Policy Issues in the United States

## LEARNING OBJECTIVES

- Describe how dietitians can become involved in setting policy at the local level.
- Identify tools the government can use to influence policy.
- Describe the United States' legislative process.
- Define the policymaking process.
- List the strategies that can be used to develop policy.
- Describe the major federal agencies that administer nutrition programs.

## ▶ Introduction

The U.S. government has created policies whose goal is to improve the general health of the public through dietary means. These policies include increasing the purchasing power of the poor, distributing surplus commodities to low-income families, and providing meals to school children and the elderly.[1] Four components form the foundation of U.S. nutrition **policy**: nutrition assistance, nutrition education, nutrition information (labeling), and nutrition research. Each of these four components is vital to promoting health, protecting against disease, and combating the obesity epidemic. Dietetic professionals can influence the food, nutrition, and health policy agenda by supporting individuals' appropriate food choices, delivering high-quality nutrition programs and services, and becoming involved with the regulatory process.[2] One example of successful policy change at the local level is the Child and Adolescent Trial for Cardiovascular Health (CATCH) study, presented in this chapter's Successful Community Strategies feature.

This chapter discusses the U.S. legislative process, policymaking processes and strategies, and the links among nutrition monitoring, nutrition research, and nutrition policy.

# ▶ Legislation and Public Policy

The government can use different tools to influence policies and the lives of citizens. Some of the tools include taxes, tax incentives, price supports for commodities, financial support, and services such as education.[3] Laws are tools that the government uses to form policies. In the United States, Congress is the main legislative body that sets policy and supplies the basic legislation that governs the people. Dietitians or public health professionals can influence the policies that affect people by providing testimony regarding the consequences of food insecurity, lack of nutrition education or nutrition services, or unavailable medical nutrition therapy to legislators who may not have the medical background or in-depth knowledge of people's needs at the local level. Also, dietitians can participate in the legislative process by asking members of Congress to sponsor a bill. For these reasons, all healthcare providers need in-depth knowledge and understanding of how a bill becomes a law.[4]

## How a Bill Becomes a Law

The three branches of the federal government are executive, judicial, and legislative. The executive branch consists of the president and presidential cabinet. The judicial branch, or court system, interprets the laws and settles legal disagreements. Congress is the legislative branch, and its major function is making laws. The U.S. Congress consists of the House of Representatives and the Senate.[3,5] The legislative branch enacts laws that initiate, modify, authorize, and appropriate funds for all programs and services that the federal government administers.[6] In Congress, most action happens in committees or subcommittees.[3,7] Several committees, such as the Committee on Agriculture, Nutrition, and Forestry and the Committee on Appropriations, consider food, nutrition, and health issues.[7] The legislative process is the same for both federal and state legislation because each level has a Senate and a House of Representatives.[8]

**Standing committees** are permanently established to create and approve legislation to authorize programs and supervise program implementation.[7] The majority of standing committees also recommend authorized levels of funds for government operations and for new and existing programs within their jurisdiction. The federal Senate and House of Representatives have a number of standing committees with jurisdiction over food, nutrition, and health-related programs.[9]

**Senate:**

- *Committee on Agriculture, Nutrition, and Forestry:* Child nutrition and other food programs
- *Committee on Appropriations:* Program funding
- *Committee on Finance:* Medicare and Medicaid programs
- *Committee on Foreign Relations:* International hunger
- *Committee on Labor and Human Resources:* Department of Health and Human Services programs—elderly nutrition, maternal and child health, and food labeling

**House of Representatives:**

- *Committee on Agriculture:* Food programs
- *Committee on Appropriations:* Program funding
- *Committee on Education and Labor:* Child and elderly nutrition programs
- *Committee on Energy and Commerce:* Food labeling
- *Committee on Ways and Means:* Medicare and Medicaid

A bill is a type of proposal used to introduce legislation. Before a bill is signed into law, both houses of Congress must approve it. However, it is very rare for both sides to pass an identical bill.[7] When the two chambers pass a bill that is similar but not identical, the differences between the versions of the bill passed by the House and the Senate are reconciled by a conference committee appointed from members of the relevant House and Senate committees. So, these joint committees have representation from both the House and the Senate.[9] Once the conferees agree on identical language, the bill is sent back to both the House and Senate for approval.[10]

After the bill has passed through the appropriate committees, it goes to the president for a signature. If the president signs the bill, it becomes law and serves as the basis for financing federal operations.[9] (See **BOX 6-1** for an example of a bill sponsored by the Academy of Nutrition and Dietetics [AND] that was approved and signed into law.) However, if the president disapproves of the bill, he or she can veto it. When that happens, the only way for the bill to become law is for both the House and the Senate to vote by a two-thirds majority to override the veto.[8] Also, if the president refuses to sign the bill within 10 days after Congress has adjourned at the end of its 2-year life span, the bill dies; this is called a "pocket veto." **FIGURE 6-1** outlines the process a bill undergoes before passage into law.

**BOX 6-1** Highlights of the Academy of Nutrition and Dietetics' Success with the Legislative Process[1,3,6-17]

An issue often requires many years before it reaches a critical mass in public support to enable a policy change. The Academy of Nutrition and Dietetics (AND) campaigned and obtained support for **medical nutrition therapy (MNT)**. MNT is the use of specific nutrition services to treat an illness, injury, or condition, and it involves two phases: 1) detailed assessment of a person's medical, psychosocial, and dietary histories and a physical examination and 2) treatment, which includes nutrition therapy, counseling, and the use of specialized nutrition supplements.

Since the 1980s, AND's government affairs program and other health-related associations have worked diligently to justify and advocate for MNT. AND's main legislative goal has been to obtain Medicare reimbursement for MNT services provided by registered dietitians. In 1992, AND began its MNT campaign by publishing a position paper proposing development of healthcare policy that guarantees affordable and accessible healthcare services for all Americans. In addition, AND proposed that nutrition assessment, therapeutic nutrition services, and intervention be included as an essential part of any healthcare reform legislation.

AND structured a grassroots lobbying network and campaigned among AND members to accomplish its goal. These efforts helped to increase the visibility of the dietetics profession on Capitol Hill and to lobby Congress to support MNT. It formed coalitions with other health-related organizations to develop a uniform position on healthcare reform. The president of AND testified at a hearing by the Health Subcommittee of the House Ways and Means Committee on Medicare and budget reconciliation issues on behalf of the Association. In addition, AND members wrote letters to legislators and met with Washington lobbyists and important members of Congress. AND also used advertisements to educate consumers and policy makers about the benefits of nutrition services and potential impact of MNT.

Finally, the Medical Nutrition Therapy Act (H.R. 2247 and S. 1964) was introduced during the 104th Congress, with the House version having 91 co-sponsors and the Senate version having 4 co-sponsors. Unfortunately, both bills expired when Congress adjourned. However, AND was not discouraged because the bill received significant support that encouraged AND to continue its efforts. AND renewed its effort by introducing the Medicare Medical Nutrition Therapy Act of 1997 (H.R. 1375 and S. 597) in the 105th Congress on April 17, 1997. This started a new endeavor to obtain a majority of congressional members as co-sponsors of the legislation by March 1998. The efforts for the passage of legislation to include MNT as part of the healthcare reform continued during the following 2 years with the help of the Honorable John E. Ensign, who introduced the bill in the House saying, "[it] will help to save Medicare and, most importantly, to save lives."

After 8 years of effort, on December 15, 2000 Congress finally passed a Medicare Part B MNT provision as part of the Benefits Improvement and Protection Act (P.L.106 to 554 [H.R. 566]). On December 21, 2000, President Clinton signed legislation (Public Law 106-554) that included the provision for creating a new Medicare MNT benefit that was limited to patients with diabetes or kidney disease (predialysis). AND President Jane White acknowledged the importance of the MNT victory, stating, "As we consider the significance of this victory, we can say without reservation that our work to bring recognition to dietetic professionals working in all settings is producing results. The ability of dietetic professionals to serve in the food and healthcare systems is growing in meaningful ways."

The implementation process for MNT benefits started as soon as President Clinton signed the legislation. The final rules that direct the application of the MNT benefits were developed by the Centers for Medicare and Medicaid Services (CMS) of the U.S. Department of Health and Human Services (DHHS) and were published in the **Federal Register** in November 2001. This process determined the payment levels, provider qualifications, and other coverage details. On January 1, 2002, registered dietitians started to register as Medicare providers and provide services to program beneficiaries.

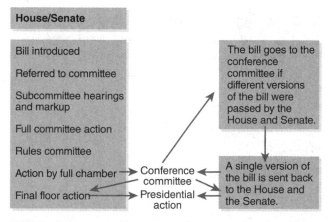

**FIGURE 6-1** How a bill becomes a law: typical path to passage of legislation.

# ▶ Implementing and Enforcing Nutrition Policy in the United States

As soon as legislation is passed and signed into law, implementation and enforcement of the law become the responsibility of the agency in the executive branch to which it is assigned. The president heads the executive branch.[7] Most of the laws enacted that affect nutrition, food, and health are passed to the U.S. Department of Agriculture (USDA) or the U.S. Department of Health and Human Services (DHHS) for implementation in public health services. Therefore, after the law is passed,

## Successful Community Strategies

### Child and Adolescent Trial for Cardiovascular Health (CATCH)[3]

Dietetics professionals who become involved in setting policy at the local level can make a significant impact on the health of individuals in the community, as demonstrated by the CATCH intervention study. The purpose of this study was to assess the outcomes of health behavior interventions, focusing on the elementary school environment, classroom curricula, and home programs for the prevention of cardiovascular disease.

Twenty-eight ethnically diverse third-grade through fifth-grade students in public schools located in California, Louisiana, Minnesota, and Texas participated in the intervention. At the school level, two primary end points were changes in the fat content of food service lunch offerings and the amount of moderate-to-vigorous physical activity in the physical education programs. At the level of the individual student, serum cholesterol change was the primary end point and was used for power calculations in the study. Twenty-eight additional schools received the dietary and physical activity intervention as well as family education.

Results showed that in the intervention school lunches, the percentage of energy intake from fat was significantly lower (from 38.7 percent to 31.9 percent) than in control lunches (from 38.9 percent to 36.2 percent). The intensity of physical activity in physical education classes increased significantly during the CATCH intervention in the intervention schools compared with the control schools. Self-reported daily energy intake from fat among students in the intervention schools decreased significantly (from 32.7 percent to 30.3 percent) compared with students in the control schools (from 32.6 percent to 32.2 percent). Intervention students reported more daily vigorous activity than control students (58.6 minutes vs. 46.5 minutes). Blood pressure, body size, and cholesterol measures, however, did not change significantly between treatment groups.

The findings of the study imply that the CATCH intervention was able to modify the fat content of school lunches, increase moderate-to-vigorous physical activity in physical education, and improve eating and physical activity behaviors in children. These changes were attributed to the policy modification in the food selections offered in the school cafeteria and the content of the physical education classes.

administrative bodies such as the USDA interpret the law and provide the detailed regulations or rules that set the policy into effect.[11] sometimes the regulations are called **secondary legislation**. The total volume of this activity is huge, confirmed by the size of the *Federal Register*. The *Federal Register* contains all regulations and proposed regulations and is published weekly. The **Code of Federal Regulations (CFR)** is a comprehensive summary of all regulations currently in operation. For example, when the Special Supplemental Nutrition Program for Women, Infants, and Children (WIC) program started, the details of the regulations were published in the *Federal Register* on July 11, 1973, about 9 months after Congress passed the law.[3] New laws and amendments to the existing law were enacted over time to increase the amount of money budgeted for the WIC program; the laws and amendments specify how the program should be implemented and approve the continuation of the program for additional budget years.[12,13]

**BOX 6-2** shows an example of the *Federal Register* notice describing the USDA's Food and Nutrition Service announcement of annual adjustments to the Income Eligibility Guidelines to be used in determining eligibility for free and reduced-price meals or free milk for the period from July 1, 2005 through June 30, 2006.

## U.S. Food and Drug Administration

The U.S. Food and Drug Administration (FDA) is a scientific, regulatory, and public health agency that oversees items accounting for 25 cents of every dollar spent by consumers. At some levels, the FDA may be the most well-known of the agencies to the general public. The FDA's policies and work affect the lives of almost every American every day because this agency is mainly responsible for determining that the food supply is safe and wholesome. Its jurisdiction encompasses items such as the following[14]:

- Human and animal drugs
- Therapeutic agents of biological origin
- Medical devices and radiation-emitting products for consumer, medical, and occupational use
- Cosmetics
- Animal feed

The FDA's jurisdiction also covers food products, including[12]:

- Labeling
- Safety of all food products (except meat and poultry)
- Bottled water

The agency has grown from a single chemist in the USDA in 1862 to a staff of about 9,100 employees

**BOX 6-2** A Portion of a Proposed Rule Published by the Department of Agriculture's Food and Nutrition Service[18]

**Federal Register: March 18, 2005 (Volume 70, Number 52)**

Notices
Pages 13160–13163
From the Federal Register Online via GPO Access
(wais.access.gpo.gov)
(DOCID: fr18mr05-35)

Department of Agriculture

Food and Nutrition Service
Child Nutrition Programs—Income Eligibility Guidelines
Agency: Food and Nutrition Service, USDA.
Action: Notice.

Summary: This Notice announces the Department's annual adjustments to the Income Eligibility Guidelines to be used in determining eligibility for free and reduced-price meals or free milk for the period from July 1, 2005 through June 30, 2006. These guidelines are used by schools, institutions, and facilities participating in the National School Lunch Program (and Commodity School Program), School Breakfast Program, Special Milk Program for Children, Child and Adult Care Food Program, and Summer Food Service Program. The annual adjustments are required by section 9 of the Richard B. Russell National School Lunch Act. The guidelines are intended to direct benefits to those children most in need and are revised annually to account for changes in the Consumer Price Index.

Reproduced from: *Federal Register.* March 18, 2005;70(52):13160-13163. Available at: http://frwebgate.access.gpo.gov/cgi-bin/multidb.cgi.

including chemists, pharmacologists, physicians, microbiologists, nutritionists, veterinarians, pharmacists, lawyers, and many others. The agency scientists evaluate applications for new human drugs and biologics, complex medical devices, food and color additives, infant formulas, and animal drugs. Also, the FDA monitors the manufacture, import, transport, storage, and sale of approximately $1 trillion worth of products yearly, which costs taxpayers about $3 per person. Investigators and inspectors visit more than 16,000 facilities a year and arrange with state governments to help increase the number of facilities checked. Although the U.S. food supply is among the safest in the world, foodborne illness has been estimated to cause approximately 76 million illnesses, 325,000 hospitalizations, and 5,000 deaths a year.[15,16] The FDA is also responsible

for the safety of 80 percent of all food consumed in the United States—the entire food supply except for meat, poultry, and some egg products, which are regulated by the USDA.

The FDA plays a significant role in protecting the nation's food against bioterrorism. Under the Bioterrorism Preparedness and Response Act of 2002, the FDA developed regulations that require all of the more than 400,000 domestic and foreign food facilities to register with the FDA. This allows the FDA to address quickly high-risk situations. Also, the new rules require importers to tell the FDA in advance about food shipments; this improves the FDA's ability to detain suspected food and require food companies to keep better records so any contamination can be traced back to its source.[17] The law not only strengthens the FDA's authority to detain suspect food, but also allows for more grants to the states to help inspect food facilities.[14]

Additionally, the Total Diet Study (TDS) is the FDA's ongoing market basket survey in which about 280 core foods (TDS foods) in the U.S. food supply are collected and analyzed to determine levels of various contaminants and nutrients in those foods. Four market baskets are usually collected each year, one in each of four geographic regions of the United States (i.e., West, North Central, South, and Northeast). For each market basket, samples of each TDS food are collected from grocery stores and fast-food restaurants in three cities within the region, prepared for consumption, and analyzed to measure the levels of selected contaminants and nutrients. The list of TDS foods is updated from time to time to reflect changing eating patterns in the United States. The target population is all age groups: infants, young children, male and female teenagers, male and female adults, and male and female older persons.[19,20] For more information on TDS visit the USDA website.

The authority and funding for many public health nutrition programs originate in Washington, D.C., but agency administrators and local and state government officials can authorize additional funds and programs to address observed community needs. Many policies originate at the program level as the nutritionist and agency administrators develop their strategies, operational plans, and protocols for delivering nutrition services and write grant proposals for innovative new programs. The two departments important for nutrition purposes at the federal level are the DHHS and the USDA.

## U.S. Department of Health and Human Services

The U.S. Department of Health and Human Services (DHHS) administers the majority of public health and nutrition programs. It is the second largest federal agency in regard to dollar amount received from the federal budget for its programs. Its organizational chart is shown in **FIGURE 6-2**. The DHHS is the U.S. government's principal agency for protecting the health of all Americans and providing essential human services, especially helping vulnerable populations (low-income families and individuals) help themselves. Its mission is to protect and advance the health of the American people. The department includes more than 300 programs covering a wide variety of activities, including the following[21]:

- Health and social science research
- Disease prevention, including immunization services
- Food and drug safety
- Medicare (health insurance for elderly and disabled Americans) and Medicaid (health insurance for low-income people)
- Health information technology
- Financial assistance and services for low-income families

- Improvement in maternal and infant health
- Head Start (preschool education and services)
- Faith-based and community initiatives
- Child abuse and domestic violence prevention
- Substance abuse treatment and prevention
- Services for older Americans, including home-delivered meals
- Comprehensive health services for Native Americans
- Medical preparedness for emergencies, including potential terrorism

DHHS's Medicare program is the nation's largest health insurer, handling more than 1 billion claims per year. Medicare and Medicaid together provide healthcare insurance for one in four Americans. The Social Security Act established both Medicare and Medicaid in 1965. The Social Security Administration (SSA) was responsible for Medicare and the Social and Rehabilitation Service (SRS) administered federal assistance to the state Medicaid programs. SSA and SRS were

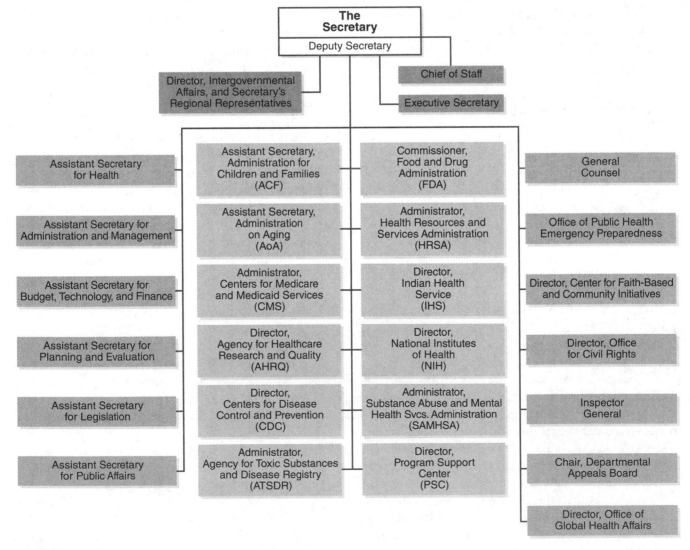

**FIGURE 6-2** Department of Health and Human Services organizational chart.

Modified from: Department of Health and Human Services website. Available at: http://www.dhhs.gov/about/index.html. Accessed February 27, 2008.

agencies in the Department of Health, Education, and Welfare (HEW). To effectively coordinate Medicare and Medicaid, the Health Care Financing Administration (HCFA) was created under HEW in 1977. In 1980, HEW was divided into the Department of Education and the DHHS. In 2001, HCFA was renamed the Centers for Medicare and Medicaid Services (CMS).

The difference between Medicare and Medicaid is that Medicare is a federal health insurance program that provides funds for medical costs to people who are 65 years of age or older, some people under 65 with disabilities, and people with permanent kidney failure. Medicaid is health insurance for low-income families funded jointly by the federal and state governments (including the District of Columbia and the Territories) to provide partial or full payment of medical costs for categories of individuals and families of any age who are too poor to pay for the care.[22] See Chapter 18 for detailed information on Medicare and Medicaid. The DHHS works closely with state and local governments, and many DHHS-funded services are provided at the local level by state or county agencies or through private sector grantees. Eleven operating divisions, including eight agencies in the U.S. Public Health Service and three human services agencies, administer the department's programs. The fiscal year 2010 budget for DHHS was $860 billion, and it employed 67,444 people. Some of these agencies and their services are presented in **TABLE 6-1**. This table does not represent an exhaustive list of nutrition education activities conducted by the federal government.

## U.S. Department of Agriculture

The USDA is another federal agency involved in healthcare, predominantly through administering the Food and Nutrition Service (FNS) programs. Its organizational chart is presented in **FIGURE 6-3**. "The mission of the USDA is to provide leadership on food, agriculture, natural resources, and related issues based on good public policy, the best available science, and efficient management."[21] The FNS oversees a variety of food assistance activities. It collaborates with state and local government welfare agencies to provide Supplemental Nutrition Assistance Program (SNAP) to low-income persons and to increase their food purchasing power. Other programs include School Breakfast and Lunch Programs, WIC, and grants to states for nutrition education training. In addition, the USDA also provides the following services[27]:

- Directs the federal antihunger effort with the Supplemental Nutrition Assistance, School Lunch, School Breakfast, and WIC Programs
- Responsible for the nation's 192 million acres of national forests and rangelands

- Plays a significant role as a conservation agency, encouraging voluntary efforts to protect soil, water, and wildlife on the 70 percent of America's lands that are in private hands
- Provides housing, modern telecommunications, and safe drinking water to rural America
- Responsible for the safety of meat, poultry, and egg products
- Conducts research in human nutrition and new crop technologies that allows the production of food and fiber using less water and pesticides
- Ensures open markets for U.S. agricultural products
- Provides food aid to people in need overseas

## ▶ The Policymaking Process

It is important for public health/community nutritionists to know the definition of policy before they can effectively initiate or change policies. "Policy is a framework that directs the actions to be followed by an individual, an organization, a government, or communities to meet the needs of society and individuals."[7,28,29] Public policies exercise a significant impact on societal behavior; they materialize when science, economics, and social and political circumstances induce government response and direction to meet a need or solve a problem.[7,28] Public policies are interpreted and implemented by public and private entities.[30] There are different types of public policies that can affect food, nutrition, and health, including the following:

- Agricultural policy influences the quantity and quality of the food supply and the costs of foods in the grocery store.[31]
- Health policy is enacted to achieve a preferred health outcome, for an individual, a family, a group, a community, or society as a whole.[32] One example of health policy is ensuring adequate healthcare (immunization, flu shots, prenatal care, etc.) for low-income families.
- Environmental policy influences consumer food intake patterns. For example, the public may perceive potential carcinogenic pollutants in foods, water, and the like as a major health problem; therefore, an effective public policy may be developed to reduce the risk of public exposure to these pollutants.
- Science policy influences funding priorities for research and for development of new food products. For example, a nutritionist may receive funding to conduct research activities that can reduce the incidence of colon cancer or develop a low-calorie food item.

**TABLE 6-1** Federal Agencies Involved in Public Health Service[21,23-26]

| U.S. Department of Health and Human Services | | |
|---|---|---|
| **Acronym** | **Agency Name** | **Services** |
| ODPHP | Office of Disease Prevention and Health Promotion | ■ Coordinates federal health promotion and disease prevention activities<br>■ Publishes *Healthy People, Promoting Health/Preventing Disease: Objectives for the Nation*, and the *Surgeon General's Report on Nutrition and Health*<br>■ Coordinates the development and implementation of the National Health Objectives for the Years 2000, 2010, and 2020 |
| FDA | Food and Drug Administration | ■ Regulates food, drugs, cosmetics, and other products<br>■ Prescribes nutrition labeling on food product packages |
| NIH<br>■ NHLBI<br><br>■ NCEP<br><br>■ NCI<br><br>■ NIA<br><br><br><br>■ NCCAM | National Institutes of Health<br>National Heart, Lung, and Blood Institute<br>National Cholesterol EducationProgram<br>National Cancer Institute<br>National Institute on Aging<br><br><br>National Center for Complementary and Alternative Medicine | ■ Manages nutrition research and education programs<br>■ Administers the National Cholesterol Education Program (NCEP) and the National High Blood Pressure Education Program (NHBPEP)<br>■ Provides services and publications to educate the public about diseases of the heart<br>■ Takes leadership in research on innovative interventions, nutrition education, and cancer prevention<br>■ Leads national programs on research on the biomedical, social, and behavioral aspects of the aging process; the prevention of age-related diseases and disabilities; and the promotion of a better quality of life for all older Americans<br>■ Explores complementary and alternative medical practices in the context of rigorous science, which involves training NCCAM researchers and disseminating authoritative information |
| CDC | Centers for Disease Control and Prevention | ■ Administers nutrition monitoring and other nutrition surveillance activities |
| NCHS | National Center for Health Statistics | ■ Administers the periodic National Health and Nutrition Examination Surveys (NHANES) and publishes and disseminates the data |
| CCDPHP | Center for Chronic Disease Prevention and Health Promotion | ■ Administers the preventive health services block grant, which covers screening and referral for many chronic diseases, manages pediatric and pregnancy surveillance programs, and administers the Behavioral Risk Factor Survey (BRFS), which includes some nutrition questions |
| OHDS | Office of Human Development Services: includes the Administration on Aging (AoA) | ■ Administers meal programs for the elderly under Title III of the Older Americans Act (OAA) |
| ACF | Administration for Children and Families | ■ Administers the Head Start Program, which provides health, food, and nutrition education for children and their parents |

| Acronym | Agency Name | Services |
|---------|-------------|----------|
| CMS | Centers for Medicare and Medicaid Services | ■ Medicare: provides insurance coverage for health services for older Americans; regulations cover nutrition and dietetic services in hospitals, nursing homes, home health agencies, hospices, and other facilities that meet the Medicare conditions of participation<br>■ Medicaid: administered through state agencies and funds health services for low-income individuals and the disabled; regulates the Early Periodic Screening, Diagnosis, and Treatment (EPSDT) program for children through partnership with states |
| HRSA | Health Resources and Services Administration | ■ Administers the maternal and child health block grant through the Division of Maternal and Child Health Resources Development<br>■ Fosters public health nutrition programs at the state and local levels by providing expert consultation through its central and regional offices, training materials, and funding for continuing education and graduate training of public health nutritionists<br>■ Administers grants for research and for innovative projects, including Special Projects of Regional and National Significance and funds for community health centers, migrant health, rural health, AIDS education, and allied health professions training |
| USDA | U.S. Department of Agriculture | ■ Responsible for food and agriculture programs |
| ■ HNIS | Human Nutrition Information Services | ■ Administers the nutrition-monitoring activities of the USDA, including the Nationwide Food Consumption Survey (NFCS), the Continuing Survey of Food Intakes by Individuals (CSFII), and the Nutrient Data Bank CSFII, which has now merged with NHANES<br>■ Produces a variety of educational materials related to the *U.S. Dietary Guidelines for Americans* |
| ■ FNS | Food and Nutrition Service | ■ Administers the National School Lunch Program, National School Breakfast Program, Summer Feeding Program, Child Care Food Program, WIC, Commodity Supplemental Food Program, and Nutrition Education and Training Program (NETP) |
| ■ FSIS | Food Safety and Inspection Service | ■ Regulates the safety of meat and poultry products and some aspects of food labeling related to those products |
| **Other Federal Departments** | | |
| FTC | Federal Trade Commission | ■ Regulates the content of food advertisements and truth-in-labeling laws |
| DE | Department of Education | ■ Responsible for working with states in relation to public education<br>■ Responsible for educational programs for handicapped children; Public Law 99-457, the Education of the Handicapped Amendments of 1986, integrated health services into early intervention programs for infants and children with special needs<br>■ Nutrition services are listed as one of the health services, with nutritionists designated as part of the early intervention team |
| DT | Department of the Treasury | ■ Regulation of the sale and labeling of alcoholic beverages by the Bureau of Alcohol, Tobacco, and Firearms |

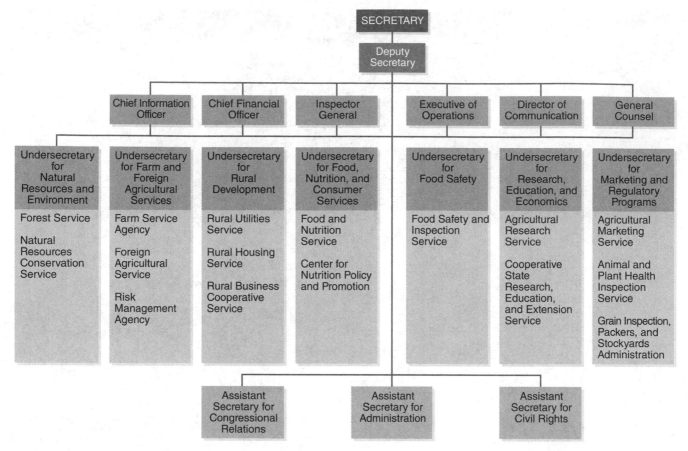

**FIGURE 6-3** Department of Agriculture organizational chart.

Modified from: U.S. Department of Agriculture website. Available at: http://www.usda.gov. Accessed March 6, 2008.

■ Socioeconomic policy influences food assistance programs for low-income individuals, creates eligibility criteria, and affects food costs.

■ Educational policy influences nutrition education programs and the capability of consumers, both youth and adults, to make educated food choices.[33]

Policies that are meticulously devised can guarantee consistent actions and prevent impulsive decisions. Mission statements, position papers, procedure manuals, protocols, office rules, and written memoranda from administrators or program managers communicate policies within an organization.[7,31]

## ▶ Policymaking Strategies

It is important for community/public health nutritionists to select the most effective strategies for a successful policy. The following section outlines some strategies for securing approval of a policy.[7,31]

### Strategy 1: Prepare a Scientific and Evidence Base

Start by studying the issue, the target audience, and the environment thoroughly; be prepared to answer questions

regarding the issues. Identify the need for the policy or legislation. Review related literature on the issue using credible professional journals such as the *Journal of the American Dietetic Association.*

### Strategy 2: Develop Broad Support

Form an alliance with various groups such as researchers, healthcare professionals, educators, farmers, consumers, religious groups, men's and women's groups, and individuals who can assist and support the issue.

It is important to be proactive, and network with nutrition experts, influential citizens in the community, friends of decision makers, and respected community groups with policy power, including the League of Women Voters, Chambers of Commerce, parent–teacher associations, and local affiliates of voluntary health agencies, such as the American Heart Association and the American Diabetes Association.

### Strategy 3: Analyze the Opposition

Policy makers need to hear strong factual arguments that refute the opponent's position. A constructive response to the opposition's arguments may contribute to the success of the policy. For example, at the local level, the discussion of whether to fluoridate drinking water in Lincoln, Nebraska, to prevent dental decay in children triggered some opposition by older adults who did not see the benefit to them. But the counterargument was that fluoridation of the water·also may prevent osteoporosis in older adults.

## Strategy 4: Develop Alternative Approaches or Compromise Positions

Listen to and analyze the opposition's viewpoint and provide an alternative solution. For example, the desire to increase nutrition service to the Hispanic community may trigger some opposition from other community members due to the increase in costs. An alternative approach or compromise might be to find volunteers from the Hispanic community who can serve as interpreters or provide other activities that can help reduce the cost of providing services to their community. Another alternative approach might be providing tax advantages to private healthcare providers such as physicians so they can significantly reduce their fees to low-income Hispanic women who need prenatal care or other healthcare services.

## Strategy 5: Estimate Needed Resources

It is important to determine the expenses involved in carrying out a legislative campaign. The expenses must be paid, so the nutritionist or policy maker must solicit the support of community members who are interested in the issue, such as special interest groups. They can help by identifying resources or contribute in-kind to the campaign. Some examples of costs are funds for media coverage, travel to various sites related to the issue, and telephone bills. It also is essential to identify the main individuals who will maintain contact with the policy makers.

## Strategy 6: Adopt Successful Strategies from Others

It is very helpful for the policy maker to identify and learn the successful strategies used by other healthcare professionals and interest groups. This step will reduce costs and save time. Review existing and established policy constantly to ensure that it is addressing the objectives of the program.

## Strategy 7: Set a Clear Direction Before Starting

Establish points for possible compromise early. In the early stage of policy formation, the direction may not be completely clear, so be amenable to changes that may be necessary during the process. Work closely with the individuals that are responsible for implementing the program and those affected by the policy.

# ▶ State and Local Policy

State health agencies may provide services through district or regional offices in states where there are no official local public health agencies. State governments are responsible for the health of their citizens.[7,34] State government policymaking structures and processes are comparable to those of the federal government. At the state level, government officials depend on state community/public health nutritionists as their experts on the nutritional status of their community.[7]

The local authorities who make policies may be executives, elected officials, federal agencies, welfare workers, public health nurses, community nutritionists, and other people working in government agencies. The population segments within rural counties that would have distinct viewpoints and interests relating to nutrition and health also may make policies. The following are many ways community nutritionists can influence policymaking processes at the grassroots level[7,35,36]:

- Evaluate the community's food, nutrition, and health needs, and present these findings to program directors, agency administrators, and boards.
- Propose programs using need assessment results.
- Supervise and report their agency's progress in meeting nutritional objectives.
- Establish policies, procedures, and protocols for nutrition services for their agency.
- Adopt national model standards for their nutrition services.
- Talk with people in the local school, such as the parent–teacher association, the principal, teachers, and parents. Get them excited about the potential to make healthy changes in the district.
- Contact the Academy of Nutrition and Dietetics ActionNet for help. Visit its website at http://www .eatright.org. It serves as a local and national contact with members of Congress.

The local political structures in the United States are diverse, so community nutritionists need to examine the structures of their local governments. Many states have strong county governments[10] with elected boards of commissioners or supervisors who pass ordinances and approve the county budget.[7] They may have a local informant, a tribal head, a director of a highly visible voluntary not-for-profit health organization, or a chamber of commerce director. In some situations the county government is responsible for public health services. The county commissioners typically appoint the county manager and the county's board of health. In large cities, a city council transmits local ordinances, budgets local revenues, and appoints the city board of health. An elected mayor or appointed city manager administers the daily activities of the city.[7,37] The county or city board of health appoints the chief health official, who may or may not be a health professional. The chief health official is responsible for local public health policy. A nutritionist can advise the chief health official and the board of health on nutrition policy.

## How Dietitians Can Become Involved in Local and National Public Policy

There are many ways in which dietitians can become involved in public policy, although it seems like an overwhelming task to some individuals. The AND periodically issues "Action Alerts" that call for members to send letters or e-mails to their senators or representatives. If the time and resources are available, people can become more involved in public policy work by volunteering as an AND **legislative network coordinator (LNC)** or a **grassroots liaison (GRL)** for a state or district. LNCs are elected by each state affiliate; they organize and mobilize AND members at the state level to become involved in federal public policy issues.[38] LNCs are the main liaisons between the state affiliate and AND government relations staff. GRLs, which represent each federal congressional district, are appointed or elected by state affiliates to serve as the principal communicator between AND members and their congresspersons. Also, the Public Policy Workshop (PPW) provided by the AND each spring in Washington, D.C., is a very good opportunity for dietitians. They can learn more about advocacy and can have the opportunity to visit the offices of the senator or representatives from their state.

If the community nutritionist does not feel comfortable writing a congressperson or does not have time to volunteer locally or attend the PPW, he or she can support the AND's public policy agenda by contributing to the AND's political action committee (ANDPAC). A **political action committee (PAC)** is a group of individuals united by similar interests. PACs represent corporations, trade associations, ideological groups, labor unions, or member associations. The purpose of a PAC is to help elect candidates whose views support the group's mission or goals. Its function is to keep the lines of communication open between

policy makers and the interest group's membership. In 1971, a campaign finance reform law legitimized PACs by granting them the status and legal authority to collect funds from individuals and make federal campaign contributions.[39,40]

The ANDPAC attempts to influence the policymaking process and its outcome. "It serves as a collective voice for dietitians by supporting candidates for federal office who are willing to support the AND's mission, vision, and principles."[38] Most importantly, "ANDPAC increases AND's visibility and access to public policy makers, consequently increasing the power of dietetics professionals' views on important legislative issues."[38] ANDPAC is nonpartisan and solicits only AND members for donations. A five-person board of directors appointed by the AND president directs ANDPAC. The ANDPAC Board selects candidates for contributions based on whether they are in a position to assist the AND on priority issues. In the 2000 election cycle, the ANDPAC was one of the top 20 contributors among healthcare professional PACs.[38]

## Initiating Policy

Community nutritionists can unite with political leaders and concerned citizens to propose a policy change for nutrition-related issues. Some examples of issues that may need policy change in the community are food safety, obesity, funding for school lunch and breakfast programs, and food security. If the community nutritionist decides to seek change for any issue, for example, food insecurity in the community, it is important to understand that there are three basic components to follow: process, projects, and policy.[41]

The process component involves building participation through community planning and collaboration. This can be accomplished by defining the community to be served, conducting a community-based needs assessment (see Chapter 2), building links with diverse groups, using the key informant process of gathering local data, developing comprehensive strategies, and incorporating a long-term strategic design.[41] The community assessment data can be presented in public meetings, legislative hearings, or other forums. An ongoing surveillance system can be developed to monitor hunger, malnutrition, obesity, diabetes, diet-related health problems, and utilization of food assistance programs.

The nutritionist and other community members can design projects, such as community gardens, farmers' markets, and food-related enterprise developments, to meet different objectives. For instance, they can work to increase the production and marketing of locally

**TABLE 6-2** Ways a Community Nutritionist Can Influence Public Policy at the Grassroots Level

| How to Influence Policy | Actions |
|---|---|
| Express your opinions. | ■ Present ideas at public meetings.<br>■ Write a letter to the editor of a newspaper, magazine, or scientific journal.<br>■ Testify at hearings at a local or state level (present oral and written information). |
| Be a political actor/cultivate public officials. | ■ Campaign for political office.<br>■ Sponsor a referendum.<br>■ Initiate a campaign to bring an issue to the attention of the general public or policy makers.<br>■ Participate in a local advisory board that can influence the political process in the community.<br>■ Organize a collection of signatures for a petition to be sent to your state legislature or city council.<br>■ Help fundraise for a local politician. |
| Participate in a PAC. | ■ Donate to the ANDPAC. |
| Network/build coalitions. | ■ Collaborate with the Academy of Nutrition and Dietetics, American Heart Association, and American Cancer Society in the local area to address different health issues.<br>■ Talk with people in the local schools, such as the parent–teacher association, principals, teachers, and parents.<br>■ Talk with people in the community, including nurses, social workers, other healthcare professionals, the mayor, campaign workers, businesses, special interest groups, church groups, and women's clubs. |
| Lobby. | ■ Advocate blocking passage of legislation that does not promote the AND's mission. Use personal contacts, letters, fax messages, telephone calls, and e-mails to express viewpoints.<br>■ Advocate for passage of legislation that promotes the AND's mission. |

grown foods and expand lower income persons' access to high-quality, nutritious foods. They can use data gathered by extension educators as discussion pieces to engage the community in a dialogue about health priorities, capacities, and future directions.[37]

Finally, government policies need to be assessed to determine whether they act as barriers or enablers to community food security projects.[41] **TABLE 6-2** presents different ways a community nutritionist can influence public policy at a grassroots level.

### ✎ Think About It

Nutrition monitoring supplies information for public policy decisions and scientific research. How do nutritionists use nutrition monitoring and examination information?

## ▶ The Links Among Nutrition Monitoring, Nutrition Research, and Nutrition Policy

Nutrition monitoring supplies information for public policy decisions and scientific research. Nutrition monitoring and examination information are used to determine dietary habits, identify high-risk population groups to plan public health intervention programs, and initiate food assistance awareness efforts; establish the national health agenda and evaluate progress toward achieving national health objectives[42-44]; establish guidelines for the prevention, detection, and management of nutritional conditions[42-45]; and evaluate the impact of nutrition initiatives for military feeding systems.[46] Data also are used to monitor food production and marketing programs and their impact on the food supply.[47,48]

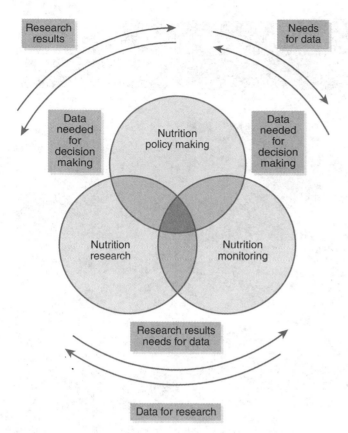

**FIGURE 6-4** Overlapping of nutrition monitoring, policy making, and research.

Modified from: the U.S Department of Agriculture/Food and Nutrition Services. Healthy Schools. Available at: http://teamnutrition.usda.gov/Healthy/wellnesspolicygoals_schoolbased.html. Accessed August 6, 2006.

Research, monitoring, and policy are intertwined through a complex set of interrelationships.[45] As shown in **FIGURE 6-4**, nutrition monitoring is vital to policymaking and research.[46,49] Monitoring provides information and a database for public policy decision making and establishes research priorities.[50,51] In an equally important role, nutrition research provides data for policymaking and for identifying nutrition-monitoring data needs.[52-54]

# ▶ Emerging Policy Issues in the United States

In the late twentieth and early twenty-first centuries, the ANDs' main legislative goal was to obtain Medicare reimbursement for medical nutrition therapy (MNT) services provided by Registered Dietitians (RDs). On January 1, 2002, RDs began to register as Medicare providers and started providing services to program beneficiaries. Other significant AND public policy efforts over the years led to the passage of the Nutrition Labeling and Education Act (NLEA), which established mandatory nutrition labeling for packaged foods. This enabled consumers to make more informed and healthier food product choices in the context of their daily diet. The NLEA also required that the FDA issue regulations that establish standards to define serving size.[55,56]

In 2005, the AND took a new approach to Medicare MNT. Representative Fred Upton and Senator Larry Craig restructured their legislation to give the CMS the authority to expand future coverage to any disease, disorder, or condition for which MNT is cost-effective using its National Coverage Determination (NCD) process. The NCD process determines the extent to which Medicare will cover specific services, procedures, or technologies on a national basis.[57] This bill does not mandate any expansion of the current MNT benefits; rather, it merely provides the CMS the authority to broaden MNT coverage through the NCD process. The MNT benefits could be expanded to cover conditions such as hypertension, dyslipidemia (abnormal blood lipids), prediabetes, obesity, or HIV/AIDS if there is evidence that nutrition intervention is effective. It allows the CMS to review the science behind recommendations to further expand the benefits without having to get Congressional approval.[58]

## Registered Dietitian Nutritionists to Order Diets

The CMS announced that Registered Dietitian Nutritionists (RDN) can now order diets in hospitals starting July 11, 2014. According to CMS, "the addition of ordering privileges increases the ability of RDNs to provide timely, cost-effective, and evidence-based nutrition services as nutrition experts on a hospital interdisciplinary team." However, the CMS rule is not a requirement for hospitals.[59]

## Farm Bill

The Farm Bill protects vital nutrition assistance programs and includes initiatives that will improve the health of the nation. The AND worked with Congress to pass a Farm Bill that supports nutrition programs and provides access to healthy food for millions of Americans. The Law was signed on February 7, 2014 and will remain in effect through 2018. In addition, the following AND recommendations were passed:

- Maintain current funding ($401 M) for SNAP education (SNAP-Ed).
- Protect and strengthen the main programs in the nutrition safety net SNAP, The Emergency Food Assistance Program (TEFAP), and the Commodity Supplemental Food Program.

- Reauthorize Senior Farmers Market Program.
- Maintain current funding for school-based Fresh Fruit and Vegetable Program.
- Support community-based initiatives that expand availability of regionally grown foods, create jobs, and promote economic growth.
- Provide $100 million for over 5 years for Food Insecurity Nutrition Incentive grants in matching funds to eligible organizations.
- Maintain funding for Specialty Crop Block Grants to support food safety and nutrition research, as well as a diversity of fruits, vegetables, and nuts.[60,61]

## Obesity

In July 2004, the DHHS announced a new Medicare coverage policy "that would remove barriers to covering antiobesity interventions if scientific and medical evidence demonstrated their effectiveness in improving Medicare beneficiaries' health outcomes."[51,52,58] Even with Medicare's policy toward obesity, MNT cannot qualify as an antiobesity intervention without specific congressional approval. However, if the AND's new bill is enacted, the CMS can review MNT evidence outcomes and make a determination as to whether coverage would be "reasonable and necessary."[57]

## Prediabetes

Another example of why a broader MNT benefit is important and can be cost-effective is in the treatment of prediabetes. In March 2002, the DHHS estimated that 16 million people have prediabetes. DHHS-supported research shows that most people with prediabetes will likely develop diabetes within a decade unless they make modest changes in their diet and level of physical activity.[61-63] A cost analysis study published in March 2004 predicted that lifestyle intervention (including diet) is more cost-effective than drugs in preventing prediabetes progression to diabetes.[19,57,62]

## Human Immunodeficiency Virus (HIV)/Acquired Immunodeficiency Syndrome (AIDS)

The nutritional management of persons infected with HIV poses a unique challenge. Malnutrition and wasting are vital issues in medical care plans because HIV-infected persons survive life-threatening infections through the use of effective medical therapies. Aggressive nutrition support can delay or reverse wasting in many cases,

and there is evidence that maintaining lean body mass may prolong the life of HIV-infected individuals.[63] Researchers have established that deficiencies of energy, protein, and micronutrients negatively affect the immune system and other normal body functions.[64] In addition, the medications taken by patients with HIV induce diabetes-like states, high blood cholesterol, and a fat storage disorder called lipodystrophy, which are best treated with MNT intervention.[57,65] In 2016, Congress passed a reauthorization of the Ryan White CARE Act, the largest federal program specifically for people with HIV and AIDS, which paid new attention to the unique dietary needs of patients.[66] With passage of the MNT bill (Public Law 106-554), a RDs can do that counseling for approved conditions or diseases. Dietitians are paid at a rate of 85 percent of what a physician would charge for the same service, so the bill will result in a net savings to Medicare.[58]

The AND's public policy agenda is established in recognition of the broad interests of AND members. Priorities are established in areas in which the association can work proactively on issues in which dietetics professionals can make a unique contribution to the policy debate. **BOX 6-3** presents the AND's 2008 public policy agenda. Some of the issues in Box 6-3 will be decided in Washington, D.C., some in individual states, some in private businesses and insurance companies, and some in hometowns.[67] For instance, the Child Nutrition Reauthorization Act 2004 (Public Law 108-265) that was passed in June 2004 required each school district in the country to develop a wellness policy to take effect by fall of 2006. This law required that, at a minimum, the wellness policies must do the following[65]:

- Include goals for nutrition education, physical activity, and other school-based activities designed to promote student wellness in a manner that the local educational agency determines appropriate
- Include nutrition guidelines for all foods available on the school campus during the school day
- Involve parents, students, and representatives of the school food authority, the school board, school administrators, and the public in the development of local wellness policies

The USDA was responsible for sending information about the implementation process to all the districts. In turn, all local districts were required to submit their wellness policy to the USDA by June 30, 2006, for implementation in the fall of 2006. **BOX 6-4** presents an example of existing state and school district policies regarding school-based activities, and **BOX 6-5** presents sources of information on federal legislation and regulations. Policies were written at the school district level.

**BOX 6-3** Academy of Nutrition and Dietetics' 2008 Public Policy Agenda[45,66]

- Medical nutrition therapy—to cover hypertension, dyslipidemia, prediabetes, and possibly obesity
- Healthy aging in the reauthorization of the Older Americans Act (OAA) and in state initiatives relating to nutrition care
- Local "wellness" policies for schools
- Disease prevention and disease management
- Reimbursement
- Research and funding for nutrition initiatives across the board

Dietitians' involvement in this process can be, but is not limited to, the following[67-70]:

- Talking with people in their community about becoming involved.
- Finding out who is in charge of food services for the district.
- Finding out if the district food service director or the local school food service director is an RD. If not, offer to serve on the wellness policy committee as a nutrition advisor or volunteer to serve on the advisory committee for the district.

**TABLE 6-3** presents how local districts can create and implement a local wellness policy, and **TABLE 6-4** describes how schools can evaluate the progress of the school's physical education policies. Finally, **TABLE 6-5** offers space to develop an action plan for quality physical education.

**BOX 6-4** An Example of Existing State and School District Policies Regarding School-Based Activities[71]

**School District of Marshfield, Wisconsin, School Nutrition Policy**

The School District of Marshfield included a school-based activities policy in its mission. This district-wide nutrition policy encouraged all members of the school community to create an environment that supports lifelong healthy eating habits. The policy emphasized that all the decisions made in all school programming must reflect and encourage positive nutrition messages and healthy food choices. Presented below is the policy of the School District of Marshfield.

1. Provide a positive environment and appropriate knowledge regarding food.
   - Ensure that all students have access to healthy food choices during school and at school functions.
   - Provide a pleasant eating environment for students and staff.
   - Allow a minimum of 20 minutes for students to eat lunch and socialize in the designated cafeteria area.
   - Enable all students, through a comprehensive curriculum, to acquire the knowledge and skills necessary to make healthy food choices for a lifetime.
2. When using food as a part of class or student incentive programs, staff and students are encouraged to utilize healthy, nutritious food choices.
3. When curricular-based food experiences are planned, staff and students are encouraged to seek out good nutrition choices whenever appropriate.
4. Reduce student access to foods of minimal nutritional value.
   - In keeping with contractual obligations to the National School Lunch/Breakfast Programs, ensure the integrity of the School Lunch Program by prohibiting food and beverage sales that are in direct conflict with the Lunch/Breakfast Programs.
   - Encourage the practice of good nutrition by reducing the sale or distribution of foods of minimal nutritional value through a 4-year plan that focuses on:
     - Reducing access to non-nutritional foods
     - Educating students about healthy foods

Modified from: U.S. Department of Agriculture/Food and Nutrition Services. Healthy Schools. Available at: http://teamnutrition.usda.gov/Healthy/wellnesspolicygoals_schoolbased.html. Accessed July 7, 2016

**BOX 6-5** Sources of Information on Federal Legislation and Regulations

- ***Congressional Handbook:*** Directory of members of Congress and Senate (annual). U.S. Chamber of Commerce, Legislative Action Department, 1615 H Street NW, Washington, DC 20062. https://www.uschamber.com/ .
- ***Congressional Quarterly:*** Documents related to legislative, executive, and judicial branch activities. *Congressional Quarterly,* 1414 22nd Street NW, Washington, DC 20037. http://www.loc.gov/flicc/svcdir/cq.html.

- **Congressional Yellow Book:** Comprehensive directories of Congress and federal agencies. Washington Monitor, 1301 Pennsylvania Avenue NW No. 1100, Washington, DC 20004. http://www.leadershipdirectories.com/products/cyb.htm.
- **Federal Register, Congressional Register:** Congressional and agency reports https://www.federalregister.gov /agencies/library-of-congress . and agency reports. Superintendent of Documents, Government https://www .federalregister.gov/documents/2017/02/06/2016-29625/copyright-office-technical-amendments
- **House and Senate Bills:** From offices of members of Congress or the Senate:
  House Document Room, H-226, U.S. Capitol, Washington, DC 20515
  Senate Document Room, SH B-04, Washington, DC 20515
  Hart Senate Office Building.
  https://www.gpo.gov/fdsys/browse/collection.action?collectionCode=BILLS and http://www.senate.gov/ pagelayout/legislative/d_three_sect ions with teasers/bills.htm.
- **Directory of Health Organization, Specialized Information System (SIS):** Specialized Information System: NLM/ NIH, 2 Democracy Plaza, Suite 510, 6707 Democracy Boulevard MSC 5467, Bethesda, MD 20892. https://www.nlm.nih.gov/pubs/factsheets/gateway.html
- **National Journal: The Weekly on Politics and Government, the Almanac of American Politics (annual):** National Journal, Inc., 17320 M Street NW, Washington, D.C. 20036. http://nationaljournal.com.
- **Reports of Congressional Audits of Federal Programs:** General Accounting Office, Information Handling and Support Facility, Document Handling and Information Service Component, P.O. Box 6015, Gaithersburg, MD 20877. http://www.gao.gov.

**TABLE 6-3** How Local Districts Can Create and Implement a Local Wellness Policy

| Step | Action |
|---|---|
| Do the initial homework. | - Identify and review existing state laws and guidelines about education, health, and/or agriculture; other school districts' policies; and your local district policies that address wellness topics before meetings start. For example, compare local wellness policies with the requirements of Section 2004 of the Child Nutrition and WIC Reauthorization Acts of 2004.<br>- At a minimum, your school district's new wellness policies must be in compliance with the federal statutory requirements, plus all relevant state and district requirements.<br>- The process may vary from one district to another. The school district superintendent's office will be helpful if you are not familiar with your district's procedures. |
| Identify a policy development team. | - Anyone can initiate a process to create a new policy or adapt an existing policy. The law requires:<br>  • Parents<br>  • Students<br>  • Representatives of the school food authority<br>  • The school board<br>  • School administrators<br>  • The public (make sure everyone who will be affected by the policy is involved)<br>- It is important to collaborate with any existing efforts in the school or community. If your school district is already working on student wellness issues and has an existing infrastructure, such as a school health council, a coordinated school health program, a local Team Nutrition team, or staff involved in the Carol M. White Physical Education Program (PEP), these people can assist in the development of the policy.<br>- The following are some resources to assist schools and school districts in establishing a new team, if needed, or in building on existing teams and partnerships:<br>  • North Carolina's Effective School Health Advisory Councils—Moving from Policy to Action<br>  • Promoting Healthy Youth, Schools, and Communities: A Guide to Community–School Health Councils from the American School Health Association (at cost)<br>  • Improving School Health: A Guide to School Health Councils, a PDF from the American Cancer Society<br>  • Team Nutrition Resources from the USDA |

*(continues)*

**TABLE 6-3** How Local Districts Can Create and Implement a Local Wellness Policy (*continued*)

| Step | Action |
|---|---|
| Assess the district's needs. | ■ Assess the current situation and the nutrition and physical activity needs of the students before making plans to develop policies.<br>■ Look for data on the education and health status of young people in your particular state. Web resources include:<br>  • The CDC's data on Obesity Trends<br>  • The CDC's Youth Risk Behavior Surveillance System (YRBS)<br>  • Action for Healthy Kids' State Profiles for Action<br>■ The following tools may help you assess your school's existing policies, programs, and areas that need improvement:<br>  • Changing the Scene Improvement Checklist is a simple checklist to help you assess the situation in your school and to help you focus on exactly what needs to be done. The State of Michigan modified this improvement checklist to measure progress as actions are taken.<br>  • School Health Index: A Self-Assessment and Planning Guide from the CDC includes information about physical activity and healthy eating. This tool enables schools to identify the strengths and weaknesses of nutrition and physical activity policies and programs and develop an action plan for improvement.<br>  • Keys to Excellence: Standard of Practice for Nutrition Integrity is a guide published by the School Nutrition<br>  • Association (SNA) that identifies the elements of a quality school nutrition program. This publication provides an easy-to-use evaluation form for assessing school meal programs' quality and tracking progress.<br>  • It's Time for Your School's Physical Education Check-Up is a checklist of physical activity measurements, created by the National Association for Sport and Physical Education (see Table 6-5). |
| Draft a policy. | ■ Based on your needs assessment, draft the initial policy statements.<br>■ Address nutrition education, physical activity, other school-based activities that promote student wellness, nutrition guidelines for all foods available on each campus, and a plan for measuring implementation, as required by Public Law 108-265, Section 2004. For more information about the components that must appear in the wellness policy, see the USDA's Health Wellness Policy Requirements.<br>■ To save time, consider adapting or adopting another district's or organization's existing policy to meet the needs of your school district. Check out the USDA's Examples: Local Wellness Policies for some ideas, available at http://teamnutrition.usda.gov.<br>■ Some state agencies that administer school meal programs offer guidance to assist local districts to create and implement local wellness policies.<br>■ Also check with professional associations and organizations for model school wellness policies and useful resources. The nongovernmental organizations that are acting as collaborators on the local wellness policy can be a good resource.<br>■ The goals that are set for nutrition education and physical activity, the nutrition guidelines, and other school-based activities must be developed in recognition of both the school district's goals and the current school wellness status.<br>■ The goals should be realistic and attainable.<br>■ Propose several policy options from which decision makers can choose. The local school board or superintendent may be interested to know the financial implications of each policy option, particularly in regard to nutrition guidelines for foods sold in vending machines or school stores. The examples of success stories in which schools improved their nutritional quality of foods offered and maintained revenue can be found in the USDA and CDC's joint publication *Making It Happen*.<br>■ Draft a plan for implementing and measuring the new policy while you are drafting the policy itself. For example, you may consider:<br>  • What indicators will be used to evaluate the progress of implementation?<br>  • Who will be responsible for monitoring the implementation of the policy?<br>  • How often will the implementation be evaluated?<br>■ Keep the school district's decision makers informed about the proposed wellness policy and obtain their support throughout the development process. |

| Step | Action |
|---|---|
| | ■ For more information on the policy development process, the following resources are available to assist you:<br>  • The USDA's Local Wellness Policy websites can help you draft policies specifically targeting nutrition education, physical activity, and nutrition guidelines for all foods available on school campuses during the school day, and other school-based activities designed to promote student wellness.<br>  • Fit, Healthy, and Ready to Learn is a school health policy guide developed by the National Association of State Boards of Education that provides sample policies on healthy eating, physical activity, and other topics.<br>  • Changing the Scene: Improving the School Nutrition Environment—A Guide to Local Action was developed by the USDA's Team Nutrition in collaboration with 16 education, health, and nutrition organizations to help schools take action in improving their nutrition environment.<br>  • CDC Guidelines for School Health Programs to Promote Lifelong Healthy Eating identifies the school-based strategies most likely to be effective in promoting lifelong healthy eating among young people.<br>  • CDC Guidelines for School and Community Programs to Promote Lifelong Physical Activity Among Young People identifies the strategies most likely to be effective in helping young people adopt and maintain a physically active lifestyle. |
| Build awareness and support. | ■ It is important to obtain support from schools and your community for the policy to be smoothly adopted and widely implemented. Student involvement also is an important component of building awareness and support. Use the resources from the USDA in Changing the Scene, available at http://teamnutrition.usda.gov to help educate various audiences about your policy initiative.<br>■ Recruit local media to spread awareness of the district's needs and community leaders to speak out in favor of the proposed solutions.<br>■ Be prepared for challenges that may arise and be sure that all the people who spoke for the policy are providing a consistent message.<br>■ When dealing with the education community, it is helpful to identify the potential benefits the policy can have on student learning and academic achievement.<br>■ Making It Happen contains many success stories of districts that built broad local support for school health policy goals. This is available at http://teamnutrition.usda.gov. |
| Adopt the policy. | ■ In most, if not all, school districts, the district board of education (the school board or school committee) must approve the wellness policy before it can be implemented.<br>■ A public hearing or presentation might be necessary. The district superintendent's office can describe the usual process and advise you on how matters are brought before the board.<br>■ Team members will have a better understanding of board procedures if they have attended board meetings prior to presenting the policy proposal.<br>■ Prepare a persuasive and concise case in support of the policy and provide supportive background information.<br>■ Invite and involve policy supporters (such as parents, school nurses, and other community members) to attend the board meeting to voice their support and/or make a presentation on behalf of the proposed policy.<br>■ For help with this process, see the USDA's PowerPoint presentation Welcome to Wellness: Putting School Nutrition Legislation into Practice. Also, check out the School Nutrition Association's PowerPoint presentation Talking to Your School Administrators: An Overview of the Local Wellness Policy (USDA). |
| Implement the policy. | ■ Implementation requires good planning and management skills, the necessary resources, consistent oversight, and widespread school staff and local community agreement.<br>■ Implementation can occur all at once or may be phased in over time. Your team is in the best position to determine which approach is likely to be most effective in your district.<br>■ The attitude of all school personnel, from individuals serving the food, to the personnel who stock vending machines, to students, coaches, teachers, and administrators, can have a significant effect on the response to the policy. A positive attitude toward new foods, new physical activity options, or other changes from everyone in the school community can make a big difference. |

*(continues)*

**TABLE 6-3**  How Local Districts Can Create and Implement a Local Wellness Policy (*continued*)

| Step | Action |
|------|--------|
| | ■ Marketing can be an important tool for policy implementation. Consider how marketing principles of product, price, placement, and promotion can work to help with policy implementation.<br>■ Implementation Tools and Resources, available at http://teamnutrition.usda.gov, provide links to specific examples of programs and activities that are helping schools fulfill their wellness policy goals. These links can help you start thinking about creative ways to implement the policies and provide resources to ease the burden of creating new curricula and learning devices. |
| Maintain, measure, and evaluate the effort. | ■ Designate one or more persons with operational responsibility for ensuring that the school is meeting the policy.<br>■ A sustained effort by each district is necessary to ensure new policies are faithfully implemented.<br>■ Periodically assess how well the policy is being managed and enforced.<br>■ Reinforce the policy goals with school staff if necessary.<br>■ Be prepared to update or amend the policy as the process moves on.<br>■ The school district or individual schools should celebrate policy success milestones (and the district team can do the same).<br>■ Evaluation and feedback are very important in maintaining a local wellness policy.<br>■ Document any financial impact to the school foodservice program, school stores, or vending machine revenues.<br>■ It also is important to assess student, parent, teacher, and administration satisfaction with the new policies.<br>■ A good evaluation plan does not need to be extensive, be formal, or put additional undue burdens on staff who are involved in the process.<br>■ Through the evaluation process, you will be able to answer some basic questions that are very important to policy makers, students, school staff, parents, and the general public:<br>• What changes to nutrition education, physical activity, the nutritional quality of foods available to students, and other aspects covered by the policy occurred in each school as a result of the district wellness policy? For example:<br>  ◆ Did the number of students participating in nutrition education change?<br>  ◆ Did the students have a different number of minutes of physical activity?<br>  ◆ Did any of the campuses change available food options?<br>  ◆ Did participation in the National School Breakfast or Lunch Program change?<br>• Did the policy and implementation address the issues identified in the needs assessment? For example:<br>  ◆ Is it making a difference?<br>  ◆ What's working?<br>  ◆ What's not working?<br>  ◆ How can the impact of the policy be increased to enhance its effect on student health and academic learning?<br>■ For more information on the evaluation process, the following resources are among those available to assist you:<br>• Evaluation Primer: An Overview of Education Evaluation. This material is excerpted from Understanding Evaluation: The Way to Better Prevention Programs.<br>• Evaluating Community Programs and Initiatives (Chapters 36 to 39 of the Community Toolbox), developed by the University of Kansas Work Group on Health Promotion and Community Development. This document contains information on developing a plan for evaluation, methods for evaluation, and using evaluation to understand and improve the initiative.<br>• Framework for program evaluation is a CDC publication, *MMWR Morb Mortal Wkly Rep*. 1999;48(No.RR-11):1-40. This outlines steps and standards for effective program evaluation.<br>• Criteria for Evaluating School-Based Approaches to Increasing Good Nutrition and Physical Activity, by Action for Healthy Kids. This outlines an array of issues to consider when evaluating school-based programs. |

Modified from: U.S. Department of Agriculture. Food and Nutrition Service/Team Nutrition. Available at: http://www.fns.usda.gov. Accessed February 22, 2011.

| **TABLE 6-4** Your School's Physical Education Check-Up: How Are You Doing? | |
|---|---|
| 1. | Is physical education taught by a qualified teacher with a degree in physical education? | Yes/No |
| 2. | Do students receive formal instruction in physical education:<br>　a) For a minimum of 150 minutes per week (elementary) and 225 minutes per week (middle and high)?<br>　OR<br>　b) At least three class periods per week for all grades the entire school year? | Yes/No |
| 3. | Is the physical education class size similar to those of other content areas to ensure safe, effective instruction? | Yes/No |
| 4. | Is there adequate equipment for every student to be active? | Yes/No |
| 5. | Is technology incorporated on a regular and continuing basis? | Yes/No |
| 6. | Are indoor and outdoor facilities safe and adequate (so that physical education classes need not be displaced by other activities)? | Yes/No |
| 7. | Is there a written mission statement and sequential curriculum based on state and/or national standards for physical education? | Yes/No |
| 8. | Are formative and summative assessments of student learning included in the physical education program, and are they related to meaningful content objectives? | Yes/No |
| 9. | Does the program provide for maximum participation for every student (e.g., inclusion, no elimination games, all students active at once, developmentally appropriate activities, etc.)? | Yes/No |
| 10. | Does the program help systematically develop the physical, cognitive, and social-emotional aspects of each student? | Yes/No |
| 11. | Do physical education teachers regularly participate in physical education professional development activities and have memberships in related professional organizations? | Yes/No |
| 12. | Do physical education teachers receive student health information and have a plan for handling emergencies? | Yes/No |
| 13. | Are there regular periodic evaluations of teacher performance by the administrators of the physical education program? | Yes/No |
| 14. | Do physical education teachers communicate with each other and parents on a frequent basis? | Yes/No |
| 15. | Do physical education teachers seek feedback for improvement from students, peers, and parents as a means for program evaluation and improvement? | Yes/No |

### How Did You Do?

If you answered "Yes" to all of the questions on the Physical Education Check-Up, your school may qualify for the NASPE STARS national recognition program for quality physical education programs. For more information, visit http://www.naspeinfo.org. If you answered "No" to one or more of the questions on the Physical Education Check-Up, please utilize this Action Plan for Quality Physical Education (see Table 6-5) to get you started improving your school physical education program. The National Association for Sport Physical Education (NASPE) has the necessary physical education standards, the opportunity to learn standards, and the appropriate instructional practices and assessment tools to help you.

| Criteria | Action | Short-Term Objectives/Goals | Long-Term Objectives/Goals | Criteria Met |
|---|---|---|---|---|
| List any questions with a "No" response from the physical education check-up. | How do you propose to change this to a "Yes" response? List action steps here. | List specific goals for the first 1–3 years. | List specific goals for the next 3–5 years. Place the date of success here. | Place the date of success here. |
| | | | | |

**TABLE 6-5** Action Plan for Quality Physical Education

Action Plan for Quality Physical Education

# Learning Portfolio

## Chapter Summary

- Many laws and regulations passed by local, state, and national officials affect the nutrition programs and nutritional status of citizens in the healthcare provider's community.
- The U.S. Congress consists of the House of Representatives and the Senate. The legislative branch enacts laws that initiate, modify, authorize, and appropriate funds for all programs and services administered by the federal government.
- Most of the laws enacted that affect nutrition, food, and health are passed to the U.S. Department of Agriculture (USDA) or the U.S. Department of Health and Human Services (DHHS) for implementation.
- The DHHS and USDA are the two federal departments important for nutrition issues.
- The government can use tools such as taxes, tax incentives, and price supports for commodities to influence policy.

- Agricultural policy initiates the nutrition policy process because it influences the quantity and quality of the food supply and the costs of foods in grocery stores.
- Individuals and organizations can testify at congressional hearings and make recommendations to modify a specific program.
- Dietetics professionals can take the lead in prevention programming because their training as counselors and educators provides skills that make them multitalented members of coalitions.
- Community nutrition professionals develop and refine leadership abilities through experience and reflection.
- Leadership refers to the influence that nutritionists exert on improving clients' health, whether clients are individuals, families, groups, or entire communities.
- Nutrition management refers to the way nutritionists manage resources when providing services.

## Critical Thinking Activities

- Determine the legislative process for your local government.
- Determine how to network with other healthcare professionals to influence a bill.
- Talk to local school districts and gather information about how they are implementing local wellness policies.
- Write letters with other community and public health professionals to influence this legislation.
- Identify city council members, the president of the Chamber of Commerce, the director of family services, the mayor, a religious leader, and other community leaders who can help them accomplish their goals.
- Create a list of questions that would help these leaders understand the major strengths and weaknesses of the community regarding infant mortality and other health issues.
- Lobbying activities: As a group, meet with the local Chamber of Commerce director in the community and ask him or her to expand public transportation to the areas that are experiencing food desert.
- Meet with the mayor of the city and ask him or her to include the issue of food desert in the agenda of the next city council meeting. Provide information to/educate the Mayor about the consequences of food desert and food insecurity.
- Educating various stakeholders: As a group, meet with people in the local school district such as the parent–teacher association and principal to educate them about the new Farm bill on school-based Fresh Fruit and Vegetable Program. Also, give them information and ideas on how to use some of the nutrition educational tools, such as MyPlate and others to develop a nutrition education program and to include more fruits and vegetable in the diet.
- Mobilizing various individuals and groups: Contact student organizations and people who are motivated to act on behalf of low-income communities, children, pregnant women, the elderly, and others to influence policymaking on ending food insecurity in the community. In addition, use grassroots activities such as writing letters, making phone calls, contacting policy makers, and demonstration to solve the problem of food insecurity in the community.

## 🔍 CASE STUDY 6-1: Preventing Fraud and Promoting Health and Adequate Prenatal Care

Two federal bills related to early intervention for pregnant women and the regulation of weight loss product fraud are at the committee level. These issues are very important because not all pregnant women receive adequate prenatal care and because many Americans are victimized by weight loss product fraud. In the meantime, people are using these products while thinking the products, and claims made about them, are regulated by the government. These products are high in fat and low in carbohydrates, protein, iron, and vitamins. A report shows the following:

- 34 percent of the public has used weight loss products whose claims are unproven.
- 63 percent are trying to improve their health.
- 54 percent think the FDA approves these products for safety.
- 46 percent think that FDA approves them for efficacy.
- 37 percent believe they are safer than prescription or over-the-counter medications.

Angelina Okoro, a public health nutrition professor, collaborated with Omari, a community nutritionist, to take action and increase the awareness of these bills because the passage of these bills is very important to the practice of

*(continues)*

## CASE STUDY 6-1: Preventing Fraud and Promoting Health and Adequate Prenatal Care (continued)

community and public health nutrition. In their community, many pregnant women are obese, with an average BMI of over 30, which increases the incidence of gestational diabetes, edema, proteinuria, and anemia. Also, some women had bright red or purple tongue and spongy, bleeding, receding gums. Angelina and Omari enlisted students enrolled in a community nutrition class to carry out some of the following activities.

### Questions

1. Knowing the foundation of the United States' nutrition policy will prepare Angelina and Omari to influence leaders about these issues. What are the four components that form the foundation of U.S. nutrition policy?
2. What is the definition of policy? What are some of the different tools the government can use to influence policies?
3. The FDA is responsible for the approval of certain health products. What are some of the things that are included in the FDA's jurisdiction?
4. What are some of the areas that the DHHSs' programs cover that Angelina and Omari must know?
5. As public health and nutrition professionals, Angelina and Omari must know the role that the USDA plays in their profession. What is the mission of the USDA? What are some of the programs or services that the USDA and Food and Nutrition Services (FNS) provide?
6. What are the strategies a dietitian can use to secure approval of a policy?
7. What are some of the ways that dietitians can become involved with and influence public policy?
8. In 2004, the Child Nutrition Reauthorization Act was passed. This act required each school district in the country to develop a wellness policy. By law, what are the requirements of these wellness policies that both Angelina and Omari must know?
9. Work in small groups or individually to discuss the case study and practice using the Nutrition Care Process chart provided on the companion website. You also can add other nutrition and health-related conditions or assessments to the case study to make the case study more challenging and interesting.

## Think About It

**Answer:** Community and public health nutritionists can use nutrition monitoring and examination information to determine dietary habits, identify high-risk population groups to plan public health intervention programs and initiate food assistance awareness efforts; establish the national health agenda and evaluate progress toward achieving national health objectives; establish guidelines for the prevention, detection, and management of nutritional conditions; and evaluate the impact of nutrition initiatives for military feeding systems. Data also are used to monitor food production and marketing programs and their impact on the food supply.

## Key Terms

**Code of Federal Regulations (CFR):** A comprehensive summary of all federal regulations currently in force.
**Federal Register:** A weekly publication that contains all regulations, proposed regulations, and the Code of Federal Regulations (CFR).
**grassroots liaison (GRL):** A position in the Academy of Nutrition and Dietetics (AND) that is appointed or elected by the state affiliate to serve as the primary

communicator between AND members and their congressperson.
**legislative network coordinator (LNC):** An elected state affiliate member of the Academy of Nutrition and Dietetics (AND) who organizes and mobilizes AND members at the state level to become involved in federal public policy issues.
**medical nutrition therapy:** A service provided by a Registered Dietitian or nutrition professional that includes counseling, nutrition support, and nutrition assessment and screening to improve people's health and quality of life.
**policy:** A framework for making decisions that guide actions to help the public.
**political action committee (PAC):** A group of individuals united by similar interests or issues.
**secondary legislation:** The action of administrative bodies such as the U.S. Department of Agriculture interpreting the law and providing the detailed regulations or rules that set a policy into effect after a law is passed.
**standing committees:** Permanently established committees that create and approve legislation, authorize programs, and oversee program implementation.

# References

1. Stewart WH. The use of government to protect and promote the health of the public through nutrition. *Fed Proc.* 1979;38(12):2557-2559.

2. Borra ST, Earl R, Gilbride JA. At a crossroads: ADA and public policy. *J Am Diet Assoc.* 2002;102(4):464-466.

3. Boyle MA, Holben D. *Community Nutrition in Action: An Entrepreneurial Approach.* 4th ed. Belmont, CA: Thomson Wadsworth; 2013.

4. Mahan KL, Escott-Stump S. *Krause's Food, Nutrition, and Diet Therapy.* 11th ed. St. Louis, MO: Mosby, 2012.

5. Luepker RV, Perry CL, McKinlay SM, et al. Outcomes of a field trial to improve children's dietary patterns and physical activity: the Child and Adolescent Trial for Cardiovascular Health—CATCH collaborative group. *JAMA.* 1996;275:768-776.

6. American Dietetic Association. Position of the American Dietetic Association: affordable and accessible health care services. *J Am Diet Assoc.* 1992;92:746-748.

7. American Dietetic Association. White paper on health care reform. *J Am Diet Assoc.* 1992;92:749.

8. American Dietetic Association. Lobbying efforts focus on health care reform. *J Am Diet Assoc.* 1993;93:754.

9. American Dietetic Association. ADA continues push for medical nutrition therapy, improved child nutrition programs and labeling of dietary supplements. *J Am Diet Assoc.* 1994;94:721.

10. American Dietetic Association. Health care reform initiatives stress grass-roots lobbying and coalition-building. *J Am Diet Assoc.* 1993;93:528.

11. American Dietetic Association. ADA mobilizes grassroots action to secure Medicare coverage for medical nutrition therapy. *J Am Diet Assoc.* 1996;96:1241.

12. Smith R. Summary of medical nutrition therapy 2005-2006. *J Am Diet Assoc.* 2006;106(3):358-361.

13. American Dietetic Association. New ADA campaign seeks more cosponsors for Medicare Medical Nutrition Therapy Act: update on child/elderly bills. *J. Am Diet Assoc.* 1997;12:1372-1373.

14. Ensign JE. Remarks on introducing the Medical Nutrition Therapy Act of 1997 in the House of Representatives. *Congr. Rec.* E6961997.

15. American Dietetic Association, Public Relations. *Team Improving Health and Saving Health-Care Dollars: Medical Nutrition Therapy Works.* Chicago, IL: American Dietetic Association; April 9, 2002.

16. Michael P. Impact and components of the Medicare MNT benefits. *J Am Diet Assoc.* 2001;101:1140-1141.

17. Winterfeldt E. Influencing public policy. *Top Clin Nutr.* 2001;16:8-16.

18. US Government Printing Office. *Fed Reg.* http://gpoaccess.gov. Accessed July 6, 2016.

19. Endres JB. *Community Nutrition Challenges and Opportunities.* Columbus, OH: Prentice Hall; 1999.

20. Enyinda CI, Ogbuehi AO. An empirical analysis of retail pricing and multimedia advertising effects on sales performance. *J Food Products Marketing.* 1997;4:3-16.

21. Kaufman M. *Nutrition in Promoting the Public's Health: Strategies, Principles, and Practice.* MA: Jones and Bartlett; 2009.

22. Stoker J. Influencing the legislative process: how a bill becomes a law. *Home Healthc Nurse.* 2003;21(5):299.

23. National Institutes of Health. NIH is the nation's medical research agency: making important medical discoveries that improve health and save lives. 2016. http://www.nih.gov/icd/. Accessed February 22, 2016.

24. Centers for Disease Control and Prevention. About the CDC. 2016. http://www.cdc.gov/cio.doc. Accessed July 7, 2016.

25. US Dept of Agriculture, Food and Nutrition Service. 2016. https://www.fns.usda.gov/. Accessed February 22, 2017.

26. US Dept of Health and Human Services. What we do. 2016. https://www.hhs.gov/ocio/about/whatwedo/what.html. Accessed July 7, 2016.

27. Austin JE, Hitt C. *Nutrition Intervention in the United States.* Cambridge, MA: Vallinger; 1979.

28. US Food and Drug Administration. FDA's counterterrorism role. 2016. http://www.fda.gov/oc/bioterrorism/role.html. Accessed August 8, 2016.

29. Spake A. FDA eyes bigger role on imported food. *U.S. News World Rep.* 1998;125(13):38.

30. Mead P, Slutsker L, Dietz V, McCaig, et al. Food related illness and death in the United States. *Emerg Infect Dis.* 1999;5(5):607-625.

31. US Food and Drug Administration. Total diet study. 2005. http://www.cfsan.fda.gov/~comm/tds-toc.html. Accessed August 8, 2006.

32. US Dept of Health and Human Services. About DHHS. 2016. http://www.dhhs.gov/about/index.html. Accessed May 13, 2016.

33. US Dept of Department of Agriculture. Nutrition Services Incentive Program. 2016. http://www.aoa.dhhs.gov/eldfam/Nutrition/Nutrition_services_incentive.asp. Accessed March 26, 2016.

34. Centers for Medicare and Medicaid Services, US Dept of Health and Human Services. Medicare and Medicaid programs programs of all-inclusive care for the elderly (PACE) program

revisions: final rule. *Fed Reg.* 2016;71(236): 71243-71337.

35. US Dept of Agriculture. About USDA. 2016. http://www .usda.gov/wps/portal/!ut/p/_s.7_0_A/7_0_1OB? navtype=MA&navid=ABOUT_USDA. Accessed May 13, 2016.

36. Sims LS. Public policy in nutrition: a framework for action. *Nutr Today.* 1993;28(2):10-20.

37. Smedley BD, Stith AY, Nelson AR. *Unequal Treatment Confronting Racial and Ethnic Disparities in Healthcare.* Washington, DC: National Academies Press; 2002.

38. Block RA, Hess LA, Timpano EV, Serlo C. Physiologic changes in the foot during pregnancy. *J Am Podiatr Med Assoc.* 1985;75(6):297-299.

39. Chapman N. Consensus and coalitions: key to nutrition policy development. *Nutr Today.* 1987;22(5):22-29.

40. Birkland TA. *An Introduction to the Policy Process: Theories, Concepts, and Models of Public Policy Making.* Armonk, NY: M.E. Sharpe; 2001.

41. Spasoff RA. The role of nutrition in healthy public policy. *Rapport.* 1989;4:6-7.

42. Oltersdorf U. Impact of nutrition behaviour research on nutrition programmes and nutrition policy. *Appetite.* 2003;41(3):239-244.

43. Wright ML. Building local knowledge for developing health policy through key informant interviews. *J Extention.* 2002;40(1).

44. Watts MML. How dietitians can make a difference through political action. *J Am Diet Assoc.* 2002;102(9):1226-1227.

45. Samour P, Ochs, M. Growing policy with grassroots activism. *J Am Diet Assoc.* 2004;104(12):1786-1787.

46. White JV, Hughes BAF. If dietetics is your profession, public policy is your business. *J Am Diet Assoc.* 2001;101(2):172.

47. Federal Election Commission. Federal campaign fianance law. 2016. http://fec.gov. Accessed July 6, 2016.

48. McCullum CC. Use of a participatory planning process as a way to build community food security. *J Am Diet Assoc.* 2002;102(7):962-967.

49. US Dept of Health, US Dept of Health and Human Services, Public Health Service. *Healthy People 2000 National Health Promotion and Disease Prevention Objectives.* Washington DC: US Dept of Health, US Dept of Health and Human Services, Public Health Service; 1990.

50. Owen A, Splett PL, Owen GM. *Nutrition in the Community: The Art and Science of Delivering Services.* 4th ed. New York, NY: McGraw-Hill; 1999.

51. US Dept of Health and Human Services. *Healthy People 2010: Understanding and Improving Health and Objectives for Improving Health.* 2nd ed. Vol 2. Washington, DC: US Dept of Health and Human Services; 2000. http://www.healthypeople. gov/2010/ Accessed February 22, 2017.

52. US Dept of Health and Human Services. *Healthy People 2010: Understanding and Improving Health.* 2nd ed. Washington DC: US Dept of Health and Human Services; 2000. http://www.healthypeople. gov/2010/About/. Accessed February 22, 2017.

53. Berdanier CD. *Handbook of Nutrition and Food.* New York, NY: CRC Press; 2013.

54. National Institutes of Health. Optimal calcium intake: NIH consensus statement. Bethesda, MD: National Institutes of Health; June 6–8, 1994.

55. US Dept of Health and Human Services. *The surgeon general's report on nutrition and health.* PHS Publication No. 88-50210. Washington, DC: US Dept of Health and Human Services; 1988.

56. National Research Council and Committee on Diet and Health. *Implications for Reducing Chronic Disease.* Washington, DC: National Academies Press; 1989.

57. Institute of Medicine, Committee on Military Nutrition Research, Food and Nutrition Board. *Military nutrition initiatives.* 91-05 report. Washington DC: Institute of Medicine; 1991.

58. US Dept of Health and Human Services Public Health Service. *Healthy People 2000 National Health Promotion and Disease Prevention Objectives.* PHS Publication 91-50212. Washington, DC: US Dept of Health and Human Services; 1991.

59. Association of Nutrition and Dietetics. FAQs: CMS final rule related to therapeutic diet orders. 2016. http://www.eatrightpro.org/resource/advocacy /quality-health-care/consumer-protection-and -licensure/faqs-cms-final-rule-related-to-therapeutic -diet-orders. Accessed February 22, 2017.

60. US Dept of Agriculture Economic Research Service. Agricultural Act of 2014: Highlights and implications. 2016. http://www.ers.usda.gov/agricultural -act-of-2014-highlights-and-implications.aspx. Accessed July 6, 2016.

61. Association of Nutrition and Dietetics. Agricultural Act, 2014: Academy recommendation. 2016. https://www.eatrightpro.org/~/media /eatrightpro%20files/advocacy/health%20food%20 systems%20and%20access/hunger%20and%20 food%20security/academy%20farm%20bill%20 recommendations%20vs%20agricultural%20 act%20of%202014.ashx. Accessed July 6, 2016.

62. Radimer K. National nutrition data: contributions and challenges to monitoring dietary supplement use in women. *J Nutr Educ.* 2007;133: 2003s-2007s.

63. Smith RE, Patrick S, Michael P, Hager M. Medical nutrition therapy: the core of ADA's advocacy efforts. *J Am Diet Assoc.* 2005;105(5 pt 1): 825-834.

64. American Diabetes Association. Final food labeling regulations. *J Am Diet Assoc.* 1993;93(2):146-148.

65. Goldfarb B. Pushing for CMS coverage of Medical Nutrition Therapy. *DOC News.* 2005;2(10):1.

66. American Dietetic Association. Medicare Medical Nutrition Therapy Act of 2005. 2005. http://www.eatright.org. Accessed February 21, 2011.

67. Smith RE. Passing an effective obesity bill. *J Am Diet Assoc.* 2006;106(9):1349-1353.

68. Kanaya AM, Narayan KM. Prevention of type 2 diabetes: data from recent trials. *Prim Care.* 2003;30(3):511-526.

69. Dalgaard M. Effects of one single bout of low-intensity exercise on postprandial lipemia in type 2 diabetic men. *Brit J Nutr.* 2004;92(3):469-476.

70. Smith RE, Patrick S, Michael P, Hager M. Medical nutrition therapy: the core of ADA's advocacy efforts. *J Am Diet Assoc.* 2005;105(6 pt 2):987-996.

71. US Dept of Agriculture, Food and Nutrition Service. Healthy schools. http://teamnutrition.usda.gov/Healthy/wellnesspolicygoals_schoolbased.html. Accessed August 6, 2016.

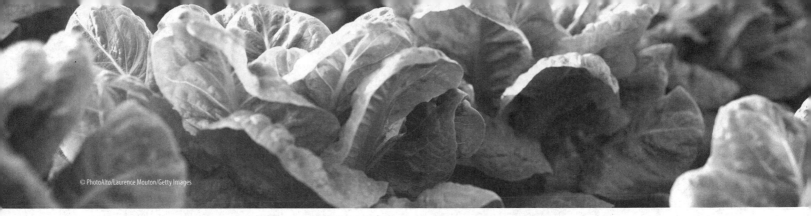

© PhotoAlto/Laurence Mouton/Getty Images

# CHAPTER 7

# Public Health Nutrition: An International Perspective

## LEARNING OBJECTIVES

- Compare the prevalence of undernutrition and overnutrition in developing and developed countries.
- Discuss the effects of undernutrition on children.
- Discuss factors that contribute to world hunger and malnutrition.
- Define food security.
- Describe women's role in preventing food insecurity.
- Identify how children become infected with human immunodeficiency virus.
- Discuss current international nutrition issues in developing and developed countries.
- Provide feeding guidelines for use during emergency relief periods.
- Discuss the different types of emergency feeding programs.
- Describe appropriate feeding methods for severely malnourished individuals.

# ▶ Introduction

Food supplies have increased significantly, especially in higher income **developed countries** that have enough to feed their population for at least the next few decades.[1,2] However, many **developing countries** experience hunger and malnutrition. It is expected that some low-income and food-insecure countries will experience lack of food in the next decade unless their population growth is matched with increased agricultural production and a growth in purchasing power.[3]

The lack of food supply leads to undernutrition. The number of chronically undernourished people has declined because many countries are using modern technologies to increase food supply. However, this number still represents about 276 million people.[1] The food supply of those individuals who are chronically undernourished is less than 2,000 calories per day.[4] The latest estimates indicate that about 790.7 million people are undernourished, 200 million of whom are in developing countries and about 19 million of whom are in developed countries.[5] The countries with the highest rates of undernutrition lack the financial resources to provide government-funded food assistance programs, such as those found in the United States.

The food assistance programs in the United States were described in earlier chapters. These include children's School Lunch and Breakfast Programs, childcare and eldercare food programs, food assistance programs for older adults such as congregate meals, and the Special Supplemental Nutrition Program for Women, Infants, and Children (WIC) that supplies low-income pregnant women and mothers with nourishing food.

# ▶ Overview of World Hunger

The most recent data show that 98 percent of the 1.02 billion people who are chronically hungry in the world are from developing countries.[5] Many developed countries, such as most European countries, Japan, Australia, New Zealand, and the United States, have enough food to provide their population with 3,400 calories per person per day. In contrast, the lowest income countries, such as Angola, Chad, Mozambique, and Somalia, have an average daily supply of less than 1,800 calories per person.[6,7]

In 1960, India, China, and other Asian countries had similar problems of hunger, but now they are among the most successful at increasing food production and consumption. Food shortages, both chronic and acute, now mainly occur in sub-Saharan Africa.[8] In Asian countries, modern technologies are used to increase food supply, and family planning programs help reduce population growth. In addition, rural agricultural economic growth generated increased incomes for the rural poor, stabilized food prices, and increased non-agricultural economic growth, which contributed to a reduction in chronic food shortages in Asia.[8] According to the Food and Agriculture Organization (FAO) of the United Nations, the number of Asians who were chronically undernourished decreased from 40 percent in 1970 to 19 percent in 1990. In China, specifically, the rate of extreme poverty decreased from 33 percent in 1990 to 16.6 percent in 2001.[9] However, the 2010 report estimated that the rate of poverty has increased to over 40 percent in China and India alone.[10]

The gap between the rich and the poor is increasing, which is one factor that contributes to chronic undernutrition and hunger. The range between the rich and the poor in Australia, Sweden, the United Kingdom, and the United States has increased over the last two decades. In the United States, about 14.7 percent of Americans, including 20.1 percent of children, live at or below the poverty level.[11] The International Food Policy Research Institute (IFPRI) has warned that at the threshold of the twenty-first century, widespread poverty, hunger, and malnutrition threaten to undermine global economic, social, political, and environmental conditions. It has been reported that the richest 20 percent of the world's population share a global income that is 86 times that of the poorest 20 percent.[12,13] In addition, industrialized countries hold 97 percent of all patents, and global corporations hold 90 percent of all technology and product patents, which makes it more difficult for developing countries to compete in the global market.[14]

During the past decades, budget deficits in many developing countries have caused governments to reexamine their polices. Many countries relaxed their agricultural markets and eliminated production and marketing controls in an effort to stimulate production. The elimination of retail price controls increased prices for domestically grown foods. Also, devaluations of exchange rates made imported foods more expensive, further increasing prices for domestically grown foods.[15] These countries' policy changes made food less affordable for many and increased nutritional vulnerability for their citizens. Rising food prices in many developing countries have not been matched by an increase in purchasing power. For example, per capita income declined between 1980 and 1992 by 2.7 percent per year in North Africa and the Near East and by 1.1 percent per year in sub-Saharan Africa. Per capita income growth in Latin America remained flat during that period. Asia was the only region with impressive performance—per capita income grew 3.3 percent per year in South Asia and 6.2 percent per year in East Asia.[16,17] Decreasing per capita incomes are not unique to developing countries.

Developed countries also experience recessions. The concern about the performance in developing countries is their low income base and the toll such declines take from those low bases. In 2013, about 2.8 billion people, half of the world population, earned less than $2.0 USD per day, and about 1.2 billion earned less than $1.00 USD per day. In 2010, worldwide, 1.3 billion people lived on less than $1.00 USD per day, 3 billion lived on under $2.00 USD a day, 1.3 billion had no access to clean water, 3 billion had no access to sanitation, and 2 billion had no access to electricity.[18] **FIGURE 7-1** presents a global map showing the levels of hunger.[19]

## ▶ Current Nutrition Issues in Developing and Developed Countries

The habit of consuming diets high in energy, saturated fat, cholesterol, and sodium and low in fiber has contributed to increases in nutrition-related chronic health conditions. Regardless of the prevalence of undernutrition in developing countries, overnutrition and its complications are emerging as major health concerns.[20] Nutrition-related chronic diseases either are appearing or are already established in every country around the world.[21,22] The incidence of chronic diseases is increasing, and infectious diseases remain a common problem in countries where urbanization is happening rapidly.[23,24]

Rapid urbanization also has contributed to a dietary change in many developing countries. It is estimated that 53 percent of the population of the developing world lived in cities in the year 2013, and 5 million will be urban dwellers by 2030.[25-27] The urban environment is usually more favorable to good nutritional status in children, but urbanization has some disadvantages, including reduced breastfeeding rates and duration, household **food insecurity** linked to the cash economy for very poor urban families, and increases in obesity associated with sedentary lifestyles.[28,29]

It has been estimated that over the next decade, 30 to 40 countries will remain in the lowest income bracket, with high incidence of infectious childhood diseases,

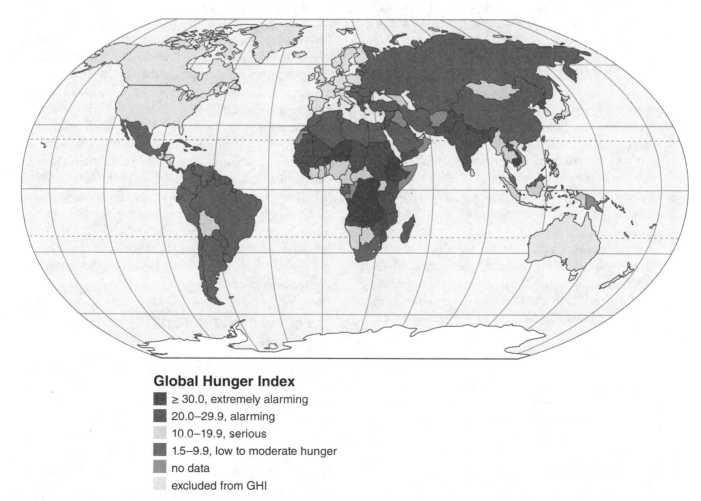

### Global Hunger Index

- ≥ 30.0, extremely alarming
- 20.0–29.9, alarming
- 10.0–19.9, serious
- 1.5–9.9, low to moderate hunger
- no data
- excluded from GHI

**FIGURE 7-1** Global map showing levels of hunger.

Source: 2006 Global Hunger Index (Wiesmann 2006). Used with permission from the International Food Policy Research Institute.

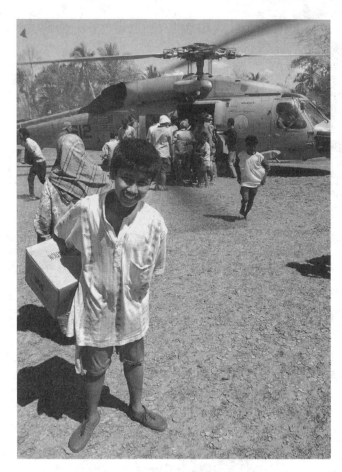

A large supply of high-quality foods can prevent malnutrition.

Courtesy of Airman Jordan R. Beesley, U.S. Navy.

undernutrition, and high fertility.[30] The major problems continue to be diarrheal diseases, acute respiratory tract illnesses in young children, HIV infection, measles, tetanus, polio, malaria, micronutrient deficiencies, parasitic diseases, and reproductive mortality.[31] In areas such as sub-Saharan Africa and South Asia, nutrition and health education need to focus on the establishment of a basic primary healthcare infrastructure: breastfeeding, maternal nutrition, **immunization** against vaccine-preventable diseases, control of diarrheal diseases, and family planning. An analysis of trends in childhood undernutrition in the 25-year period between 1970 and 1995 showed a 15.5 percent reduction in the rates of underweight children due to an improvement in formal nutrition education, national food availability, and basic sanitation and health services.[29]

In a group of moderately higher income countries in East Asia, Latin America, and the Middle East, infectious diseases, malnutrition, and reproductive health problems remain high and rapid urbanization, industrialization, and economic development are causing new health problems, including occupational injuries and preventable chronic diseases.[32,33]

In high-income countries, diet-related chronic diseases dominate the public health nutrition agenda.

Problems of undernutrition and access to food primarily affect lower income groups. In the United States and the United Kingdom, obesity and its complications also are prevalent among poorer segments of the population. So-called diseases of affluence are actually diseases of poverty in some of the richer countries.[34,35]

Nations in Eastern Europe and the former Soviet Union present special cases. These have been categorized as "industrialized, non-market economies."[34] They have passed through demographic, epidemiological, and nutrition transitions, but are undergoing an epidemic of high mortality from preventable causes among young adults.[36] These include high alcohol consumption, trauma, poisoning, respiratory diseases (often secondary to smoking), and complications of pregnancy and childbirth. Also, the very high cost of foods contributed to dietary and nutritional problems, such as inadequate fruit and vegetable intake; micronutrient deficiencies in some groups, including iodine deficiency disease; and undernutrition in the elderly.[37-39]

# ▶ Malnutrition, Food Insecurity, and Hunger

**Food security** means "access at all times by all people to an adequate amount of safe, nutritious, and culturally appropriate foods for active and healthy lives."[40] A significant number of people are food insecure or hungry worldwide. The FAO reported that over 795 million people in the world do not have enough to eat.[41] More than half of all child deaths worldwide are associated with malnutrition.[31,42] **Malnutrition** is poor nutritional status due to dietary intake either above or below the optimal level. Micronutrient deficiencies are especially widespread. In the developing countries, about 20 percent of the population suffer from iodine deficiency, about 25 percent of children have a subclinical vitamin A deficiency, and more than 40 percent of women are anemic.[30,43]

## The Effect of Hunger and Malnutrition on Health

Hunger is defined as a condition in which people lack the basic food intake needed to provide them with the energy and nutrients for fully productive, active lives.[44] In developing countries, hunger and poverty are more prevalent than acute hunger caused by **famine**, which is a widespread lack of access to food due to a disaster, drought, political conflict, or war that causes a collapse in the area's food production and marketing systems. Approximately 33 percent of children younger than 5 years of age in developing countries experience **stunting** (malnourished based on height for age), signifying long-term, cumulative effects of inadequate nutrition and/or poor health conditions.[45] Approximately 27 percent of children ages 3 to 5 years in developing countries are wasted (malnourished based on weight for age).[45] Impairment of growth can have both immediate and long-term negative effects on a child's health, impairing their ability to learn and their potential for future achievement, and increasing their risk for developing chronic diseases later in life. The United Nations International Children's Fund (UNICEF) stated that the mortality rate of those younger than 5 years is a good measure of the mother's knowledge of many important public health services, such as immunization; the availability of prenatal and other health services; income; the availability of food, clean water, and safe sanitation; and the overall safety of the child's environment.[46]

Good nutrition is an essential part of good health. An extensive network of food assistance programs provides nutritious foods daily to millions of U.S. citizens.[47] One of every six Americans receives food assistance of some kind at a total cost of almost $33 billion per year.[48] Despite that, the programs are not fully successful in preventing hunger, even among those who receive their benefits. In the United States from 2009 to 2010, the prevalence of food insecurity decreased slightly from 14.7 percent to 14.5 percent and the prevalence of food insecurity with hunger from 5.7 percent to 5.4 percent.

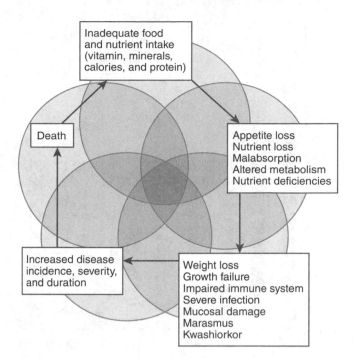

**FIGURE 7-2** Inadequate dietary intake and the cycle of disease.

Inadequate food intake and infection operate in a vicious cycle that accounts for the high morbidity and mortality rate in developing countries. When children's dietary intake is inadequate, their immune system defenses decrease, causing higher incidence, severity, and duration of diseases. In turn, many diseases suppress appetite and increase nutrient loss, thus continuing the cycle. **FIGURES 7-2** and **7-3** present the inadequate dietary intake/disease cycle and the effect of malnutrition on child mortality, respectively.[49]

In addition to causing human suffering, hunger and malnutrition have negative effects on cognitive development, growth, and health.[50-52] Hunger and malnutrition also have negative effects on labor productivity and a nation's development. According to the World Bank, the global loss of social productivity in one year alone, caused by three overlapping types of malnutrition—nutritional stunting and wasting, iodine deficiency disorders, and deficiencies of iron and vitamin A—is equivalent to 46 million years of productive, disability-free life.[53,54] Hence, a significant effort to eliminate hunger could yield positive benefits for individuals, nations, and the world community.

## ▶ Women's Contribution to Food Security

Women contribute significantly to prevent food insecurity and malnutrition worldwide, especially in developing countries.[55] However, this contribution is overlooked and

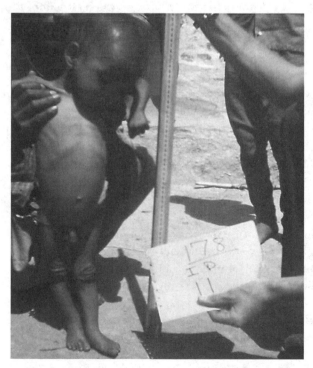

Marasmic-kwashiorkor is a condition in which there is a deficiency of both calories and protein, with severe tissue wasting, loss of subcutaneous fat, and dehydration.
Courtesy of Dr. Edward Brink/CDC

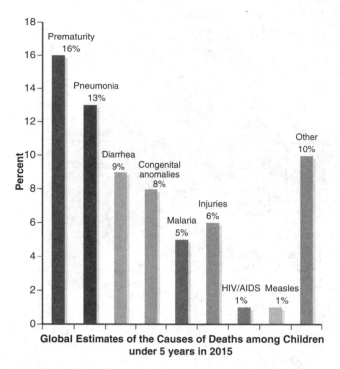

**FIGURE 7-3** The effects of malnutrition on child mortality.

Data from Müller O, Krawinkel M. Malnutrition and health in developing countries. *Can Med Assoc J.* 2005;173(3):279–286.

mostly uncompensated. Women represent 50 percent of the adult population, make up one third of the official labor force, perform nearly two thirds of all working hours, receive only one tenth of the world's income, and own less than 1 percent of property.[56] To illuminate the roles of women in national and international development, the United Nations declared the United Nations Women's Decade from 1975 to 1985. This recognition contributed to an appreciation of rural women as energizers of any nation's economy, especially in countries whose economies are agriculture-based, such as developing countries.[57]

Poverty has become a women's issue. In the United States, almost 35 percent of households with children headed by single women live below the poverty level. Seven of ten hungry people in the world are women and girls, yet they receive only about half of the available food aid and often use it to feed their children as well as themselves. Even starving women are more likely to give food they receive to their hungry children first. In Asia and Africa, approximately 60 to 80 percent of women are engaged in farming, have less access to jobs in a formal labor market, have fewer opportunities to enroll in primary and secondary schools, and have fewer opportunities to own and control land and housing. In one third of households worldwide, women are the sole breadwinners.[58-60] Malnourished women in poverty bear sickly infants who cannot resist the diseases of poverty, and many die within the first years of life.[60] One child in six is born underweight, and 10 million die by age 5, half from malnutrition-related causes.[61]

In the United States, President Clinton signed the Personal Responsibility and Work Opportunity Reconciliation Act in 1996, initiating a major reform of the U.S. welfare system. One of the main objectives of the reform was to move mothers permanently from welfare to employment. Data show that less-educated mothers are disproportionately represented in occupations with low wages and high rates of **nonstandard work schedules** (irregular days, rotating hours or days, weekend days, and regular evening or night hours). Many of these women who work nonstandard hours do so mainly because of the labor market rather than from personal choice. In addition, job characteristics rather than family characteristics are more likely to cause employment during nonstandard times.[62,63] Thus, less-educated mothers are drawn into working nonstandard hours by a lack of options. The most common occupations held by these women include cashiers, nursing aids, and waitresses, and at least 40 percent of them work nonstandard hours. Welfare reform has created a group called the "working poor," people who are employed, but earn low wages that cause food insecurity and homelessness, which affect children as well as adults.[64]

Caregiving is a major role for women throughout their lives. About 72 percent of unpaid family caregivers are women, the majority of whom are middle-aged daughters or daughters-in-law.[63] For many women, caring for family members is informal care that they provide in addition to paid employment outside the home. Mothers assume the primary responsibility for the health and illness of their young families, wives often care for their aging and ill husbands, and daughters and daughters-in-law care for aging parents or in-laws. Unfortunately, in today's society, the role of the caregiver is devalued. In a family with three or more children, women spend about 90 hours a week in paid and unpaid work, while men typically spend only 60 hours.[62] The added responsibility and financial strain of the caregiver role can lead to caregiver burden and increased stress.

Maternal and women's health issues are critical to examine from a global perspective. Ninety nine percent of deaths during childbirth occur in developing countries and most of them are preventable. Infectious diseases, blood loss, and unsafe abortions account for most of the deaths[65,66] In the developing countries, an estimated 303,000 women died during pregnancy and childbirth in 2015, over 800 women die each day from pregnancy and childbirth complications, and many millions more suffered without treatment. Annual maternal mortality rates vary widely among the regions of the world; it is low in Latin America (670,000) but very high in Sub-Sahara Africa (546,000) and South Asia (200,000).[67] In many of the poor African countries, one mother dies from pregnancy complications and delivery per every 100 live births.[68,69]

One of the objectives of the World Bank and the United Nations is the Millennium Development Goals (MDGs). The purpose of the MDGs is to promote poverty reduction, education, maternal health, and gender equality; to combat child mortality, AIDS, and other diseases; and to reduce maternal death rates by three quarters by 2015. Information on MDGs can be obtained from the U.N. Development Programme website at http://www.undp.org.

## Prevalence of HIV/AIDS in Women and Children

In addition to hunger, poverty, and malnutrition, women and children also experience a high rate of HIV infection. In 2014, approximately 2.6 million children under the age of 15 became infected with HIV, mainly through mother-to-child transmission (MTCT). MTCT occurs when an HIV-positive woman passes the virus to her baby. This can occur during pregnancy, labor and delivery, or breastfeeding. Without treatment, approximately 15 to 30 percent of babies born to HIV-positive women will become infected with HIV during pregnancy and delivery, and 5 to 20 percent will become infected through breastfeeding.[70]

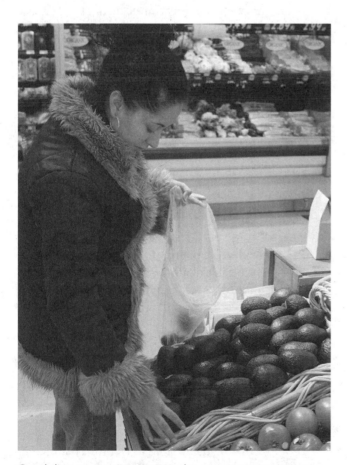

Good dietary practices start at the grocery store.
© Robert Nystrom/ShutterStock, Inc.

HIV is responsible for the development of AIDS, a devastating illness that was first recognized in 1981.[71] A retrovirus, HIV infects a cell and uses an enzyme called reverse transcriptase to transcribe the viral genome onto the cell's DNA, resulting in viral replication by the infected cell.

The following threefold strategy is needed to prevent babies acquiring HIV from their infected mothers[72,73]:

A. Prevent HIV infection among prospective parents.

B. Avoid unwanted pregnancies among HIV-positive women.

C. Prevent the transmission of HIV from HIV-positive mothers to their infants during pregnancy, labor and delivery, and breastfeeding. This can be achieved through the use of antiretroviral drugs, safer feeding practices, and other interventions.

At the end of 2014, young women 15 to 24 years old accounted for 18.6 million of all adults living with HIV worldwide and 70 percent in sub-Saharan Africa.

It is the position of the American Dietetic Association and Dietitians of Canada that efforts to optimize nutritional status, including medical nutrition therapy and nutrition-related education, should be components of the total health care provided to people infected with HIV.[74]

## Nutrition Education and Counseling for Those with HIV/AIDS

Specific counseling guidelines and recommendations address the following areas, as appropriate, for the client with HIV/AIDS[74-76]:

- Provide a healthful eating plan and principles to ensure adequate nutrient intake using recommended foods and amounts.
- Enforce food and water safety issues, including food shopping, storage, preparation, and dining away from home.
- Integrate perinatal nutrition and breastfeeding recommendations for HIV-infected mothers of newborn children. Ensure access to infant formula and food as an alternative to breastfeeding.
- Consider cultural and ethnic beliefs related to diet and food.
- Establish nutrition strategies for symptom management, such as anorexia, early satiety, swallowing problems, nausea and vomiting, diarrhea, food intolerances, and other barriers to food intake.
- Observe food–medication interactions, including meal timing for optimal medication efficacy and supplementation and foods to emphasize or avoid

unwanted interactions (such as reduced medication absorption, nutrient depletion, or altered laboratory values).

- Reconcile psychosocial and economic issues that may prevent appropriate nutrient intake, including referral and access to community resources that help support nutrition, and health-related parenting classes or other support groups.
- Establish alternative feeding methods (supplementation, tube feeding, or parenteral nutrition) or special diets, individual vitamin and mineral supplementation, and other complementary nutrition practices.
- Seek additional therapies that support nutrition, including physical activity and exercise; medications for symptom management, inflammation, and hormonal modulation; and disease management.
- Establish strategies for treatment of altered fat metabolism and deposition, including diet and exercise, lipid-lowering medication, glycemic control, hormonal normalization, and anabolic medications.
- Conduct community-based nutrition research to determine how many individuals with HIV/AIDS need to participate in home-delivered meal programs.

## ▶ Causes of Hunger and Malnutrition

Poverty is the major cause of hunger and malnutrition. The causes of poverty include lack of resources, unequal income distribution around the world and within specific countries, and conflict. An estimated 1.3 billion poor people in developing countries live on $1 USD per day or less.[77,78] Of these, an estimated 925 million suffer from chronic hunger, which means that their daily intake of calories is not enough for them to lead active and healthy lives.

Conflict is another cause of hunger and poverty and, subsequently, malnutrition. The United Nations High Commissioner for Refugees (UNHCR) reported that at the end of 2015, there were 21.3 million refugees.[77] The incidence of malnutrition is widespread at the early stages of refugee emergencies, which increases the risk for disease and death.[61] The causes of hunger and malnutrition comprises a wide variety of problems that include, but are not limited to, the following[61,78]:

- Maternal undernutrition
- Iodine, vitamin A, iron, and zinc deficiencies
- Diarrhea, HIV, and other infectious diseases
- Inadequate infant and child feeding practices
- Female time constraints

- Limited household income and agricultural production
- Food insecurity
- Environmental degradation and urbanization

## ▶ Solving World Hunger and Malnutrition

Solving world hunger is a daunting task. It involves controlling population growth, increasing food production and economic opportunity, and providing for and maintaining adequate, culturally acceptable food and nutritional supplies for a large and diverse population. In addition, the solutions involve economic policies that promote sustainable agriculture, technological advancement, education, maintaining the global ecosystem, and legislative measures. In addition, the input of politicians, nutrition scientists, economists, and the food industry is essential to solving the problem of world hunger and malnutrition.

Another way to decrease world hunger is to maintain the world's food supply for the long term by developing policies that promote sustainable agriculture. Three general areas of concern inspire the concept of sustainable agriculture[79-81]:

- Economic concerns (economic justice) to increase or maintain the number, quality, and long-term economic possibility of farming and other agricultural business opportunities in a community or region. This would foster the continued existence of owner-operated farms and the long-term profitability of agriculture by embedding local agricultural and food production into the community.
- Environmental concerns to increase, rather than diminish, the integrity, diversity, and long-term productivity of both the managed agricultural ecosystem and the surrounding natural ecosystems. This would reduce the undesirable impact of agriculture on land, water, and wildlife resources.
- Public welfare concerns to increase rather than threaten the health, safety, and aesthetic satisfaction of agricultural producers and consumers. This would increase food quality and reduce human exposure to toxic chemicals.

Linking these efforts explicitly to sustainable agriculture and promoting more engagement between ecologically oriented farmers and their communities could stimulate more economic and political support for these farmers and help them and their communities achieve greater sustainability.

In addition to sustainable agriculture, sufficient energy and adequate nutrients in the diet ensure the nutritional health of a population. If the foods and crops grown or imported do not meet all nutrient needs, the quality of the diet will be poor and malnutrition will occur. **Nutrification** of foods may be the solution to this problem. Nutrification is the process of adding one or more nutrients to commonly consumed foods with the goal of increasing the nutrient intake.[82] The foods selected for nutrification should be those the majority of the population consumes.

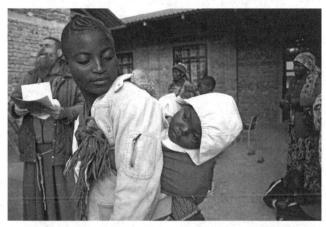

Women and children are most affected by HIV/AIDS.
© Franco Volpato/Shutterstock

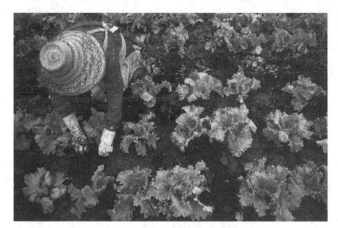

Women contribute to food security worldwide.
© AbleStock

## ▶ Global Initiatives

A major focus of health and nutrition policies and programs in developing nations is to prevent undernutrition by improving food security, the availability of health services, and economic status. A problem facing international development agencies is how to promote economic growth and at the same time prevent the undesirable effects of nutrition transition. **Nutrition transition** is a shift in dietary habit from a diet high in complex carbohydrates and fiber to a diet higher in fat, saturated fat, and sugar; this occurs as incomes increase. To address growing concerns about this problem,

individual countries have developed public health campaigns and policies that also include strategies to prevent overnutrition and promote healthy lifestyles.[83]

International campaigns also target the prevention and control of chronic diseases. One of these programs is the World Health Organization International Code of Marketing of Breast-Milk Substitutes (WHO Code), which aims to protect and promote breastfeeding. Data collected between 1990 and 2000 show that exclusive breastfeeding in developing countries increased among infants younger than 4 months (from 46 percent to 53 percent) and among infants older than 6 months (from 34 percent to 39 percent).[84] Another program is Interhealth, developed by WHO. Each country involved in Interhealth must assess its nutritional behaviors and intakes, physical activity levels, blood pressures, blood cholesterol levels, and other chronic disease risk factors, such as smoking, alcohol consumption, and obesity. Then they must implement strategies to reduce these risk factors, monitor trends in mortality, and evaluate the success of their programs. Programs directed toward feeding people are emphasized in countries where chronic disease rates are low and infectious disease rates and undernutrition are high. For countries with high chronic disease risks, nutrition recommendations similar to the *Dietary Guidelines for Americans* encourage maintenance of appropriate body weight; decreased consumption of total fat, saturated fat, cholesterol, and sodium; increased consumption of fiber-rich foods and complex carbohydrates; and moderate alcohol intake.[85,86]

## ▶ Emergency Relief Efforts

Emergency food and feeding programs have existed throughout history. References to this are seen in Babylonian records and the Old Testament (such as the Joseph story). However, in the past century, relief efforts have been continuous. Several organizations have been established to anticipate immediate and future disasters and address ongoing situations. Several countries have organized emergency response agencies for domestic relief, and international agencies have been established by international agreements to address transnational emergency concerns. In addition, many nongovernmental organizations are interested in and conducting relief services.[87] Persistent high mortality rates among refugee populations were observed in the last two decades. Studies show the problem of extremely high mortality rates for populations in camps persists for months after people's arrival at the camps.[88,89] Logically, even if the initial high death rates could not be avoided, once people are in camps and in touch with assistance, the continuing large numbers of deaths should be preventable.

## Food Supplies

Estimates of overall food supplies provided to refugee camps, accumulated in the mid-1990s, showed that in many cases the supplies were inadequate; for example, in one survey, about a quarter of the camps were receiving less than 1,000 kcal/person per day and almost all were receiving less than 2,000 kcal.[90] In many camps, the mortality rate was extraordinarily high. It was determined that a camp would not have a normal mortality rate if the inhabitants received below 1,500 kcal/day. In 1989, a "minimal level" of 1,900 kcal/person/day replaced the 1,000 kcal/person per day standard.[91]

More realistic estimates of energy requirements of approximately 2,000 kcal/person per day are now being enforced. In 1995, the U.S. National Academy of Sciences Committee recommended a minimum of 2,100 kcal/person per day.[92] This level was endorsed by the UNHCR and the World Food Programme (WFP) in 1997.[93] In 2000, the WHO recommended 2,100 kcal/person per day, with a range of 1,900 to 2,300 kcal/person per day.[94]

## Types of Emergency Food Programs

Ensuring an adequate general food supply during a disaster is a major public health priority. Two common types of programs are general and selective. Selective programs are of two types: 1) therapeutic feeding programs for treatment of the severely malnourished and 2) supplementary feeding programs.

Supplementary feeding programs often are targeted either toward the moderately malnourished alone or toward the moderately malnourished plus other groups. When the supplementary feeding becomes wide enough, it is then referred to as a blanket supplementary feeding program; this type of program covers the needs of a specified vulnerable group (e.g., all mothers and young children).[95]

Therapeutic feeding programs are now well established. They began by treating children in experimental wards and continued with the transference of expensive hospital diets to refugee situations.[96] Casein was used instead of milk products alone because of concerns for lactose intolerance, but the need to have available and inexpensive mixtures minimized the concern.[95] Therefore, the procedure of frequent feeding with high-energy milk-based diets was successfully introduced into refugee situations in the 1970s. In fact, the procedures described by the WHO in 2000[45] were practically the same as those used 22 years earlier.[97]

One early example of a therapeutic diet was reported by Mason et al.[97] They found that very rapid nutritional catch-up could be achieved using a simple dry skim milk/sugar/oil/micronutrient mix, fed in a milk-like preparation. The formula concentration is 1 kcal/g at an intake of 150 kcal/kg body weight per day in a refugee setting. The growth rates were such that children could recover within a few weeks, and the mortality rates, even under the difficult circumstances of a refugee camp, were not as high as those in a hospital setting. However, mortality rates of 10 to 20 percent have persisted for many years, and the next stages of treatment for severe malnutrition should involve reducing this mortality and at the same time maintaining high recovery rates.[99]

## Oral Rehydration Therapy

Oral rehydration therapy (ORT) has been very helpful in reducing the mortality rate in malnourished individuals. As mentioned earlier, the relationship between malnutrition and infection is cyclical. Infection predisposes children to malnutrition, which impairs the immune defense system and, subsequently, predisposes children to infection.[100] Diarrhea also is a major cause of childhood malnutrition and death, and it is common during emergency feeding periods (due to infections). Diarrheal illnesses are persistent worldwide, and they have a large impact in developing countries. Children younger than 5 years are affected most, with over 7.6 million deaths per year due to dehydration associated with diarrheal illness. ORT involves the replacement of fluids and electrolytes lost during an episode of diarrheal illness.[101] The WHO estimates that over 1 million deaths are prevented annually by ORT.[102]

The WHO and UNICEF are the principal sponsors of global rehydration projects.[103] These projects involve the development and distribution of prepackaged solutions, combined with education efforts for instruction in home preparation and delivery. There is some variation among packaged solutions, but the principal ingredients are glucose, sodium, and potassium. The UNICEF recipe for a simple homemade solution contains 5 cups of boiled water, 8 teaspoons of sugar, and 1 teaspoon of salt, resulting in 1 liter of solution. In addition, fruit juices, coconut water, and other indigenous solutions can adequately substitute for oral rehydration solution.

## ☑ Think About It

A community in Asia was evacuated due to flood. They are now living in refugee camps. They have been displaced for almost 3 months, and they are not likely to be able to return to their homes soon. The living conditions in the camp are very difficult because of insufficient nutritious foods and lack of clean water, and some of the children are dying from diarrhea due to infection.

What is the effect of diarrhea on children? What is the purpose of ORT? What are the main ingredients in ORT? What is the UNICEF recipe for a simple homemade rehydration solution?

## Other Types of Emergency Foods

The foods provided during emergency situations are mostly unprocessed grains, although processed foods are critical for meeting micronutrient needs and helping in situations where local processing capability is absent. Processed foods that are distributed in significant quantities include wheat flour, bulgur wheat, cornmeal, vegetable oil (usually from soybeans), and various forms of soy-fortified cereals and cereal blends. All of these processed grains are fortified with micronutrients.[85]

Foods of interest designed for young children include blended foods, corn–soy blends (CSBs), and wheat–soy blends (WSBs). These are the richest sources of micronutrients for emergency feeding programs. The micronutrient premixes consist of 17 minerals and vitamins important to the growth and health of young children and other physiologically vulnerable groups, such as pregnant and lactating women.[85]

The U.S. Department of Agriculture (USDA) and U.S. Agency for International Development (USAID) developed these foods with assistance from the National Institutes of Health (NIH).[104] They are intended to complement the supply and acceptance of dry milk as a protein source, which was widely distributed and a common U.S. agricultural surplus.

The protein source provided during an emergency must be of high biological value and easily digested. Cow's milk is mostly available, but as mentioned earlier, some clinicians worry about the possibility of lactose malabsorption in severely malnourished people. However, cow's milk is typically well tolerated and assimilated by severely malnourished children and can be safely promoted. Goat's, ewe's, buffalo's, and camel's milk also can be used.[105,106] Human, mare's, and donkey's milk have very low protein concentrations. Cow's dried skimmed milk has very low energy density, which must be restored by adding sugar and/or vegetable oil. Eggs, meat, fish, soy isolates, and some vegetable protein mixtures also are sources of protein.[106]

## Introduction of Traditional Foods

Other foods, especially those available at home, can gradually be introduced into the diet in combination with the high-energy, high-protein formulas. This procedure should be carried out when edema is not present, skin lesions are improved, the client is active and interacts with the environment, the appetite is restored, and adequate rates of catch-up growth have been achieved. Local traditional foods can then be used in appropriate combinations in addition to the liquid formula.[107,108] This information is presented in **BOX 7-1**. The foods can be served as separate dishes or the parts can be mashed or blended and fed as paps/custards to infants and young children.

---

**BOX 7-1** Appropriate Combination of Foods[109]

- One part of a dry legume or its flour (e.g., black beans, soybeans, kidney beans, cowpeas) and three parts of a dry cereal or flour (e.g., corn, rice, wheat). Fat or oil should be added to the mashed or strained legume during or after cooking in amounts equal to the weight of the dry legume or flour and to the cereal preparations in amounts of 10 to 30 mL (2 to 6 teaspoons) oil/100 g dry cereal product, depending on the type of preparation.
- Four parts of a dry cereal (e.g., rice or wheat) and one part of fresh fish, fowl, or meat. Fat or oil should be added in amounts equal to 20 to 40 percent of the dry weights.

---

# ▶ Refeeding Severely Malnourished Individuals

Refeeding syndrome may develop in severely malnourished clients during the first week of nutritional repletion.[110-112] During refeeding, extracellular fluid volume expands rapidly and often causes dependent edema. This is due to increased sodium intake combined with sodium retention caused by the effect of insulin stimulated by the increased carbohydrate consumption. A low-sodium diet during refeeding can reduce this aspect of the syndrome.[113] The specific changes in body composition due to refeeding are determined by the existing metabolic state, body composition, and, most importantly, the composition of the refeeding diet.[114-116] The following criteria have been observed[117-119]:

- A diet high in sodium and carbohydrate predisposes the client to increases in extracellular volume and edema.
- A low-protein, high-energy refeeding diet produces fat gain without an increase in lean tissue mass.
- A high-protein diet (e.g., 2 g/kg body weight per day) can stop ongoing nitrogen losses, even when energy balance is negative.
- A high-energy, high-protein diet will replete both fat and lean tissue stores at a rate that can be predicted with reasonable accuracy from the resulting energy and nitrogen balances, both of which can be measured or estimated.
- Malnourished patients with limited mobility will increase their central protein stores, which confer an important benefit, but they cannot be expected to gain muscle mass unless their muscles are exercised. Therefore, physical activity is a factor because it increases energy needs and, more importantly, exercises muscles.

Generally, the best steps in refeeding severely malnourished individuals are normalizing fluid and electrolyte parameters and maintaining them, continuing supplementation, and providing a mixed diet at the maintenance energy level to establish tolerance and avoid refeeding syndrome.[108]

## Mortality

The mortality rate of refugees in hospitals due to severe malnutrition has not changed in about 40 years. Currently it is approximately 20 to 40 percent,[105] despite the fact that under refugee camp conditions, mortality rates of 5 to 10 percent are achieved.[120] This mortality rate is due to poor case management of edematous protein-energy malnutrition (PEM).[121] It has been reported that low mortality is attainable with adequate treatment, and, in some centers, it is as low as 4 to 6 percent for both edematous and nonedematous forms.

## Refugees and Famine Relief

The methods for treating clients en masse, or without highly trained nursing staff, have not been adopted in resource-poor settings. The lack of a clear method to manage refugees may contribute to malnutrition and, subsequently, the high mortality rate associated with refugee camps. The humanitarian movement during the Biafran war of independence in Nigeria five decades ago used dietary methods that were mostly experimental. During this time, the Medicines sans Frontiers (MSF; Doctors without Borders) was formed; the International Committee of the Red Cross (ICRC) added a nutrition department; and the Oxford Committee for Famine Relief (Oxfam) expanded and formed an effective nutrition department. These three organizations and their advisors developed the K-mix 2 diet. The diet that UNICEF was advocating for treatment of severe malnutrition in 1996 was the same K-mix 2 diet.[88] Hence, it is important to update the management method used with refugees.

Internet resources for more information about hunger and malnutrition can be found at http://nutrition.jbpub.com/communitynutrition. Also available online are the nutritional characteristics of Wheat-soy blends (WSB) and Corn-soy blends (CSB) and formulations for high-protein, high-energy liquid foods. Recommendations include the use of Ready to Use Therapeutic Food (RUTF) fortified with vitamins and minerals. The diet should contain 520 to 550 kcal/100 g, fat 45 to 60 percent, and protein 10 to 12 percent (half of the protein from milk product) of the total energy for severe acute malnourished children.

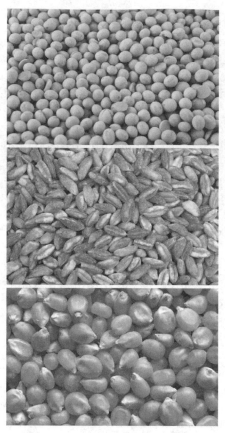

Variety is important to good dietary practice (shown here: soy, wheat, and corn).
© Jovan Nikolic/ShutterStock, Inc. © Wendy T. Davis/ShutterStock, Inc. © ajt/ShutterStock, Inc.

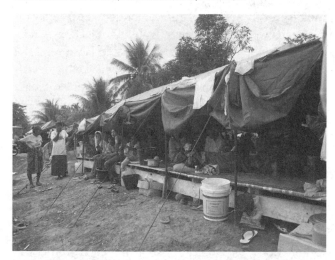

Intervention relief during emergency periods can save lives.
© A.S. Zain/ShutterStock, Inc.

## ▸ The Role of Community Nutritionists

Community nutritionists can play important leadership roles in preventing hunger and malnutrition at the international level. They also can collaborate with policy makers, government and community leaders, health departments, antihunger organizations, and community-based organizations, including emergency food providers, to reduce food insecurity, hunger, and subsequently malnutrition.

To assist in preventing the causes of poverty and malnutrition, community nutritionists need to work directly with the poor and do fieldwork. There are three possible levels of involvement in fieldwork for community nutritionists. First, nutritionists can seek community participation in a given project. Second, they can raise awareness of the situation among the population. Finally, they can help mobilize the masses to effectively empower the poor. Because village/local problems often are not the governments' problems, the nutritionist must convert local needs into concrete issues so a course of action can be mapped out. In addition, the nutritionist can use already successful part of the goals that the USDA's Community Food Security Initiative developed to reduce hunger by half by 2015. These goals include, but are not limited to, the following[122]:

- Improve coordination among existing antihunger programs.
- Increase public awareness of the causes and consequences of food insecurity.
- Highlight innovative community solutions to hunger.

This chapter's Successful Community Strategies presents successful community efforts to reduce malnutrition.

# Successful Community Strategies

## Fighting Malnutrition in Senegal and Madagascar[122]

Two successful large-scale community nutrition projects in Africa used a contracting approach in rural and urban areas to prevent malnutrition. The two case studies were the Food Security and Nutrition Project (SECALINE) in Madagascar and the Community Nutrition Project (CNP) in Senegal. The projects were very similar in the types of services they provided and in combining private administration with public finance.

In Senegal, the CNP started in 1996 in poor peri-urban areas and served 100,000 children up to 3 years of age, plus 131,000 women in 14 cities. The Madagascar (SECALINE) project started in 1994; this project was similar to the CNP, but it aimed at rural areas in two of the most vulnerable regions of the country, serving 241,000 children under 5 years of age and their mothers in 534 villages for over 4 years. Both projects were executed outside the Ministry of Health but followed the national health policy. In Senegal, the project was managed by Agetip, a nongovernmental organization that works on the principles of delegated contract management and signed a convention with the government to execute the project. The Inter-ministerial National Commission against Malnutrition, located within the Presidency of the Republic, closely monitored this project. In Madagascar, a project staff was linked to the office of the prime minister, whose workers managed the project. Agetip and SECALINE's project units managed contracts for the government, monitored them, and were fully responsible for project implementation and results.

Children stayed in the program for 6 months in Senegal and 4 months in Madagascar. Both projects provided the following services at the community level:

- Monthly growth monitoring of the children.
- Weekly nutrition and health education sessions for women.
- Referral to health services for unvaccinated children, pregnant women, severely malnourished children, and sick beneficiaries
- Home visits to follow beneficiaries who were referred or who did not go to the services.
- Food supplementation to malnourished children (in Senegal, a flour mix made of local ingredients; in Madagascar, locally bought nonmanufactured food).
- Improved access to water standpipes (in Senegal) or referral to a social fund for income-generating activities (in Madagascar).

In urban Senegal these services were provided in a rented building called the Community Nutrition Center; in rural Madagascar, they were provided in a thatch and bamboo structure.

## Impact on the Nutritional Status of Children

In both projects, malnutrition rates decreased rapidly among the children reached by the projects. In Madagascar, the project's coverage rate in the targeted zones increased from 50 percent to 87 percent by September 1997, and malnutrition rates among beneficiary children diminished significantly.

In Senegal, a similar trend was observed and a community-based study in one city confirmed with two cross-sectional surveys that malnutrition rates decreased throughout all the neighborhoods. The study showed that after 17 months of project implementation, severe malnutrition disappeared among children of 6 to 11 months, and moderate malnutrition among those of 6 to 35 months decreased from 28 to 24 percent. The impact seems directly linked to the project because there was no significant change in socioeconomic characteristics between the baseline

*(continues)*

## Successful Community Strategies *(continued)*

and impact studies and also because the study showed that malnutrition rates were lower among children who participated in the project previously compared to those who never participated. For example, the rate of malnutrition was 23 percent among children of 12 to 17 months who participated in the previous project, compared to 30 percent for those who did not participate in the project.

These projects illustrate that contracting out is a feasible option for organizing large-scale prevention programs. The projects show strong indications of success in terms of reducing malnutrition and increasing community involvement. When choosing this type of option, a government can tap available private local human resources through contracting out, rather than delivering those services using public sector resources.

# Learning Portfolio

## Chapter Summary

- Nutrition-related chronic diseases are either appearing or are already established in every country around the world.
- It has been estimated that, over the next decade, about 30 to 40 countries will remain in the lowest income bracket, with high incidences of infectious childhood diseases, undernutrition, and high fertility.
- The International Food Policy Research Institute (IFPRI) has warned that at the threshold of the twenty-first century, widespread poverty, hunger, and malnutrition threaten to undermine global economic, social, political, and environmental conditions.
- In addition to human suffering, hunger and malnutrition have negative effects on cognitive development, growth, and health.
- Food security means access at all times by all people to adequate amounts of safe, nutritious, and culturally appropriate food for an active and healthy life.
- Ninety-nine percent of maternal deaths occur in developing countries, and most of them are preventable.
- Women represent 50 percent of the adult population, make up one third of the official labor force, perform nearly two thirds of all working hours, receive only one tenth of world income, and own less than 1 percent of the world's property.
- The refeeding syndrome may develop in severely wasted clients during the first week of nutritional repletion.
- The specific changes in body composition induced by refeeding are determined by the existing metabolic state, body composition, and, most importantly, the composition of the refeeding diet.
- The mortality rate in hospitals from severe malnutrition has not changed in about 40 years. Currently, it is at approximately 20 to 40 percent, despite the fact that under refugee camp conditions mortality rates of 5 to 10 percent are achieved.

## Critical Thinking Activities

- Choose three to four countries and compare the rate of income per capita for each country.
- Identify the different types of grains grown in three different countries and discuss how these grains can be utilized to prevent malnutrition. Prepare a blend of grains that will provide adequate calories and protein.
- Choose a country and determine the labor force composition.
- Interview a welfare-to-work mother and determine the advantages and disadvantages of working instead of being on welfare. Determine the possibility of obtaining a job that does not have a nonstandard work schedule.
- Prepare a low-cost meal (lunch and dinner) on a $1 USD budget.
- Read and summarize an article on food insecurity, world hunger, and relief efforts.
- Determine the nutrient content of a blended diet for the management of malnutrition.
- Brainstorm how to solve world hunger.
- List at least five ideas for campus-wide programs to increase awareness of global hunger and nutrition issues during World Food Day, October 16.
- Select two areas in the world (Asia, Africa, Europe, etc.) where hunger and undernutrition are major problems. List and discuss the causes of undernutrition in these areas. Discuss the solutions that are in place or proposed to solve these problems.

- Volunteer at a local soup kitchen or homeless shelter once a month.
- Someone dies of hunger every day. Go to http://www.thehungersite.com and click on Click Here to Give—It's Free to send a meal to someone in need. This site is affiliated with the U.N. World Food Program,

which tracks the number of clicks and then sends a bill to one of its corporate or nonprofit sponsors.

- Go to the Power to End Hunger website at http://www.action.org to learn how to speak powerfully about ending world hunger, and then write to your senator or representative.

## 🔍 CASE STUDY 7-1: Food Insecurity, World Hunger, and Malnutrition

Five undergraduate students who enrolled in a community nutrition course were assigned to appeal to businesses and churches in the community for foods to feed homeless persons. They also were asked to prepare and serve at least two meals to feed men who were underweight and had bleeding gum and chapped, red, swollen lips; pregnant women with symptoms of anemia; and children in a homeless shelter with symptoms of PEM. They were asked to read about food insecurity, world hunger, sustainable agriculture, and the efforts by various relief organizations that help undernourished people in developing countries. Some of the assigned international relief organizations included Catholic Charities USA, UNICEF, USAID, and WHO. After they had completed the assignments, the students became concerned about the high rate of hunger and malnutrition in developing countries. Although they are college students who cannot afford to make significant monetary contributions to relief organizations, they decided to contribute in other ways. They wrote letters to their state representatives and senators about proposing policies that would reduce world hunger. They also involved their friends in creating awareness of the prevalence of hunger and malnutrition in the world.

### Questions

1. What are the differences between developing and developed countries?
2. What are some of the current nutrition issues in developing and developed countries?
3. The students prepared information on how to prevent HIV infection. What strategy is needed to prevent babies acquiring HIV from their infected mothers?
4. What are some of the causes of hunger and malnutrition worldwide?
5. What are the three general areas of concern that inspire the concept of sustainable agriculture that the students must know? Provide a description of each area.
6. What are the different types of emergency feeding programs that these clients may need?
7. The students learned about refeeding syndrome. What is refeeding syndrome and when does it occur? What criteria have been observed in individuals with refeeding syndrome?
8. What role can community nutritionists play in the prevention of hunger and malnutrition?
9. Work in small groups or individually to discuss the case study and practice using the Nutrition Care Process chart provided on the companion website. You can also add other nutrition and health-related conditions or assessments to the case study to make the case study more challenging and interesting.

## Think About It

**Answer:** Diarrhea is associated with dehydration. ORT involves the replacement of fluids and electrolytes lost during an episode of diarrheal illness. The main ingredients in ORT are glucose, sodium, and potassium. The UNICEF recipe for a simple homemade solution is 5 cups of boiled water, 8 teaspoons of sugar, and 1 teaspoon of salt, resulting in 1 liter of solution. In addition, fruit juices, coconut water, and other indigenous solutions can adequately substitute for oral rehydration solution.

## Key Terms

**developed countries:** Countries that have reached a stage of economic development characterized by the growth of industrialization. The amount of money made

by the population (national income) is enough to pay for schools, hospitals, and other services (domestic savings).

**developing countries:** Countries that have not reached the stage of economic development characterized by the growth of industrialization. The amount of money made (national income) is less than the amount of money needed to pay for schools, hospitals, and other services (domestic savings).

**famine:** Widespread lack of access to food due to a disaster or war that causes a collapse in the food production and marketing systems.

**food insecurity:** The inability to obtain sufficient food for any reason.

**food security:** To have access to an adequate amount of food at all times that is safe, nutritious, and culturally appropriate for an active and healthy life.

**immunization:** Injection of a killed or inactivated organism into the body to stimulate the immune system to develop antibodies against an active disease-causing organism.

**malnutrition:** Poor nutritional status due to dietary intake either above or below the optimal level.

**nonstandard work schedule:** Working irregular hours, irregular days, rotating hours or days, weekend days, and regular evening or night hours.

**nutrification:** The process of adding one or more nutrients to commonly consumed foods in an attempt to increase their nutrient content.

**nutrition transition:** A shift in dietary habit from a diet high in complex carbohydrates and fiber to a diet higher in fat, saturated fat, and sugar; this occurs as incomes increase.

**stunting:** A decrease in linear growth rate that is an indicator of inadequate nutrient intake in children.

# References

1. Missiaen M, Shapouri S. Food shortages in developing countries continuing. *Food Rev.* 1995;18(1):24-31.
2. Johnson DG. Population, food, and knowledge. *Am Econ Rev.* 2000;90(1):1-15.
3. Alexandratos N. Countries with rapid population growth and resource constraints: issues of food, agriculture, and development. *Popul Dev Rev.* 2005;31(2):237-258.
4. Ge KY. Definition and measurement of child malnutrition. *Biomed Environ Sci.* 2001;14(4):283-291.
5. Food Insecurity and Vulnerability Information Mapping System. What is meant by food insecurity and vulnerability? 2006. http://g4aw.spaceoffice .nl/en/Projects/International/International -Initiatives/Food-Insecurity-and-Vulnerability -Information-and-Mapping-Systems-FIVIMS/. Accessed February 26, 2017.
6. Putnam J, Allshouse J, Kantor LS. U.S. per capita food supply trends: more calories, refined carbohydrates, and fats. *Food Rev.* 2002;25(3):1-15.
7. US Dept Agriculture, Economic Research Service. Food security assessment. 2005, 2006. 2005/GFA-2017. http://science.sciencemag.org /content/sci/327/5967/825.full.pdf?ijkey=cCTDX tM63n75.&keytype=ref&siteid=sci. Accessed February 26, 2017.
8. Herdt RW. Food shortages and international agricultural programs. *Crit Rev Plant Sci.* 2004;23(6):505-517.
9. United Nations. *Review of the first United Nations Decade for the Eradication of Poverty (1997-2006).* E/CN.5/2006/3. New York, NY: United Nations; 2006.
10. Food and Agriculture Organization. *The State of Food Insecurity in the World. 2002.* Rome, Italy: Food and Agriculture Organization of the United Nations; 2002.
11. US Dept of Agriculture, Foreign Agricultural Service. Discussion paper on domestic food security. 2016. http://www.fas.usda.gov/. Accessed February 16, 2016.
12. Journey Forever. Community development. http:// journeytoforever.org/community2.html. Accessed February 16, 2016.
13. Joachim von Braun M, Rosegrant W, Pandya-Lorch R, et al. *New Risks and Opportunities for Food Security Scenario Analyses for 2015 and 2050.* Washington, DC: International Food Policy Research Institute; 2005.
14. United Nations Organization. *Development Programme: Human Development Report 2000.* New York, NY: Oxford University Press; 2000.
15. United Nations Conference on Trade and Development. *The Least Developed Countries Report 2002: Escaping the Poverty Trap.* New York, NY: United Nations; 2002.
16. Hartwig de Haen KS, Shetty P, Pingali P. The world food economy in the twenty-first century: challenges for international co-operation. *Dev Policy Rev.* 2003;21(5-6):683-696.
17. Pinstrup-Andersen P. The future world food situation and the role of plant diseases. In: *The Plant Health Instructor.* Washington, DC: International Food Policy Research Institute; 2001.
18. Global Issues Home. Causes of poverty: poverty facts and stats. 2006. http://www.globalissues .org/. Accessed February 16, 2011.
19. United Nations Organization. Global hunger. http://www.un.org/sustainabledevelopment/. Accessed February 26, 2017.
20. Shi Z. The sociodemographic correlates of nutritional status of school adolescents in Jiangsu Province, China. *J Adolesc Health.* 2005;37(4):313-322.
21. Smith SC Jr, Jackson R, Pearson TA. Principles for national and regional guidelines on cardiovascular disease prevention. *Circulation* 2004;109:3112-3121.
22. Soowon K, Symons M, Popkin B. Contrasting socioeconomic profiles related to healthier lifestyles in China and the United States. *Am J Epidemiol.* 2004;159:184-191.
23. Vorster H, Bourne LT, Venter CS, Oosthuizen W. Contribution of nutrition to the health transition in developing countries: a framework for research and intervention. *Nutr Rev.* 1999;57:341-349.
24. McMichael AJ. Environmental and social influences on emerging infectious diseases: past, present and future. *Phil Trans R Soc B.* 2004;359(1447):1049-1058.

25. Cohen B. Urbanization in developing countries: current trends, future projections, and key challenges for sustainability. *Technol Soc.* 2006; 28:63-80.

26. United Nations Organization. The millennium development goals report 2015 summary. 2016. http://www.un.org/millenniumgoals/2015_MDG_Report/pdf/MDG%202015%20Summary%20web_english.pdf. Accessed February 24, 2016.

27. Royal Geographical Society. Megacities, urbanisation and development. 2016. http://www.rgs.org/OurWork/Schools/Teaching+resources/Key+Stage+3+resources/Global+Learning+Programme/Megacities.htm. Accessed July 9, 2016.

28. Mendez MA, Monteiro CA, Popkin BM. Overweight exceeds underweight among women in most developing countries. *Am J Clin Nutr.* 2005;81(3):714-721.

29. Smith L, Haddad L. *Explaining Child Malnutrition in Developing Countries: A Cross-Country Analysis.* Washington, DC: International Food Policy Research Institute; 2000.

30. Black R, Morris S, Bryce J. Where and why are 10 million children dying every year. *Lancet.* 2003;361(9376):2226-2234.

31. Caulfield LE, Mercedes de Onis, Monika B, Black RE. Undernutrition as an underlying cause of child deaths associated with diarrhea, pneumonia, malaria, and measles. *Am J Clin Nutr.* 2004;80(1):193-198.

32. Ruel MT. Urbanization in Latin America: constraints and opportunities for child feeding and care. *Food Nutr Bull* (Special Issue on Processed Complementary Foods in Latin America. 2000;21(1):12-24.

33. Barba CVC, Rabuco LB. Overview of ageing urbanization and nutrition in developing countries and the development of the reconnaissance project. http://www.unu.edu/unupress. Accessed February 18, 2016.

34. Banks J, Marmot M, Oldfield Z, Smith JP. Disease and disadvantage in the United States and in England. *JAMA.* 2006;295(17):2037-2045.

35. Taylor WC, Poston WSC, Jones L, Kraft MK. Environmental justice: obesity, physical activity and healthy eating. *J Health Polit Policy Law.* 2006;31(1):S30-S54.

36. Popkin B. An overview on the nutrition transition and its health implications: the Bellagio meeting. *Public Health Nutr.* 2002;5(1A):93-103.

37. Tamara M, Brennan P, Boffetta P, Zaridze D. Russian mortality trends for 1991-2001: analysis by cause and region. *BMJ.* 2003;327:7421-7964.

38. Döbróssy L. Epidemiology of head and neck cancer: magnitude of the problem. *Cancer Metastasis Rev.* 2005; 24(1):9-17.

39. Shahar D, Shai I, Vardi H, Shahar A, et al. Diet and eating habits in high and low socioeconomic groups. *Nutrition.* 2005;21(5):559-566.

40. Coates J, Frongillo EA, Rogers BL, Webb P, et al. Commonalities in the experience of household food insecurity across cultures: what are measures missing? *J Nutr.* 2006;136(5):1438S-1448S.

41. United Nations Food and Agriculture Organization. *The State of Food Insecurity in the World.* Rome, Italy: United Nations Organization; 2002.

42. Mulholland EK, Adegbola RA. Bacterial infections a major cause of death among children in Africa. *N Engl J Med.* 2005;352:75-77.

43. Jackson RT, Pellett PL. Introductory observations: the region, nutrition, and health. *Ecol Food Nutr.* 2004;43(1):3-6.

44. Struble MB, Aomari LL. Position of the American Dietetic Association: addressing world hunger, malnutrition, and food insecurity. *J Am Diet Assoc.* 2003;103(8):1046-1057.

45. Cole M, Neumayer E. The impact of poor health on total factor productivity. *J Dev Stud.* 2006;42(6):918-938.

46. United Nations Children's Fund. *The State of the World's Children: 2001.* New York, NY: United Nations Children's Fund; 2001.

47. Nord M, Andrews M, Carlson S. *Household Food Security in the United States, 2002.* United Nations Children's Fund; 2003.

48. US Dept of Agriculture. Briefing room 2000. 2000. http://www.usda.gov/. Accessed February 18, 2011.

49. Podewils L, Mintz E, Nataro J, Parashar U. Acute, infectious diarrhea among children in developing countries. *Semin Pediatr Infect Dis.* 2004;15(3):155-168.

50. Pelletier D, Frongillo EA. Changes in child survival are strongly associated with changes in malnutrition in developing countries. *J Nutr.* 2003;133:107-119.

51. Beaton GH, Martorell R, Aronson KJ, et al. *Effectiveness of Vitamin A Supplementation in the Control of Young Child Morbidity and Mortality in Developing Countries.* Nutrition Policy Discussion Paper No. 13; Geneva, Switzerland: Administrative Coordinating Committee, Subcommittee on Nutrition; 1993.

52. Vozoris N, Tarasuk VS. Household food insufficiency is associated with poorer health. *J Nutr.* 2003;133:120-126.

53. Kouhkan A, Pourpak Z, Moin M, Reza M, et al. Study of malnutrition in Iranian patients with primary antibody deficiency. *Iran J Allergy Asthma Immunol.* 2004;3(4):189-196.

54. Djazayery A. Regional overview of maternal and child malnutrition: trends, interventions and outcomes. *East Mediterr Health J.* 2004;10(6):731-736.

55. Kotzé DA. Role of women in the household economy, food production and food security: policy guidelines. *Outlook Agric.* 2003;32(2): 111-121.

56. Hindin MJ. Women's input into household decisions and their nutritional status in three resource-constrained settings. *Public Health Nutr.* 2006;9(4):485-493.

57. Fonchingong CC. Negotiating livelihoods beyond Beijing: the burden of women food vendors in the informal economy of Limbe, Cameroon. *Int Soc Sci J.* 2005;57(184):243-253.

58. Ganguli I, Terrell K. Institutions, markets and men's and women's wage inequality: evidence from Ukraine. *J Coop Econ.* 2006;C14:1-33.

59. Gupta GR, Malhotra A. Empowering women through investments in reproductive health and rights. http://www.packard.org. Accessed February 18, 2016.

60. Oldewage-Theron WW. A community-based integrated nutrition research programme to alleviate poverty: baseline survey. *Public Health.* 2005;119(4):312-320.

61. World Health Organization. Nutrition risk factors: meeting of interested parties. 2001. http://www.who.int/. Accessed February 18, 2016.

62. American Psychological Association. Working mothers: happy or haggard? http://www.apa.org/psychnet. Accessed July 9, 2016.

63. Robinson K. Family care giving: who provides the care, and at what cost? *Nurs Econ.* 1997;15(5):243-247.

64. Furness BBW. Prevalence and predictors of food insecurity among low-income households in Los Angeles County. *Public Health Nutr.* 2004;7(6):791-794.

65. Mutharayappa R. Reproductive morbidity of women in Karnataka. *J Healthc Manag.* 2006;8(1):23-50.

66. Radda G, Michael T, Meade D. Suicide rates in China. *Lancet.* 2002;359(9481):2274-2282.

67. United Nations International Children's Fun http://data.unicef.org/topic/maternal-health/maternal-mortality/. Accessed February 26, 2017.

68. United Nations Organization for Economic Co-operation and Development, International Monetary Fund, World Bank 2000. *A Better World for All.* Washington, DC: Grundy & Northedge; 2000.

69. Hill K, Arifeen SE, Koenig M, Al-Sabir A, et al. How should we measure maternal mortality in the developing world? A comparison of household deaths and sibling history approaches. *Bull WHO.* 2006;84(3):173-180.

70. De Cock KM, Fowler MG, Mercier E. Prevention of mother-to-child HIV transmission in resource-poor countries: translating research into policy and practice. *JAMA.* 2000;283(9):1175-1182.

71. Chin J. *Control of Communicable Diseases Manual.* 17th ed. Washington, DC: American Public Health Association; 2000.

72. United Nations Joint Programme on HIV/AIDs. Questions and answers. III. Selected issues: prevention and care. http://data.unaids.org/pub/InformationNote/2006/qa_partii_en_nov06.pdf. Accessed February 26, 2017.

73. Duerr A, Hurst S, Kourtis AP, Rutenberg N, et al. Integrating family planning and prevention of mother-to-child HIV transmission in resource-limited settings. *Lancet* 2005;366(9481):261-263.

74. Fields-Gardner C, Ayoob, K. Position of the American Dietetic Association and Dietitians of Canada: nutrition intervention in the care of persons with human immunodeficiency virus infection. *J Am Diet Assoc.* 2000;100(6):708-717.

75. Nerad J, Romeyn M, Silverman E, et al. General nutrition management in patients infected with human immunodeficiency virus. *Clin Infect Dis.* 2003;36:S52-S62.

76. Kraak VI. Home-delivered meal programs for homebound people with HIV/Aids. *J Am Diet Assoc.* 1995;95(4):476-481.

77. United Nations High Commissioner for Refugees. Refugee populations: new arrivals and durable solutions in 84, mostly developing, countries. 2005. http://www.unhcr.ch/statistics. Accessed July 9, 2016.

78. Grosvenor B, Smolin L. *Nutrition From Science to Life.* New York, NY: Harcourt; 2002.

79. William NM. Green chemistry and the path to sustainable agriculture. *Am Chem Soc.* 2004; 887:7-21.

80. Fish R, Seyour S, Watkins C. Sustainable farmland management as political and cultural discourse. *Geogr J.* 2006;172(3):183-189.

81. Brodt S, Feenstra G, Kozloff R, Klonsky K, et al. Farmer-community connections and the future of ecological agriculture in California. *Agric Human Values.* 2006;23(1)75-88.

82. Koplan JP, Jeffrey P, Puska P, Cahill K, et al. Improving the world's health through national public health institutes. *Bull WHO.* 2005;83(2):154-157.

83. Labbok MH, Blanc A, Clark D, Terreri N. Trends in exclusive breastfeeding: findings from the 1990s. *J Hum Lact.* 2006;22(3):272-276.

84. Birch M, Miller S. Humanitarian assistance: standards, skills, training, and experience. *BMJ.* 2005;330(7501):1199-1201.

85. Marchione T. Foods profided through U.S. government emergency food aid programs: policies and customs governing their formulation, selection and distribution. *J Nutr.* 2002;132: 2104s-21111s.

86. James R, Hargreaves M, Collinson A, Kahn K, et al. Childhood mortality among former Mozambican refugees and their hosts in rural South Africa. *Int J Epidemiol.* 2004;33(6):1271-1278.

87. Thomas JL, Luke C, Adam K, Kuiper HK, et al. Mortality rates in conflict zones in Karen, Karenni, and Mon states in eastern Burma. *Trop Med Int Health.* 2006;11(7):1119-1127.

88. Golden M. The development of concepts of malnutrition. *J Nutr.* 2002;132(7):2117s-2122s.

89. US Dept of Health and Human Services, Public Health Service: Famine affected refugee and displaced populations recommendations for public health issues. *MMWR Morb Mortal Wkly Rep.* 1992;41: RR(13):11.

90. Posner B, Franz M, Quatromoni PL, INTER-HEALTH Steering Committee. Nutrition and the global risk for chronic diseases: the INTER-HEALTH Nutrition Initiative. *Nutr Rev.* 1994;52(6): 201-207.

91. National Academy of Sciences. *Estimated Mean per Capita Energy Requirements for Planning Emergency Food Aid Rations.* Washington, DC: National Academy Press; 1995.

92. United Nations High Commissioner for Refugees. *World Food Programme Guidelines for Estimating Food and Nutrition Needs in Emergencies.* Geneva, Switzerland: United Nations; 1997.

93. World Health Organization. *The Management of Nutrition in Major Emergencies.* http://www.who .int/features/qa/. Accessed July 9, 2016.

94. Ville de Goyet C, Seaman J, Geijer U. *The Management of Nutrition Emergencies in Large Population.* Geneva, Switzerland: World Health Organization; 2004.

95. Mason J. History of food and nutrition in emergency relief: lesson on nutrition of displaced people. *J Nutr.* 2002;132:2096s-2103s.

96. Spiegel PB, Paul B, Salama P, Maloney S, van der Veen S. Quality of malnutrition assessment surveys conducted during famine in Ethiopia. *JAMA.* 2004;292(5):613-618.

97. Mason J, Hay R, Leresche J, Peel S, et al. Treatment of severe malnutrition in relief. *Lancet.* 1974;2:332-335.

98. World Health Organization. Management of severe malnutrition: a manual for physicians and other senior helath workers. Geneva, Switzerland: World Health Organization; 1999.

99. Bhatia R, Thorne-Lyman A. Food aid in emergencies and public health nutrition. *Forum Nutr.* 2003;56:391-394.

100. Centers for Disease Control and Prevention. Managing acute gastroenteritis among children: oral rehydration, maintenance, and nutritional therapy. *MMWR Morb Mortal Wkly Rep.* 2003; 52(RR16)1-16.

101. World Health Organization. Protecting, promoting, and supporting breastfeeding: the management of bloody diarrhoea in young children. Geneva, Switzerland. http://www.who.int/nutrition/publications/infantfeeding/inf_assess_nnpp_eng.pdf. Accessed February 26, 2017.

102. World Health Organization. Oral rehydration salts (ORS): a new reduced osmolarity formulation. Geneva, Switzerland: World Health Organization; 2002.

103. Senti FR. Guidelines of the nutrient composition of processed foods. *Cereal Sci Today.* 1972;17:157-161.

104. Grant CC, Rotherham BB, Sharpe SS, et al. Randomized, double-blind comparison of growth in infants receiving goat milk formula versus cow milk infant formula. *J Paediatr Child Health.* 2005;41(11):564-568.

105. Brewster DR. Critical appraisal of the management of severe malnutrition: epidemiology and treatment guidelines. *J Paediatr Child Health.* 2006;42(10):568-574.

106. Kukuruzovic H, Brewster DR. Milk formulas in acute gastroenteritis and malnutrition: a randomized trial. *J Paediatr Child Health.* 2002;38(6):571-577.

107. Colecraft EK, Esi K, Marquis GS, et al. Longitudinal assessment of the diet and growth of malnourished children participating in nutrition rehabilitation centres in Accra, Ghana. *Public Health Nutr.* 2004;7(4):487-494.

108. Shils M, Olson JA. *Modern Nutrition in Health and Disease.* 11th ed. Baltimore, MD: Lippincott Williams & Wilkins; 2012.

109. Flesher ME, Archer ME, Katharine KA, et al. Assessing the metabolic and clinical consequences of early enteral feeding in the malnourished patient. *JPEN J Parenter Enteral Nutr.* 2005;29(2):108-117.

110. Hearing SD. Refeeding syndrome. *BMJ.* 2004;328: 908-909.

111. Fotheringham J, Jackson K, Kersh R, Gariballa SE. Refeeding syndrome: life-threatening, underdiagnosed, but treatable. *QJM.* 2005;98:318-319.

112. Tsintzas K, Jewell K, Kamran M, et al. Differential regulation of metabolic genes in skeletal muscle during starvation and refeeding in humans. *J Physiol.* 2006;575(Pt 1):291-303.

113. Hoppe C, Mølgaard C, Michaelsen KF. Cow's milk and linear growth in industrialized and developing countries. *Ann Rev of Nutr.* 2006;26:131-173.

114. Kerruish KP, O'Connor KP, Humphries JJ, et al. Body composition in adolescents with anorexia nervosa. *Am J Clin Nutr.* 2002;75(1):31-37.

115. Hoppe C, Mølgaard C, Juul A, Michaelsen KF. High intakes of skimmed milk, but not meat, increase serum IGF-I and IGFBP-3 in eight-year-old boys. *Eur J Clin Nutr.* 2004;58(9):1211-1216.

116. Thapar NN, Sanderson IR, Ian R. Diarrhoea in children: an interface between developing and developed countries. *Lancet.* 2004;363(9409):641-653.

117. Amadi BB, Mwiya MM, Thomson MM, Chintu CC, et al. Improved nutritional recovery on an elemental diet in Zambian children with persistent diarrhoea and malnutrition. *J Tropic Pediatr.* 2005;51(1):5-10.

118. Manary MJ, Yarasheski KE, Smith S, Abrams ET, et al. Protein quantity not protein quality accelerates whole-body leucine kinetics and the acute-phase response during acute infection in marasmic Malawian children. *Brit J Nutr.* 2004;92(4):589-595.

119. Ashworth AA, Chopra MM, McCoy DD, et al. WHO guidelines for management of severe malnutrition in rural South African hospitals: effect on case fatality and the influence of operational factors. *Lancet.* 2004;363(9415):1110-1115.

120. Jahoor FF, Badaloo A, Reid MA, Forrester M, et al. Protein kinetic differences between children with edematous and nonedematous severe childhood undernutrition in the fed and postabsorptive states. *Am J Clin Nutr.* 2005;82(4):792-800.

121. National Center for Appropriate Technology. Community food security initiative. http://attra.ncat.org/. Accessed February 18, 2016.

122. Mark T, Diallo I, Ndiaye B, Rakotosalama J. Successful contracting of prevention services: fighting malnutrition in Senegal and Madagascar. In: World Bank WD, USA, SED, Senegal, Agetip, Senegal, and SECALINE, Madagascar. Vol 14. Oxford: Oxford University Press: Health Policy and Planning; 1999:382-389.

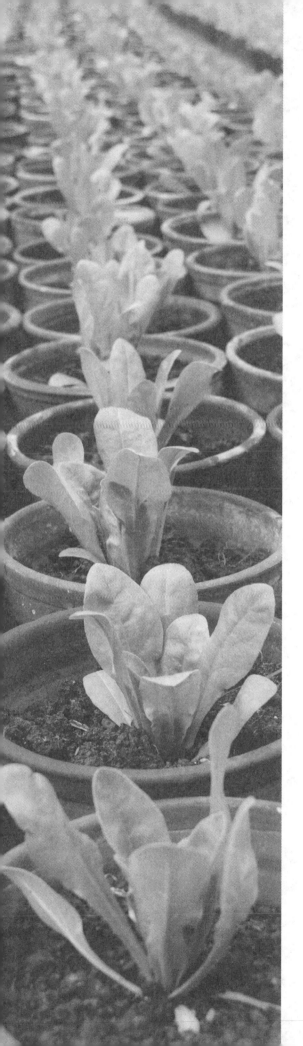

# PART II

# Nutrition Interventions for Vulnerable Populations

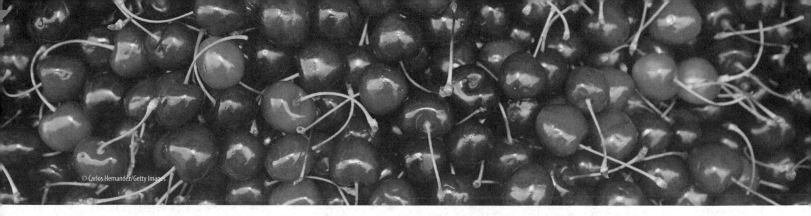

© Carlos Hernandez/Getty Images

# CHAPTER 8

# Nutrition During Pregnancy and Infancy

## CHAPTER OUTLINE

- Introduction
- Progress Report Toward Healthy People 2010 and 2020 Objectives
- Physiological Events of Pregnancy and the Mother's Health
- Preconception Health
- Factors That Can Influence the Outcome of a Pregnancy
- Diet-Related Complications of Pregnancy
- Nutrition Assessment During Pregnancy
- Adolescent Pregnancy
- Physical Activity During Pregnancy
- Nutrition in Infancy
- Nutrient Needs During Infancy
- Nutrition-Related Health Concerns During Infancy
- Methods of Feeding Infants
- Management and Techniques for Successful Breastfeeding
- Supplemental Nutrition Programs During Pregnancy, Infancy, and Lactation

## LEARNING OBJECTIVES

- Identify stages of development for the fetus.
- List the maternal weight gain recommendations.
- Discuss the nutritional complications of pregnancy.
- Identify common nutrition issues that affect infants.
- Identify different screening and assessment methods for infants.
- Discuss the nutritional needs of infants and pregnant and lactating women.
- Discuss the benefits of breastfeeding.
- List the guidelines for successful breastfeeding
- List the food assistance programs and services available for children and pregnant women.

# ▶ Introduction

A mother's previous life experiences, general health and fitness, life-long dietary habits, and genetic heritage are part of each pregnancy. A woman's nutritional habits prior to pregnancy are as important to the success of the pregnancy as her diet during the 9 months of gestation.[1] Enabling pregnant women to meet their nutrient needs is a public health priority in the United States and many other countries. This priority is based on the fact that malnutrition during pregnancy has serious, long-term effects on the mother and child. For example, two international studies done by the Institute of Nutrition of Central America and Panama (INCAP) and the Nutrition Collaborative Research Support Program (NCRSP) found that marginal malnutrition during pregnancy caused stunted growth and functional impairments early in life.[2] The consequences of early malnutrition persisted even later in life. The NCRSP study also showed that multiple micronutrient deficiencies were associated with poor growth and function. The researchers' overall conclusion was that attention should be directed to determining the adequacy of micronutrient status during the **prenatal** period and to developing approaches that can prevent early growth failure. One way for women to prevent birth defects is by maintaining adequate vitamin and mineral intake at least 2 months before pregnancy.

# ▶ Progress Report Toward Healthy People 2010 and 2020 Objectives

In the United States, national goals to increase the number of pregnant women who receive prenatal care have been established (see **TABLE 8-1**). Of the maternal and infant health objectives included in Healthy People 2010, progress was made toward the target in 25 objectives and direction was made away from the target in 9 objectives. However, progress was made toward one of the 2020 objectives (see **TABLE 8-2**). Three objective exceeded their 2010 targets. Observable gains were made in the areas of decrease in infant deaths, decrease in fetal deaths, and increase in breastfeeding, with a slight increase in early use of prenatal care. However, the decrease in hospitalization for complications of pregnancy was not statistically different from that of the baseline. In addition, an increase in abstinence from tobacco use during pregnancy was reported. The increase in **cesarean sections** from 18 percent to 26 percent moved away from 2010 target of 15 percent. The proportion of repeat cesarean births increased from 72 percent to 91 percent, which did not meet the target of 63 percent. In addition, no progress was made toward a decrease in **low birth weight (LBW)**. Progress was

| TABLE 8-1 | Healthy People 2010 Maternal and Infant Health Objectives | | | | |
|---|---|---|---|---|---|
| HP 2010 Objective Number | Healthy People 2010 Objective | Baseline (Year) | 2010 Target | Progress Review |
| 16.1c | Reduce infant mortality (i.e., within 1 year of birth) to no more than 4.5 per 1,000 live births. | 7.2 (1998) | 4.5 | 6.8 |
| | a. African Americans | 13.8 (1998) | 4.5 | 13.2 |
| | b. Hispanics | 5.8 (1998) | 4.5 | 5.5 |
| | c. Native American/Alaskan Natives | 9.3 (1998) | 4.5 | 8.4 |
| 16.4 | Decrease the number of maternal deaths to 3.3 per 100,000 live births. | 9.9 (1999) | 3.3 | 13.1 |
| | a. African American women | 25.4 (1999) | 3.3 | 34.7 |
| 16.6 | Increase the number of pregnant women who receive prenatal care in the first trimester of pregnancy. | 83% of live births (1998) | 90% | 84% |

| HP 2010 Objective Number | Healthy People 2010 Objective | Baseline (Year) | 2010 Target | Progress Review |
|---|---|---|---|---|
| 16.10 a and b | Reduce low birth weight to an incidence of no more than 5 percent of live births and very low birth weight to no more than 0.9 percent of live births. | 7.6% (1998) 1.4% (1998) | 5.0% 0.9% | 8.1% 1.5% |
| | African American infants | | | |
| | (a) Low birth weight | 13.0% (1998) | 5.0% | 13.4% |
| | (b) Very low birth weight | 3.1% (1998) | 0.9% | 3.1% |
| 16.13 | Increase the percentage of healthy full-term infants who are put down to sleep on their backs. | 35% (1996) | 70% | 70% |
| 16.15 | Reduce the occurrence of spina bifida and other neural tube defects to 3 per 10,000 live births. | 6 (1996) | 3 | 5.6 |
| 16.17a | Increase abstinence from alcohol use by pregnant women to 94 percent. | 86% (1996-1997) | 94% | 80% |
| 16.17c | Increase abstinence from tobacco use by pregnant women to at least 99 percent. | 87% (1998) | 99% | 90% |
| 16.17d | Increase abstinence from illicit drugs (cocaine and marijuana) by pregnant women to 100 percent. | 98% in (1996-1997) | 100% | 96% |
| 16.18 | Reduce the occurrence of fetal alcohol syndrome to no more than 0.12 per 1,000 live births. | 0.67 (1993) | 0.12 | Data not available |
| 16.19a | Increase the number of mothers who breastfeed their babies in the early postpartum period to at least 75 percent. | 64% (1998) | 75% | 74% |
| 16.19b | Increase the proportion who breastfeed for 5 to 6 months after birth to at least 50 percent. | 29% (1998) | 50% | 56% |
| 19.12c | Reduce the incidence of iron deficiency to less than 7 percent for ages 12 to 49 years. | 11% (1988-1994) | 7% | 13% |
| 19.13 | Reduce the incidence of anemia in low-income pregnant women in the third trimester to 20 percent. | 29% (1996) | 20% | 31% |

Modified from: National Center for Health Statistics, Department of Health and Human Services. *Healthy People Progress Review*. Hyattsville, MD: Public Health Service; 2004. http://www.healthypeople.gov/2010/data/midcourse/html/focusareas/FA16TOC.htm. Accessed October 8, 2011.

made in the areas of decrease in maternal deaths and in the incidence of **fetal alcohol syndrome (FAS)**. Child health objectives were not included in the maternal and infant focus area in Healthy People 2010.[3]

Many of these conditions and risk factors disproportionately affected certain racial and ethnic groups. The disparities between European American and non-European American groups in infant death, maternal death, and low birth weight were wide and, in many cases, growing. Specifically, African American and Hispanic women were less likely than European Americans to participate in early prenatal care. For both African American and European American women, the proportion entering prenatal care in the first trimester rose with maternal age until the late thirties and then began to decline. For example, in 2005, 76 percent of

**TABLE 8-2** Healthy People 2020 Maternal and Infant Health Objectives

| HP 2020 Objective Number | Healthy People 2020 Objective | Baseline (Year) | 2020 Target | Progress Review |
|---|---|---|---|---|
| MICH 1.3 | Reduce the rate of all infant deaths (i.e., within 1 year of birth) | 6.7 infant deaths per 1000 live births (2006) | 6.0 infant deaths per 1,000 live births* | 6.0 (2013) |
| MICH 5 | Reduce the rate of maternal mortality | 12.7 maternal deaths per 100,000 live births (2007) | 11.4 maternal deaths per 100,000 live births* | NA |
| MICH 8 | Reduce low birth weight (LBW) and very low birthweight (VLBW) | 8.2% of live births were LBW in (2007) | 7.8% | 8.0% (2013) |
| MICH 8.1 | Low birth weight | | | |
| MICH 8.2 | Very low birth weight | 1.5% of live births were VLBW | 1.4% | 1.4% (2013) |
| MICH 10 | Increase the proportion of pregnant women who receive early and adequate prenatal care | | | |
| MICH 10.1 | Prenatal care beginning in first trimester | 70.8% in (2007)* | 77.9% | NA |
| MICH 11 | Increase abstinence from alcohol, cigarettes, and illicit drugs among pregnant women | | | |
| MICH 1.1 | Alcohol | 89.4% of pregnant females reported abstaining from alcohol in the past 30 days (2007-2008) | 98.3%* | 90.6% (2013 |
| MICH 11.2 | Binge drinking | 95% of pregnant females reported abstaining from binge drinking during the past 30 days (2007-2008) | 100%* | 97.2% (2013) |
| MICH 11.3 | Cigarette smoking | 89.6% of females reported abstaining from smoking cigarettes during pregnancy (2007) | 98.%* | NA |
| MICH 11.4 | Illicit drugs | 94.9% of pregnant females reported abstaining from illicit drugs in the past 30 days (2007-2008) | | |
| MICH 13 | (Developmental) Increase the proportion of mothers who achieve a recommended weight gain during their pregnancies | TBD† | TBD* | NA |

| HP 2020 Objective Number | Healthy People 2020 Objective | Baseline (Year) | 2020 Target | Progress Review |
|---|---|---|---|---|
| MICH 14 | Increase the proportion of women of childbearing potential with intake of at least 400 μg of folic acid from fortified foods or dietary supplements | 23.8%. (3003-2006) | 26.2%* | 22.8% (2007-2010) |
| MICH 15 | Reduce the proportion of women of childbearing potential who have low red blood cell folate concentrations | 24.5% (2003-2006) | 22.1%* | 24.9% (2007-2010 baseline revised) |
| MICH 16 | Increase the proportion of women delivering a live birth who received preconception care services and practiced key recommended preconception health behaviors | | | |
| MICH-16.2 | Increase the proportion of women delivering a live birth who took multivitamins/folic acid prior to pregnancy | 30.3%* of females delivering a recent live birth took multivitamins/folic acid every day in the month prior to pregnancy (2007) | 33.1% | NA |
| MICH 16.5 | Increase the proportion of women delivering a live birth who had a healthy weight prior to pregnancy | 52.5%* of females delivering a recent live birth had a normal weight (i.e., a BMI of 18.5 to 24.9) prior to pregnancy (2007) | 57.8% | NA |
| MICH-20 | Increase the proportion of infants who are put to sleep on their backs | 68.9%* of infants were put to sleep on their backs (2007) | 75.8% | |
| MICH-28 | Reduce occurrence of neural tube defects | | | |
| MICH 28.1: | Reduce the occurrence of spina bifida | 34.2* cases of spina bifida per 100,000 live births in (2005-2006) | 30.8 cases of spina bifida per 100,000 live births | 30.5 (2010) |
| MICH-28.2 | Reduce the occurrence of anencephaly | 24.6* cases of anencephaly per 100,000 live births (2005-2006) | 22.1 cases of anencephaly per 100,000 live births | 12.8 (2010) |

Modified from: National Center for Health Statistics, Department of Health and Human Services. *Healthy People Progress Review*. Hyattsville, MD: Public Health Service; 2004. https://www.healthypeople.gov/2020/topics-objectives/topic/maternal-infant-and-child-health/objectives. Accessed July 8, 2016.

*Target-Setting Method: 10% improvement.
†Target is not applicable for this population group.

African American women compared with 85 percent of European American women of the same age, participated in prenatal care in the first trimester.[4]

According to the most current review of Healthy People 2010, some progress has been made toward reduction in the **infant mortality rate** from 7.2 deaths per 1,000 live births in 1998 to 6.7 per 1,000 in 2010. A decline of 6.9 percent overall is needed to reach the targeted infant mortality rate of 4.5 infant deaths per 1,000 live births in 2010, and even greater declines are required for certain racial/ethnic populations to reach the target. Although a reduction in infant mortality rates was observed in Asians (4.5), Hispanic infant mortality rate was 11.1 per 1,000 live births and that of African Americans was 13.4 per 1,000 live births.

In addition, there was a decrease of new cases of the incidence of spina bifida from 60 to 48 per 100,000 live births in 2010. The Healthy People 2010 target is 30 per 10,000 live births. This decline can be attributed to public health awareness programs geared toward educating young women to increase their consumption of folic acid from various sources such as dietary supplements and fortified foods.[5]

## ▶ Physiological Events of Pregnancy and the Mother's Health

Maternal nutritional needs are based on the mother's physiological demands and those of fetal growth and development. Therefore, understanding the physiological changes during pregnancy is important when assessing the nutritional and educational needs of pregnant women. **TABLE 8-3** briefly reviews the prenatal events that cause the varying nutritional needs of the mother.[6]

During weeks 8 to 40 of gestation, the mother reserves additional nutrients in preparation for childbirth and lactation. Optimal nutritional reserves and continuing support are essential at every stage of pregnancy, however. Pregnancy requires an abundant maternal nutrient base, making preconception nutrition essential.

### Physiological and Metabolic Changes in Pregnancy

Many physiological and biochemical changes occur during a normal pregnancy. Some of the changes are as follows[7,8]:

- Blood volume expands by 50 percent, resulting in a decrease in hemoglobin levels, blood glucose values, and serum level of albumin.

- Increased cardiac output increases oxygen requirements and the threshold for carbon dioxide is lowered, which makes breathing more difficult.
- Increased progesterone level relaxes the uterine muscle.
- Gastrointestinal motility diminishes to allow for increased absorption of nutrients.[6]

Pregnancy is a normal physiological process that is associated with significant changes in every maternal organ system and metabolic pathway. Every single blood and urine measurement of nutrients is significantly altered from nonpregnant values because of these changes. Values change as the pregnancy advances from the first to the third trimester, to delivery, and then returns toward normal during the postpartum period. The major physiological changes are[7,8]:

- A 50 percent expansion of plasma volume with a 20 percent increase in hemoglobin mass
- Increasing levels of estrogen and progesterone as well as other placenta-related hormones
- Increase in red blood cell volume
- Increase in body water
- Increase in renal glomerular filtration rate
- Increase in respiratory tidal volume

These changes have an impact on maternal lipids, cholesterol, carotene, vitamin E, and blood clotting factors. The first major physiological changes include decreased biochemical levels of substances in the blood such as albumin and hemoglobin during pregnancy, which return to normal within 8 to 10 weeks postpartum. The second is the estrogen–progesterone placental hormone changes that cause lipid levels to increase during pregnancy and return to baseline levels postpartum.[7,9]

The mother also must adapt to progressive increases in cardiac output to a peak at 28 weeks, accumulation of body water, and changes in renal, respiratory, gastrointestinal, and genitourinary functions. These physiological adaptations during pregnancy alter the blood levels of many nutritional components.

In general, nutrients that are water-soluble (such as vitamin C, folic acid, vitamin $B_6$, and vitamin $B_{12}$) decrease as serum albumin and ferritin levels decrease and white blood cells increase.[7,9,10] In addition, urinary excretion of the end products of folate, niacin (N'methylnicotinamide), and pyridoxine metabolism and of intact riboflavin increases. In contrast, the serum levels of several fat-soluble nutrients such as carotene and vitamin E (tocopherol) increase as much as 50 percent during pregnancy; however, vitamin A levels seem unchanged.[7]

Public health and community nutritionists need to interpret the laboratory results of pregnant clients against gestational norms, not against the nonpregnant

**TABLE 8-3** Nutrient Needs Throughout Fetal Growth and Development

| Stages of Development | Events and Types of Tissue Development | Major Nutrients Needed | Dietary Reference Intake/Day (19-50 Years) |
|---|---|---|---|
| First stage: 1-2 weeks after fertilization of the egg. The first stage of fetal development is the implantation stage. | The special cells develop within 9-10 days. The **trophoblast** attaches the ovum to the uterine wall and supplies nutrients to the embryo. The trophoblast later becomes the placenta. Rapid fetal development and growth occur. Neural tube forms. Heart and primitive circulatory system rapidly form. | Calories<br>Protein<br>Iron<br>Calcium<br>Folic acid<br>Thiamin<br>Riboflavin<br>Niacin<br>Vitamin C<br>Vitamin D<br>Vitamin A | –<br>60 g<br>27 mg<br>1,000 mg<br>600 µg<br>1.4 mg<br>1.4 mg<br>18 mg<br>85 mg<br>5 µg<br>770 µg |
| Second stage: 2-8 weeks after fertilization. Differentiation of major organs and tissues. | Cell differentiation occurs to develop the embryo. Three basic layers of tissue form and develop into three different organs (ectoderm, mesoderm, and endoderm). Ectoderm (outer layer) becomes the brain, nervous system, skin, hair, nose, epidermis, and eye lens. Mesoderm (middle layer) produces all the bones, voluntary muscles, spleen, all parts of the cardiovascular and excretory systems, and blood. Endoderm (inner layer) forms all the glands and all parts of the respiratory and digestive systems, lungs, liver, and pancreas. Cartilage and bones begin to form. | Calories<br>Protein<br>Iron<br>Calcium<br>Folic acid<br>Thiamin<br>Riboflavin<br>Niacin<br>Vitamin C<br>Vitamin D<br>Vitamin A | 340 kcal* extra per day<br>60 g<br>27 mg<br>1,000 mg<br>600 µg<br>1.4 mg<br>1.4 mg<br>18 mg<br>85 mg<br>5 µg<br>770 µg |
| Third stage: 8-40 weeks (term). | Intensive maternal physiological growth occurs. Most of the fetus joints are formed. | Calories<br>Protein<br>Iron<br>Calcium<br>Folic acid<br>Thiamin<br>Riboflavin<br>Niacin<br>Vitamin C<br>Vitamin D<br>Vitamin A | 452 kcal* extra per day<br>60 g<br>27 mg<br>1,000 mg<br>600 µg<br>1.4 mg<br>1.4 mg<br>18 mg<br>85 mg<br>5 µg<br>770 µg |

*Pregnant women need extra kilocalories per day.
Data from: Williams SR. *Nutrition and Diet Therapy*. 7th ed. St. Louis, MO: Mosby; 1993.

female standards. It also may be necessary to conduct biochemical assessments throughout gestation.[10]

## ▶ Preconception Health

Preconception counseling is a type of preventive medicine that consists of risk assessment, health promotion, and intervention. Therefore, it may be the most critical aspect of prenatal care for the prevention of birth defects. All women of childbearing age should be considered at risk for birth defects and be advised about preventive activities. This includes folic acid supplementation; rubella and hepatitis B immunization; avoiding tobacco use, alcohol use, and substance abuse; following instructions for appropriate nutrition and weight gain;

avoiding pesticides; and undergoing genetic carrier screening (e.g., **phenylketonuria [PKU]**, sickle cell anemia, etc.), depending on ethnicity. Genetic screening is important because approximately 3,000 to 4,000 U.S.-born women of childbearing age have had babies with PKU but without severe mental retardation thanks to the strict medical nutrition therapy they received during pregnancy.[11-13] Infants are at very high risk for mental retardation if women with PKU do not maintain a low phenylalanine diet during pregnancy. PKU is an inherited disorder in phenylalanine metabolism, primarily caused by a deficiency of phenylalanine hydroxylase, which converts the amino acid phenylalanine to tyrosine. Blood phenylalanine levels before and throughout the pregnancy must be maintained to prevent an undesirable outcome.[11]

Women with chronic diseases such as diabetes should be evaluated about their effect on pregnancy and should receive the best therapy for a better pregnancy outcome.[14]

## The Importance of Folate

Preconception folate status is an important concern because inadequate folate very early in the pregnancy can cause **neural tube defects (NTDs)**, including spina bifida and anencephaly.[14,15] Women of childbearing age should be aware of the importance of folate on fetus development.

In the United States, approximately 4,000 pregnancies each year are affected by the incidence of NTDs.[16] Daily intake of 400 μg of folic acid throughout the period before and after conception could prevent 50 to 70 percent of the incidences.[17] Krishnaswamy and Madhavan Nair[18] reported that the incidence of NTDs could be cut in half if all women have an adequate folate intake during the preconception period.

Women can obtain enough folate by consuming a good basic diet and a fortified breakfast cereal (e.g., Smart Start, Total, or Product 19) or a regular breakfast cereal (e.g., Cheerios, corn flakes, or raisin bran). Prior to cereal fortification, mean total folate intake in U.S. women was approximately 250 μg per day.[16] Cereal fortification is estimated to increase folate intake in most women by an average of 80 g per day. Efforts to prevent birth defects should include more than cereal fortification, for example, including other folate sources such as orange juice, cooked asparagus, lentils, and lettuce. Vegans and other strict vegetarians also should take a supplement of vitamin B$_{12}$ because their diets contain no animal products, which are the main source of B$_{12}$. Low folate and vitamin B$_{12}$ levels are independent risk factors for NTDs.[16,19] **TABLE 8-4**

provides more information about the Dietary Reference Intake (DRI) recommendations for specific nutrients before and during pregnancy. **BOX 8-1** presents a case study on preconception health.

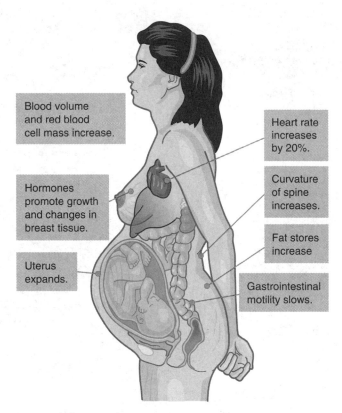

Blood volume and red blood cell mass increase.

Heart rate increases by 20%.

Hormones promote growth and changes in breast tissue.

Curvature of spine increases.

Fat stores increase

Uterus expands.

Gastrointestinal motility slows.

Maternal changes during pregnancy.

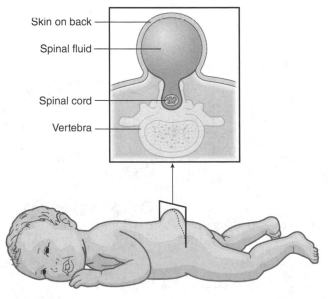

Skin on back

Spinal fluid

Spinal cord

Vertebra

Spina bifida is a neural tube defect.

**TABLE 8-4** Nutrient Requirements Before and During Pregnancy

| Nutrient | Pregnant | Nonpregnant | Importance in Pregnancy | Risk Factors for Deficiency | Concerns |
|---|---|---|---|---|---|
| Iron | 27 mg | 14–18 y: 15 mg<br>19+ y: 18 mg | ■ Iron "costs" of pregnancy are approximately 1 g.<br>■ Needed for maternal red blood cells.<br>■ Incorporated into the placenta and the developing fetus.<br>■ Anemia raises maternal cardiac workload and may place the fetus at risk for preterm birth. | ■ Pregnancy<br>■ Heavy menstrual blood loss prior to conception<br>■ Frequent blood donation<br>■ Multiple gestations<br>■ Vegetarian diet<br>■ Low intake of vitamin C<br>■ Chronic aspirin use | ■ Few women can meet the demand for iron with diet alone.<br>■ Encourage vitamin C intake to enhance absorption of iron.<br>■ Milk, coffee, and tea inhibit iron absorption and should not be consumed with iron supplements. |
| Folate (DFE) | 600 μg | 400 μg | ■ Essential for cell metabolism and replication.<br>■ Needed for hemoglobin synthesis.<br>■ Plays role in DNA and RNA synthesis.<br>■ Deficiencies present with elevated homocysteine levels and macrocytic anemia. | ■ Diet poor in foods that supply folic acid: add fortified whole grain bread and cereal, legumes, leafy vegetables, fruit, and yeast<br>■ Cigarette smoking<br>■ Alcohol abuse<br>■ Oral contraceptive use<br>■ Malabsorption syndrome | ■ Teach the importance of adequate folic acid intake to lower the risk for neural tube defects.<br>■ Supplementation should begin prior to conception because closure of the neural tube occurs by the 28th day of gestation. |
| Vitamin C | 14–18 y: 80 mg<br>19+ y: 85 mg | 14–18 y: 65 mg<br>19+ y: 75 mg | ■ Promotes collagen synthesis for use in connective tissue.<br>■ Has antioxidant properties.<br>■ Assists in the absorption of other nutrients and drugs. | ■ Poor dietary intake<br>■ Cigarette smoking<br>■ Drug and alcohol abuse<br>■ Aspirin use<br>■ Oral contraceptive use | ■ No known link of deficiency to pregnancy outcome.<br>■ Transports easily to the fetus; high doses during pregnancy may cause dependency and scurvy symptoms in babies. |
| Vitamin B$_6$ | 1.9 mg | 14–18 y: 1.2 mg<br>19+ y: 1.3 mg | ■ Required for protein, lipid, and carbohydrate metabolism.<br>■ Helps form nonessential amino acids and neurotransmitters.<br>■ Theories suggest a potential link between B$_6$ and problems related to pregnancy: nausea and vomiting, preeclampsia, and depression. | ■ Inadequate dietary intake | ■ Pregnant women may need help to evaluate scientific claims of a role for B$_6$ supplementation<br>■ Although fetal growth increases B$_6$ needs during pregnancy, no clear evidence exists to support its use in treating problems related to pregnancy. |

*(continues)*

**TABLE 8-4** Nutrient Requirements Before and During Pregnancy *(continued)*

| Nutrient | Pregnant | Nonpregnant | Importance in Pregnancy | Risk Factors for Deficiency | Concerns |
|---|---|---|---|---|---|
| Thiamin | 1.4 mg | 14-18 y: 1.0 mg<br>19+ y: 1.1 mg | ▪ These B complex vitamins function primarily to release energy from cells.<br>▪ Deficiencies harm fetuses in animal studies, but similar effects in humans have not been identified. | ▪ Women in the United States take insufficient quantities of thiamin and riboflavin from dietary sources to meet needs during pregnancy. | ▪ Thiamin and riboflavin have a low potential for toxicity.<br>▪ High doses of nicotinic acid (a form of niacin) may cause flushing and gastrointestinal problems. |
| Riboflavin | 14 mg | 14-18 y: 1.0 mg<br>19+ y: 1.1 mg | | | |
| Niacin (NE) | 18 mg | 14 mg | | | |
| Vitamin B$_{12}$ | 2.6 µg | 2.4 µg | ▪ Needed for normal cell division and protein synthesis. | ▪ History of gastric resection or malabsorption<br>▪ Strict vegetarian diet | ▪ Supplementation is normally not necessary during pregnancy.<br>▪ Monitor for signs of deficiency in vegans.<br>▪ Nontoxic, but the effects of high doses on the fetus are not known. |
| Pantothenic acid | 6 mg | 5 mg | ▪ Regulates adrenal activity, essential for gluconeogenesis and carbohydrate and lipid metabolism. | ▪ Deficiency is rare; needs may increase with malabsorption. | ▪ Supplementation is generally not needed during pregnancy. |
| Vitamin A (RAE) | 14-18 y: 750 µg<br>19+ y: 770 µg | 700 µg | ▪ Poor maternal vitamin A status in undernourished populations increases preterm birth, intrauterine growth retardation and low birth weight. | ▪ Deficiency is rare in the United States but widespread in developing countries.<br>▪ Fat malabsorption. | ▪ Excess vitamin A causes a variety of fetal abnormalities in animals.<br>▪ Inform women of reproductive age to avoid high doses of vitamin A, including the derivative found in some acne medications. |
| Vitamin D* | 5.0 µg | 5.0 µg | ▪ Regulates the use of calcium in mother and baby.<br>▪ Deficiencies are linked to neonatal hypocalcemia and maternal osteomalacia. | ▪ Northern climates with low exposure to sunlight<br>▪ Darkly pigmented skin<br>▪ Low intake of vitamin D–fortified milk | ▪ Supplementation is not needed during pregnancy if milk consumption is adequate.<br>▪ Toxicity may cause excess calcium absorption in fetus. |
| Vitamin E | 15 mg | 15 mg | ▪ Acts primarily as an antioxidant.<br>▪ Deficiency is associated with spontaneous abortion in animals, but human effects are not clear. | ▪ Fat malabsorption<br>▪ Impaired bile secretion or pancreatic function | ▪ Deficiencies are common among premature infants but this may not reflect maternal vitamin status. |

| Nutrient | Intake | Intake | Function | Deficiency | Clinical considerations |
|---|---|---|---|---|---|
| Vitamin K* | 14-18 y: 75 µg<br>19+ y: 90 µg | 14-18 y: 75 µg<br>19+ y: 90 µg | ■ Essential for blood clotting.<br>■ Transfer of maternal vitamin K to the fetus is limited. | ■ Fat malabsorption<br>■ Long-term antibiotic therapy | ■ Most newborns in the United States receive vitamin K by injection shortly after birth. |
| Calcium* | 14-18 y: 1,300 mg<br>19+ y: 1,000 mg | 14-18 y: 1,300 mg<br>19+ y: 1,000 mg | ■ Essential for formation of fetal skeleton and teeth. | ■ Diet lacking in milk products | ■ Supplement pregnant women who do not consume dairy foods. |
| Phosphorus | 14-18 y: 1,250 mg<br>19+ y: 700 mg | 14-18 y: 1,250 mg<br>19+ y: 700 mg | ■ Essential for formation of fetal skeleton and teeth. | ■ Deficiency is rare because phosphorous is found in a variety of foods. | ■ Studies suggest that an imbalance of phosphorus and calcium causes leg cramps during pregnancy. |
| Magnesium | 14-18 y: 400 mg<br>19-30 y: 350 mg<br>31 y: 360 mg | 14-18 y: 360 mg<br>19-30 y: 310 mg<br>31 y: 320 mg | ■ Used for tissue growth and cell metabolism | ■ Deficiency is rare because magnesium is widely distributed in food.<br>■ Absorption increases when intake is low. | ■ Routine supplementation during pregnancy is not necessary. |
| Iodine | 220 µg | 150 µg | ■ Acts as an essential component of thyroid hormones.<br>■ Iodine deficiency causes cretinism in newborns.<br>■ Also may cause more subtle cognitive and developmental impairments. | ■ Deficiency is not prevalent in the United States. | ■ Pregnant women should use iodized salt to avoid deficiency.<br>■ Excessive doses may cause congenital goiter. |
| Zinc | 14-18 y: 12 mg<br>19+ y: 11 mg | 14-18 y: 9 mg<br>19+ y: 8 mg | ■ Used in forming DNA and RNA.<br>■ In animal models, deficiency causes fetal malformation; human studies show poor pregnancy outcomes with zinc deficiency. | ■ Deficiency may occur in women taking iron supplementation for anemia. | ■ Suggest zinc supplementation for pregnant women taking more than 30 mg of iron daily.<br>■ Excessive zinc has been associated with preterm labor and stillbirth. |

Dietary Reference Intakes: recommended intakes of vitamins and minerals for individuals.

DFE, dietary folate equivalent; NE, niacin equivalent; RAE, retinol activity equivalents, alpha-tocopherol.

*Note:* Values are presented as Recommended Dietary Allowance (RDA), which are set to meet the needs of 97 to 98 percent of individuals in a group. Nutrients followed by * are listed as adequate intake (AI), indicating that some uncertainty exists regarding the percentage of individuals covered by this intake.

Modified from: Worthington PH. *Practical Aspects of Nutritional Support: An Advanced Practice Guide.* Philadelphia, PA: Saunders; 2004. Reprinted with permission.

## BOX 8-1 Case Study on Preconception Health

Angela, a 22-year-old college student, visited the student health center with complaints of stress, heavy menstrual blood loss, and tiredness. During the nutrition assessment with the university dietitian, she disclosed that she does not like to drink milk or eat other dairy products. She likes to drink at least 5 cups of coffee (brewed, regular) a day and eats breakfast only on weekends. The psychosocial evaluation revealed that Angela works 30 hours a week as a bartender in a local pub where smoking is allowed and lives in an apartment with her recently unemployed husband, Andrew. Both Angela and her husband are full-time students. They have discussed starting a family after graduating from college, but their parents want grandchildren now. They currently are not practicing any birth control methods. Further interviews revealed that Angela has minimal knowledge of preconception nutrition; she consumes a diet of take-out foods that is high in fat, sodium, and sugar, with infrequent consumption of fresh fruits or vegetables. She drinks three or four cans of beer on weekends with Andrew and smokes one pack of cigarettes a week. She does not do any physical activity because she is very busy and does not like to exercise. Their yearly income is below 130 percent of the U.S. poverty guidelines.

### Questions

1. Angela has minimal knowledge of preconception nutrition, and she is not using any birth control method, so the dietitian decided to explain the stages of fetal growth to her. What are the different stages of fetal growth and development? In each stage, what are the events and types of tissue that are developing?
2. What is preconception counseling? What preventive activities do nutritionists encourage?
3. The dietitian explained the importance of health screening before and during pregnancy. What is phenylketonuria (PKU)? Why is it important to conduct a genetic screening before pregnancy?
4. The dietitian emphasized to Angela the importance of consuming foods that are high in folate. Why is folate status such an important part of preconception health? What are some good sources of folate?
5. What are the recommended amounts of calories, protein, iron, calcium, and vitamin C during pregnancy that the dietitian should include in her nutrition counseling, and what is the importance of these nutrients during pregnancy?

6. What are the amounts of servings recommended for pregnant or lactating women for grains; vegetables; fruits; dairy products; meats, poultry, and fish; and nuts, seeds, and legumes that Angela should know?
7. The dietitian included information about pica during the preconception counseling. What is pica and why is it a concern during pregnancy?
8. What are some of the factors that can influence the outcome of a pregnancy that may have a direct effect on Angela if she were to become pregnant?
9. What are the physical activity guidelines for pregnancy? What are the warning signs to stop physical activity if Angela were to become pregnant?
10. Work in small groups or individually to discuss the case study using the Nutrition Care Process chart provided on the companion website. You also can add other nutrition and health-related conditions or assessments to the case study to make the case study more challenging and interesting.

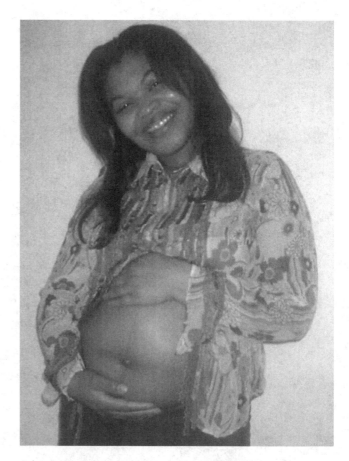

Adequate preconception nutrition is essential to a successful pregnancy.

# ▶ Factors That Can Influence the Outcome of a Pregnancy

Many factors affect the health of a mother and her **fetus** and require special sensitive counseling.[6] These factors include, but are not limited to, socioeconomic status, age and parity of the mother, inadequate prenatal care, use of illegal or over-the-counter (OTC) medications, prenatal **ketosis**, caffeine, alcohol, cigarette smoking, and pica. These and other factors are discussed in the following sections. **BOX 8-2** lists the modifiable practices or conditions that are harmful to the developing fetus.

## Low Socioeconomic Status

Community and public health nutritionists need to pay close attention to low-income or poor women and young girls. Some of the socioeconomic situations that can cause problems during pregnancy include inadequate health care, poor health practices, and lack of education.[20]

Community nutritionists should refer low-income pregnant women to government programs such as the Special Supplemental Nutrition Program for Women, Infants, and Children (WIC), the WIC Farmers' Market Nutrition Program (FMNP), and other state and federal programs so they can get help with food, housing, and health insurance (Medicare or Medicaid). The WIC program provides vouchers for specified nutritious foods along with nutrition education to low-income pregnant or postpartum women, infants, and children younger than 5 years of age who are nutritionally at risk. The FMNP can play an important role in reducing nutrition-related complications in low-income pregnant women.[21] It builds on the WIC program by providing additional vouchers to selected WIC recipients to help them buy fresh produce at local farmers' markets. This can reduce nutrition-related problems such as iron-deficiency anemia and NTDs.

## Age and Parity

Pregnancy at very early or later age of the reproductive cycle creates high-risk situations. The obstetric history of a woman is expressed in terms of number and order of pregnancies, or the gravida status. But a pregnant 15-year-old or younger is at high risk because she has not completed her own growth; therefore, adequate weight gain and the quality of her diet are essential and need special attention.[22] However, a primigravida (first pregnancy) older than 35 years also needs special attention because of the complications associated with bearing children later in the reproductive cycle. These complications include, but are not limited to, hypertension, either preexisting or pregnancy-induced; obesity; diabetes; and having a child with Down syndrome.[6,7,20]

In addition, having children too close together can deplete a mother's nutritional stores, making each successive pregnancy a higher risk.[6] Infants born less than a year apart are more likely to be born with a low birth weight than those further apart in age. In Zhu's study,[23] the risks of low birth weight, preterm birth, or small size for gestational age were higher for infants conceived fewer than 6 months apart compared to those conceived 18 to 23 months apart. Both shorter and longer interpregnancy intervals were associated with higher risks. Infants conceived 18 to 23 months after a live birth had the lowest risk.[23] This risk was more prevalent among younger and Hispanic women. Community and public health nutritionists should pay close attention to these risk factors, especially in women who have other risk factors (e.g., use of tobacco or alcohol, and those at a younger or older maternal age).

## Inadequate Prenatal Care

Inadequate, absent, or delayed prenatal care is associated with potential negative pregnancy outcomes.

---

**BOX 8-2** Modifiable Practices That Are Harmful to the Developing Fetus[153-155]

- Drinking alcohol (causes birth defects)
- Heavy use of aspirin (causes bleeding)
- Using illegal drugs such as cocaine or using over-the-counter medications (causes birth defects)
- Smoking (causes low-birth-weight infants and other problems)
- Inadequate diet such as few or no fruits and vegetables or dairy products or a great deal of high-fat and high-sugar food (may cause anemia, birth defects, obesity, etc.)
- Excessive vitamin A intake (above 10,000 IU [3,000 RAE/day]) and megadose use of other nutrient supplements (may cause birth defects)
- Excessive caffeine intake—more than one cup of coffee or 12 ounces of caffeinated beverages per day, such as soda, tea, chocolate, and coffee (affects fetal heart rate and breathing, can cause low-birth-weight infants)

The negative outcomes include anemia, gestational diabetes, and nutritional deficiencies in the fetus; for mothers with chronic diseases, such as hypertension or diabetes, the risk for fetal damage can increase.[24,25] Prenatal care includes physical examinations, laboratory tests, nutritional counseling, and regular checkups, which can help detect preexisting conditions and possible complications, as well as help women know what to expect during their pregnancy. Lack of prenatal care can cause a woman to deliver a low-birth-weight baby, and the baby is more likely to die during the first 4 weeks of life than a normal-birth-weight infant.[26] The ideal time to start prenatal care is before conception. Yet, approximately 20 percent of women in the United States receive no prenatal care in the first trimester.[6]

## Illegal or Over-the-Counter Drug Use

Drug use, both recreational and medicinal, also poses numerous problems.[27] The use of over-the-counter (OTC) medications poses potential adverse effects. For example, OTC medications contain both active and inactive ingredients (colorings, sweeteners, flavorings, and preservatives) that are often combined, which may cause unfavorable interactions.[28] The most frequently used OTC medications are cold remedies that typically contain 15 inactive ingredients plus active ingredients, any of which could have interactions.[29] Pregnant women are discouraged from using OTC medications without medical advice. However, in a retrospective study of 2,752 mothers who gave birth to normal infants, results showed that two thirds of these mothers used OTC medication 1.5 times more often than prescribed medication.[29] Results also showed that the use of OTC medications correlated positively with multiple illnesses, higher socioeconomic status, and European American women. In another study, pregnant women also reported they used between 2.3 and 2.6 OTC medications during pregnancy.[30,31]

In addition, mega-dosing with basic nutrients such as vitamin A during pregnancy may cause fetal damage. In particular, drugs made from vitamin A compounds—retinoids such as Accutane or etretinate prescribed for severe acne—are harmful to the fetus. Reports show they have caused spontaneous abortions of malformed infants in women who conceived during such acne treatment.[6,32]

The use of street drugs is especially hazardous, exposing the developing fetus to the risks for addiction and possibly AIDS due to the mother's use of contaminated needles. Cocaine has the most devastating consequences for developing fetuses.[33,34] As cocaine use has become more common, the number of infants born to cocaine-using women has increased.[35] Maternal use of cocaine during pregnancy is linked to preterm birth, low birth weight, and physical malformations in newborns. Community nutritionists should explain to pregnant women that exposure of the fetus to cocaine disrupts the development of the brain and nervous system and may reduce interactive behaviors and responses to environmental stimuli.[36]

## Caffeine During Pregnancy and Lactation

Information on the effects of caffeine consumption during pregnancy on the fetus is mixed. The U.S. Food and Drug Administration (FDA) recommendation for pregnant women is to avoid caffeine or consume it sparingly because caffeine can enter the bloodstream through the placenta and the developing fetus has a limited ability to metabolize it. Caffeine is also known to decrease the availability of calcium, iron, and zinc.[37] It can affect fetal heart rate and breathing.[38] The recommendation is to limit intake to one cup of coffee or 12 ounces of caffeinated beverages per day. **TABLE 8-5** shows the caffeine content per serving of some common foods.[37,39] Caffeine does pass into breast milk; therefore, consumption during lactation also should be limited.

## Alcohol and Cigarette Smoking

Consumption of alcohol during pregnancy may cause irreversible brain damage, growth retardation, mental retardation, facial abnormalities, and vision abnormalities.[40] Results of one research study showed that excessive consumption of alcohol affects fetal development and causes FAS, irreversible damage to the brain, and mental and physical retardation in the fetus.[40] Community nutritionists should discourage the use of alcohol during pregnancy and explain to clients that FAS is preventable by abstaining from alcohol during pregnancy.

Dietitians should explain that alcohol does not increase milk volume and that chronic consumption can inhibit the milk ejection reflex. The American Academy of Pediatrics (AAP) recommends that the breastfeeding mother should avoid drinking alcohol because it can pass to the baby through the breast milk. However, the AAP recommends that if breastfeeding mothers choose to drink alcohol, they should do so just after breastfeeding rather than just before. The allowable alcohol consumption while breastfeeding is no more

**TABLE 8-5** Caffeine Content of Selected Foods per Serving

| Food Name | Serving Portion | Caffeine Content (mg) |
|---|---|---|
| Candy, semisweet chocolate | 1 oz | 17.58 |
| Candy, sweet chocolate | 1 oz | 18.71 |
| Cocoa powder, unsweetened | 1 Tbsp | 12.42 |
| Coffee, brewed, regular | 6 fl oz | 103.24 |
| Coffee, brewed, espresso | 6 fl oz | 377.54 |
| Coffee, instant, regular, prepared | 6 fl oz | 57.28 |
| Coffee, instant, decaffeinated, prepared | 6 fl oz | 1.79 |
| Coffee, instant, cappuccino flavor, prepared | 6 fl oz | 74.88 |
| Coffee, instant, French flavor, prepared | 6 fl oz | 51.03 |
| Coffee, instant, mocha flavor, prepared | 6 fl oz | 33.84 |
| Cola beverage, regular | 12 fl oz | 37.00 |
| Cola beverage, diet | 12 fl oz | 49.70 |
| Ice cream, chocolate | 0.5 cup | 40.92 |
| Milk, chocolate | 8 fl oz | 5.00 |
| Tea, brewed | 6 fl oz | 35.60 |
| Tea, instant, unsweetened, prepared | 6 fl oz | 23.14 |
| Tea, instant, unsweetened, lemon flavored, prepared | 6 fl oz | 19.64 |

Reproduced from: The U.S. Department of Agriculture Nutrient Database for Standard Reference, release 11-1; and The Nutrition Coordinating Center, University of Minnesota, Nutrition Data System for Research, database version 38. *Table Caffeine Content of Selected Common Foods per Serving.* The Nutrition Coordinating Center, University of Minnesota; 2007. Reprinted with permission.

than 2 to 2.5 ounces of liquor, 8 ounces of wine, or 2 cans of beer on any day.[41]

Cigarette smoking is responsible for 20 to 30 percent of all low-birth-weight deliveries in the United States and increases the risk for infant mortality.[42] Carbon monoxide and nicotine from smoking increase fetal carboxyhemoglobin, reduce placental blood flow, and limit the oxygen supply to the fetus. In addition, women who smoke cigarettes are at risk for delivering low-birth-weight infants.

## Pica

**Pica** is a persistent compulsive consumption of non-food items. It is an unusual type of craving that is more common during pregnancy. Pica is more common in African American than European American women, in rural rather than urban women, and in women with a family history of the practice.[43] It is a recognized complication of pregnancy because it contributes little or no nutritional value. Pica occurs worldwide and is found

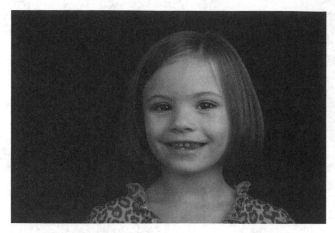

Consumption of alcohol during pregnancy may cause irreversible brain damage, mental retardation, and facial abnormalities.

© Rick's Photography/Shutterstock

in both genders and all ages and races. It is of special concern because pregnant women and their children may absorb toxic substances, such as lead, from the material they consume. Fecal impaction and parasite infections (from ingested soil) also may occur in women and children who experience pica.[44]

Pica is classified into four categories distinguished by the substance consumed. Geophagia is the consumption of earth and clay, amylophagia is the consumption of starch, and pagophagia is excessive eating of ice. The fourth (miscellaneous) category includes consumption of ash, chalk, antacids, paint chips, baking soda, mothballs, wax, charcoal, burnt matches, hair, and other substances.[45]

The origin of this practice is not well understood. The nutritional hazards most frequently linked with pica are lead poisoning and iron-deficiency anemia, but it is not clear whether pica is a cause of these problems.

## Mother and Father's Health

Adequate nutrient intake is important for a successful pregnancy. During pregnancy, eating healthfully is essential for a positive outcome for both the fetus and the mother. Pregnant women should be encouraged to plan their food intake using the dietary food guide presented in **TABLE 8-6**.

Community nutritionists also should advise fathers-to-be to consider their eating and other habits. Limited evidence suggests that men who consume too few fruits and vegetables containing vitamin C or who drink too much alcohol in the weeks before conception may sustain damage to their sperm's genetic material. This damage can cause birth defects in future children.[48] In addition, if they practice eating nutritiously, it can encourage the mother-to-be to eat nutritiously.

## Maternal Weight Gain During Pregnancy

Appropriate weight gain during pregnancy is necessary for a successful pregnancy outcome. For this reason, health professionals have adopted the Institute of Medicine (IOM) guidelines regarding weight gain. A review found that the best pregnancy outcomes were obtained when the weight-gain guidelines (shown in **TABLE 8-7**) were followed.[49] Weight gain below the recommendations was associated with a risk for preterm delivery and low birth weight; those above the suggested range had a higher risk for cesarean delivery and excessive postpartum weight retention.

Although African American women are at greater risk for delivering low-birth-weight babies, an empiric evaluation of the IOM's pregnancy weight-gain guidelines by race does not support a recommendation that these women should strive for weight gains in the upper half of the IOM recommended range[52] because the data show questionable benefits in the reduction of risk for low-birth-weight babies.

Obese women have a greater risk for pregnancy complications, including **gestational diabetes mellitus**, hypertensive disorders, cesarean deliveries, postoperative morbidity, gestational hypertension, preeclampsia, fetal death, and possible birth defects.[50,51] Infants of obese women also may be at greater risk for perinatal death

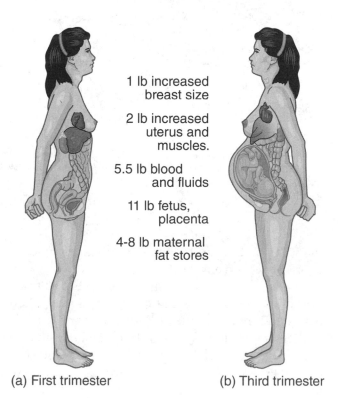

1 lb increased breast size

2 lb increased uterus and muscles.

5.5 lb blood and fluids

11 lb fetus, placenta

4–8 lb maternal fat stores

(a) First trimester

(b) Third trimester

Components of maternal weight gain.

**TABLE 8-6** Diet Planning Guide for Pregnant, Lactating, and Nonpregnant Women[*,46,47]

| Food Groups | Nonpregnant Women | Pregnant or Lactating Women | 1,600 Calories | 2,000 Calories | 2,600 Calories | 3,100 Calories | Serving Sizes | Examples of Foods | Major Source of |
|---|---|---|---|---|---|---|---|---|---|
| Grains[†] | 6-11 servings | 7-11 (7+) servings | 6 servings | 7-8 servings | 10-11 servings | 12-13 servings | 1 slice bread 1 oz dry cereal ½ cup cooked rice, pasta, or cereal | Whole wheat bread, English muffin, pita, bagel, cereals, grits, oatmeal, crackers, unsalted pretzels, and popcorn | Energy and fiber |
| Vegetables | 3-5 servings | 4-5 (5+) servings | 3-4 servings | 4-5 servings | 5-6 servings | 6 servings | 1 cup raw leafy vegetables ½ cup cooked vegetables 6 oz vegetable juice | Tomatoes, potatoes, carrots, green peas, squash, broccoli, turnip greens, collards, kale, spinach, artichokes, green beans, lima beans, and sweet potatoes | Rich sources of potassium, magnesium, and fiber Vitamins A and C |
| Fruits | 2-4 servings | 3-4 (4+) servings | 4 servings | 4-5 servings | 5-6 servings | 6 servings | 6 oz fruit juice 1 medium fruit ¼ cup dried fruit ½ cup fresh, frozen, or canned fruit | Apricots, bananas, dates, grapes, oranges, orange juice, grapefruit, grapefruit juice, mangoes, melons, peaches, pineapples, prunes, raisins, strawberries, and tangerines | Important sources of potassium, magnesium, vitamin C, and fiber |
| Dairy products, low-fat or fat-free dairy foods | 2 servings | 3-4 (4+) servings | 2-3 servings | 2-3 servings | 3 servings | 3-4 Servings | 8 oz milk 1 cup yogurt 1½ oz cheese | Fat-free or low-fat milk, fat-free or low-fat buttermilk, fat-free or low-fat regular or frozen yogurt, and low-fat and fat-free cheese | Major sources of calcium, vitamin D, and protein |

(continues)

**TABLE 8-6** Diet Planning Guide for Pregnant, Lactating, and Nonpregnant Women *,46,47 *(continued)*

| Food Groups | Nonpregnant Women | Pregnant or Lactating Women | 1,600 Calories | 2,000 Calories | 2,600 Calories | 3,100 Calories | Serving Sizes | Examples of Foods | Major Source of |
|---|---|---|---|---|---|---|---|---|---|
| Meats, poultry, fish | 2-3 servings | 3 (3+) servings | 1-2 servings | 2 or fewer servings | 2 servings | 2-3 Servings | 3 oz cooked meat, poultry, or fish | Select only lean; trim away visible fats; broil, roast, or boil instead of frying; remove skin from poultry | Rich sources of protein, vitamin D, and magnesium |
| Nuts, seeds, legumes | 2-3 servings ¼ cup of cooked dry beans or peas equals 1 oz of products in the meat and beans group) | 3 (3+) servings | 3-4 servings/ week | 4-5 servings/ week | 1 serving | 1 serving | 1/3 cup or ½ oz nuts 2 Tbsp or ½ oz seeds ½ cup cooked dry beans or peas | Almonds, filberts, mixed nuts, peanuts, walnuts, sunflower seeds, kidney beans, and lentils | Rich sources of energy, magnesium, potassium, protein, and fiber |

*This plan is based on 1,600, 2,000, 2,600, and 3,100 calories. The number of daily servings in a food group and amounts vary to accommodate a participant's caloric and nutritional needs or food preferences. This table can help in planning menus and food selection in homes, restaurants, and grocery stores.

†Whole grains are recommended for most servings to meet fiber recommendations.

‡Equals ½ to 1¼ cups, depending on cereal type. Check the product's Nutrition Facts Label.

§Fat content changes serving counts for fats and oils. For example, 1 Tbsp of regular salad dressing equals 1 serving; 1 Tbsp of low-fat dressing equals ½ serving; 1 Tbsp of fat-free dressing equals 0 servings.

**TABLE 8-7**   Recommended Range of Weight Gain for Pregnant Women[50,51]

| Prepregnancy Weight-for-Height Body Mass Index (BMI) | Weight Category | Total Weight Gain (Pounds) | Total Weight Gain (Kilograms) | Weight Gain First Trimester (Pounds) | Weight Gain Second and Third Trimesters (Pounds Week) |
|---|---|---|---|---|---|
| < 19.8 | Underweight | 28-40 | 12.5-18.0 | 5.0 | 1.07 |
| 19.8-26.0 | Normal weight | 25-35 | 11.5-16.0 | 3.5-5.0 | 0.97-1.0 |
| 26.0-29.0 | Overweight | 15-25 | 7.0-11.5 | 2.0 | 0.67 |
| > 29.0 | Obesity | 15-25 | 7.0 | | 0.50 |

*The range for women with twins is 35 to 45 lb (16.0-20.5 kg). The range for women with triplets is 45 to 55 pounds (20.5-25.0 kg). Young adolescents (< 2 years after menarche) and African American women should strive to gain at the upper end of the range. Short women (< 62 inches tall [< 157 cm]) should strive to gain at the lower end of the range. Weight gain varies widely, and these values are suggested only as guidelines for identifying individuals whose weights may be too high or low for health.

and are twice as likely to be obese and develop type 2 diabetes later in life.[53]

## Rate of Weight Gain

The recommendation for pregnancy weight gain is to gain a total of 3 to 5 pounds during the first trimester and 1 pound per week for the second and third trimesters. In 1996, the Maternal Weight Gain Expert Group of the National Academy of Sciences suggested a weight gain of 1.5 pounds per week for normal weight women during the second half of a twin pregnancy.[54]

The weight gain of pregnant women consists of water, protein, and fat. The measurements of maternal water gain may predict birth weight better than measurements of composite weight gain. The total amount of weight gained, the composition of gain, and the rate of energy metabolism differ among healthy pregnant women. **TABLE 8-8** presents typical weight-gain distribution.[37] Many women express concern regarding the weight they gain during pregnancy; community nutritionists should advise them that only a small amount of fat is stored and that the stored fat will be a source of energy for breastfeeding.

Pregnant women should avoid dieting to lose weight because pregnancy is an anabolic state that requires additional calories to support the growth and metabolic activity of the fetus, **placenta**, and maternal tissues. In addition, pregnancy uses calories to build maternal fat stores that supply the energy needed to meet the metabolic demands of late pregnancy and lactation.[55] Women's energy needs increase 340 kcal/day during the second trimester and 452 kcal/day above nonpregnant

**TABLE 8-8**   Typical Weight Distribution During Pregnancy

| Source | Pounds | Kilograms |
|---|---|---|
| Amniotic fluid | 2.0-2.6 | 4.4-5.7 |
| Fetus | 7.0-8.5 | 15.4-18.7 |
| Fat/breast tissue stores for breastfeeding | 1.0-4.0 | 2.2-8.8 |
| Increased blood volume | 4.0-5.0 | 8.8-11.0 |
| Increased weight of uterus | 2.0 | 4.4 |
| Maternal fat stores | 4.0-7.0 | 8.8-15.4 |
| Placenta | 2.0-2.5 | 4.4-5.5 |
| Extra tissue fluid | 3.0-5.0 | 6.6-11.0 |
| **Total** | **25-36.6** | **55-80.5** |

Modified from: Berdanier CD, Feldman EB, Flatt WP. *Handbook of Nutrition and Food*. Washington, DC: CRC Press; 2002.

period during the third. This extra energy can be obtained from milk, vegetables, and grains. Energy needs during the first trimester are the same as for nonpregnant women.[6,50] Dietitians working with pregnant women

**BOX 8-3** The Effects of Prenatal Ketosis[37,99]

The fetal brain uses **ketone bodies** poorly. Crash diets or fasting for more than 12 hours during pregnancy is not advisable. A pregnant woman can develop significant ketosis after only 20 hours of fasting. Eating about 100 g of carbohydrates every day prevents ketosis. Even nonpregnant women usually eat twice this amount. Community nutritionists should discourage mothers from skipping meals or dieting, especially during pregnancy.

**BOX 8-4** Remedies for Nausea and Vomiting[6,37]

- Eat small, frequent meals.
- Eat dry/cold foods.
- On waking, arise slowly.
- Chew gum or suck on hard candies.
- Take prenatal vitamins and iron supplements on a full stomach or at a time of day when feeling well.
- Avoid caffeine.
- Eat combinations of foods that are salty and tart.
- Avoid spicy foods, acidic foods, and strong odors.
- Sniff lemon.

should explain to their clients that adequate weight gain reduces the risk for low-birth-weight infants and that crash diets may cause prenatal ketosis and slow down the fetus's brain development (see **BOX 8-3**). They should encourage their clients to plan their food intake using the dietary guidelines presented in Table 8-6.

## ▶ Diet-Related Complications of Pregnancy

Several complications of pregnancy may have an impact on nutritional status. Some of these include nausea and vomiting, **hyperemesis gravidarum** (severe nausea, dehydration, and vomiting during pregnancy), constipation, and gestational diabetes.

### Nausea and Vomiting/Morning Sickness

Approximately 70 percent of pregnant women experience nausea during the first 14 to 16 weeks of pregnancy, and 37 to 58 percent of them experience vomiting. This is due to the hormonal changes that occur early in pregnancy. The incidents range from mild queasiness to unbearable nausea. Many women complain that smells—mainly cooking smells—make them sick. The remedies for this condition may include diet changes, the use of ginger extract, increased fluids, and reassurance.[36,55] **BOX 8-4** provides suggestions that may help combat nausea.

### Heartburn, Constipation, and Hemorrhoids

Heartburn is a burning sensation in the lower esophagus near the heart. This is common during pregnancy because a hormone produced by the placenta, progesterone, relaxes the muscles in both the uterus and the intestinal tract. This often causes heartburn as stomach acid flows back into the esophagus.[48] The remedies are to not lie down after eating, to eat less fat so the foods pass more quickly from the stomach into the small intestine, and to avoid spicy foods.

Constipation is common in pregnancy due to decreased motility of the gastrointestinal tract caused by the relaxing hormone of the placenta (progesterone). Iron supplementation also increases the incidence of constipation, as do low fiber and low fluid intake. The recommendation is to consume 20 to 30 grams of dietary fiber daily, perform exercise regularly, and eat dried fruits, such as dried apricots and plums.[36,56] Straining during elimination can lead to hemorrhoids, and it may be necessary to reevaluate the need for and dose of iron supplementation and the dietary patterns of the client.[57]

### Anemia

Blood volume increases during pregnancy; this leaves proportionately fewer red blood cells in a pregnant woman's bloodstream.[58] The lower ratio of red blood cells to total blood volume is a condition known as physiological anemia. It is a normal response to pregnancy; however, anemia also may result from inadequate iron stores and a low dietary iron intake and may be a condition that requires medical attention.[59]

In some cases, iron-deficient women have normal hemoglobin values. However, such women do not have iron stores to draw from during illness, injury, or pregnancy. The consequences of iron deficiency are iron-deficiency anemia and low blood volume. Iron-deficiency anemia at the beginning of pregnancy is linked to a risk for preterm delivery and low-birth-weight infants.[60,61] In addition, iron deficiency during pregnancy is very dangerous because it increases the risk for maternal and infant death significantly and may contribute to low iron status in the infant. Iron deficiency has been attributed to low scores on intelligence, language, gross motor development, and attention tests in affected children at the age of 5 years.[61-63]

Pregnant women should be encouraged to eat iron-rich foods such as lean red meat, fish, poultry, dried fruits, and iron-fortified cereals. It has been reported that meat and ascorbic acid–rich fruits increase non-heme iron absorption. Whole grain cereals, unleavened whole grain breads, legumes, tea, and coffee should be consumed separately from iron-fortified foods and iron supplements because they reduce iron absorption.[60,61,64]

## Pregnancy-Induced Hypertension

Another serious disorder whose symptoms may include high blood pressure, edema, and protein in the urine is pregnancy-induced hypertension. In very severe form, kidney failure, seizures, and even death of the mother and fetus may occur. In its mild forms it is known as preeclampsia and in severe forms as **eclampsia**. The exact cause is not known, but calcium, magnesium sulfate supplements, and bed rest may lower the risk for preeclampsia.[65]

## Gestational Diabetes Mellitus

Gestational diabetes mellitus (GDM) is glucose intolerance during pregnancy. Individuals who were diagnosed as diabetic before pregnancy are not classified as having gestational diabetes. Screening for gestational diabetes is recommended between 24 and 28 weeks of pregnancy using a 50-gram, 1-hour oral glucose challenge.[66] GDM occurs in approximately 3 to 4 percent of all pregnancies, resulting in approximately 135,000 cases annually in the United States, but it disappears at the end of the pregnancy. Women who have had gestational diabetes mellitus are at increased risk for developing type 2 diabetes later, however. Some studies have reported that approximately 40 percent of women with a history of GDM were subsequently diagnosed as having diabetes.[67] The risk factors for GDM include pregnancy after age 30, obesity, previous congenital abnormalities, previous stillbirth, and family history of type 2 diabetes.[67] The major concerns for the fetus of gestational diabetic individuals are high birth weight (9 pounds at term or in the 90th **percentile** in weight for gestational age), hypoglycemia at birth, and increased incidence of obesity.

## Foodborne Illness During Pregnancy

Pregnant women are at high risk for foodborne illness.[68,69] The most common causes of diarrhea during pregnancy are several foodborne or waterborne pathogens such as bacteria, protozoa, or viruses, including the *Salmonella* species, *Helicobacter pylori*, *Shigella*, *Escherichia coli* (*E. coli* O157:H7), and cryptosporidium.[70] Hepatitis A also is a foodborne or waterborne pathogen of concern. During pregnancy, listeriosis, caused by *Listeria monocytogenes*, can result in premature delivery, stillbirth, or infection in the newborn.[71] *Toxoplasma gondii* is a protozoan that can be passed from the mother to the fetus and can result in infant death or mental retardation.[72] The following are guidelines for pregnant women to avoid foodborne illnesses.[73-75]

- Do not consume unpasteurized juices, raw sprouts, or raw (unpasteurized) milk products.
- Avoid raw or undercooked meat, poultry, eggs, fish, or shellfish.
- Cook leftovers and ready-to-eat food (e.g., hot dogs) until steaming hot, and avoid homemade cheese, cheese purchased from street vendors, and soft cheeses such as Brie, feta, blue, and Camembert to avoid listeriosis.
- To avoid toxoplasma, wash hands thoroughly after handling cat feces and cleaning the cat litter box.
- Handle all foods safely by washing hands with warm soapy water and cook food thoroughly.

The FDA also advises pregnant women to avoid consuming large fish, including shark, swordfish, king mackerel, and tilefish, because these fish accumulate unsafe levels of methylmercury.[76] A moderate amount (6 to 12 ounces or less per week) of other fish (tuna steaks, halibut, snapper, canned albacore, or chunk white tuna) may be safe during pregnancy. Pregnant women should contact their state or local health departments for more information or advisories on fish caught or sold in their local markets. See **BOX 8-5** for additional risk factors in pregnancy.

## ☑ Think About It

The community outreach health professionals organized their annual health fair at a center that serves a mainly Hispanic community in an urban city. The majority of the participants were pregnant, with an annual income of less than 185 percent of the poverty guidelines for prenatal and postpartum care. Mary, the nutritionist serving in this city, was asked to assess the pregnant women's rate of weight gain and provide recommendations for addressing any of the risks associated with underweight and/or obesity. Of the pregnant women, 20 percent were underweight and 50 percent were obese. What are the complications associated with underweight and obesity during pregnancy? Which food assistance programs can Mary recommend to these pregnant women?

**BOX 8-5** Pregnancy Risk Factors[72,77]

### Risk Factors Present at the Onset of Pregnancy

- Age younger than 15 years or older than 35 years
- Frequent pregnancies: three or more during a 2-year period
- Poor obstetric history or poor fetal performance
- Poverty
- Abuse of nicotine, alcohol, or drugs
- Therapeutic diet required for a chronic disorder
- Weight < 85 percent or > 120 percent of standard weight
- Level of education (less than high school education)

### Risk Factors Occurring During Pregnancy

- Low hemoglobin (< 12 g) or hematocrit (< 35 mg/dl)
- Inadequate weight gain: any weight loss or weight gain of less than 1 kg (2 lb)/month after the first trimester
- Excessive weight gain: more than 1 kg (2 lb)/week after the first trimester
- Late prenatal care
- Genetic make-up

## ▶ Nutrition Assessment During Pregnancy

Nutrition assessment is an essential component of the nutritional care of a pregnant woman. It provides the foundation for planning a woman's education, individualized care, and direction throughout the pregnancy, which is necessary for a positive outcome for both the mother and baby. The nutrition assessment during pregnancy addresses the three stages of gestation and the postpartum stage. Preferably, the first prenatal visit should be a follow-up of the preconception visit. However, preconception visits are not yet common. The assessment performed during the first prenatal visit is influenced by the stage of gestation.[37,71]

Nutrition assessment during pregnancy should include the use of the Daily Food Checklist Tool provided in **TABLE 8-9**. In addition, the Nutritionist can use the Nutritional Risk Score, which shows a quantitative

method for assessing a client's diet.[36,37] The client's usual intake is determined for each of the food groups with a maximum score of:

> Meats and alternatives, 40 points
> Dairy Products, 15 points
> Bread and cereal, 15 points
> Fruits and vegetables, 15 points

A client with less than 80 points is at nutritional risk. Clients with a score less than 50 should receive dietary counseling. The dietitian also should determine whether the client has problems such as nausea, vomiting, lactose intolerance, constipation, or cravings for nonfood items. The nutritionist can also assess for risk factors that can be used for referral, counseling, and nutrition intervention programs.[37] The techniques for assessing a pregnant woman's needs are outlined in **TABLE 8-10** and may include personal history (demographic, social, etc.), dietary assessment, clinical observations and physical examination, anthropometry, and laboratory data. These criteria may be used for assessing and monitoring nutritional status, planning care, and promoting the health of pregnant women.

## ▶ Adolescent Pregnancy

In the United States, approximately 1 million adolescent girls between the ages of 12 and 19 become pregnant each year.[72] Many teenage women, especially the youngest ones, have not had time to store the nutrients needed to support their own rapid growth and development, much less store nutrients needed to support pregnancy and a developing fetus. Adolescents have more miscarriages, premature births, stillbirths, and low-birth-weight infants than adult women.[51,79] Undoubtedly, teenage pregnancy is a major public health problem.

The personal and societal impact of teenage pregnancy in the United States is huge; an estimated 84 percent of teenage pregnancies are unintended (i.e., they occur sooner than desired or are not wanted at the time).[80]

Research shows that postneonatal mortality rates were higher for mothers ages 12 to 17 years after adjusting for socioeconomic and other known risk factors. The high postneonatal mortality rate observed in this study was attributed to increased risk for accidental and infectious deaths in these infants. These incidences could be due to maternal maturity and ability adequately supervise these developing

| **TABLE 8-9** Daily Food Checklist | | | |
|---|---|---|---|
| **Foods Group** | **First Trimester** | **Second & Third Trimester** | **What Counts as 1 Cup or 1 Ounce** |
| **Fruits** | 2 cups | 2 cups | 1 cup fruit or 100% juice<br>½ cup dried fruit |
| **Vegetables** | 2½ cups | 3 cups | 1 cup raw or cooked vegetables or 100% juice<br>2 cups raw leafy vegetables |
| **Grains** | 6 ounces | 8 ounces | 1 slice bread<br>1 ounce ready-to-eat cereal |
| **Protein Foods** | 5½ ounces | 6½ ounces | 1 ounces lean meats, seafood, or poultry ¼ cooked beans<br>½ ounces nuts or 1TSP peanut butter<br>1 egg |
| **Dairy** | 3 cups | 3 cups | 1 cup milk<br>8 ounces yogurt<br>1½ ounces natural cheese<br>2 ounces processed cheese |

If the clients is not gaining weight or gaining too slowly, you may recommend that they increase the amount they consume from each food group a little.

If the clients is gaining weight too fast, you may recommend they reduce the amount or change the types of food they are eating.

Reproduced from United States Department of Agriculture. Tips for Pregnant Moms. Accessed March 25, 2017 at https://wicworks.fns.usda.gov/wicworks/Topics/PregnancyFactSheet.pdf.

infants. Results also showed that participation in WIC and Medicaid was helpful in reducing the neonatal mortality rate.[78]

More than 70 national health and social welfare organizations support age-appropriate comprehensive school health-education programs to reduce teenage pregnancy.[81] These programs counsel abstinence as well as provide teenagers with the knowledge and skills they need to avoid unplanned pregnancies. In addition to health education efforts, family-planning services for sexually active teenagers are essential for reducing teenage pregnancy.

The pregnant adolescent is viewed as a high-risk individual who is highly susceptible to poor pregnancy outcomes. Identification of pregnant adolescents and management of their problems and concerns should be a primary goal of community health organizations. The following are issues in adolescent pregnancy that influence nutritional well-being and that need to be addressed in intervention strategies.[51]

- *Acceptance of the pregnancy:* The desire to carry out a successful pregnancy and acceptance of responsibility

- *Food resources:* Family meals (timing, quantity, quality) and food assistance (willingness to participate in WIC)
- *Body image:* Degree of acceptance of an adult body, maturity in facing bodily changes throughout pregnancy
- *Living situation:* Acceptance by partners and extended family, financial support, and ethnic group (religious, cultural, and social patterns)
- *Relationship with the father of the child:* Presence or absence of the father, quality of relationship, influence on mother's nutritional habits, tolerance of physical changes in pregnancy, and physical needs of mother and child
- *Peer relationship:* Support from friends and their influence on general lifestyle
- *Nutritional state:* Weight-for-height proportion, tissue stores of nutrients, history of dietary patterns and nutritional status, substance use, and activity patterns
- *Prenatal care:* Initiation of and compliance with prenatal care and dependability of supporting resources.

**TABLE 8-10** Criteria for Assessing and Monitoring Nutritional Status During Pregnancy and Postpartum[6,51,78]

| Stages/ Visits | Personal History Data | Dietary Assessment | Clinical and Physical Examination | Anthropometric Assessment | Laboratory Measures |
|---|---|---|---|---|---|
| First trimester | **Age**<br>**Medical records:**<br>■ Review previous obstetric history<br>■ Medical condition<br>■ Genetic disorder<br>■ Medications/supplements<br>■ Number of pregnancy<br>■ Parity (number of children born alive)<br>■ Breastfeeding experience<br>■ Socioeconomic status:<br>　• Low income<br>　• Inadequate access to food<br>■ Education level<br>■ Substance abuse<br>■ Cigarette use<br>■ Living situation<br>■ Cultural background<br>■ Sleep pattern (7-8 hours) | Dietary history:<br>Pica practice<br>Lactose intolerance<br>Food allergies and intolerances<br>PKU | General examination of gums, teeth, tongue, eyes, and hair<br>History of pregnancy-induced hypertension (PIH), gestational diabetes, or iron-deficiency anemia | Measurements of height, weight, body mass index (BMI), and skinfold measurements (as needed) | Hemoglobin and hematocrit<br>Screen for anemia, urine analysis for ketone bodies, glucose, and protein levels |
| Second trimester/ follow-up visits | Review medical records<br>Discuss food assistance programs (WIC, Supplemental Nutrition Assistance Program, etc.) | Dietary history<br>Additional probing of dietary practice<br>Dietary supplements (iron, folate) and nutrients deficiency | Screen for anemia, dental health<br>Iron, $B_{12}$, and folate deficiency | Weight gain using BMI measures | Hemoglobin and hematocrit<br>Urinalysis for ketone bodies, protein, and glucose levels |
| Third trimester/ follow-up visits | Review medical records<br>Discuss food assistance programs (WIC, Supplemental Nutrition Assistance Program, etc.) | Additional probing of dietary practice<br>Dietary supplements (iron, folate) | Screen for anemia, dental health<br>Iron, folate, and $B_{12}$ deficiency | Rate of weight gain | Hemoglobin and hematocrit<br>Urinalysis for ketone bodies, protein, and glucose levels |
| Postpartum visits | Review medical records<br>Support at home<br>Assistance with initiating breastfeeding<br>Avoidance of harmful substances<br>Adequate rest | Dietary history<br>Availability of food<br>Review the need for food assistance programs (WIC, Supplemental Nutrition Assistance Program, etc.) | Screen for anemia, dental health<br>Iron, folate, and $B_{12}$ deficiency | Weight management method after delivery | Check for postpartum anemia if heavy blood loss occurred at delivery |

# ▶ Physical Activity During Pregnancy

Research shows that physical activity can facilitate labor and reduce psychological stress. Women who remain active during pregnancy report fewer discomforts throughout their pregnancies and gain less weight than those who are not physically active.[84] Studies show that structured exercise three or four times per week during the third trimester produced lower infant birth weights.[82] The odds of a lower infant birth weight were substantially increased for those who exercised five or more times per week and modestly increased for those at the other extreme, who engaged in structured exercise two or fewer times per week.[83] Physical activities during pregnancy should be chosen with care. See **BOX 8-6** for

---

**BOX 8-6**  Guidelines and Warnings for Pregnant Women While Undertaking Physical Activity

During pregnancy, physical activity is important for building energy and stamina for childbirth. However, excessive and high intense exercise may be harmful. It is important to follow exercise guidelines and consult your physician if you observe any of the following warning signs:

**Warning Signs to Stop Physical Activity**
- Vaginal bleeding
- Uterine contractions
- Nausea, vomiting
- Dizziness or faintness
- Difficulty walking
- Decreased fetal activity
- Palpitations or rapid heart rate
- Numbness in any part of the body
- Problems with vision

**Guidelines to Follow While Exercising**
- Reduce the intensity of exercise by 25 percent of what would be a normal workout.
- Do not exceed 140 beats per minute.
- Do not go above 101° F (38.3° C).
- Moderate activity should not exceed 30 minutes; intersperse with low-intensity exercise and rest periods.
- Avoid lying on back for more than 5 minutes after entering the second trimester.
- Exercise should be performed consistently at least three times per week and include a warm-up and a cool-down period.

Data from: Berdanier CD, Feldman EB, Flatt WP. *Handbook of Nutrition and Food.* Washington, DC: CRC Press; 2002.

---

physical activity guidelines and the warning signs to stop physical activity.

# ▶ Nutrition in Infancy

**Infancy** is defined as the period between birth and 1 year of age. Early infancy from birth to 6 months of age is when the most rapid growth happens. Middle infancy is from 6 to 9 months, when growth slows but is still rapid, and late infancy is 9 to 12 months, when growth slows and babies' maturation and activity allow them to eat a wider variety of foods. The average weight of a healthy term infant is 7.7 pounds (3.5 kg).[82] Full-term newborns who weigh less than 5.5 pounds (2.5 kg) are **small for gestational age (SGA)**. A research study reported that vitamin D deficiency was associated with SGA babies in European American women and a more modest increased risk also may exist for higher serum 25(OH)D levels.[37] Infants lose about 10 percent of their body weight in the first week of life, but both breastfed and formula-fed infants should regain it within 2 weeks of age. This first year of life is critical for the rapid growth of all major organ systems. This rapid growth rate makes nutrition a critical element of caring for infants. Nutrition during this time influences how an infant will grow and thrive.

WIC is a federal health, nutrition, and prevention program with a successful record of improving diet and reducing infant mortality and morbidity. The infant mortality rate in the United States has decreased slightly from 6.84 in 2003 to approximately 6.14 in 2010.[84] However, the U.S. infant mortality rate remains higher than that of many other industrialized countries. Infant mortality rates vary widely by racial and ethnic group and geographically, with the highest rate among infants born to African American mothers in the largest U.S. cities. It also has been reported that infant mortality rates are higher for infants born preterm or with a low birth weight.[85]

Nutritionists and other healthcare professionals can use different intervention strategies to help reduce the incidence of infant mortality and improve the health of mothers. For example, the Infant Health and Development Program examined the effect of regular home counseling, free daycare center programs, and participation in a parental support group on more than 1,000 infants and families. The mothers of 377 infants received the 3-year intervention; the control group was closely monitored and mothers were referred to all appropriate community services. Results showed that the intervention made a significant difference in the development of the premature and low-birth-weight infants and their mothers. The intervention group infants had significantly higher IQs, fewer behavioral problems, and no major illness; in addition, their mothers were less depressed and less likely to smoke compared to the control group. After 5 years, the differences between the intervention and control groups lessened.[86]

## Physical Growth and Development Assessment

Community and public health dietitians use anthropometric measurements as well as **growth charts** to monitor children's growth and development. Infants double their birth weight by 4 to 6 months and gain approximately 5 to 7 ounces a week. They typically triple their birth weight in 1 year.[87,88] Body weight is measured with an electronic scale or a beam balance without detachable weights. Infants gain approximately 1 inch per month from birth to 6 months and gain ½ inch per month from 6 to 12 months. They typically increase their **length** by 50 percent in their first year.[88,89] The measurement of length requires two examiners using a calibrated length board with a fixed headpiece and movable footboard.

**Head circumference** is measured with a narrow flexible steel or paper tape applied to the head above the eye ridges and encircling the most prominent parts of the forehead and the back part of the head or skull. A maximum of three measurements are used to determine the maximal circumference.

Normal growth is a strong indicator of nutritional adequacy and the overall health of an infant. During routine checkups throughout childhood and adolescence, nutritionists and other healthcare professionals measure weight, height (or length), and head circumference and plot these values on growth charts. Each growth chart consists of a set of curves called percentiles that show the distribution of values for U.S. children based on a certain measurement.[37,90,91] The latest growth charts can be obtained on the Centers for Disease Control and Prevention website at http://www.cdc.gov.

Length and head circumference are more sensitive measures than weight for assessing a baby's growth and nutritional status. Weight alone reflects recent nutritional intake. Head circumference measures brain growth and development. Chronic malnutrition can limit brain growth and is reflected in inadequate gains in head size. Head circumference measurements are more useful in infants and children up to 2 years of age.[91,92]

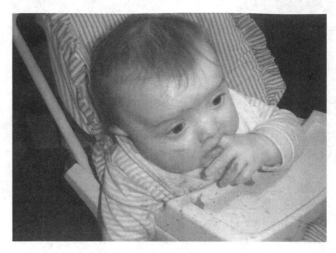

Eating solid foods after months of liquids is enjoyable.

## Introduction to Solid Food

Weaning is the ending of breastfeeding or bottle-feeding and substitution of food for breast milk or infant formula. The AAP recommends that solid foods be introduced between the ages of 4 and 6 months.[93] This range allows for differences in growth and development among babies. **TABLE 8-11** presents suggestions for adequate supplemental foods for infants.

## Water

Infants have higher **insensible water losses** (the continual loss of body water by evaporation from the respiratory tract and diffusion through the skin) as well as a higher overall metabolic rate. They are more susceptible to developing dehydration from vomiting and diarrhea, especially if solute intake is high, as it is in cow's milk. Infants need 1.5 ml of water per kilocalorie consumed. Human milk fulfills this need, and properly prepared formula accomplishes the same task. Foods high in protein or electrolytes, such as meat and eggs, may cause dehydration if offered without water.[96] Water should be offered to infants regularly once they are eating solid food (2 to 4 oz twice a day). **TABLE 8-12** presents some rules for introducing solid foods.

## ▶ Nutrient Needs During Infancy

### Energy

Because of the rapid growth that occurs during infancy, babies' energy and nutritional requirements are always changing. As mentioned earlier, infants usually double their birth weight by 4 to 6 months and triple it by 1

**TABLE 8-11** Age-Specific Introduction of Food[91,92,94,95]

| Food | Amounts | Age of Introduction |
|---|---|---|
| Breast milk or formula | 16-32 oz/day | 0-4 months |
| Iron-fortified baby cereal, rice, barley, oatmeal (start with rice cereal) Human milk or formula | 1 Tbsp cereal mixed with human milk or formula; gradually increase the amount of cereal to 3-4 Tbsp once or twice per day 24-32 oz per day | 4-6 months |
| Strained or pureed vegetables plus fruits such as mashed bananas, pears, applesauce, and fruit juices Toast or teething biscuits, iron-fortified cereal Human milk or formula Water | Vegetables, 2 Tbsp twice per day and fruits, 2 Tbsp twice a day; fruit juices 1-2 oz twice per day 2-4 Tbsp twice per day 24-32 oz per day 2-4 oz twice per day | 6-8 months |
| Strained meats | 1-2 Tbsp twice a day | 6-8 months |
| Egg yolk, yogurt | 1-2 Tbsp per day | 6-8 months |
| Well-cooked, soft, bite-sized pieces of meats Fruit juices Vegetables, carrots, banana, applesauce, spinach, squash Soft breads, infants' cereal, creamed rice, and other finger foods Human milk or formula Water | 2-3 Tbsp per day 1-2 oz twice per day 2-4 Tbsp twice per day 2-3 Tbsp twice per day 16-32 oz per day 2-4 oz per day | 9-10 months |
| Egg white; small tender pieces of meat, chicken, or fish; mild cheese; cooked dried beans Infants' cereals, bread, rice, noodles Cooked vegetable pieces and all fresh fruits, peeled and seeded Human milk or formula Water | 1 oz or ¼ cup twice per day 2-4 servings per day ¼ cup twice per day 16-32 oz per day 2-4 oz per day | 12 months |

year.[88,91,96] Infants require approximately 108 kcal/kg of body weight per day from birth to 6 months, approximately 650 kcal/day. The recommended amount of calories for infants 6 to 12 months is 98 to 100 kcal/kg body weight, approximately 850 kcal/day.[80] Infants need a higher energy intake than adults because the resting metabolic rates of infants and their needs for growth and development are very high. A normal infant pulse rate is 120 to 150 beats per minute, and their normal respiratory rate is 30 to 50 breaths per minute.[94] Because of the large proportion of skin surface to body size, temperature regulation takes significant energy.

In addition, an activity such as crying may double the infant's energy expenditure.[90,94]

## Protein

The recommended amount of protein for infants birth to 6 months is approximately 2.2 g/kg body weight, and for 6 to 12 months is 1.6 g/kg body weight. It is important to include the nine essential amino acids; any deficiency in any of the amino acids can cause growth retardation.[95] The protein in breast milk is easy to digest and contains all the essential amino acids infants need.

| **TABLE 8-12** Some Rules for Introducing Solid Foods[6,38,95,102] | |
|---|---|
| **Actions** | **Alternative Actions** |
| ▪ Introduce one new food at a time for 3 to 5 days, and check for reactions such as stomachaches, diarrhea, skin rashes, or wheezing. Then start with the next food. | ▪ If the child rejects it, try the same food later.<br>▪ Keep diapering areas separate from food preparation areas. |
| ▪ The best first food is iron-fortified infant rice cereal mixed with breast milk or formula. It provides a good source of iron as well as a good distribution of calories, protein, fat, and carbohydrate. Rice cereal is less likely to cause an allergic reaction than other foods. Offer cereal on a spoon, not in a feeding bottle. | ▪ Delay introduction of allergenic foods such as cow's milk, eggs, peanuts, fish, shellfish, soy, and wheat, especially in families with a strong history of allergies.<br>▪ Start with one cereal feed daily until the child is taking two meals daily and getting a daily total of 1/3 to ½ cup. |
| ▪ Avoid adding salt, sugar, and other seasonings or using foods such as hot dogs, canned spaghetti dinners, and canned soups because their high salt content can put an additional load on the infant's kidneys. | ▪ Provide a wide variety of foods. Feeding infants a variety of foods enhances their acceptance of new foods.<br>▪ Offer cereal on a spoon unless medically indicated by conditions such as esophageal reflux. |
| ▪ Avoid putting solid foods in the bottle.<br>▪ Parents should be the first ones to introduce new foods and changes in a child's feeding routine.<br>▪ Wash all fruits and vegetables, and cook meat until juices run clear and no pink remains.<br>▪ Infants younger than 12 months of age should not consume honey or corn syrup because these products can cause a potentially fatal form of food poisoning (spores of clostridium). | ▪ Do not force-feed.<br>▪ Parents should decide and determine how the child will be fed.<br>▪ Delay introducing foods that the child cannot break down easily in the mouth such as popcorn, nuts, hard candy, hot dogs, and raw fruits and vegetables (such as grapes and carrots) because they can lead to choking, especially in children younger than 3 years old. Also avoid peanut butter on bread; it can form a sticky bolus and block the child's airway |

Human milk contains approximately 70 percent whey and 30 percent casein (phosphorus-containing proteins). The whey portion of milk consists of soluble proteins that are easily digested. The major whey protein in breast milk is alpha-lactalbumin, which has an amino acid prototype much like that of the body's tissues. The infant's body can absorb it easily and without much processing; infants use it for building tissue.[94] In comparison, cow's milk contains approximately 18 percent whey and 82 percent casein. Casein forms hard curds in infants' stomach that they cannot digest or absorb.[95]

## Carbohydrates and Fats

Carbohydrates and fats contribute the majority of an infant's energy. The carbohydrate in human milk and in infant formulas made from cow's milk is lactose.[95] Infants digest lactose easily and tolerate it well. Breast milk contains amylase, which is 40 to 60 times more active than in cow's milk.[92] The lactose in milk supplies galactose, which is important for the formation of brain cells.[94]

Fat is important for the development of the central nervous system and provides most of the infant's energy source. Human milk contains alpha-linolenic acid, an essential omega-3 fatty acid that can be converted to eicosapentaenoic acid (EPA) and docosahexaenoic acid (DHA). Research shows that visual acuity and learning abilities correlate with the amount of DHA in the retina and brain phospholipids.[97] Approximately 95 to 98 percent of the fat in human milk is absorbed because breast milk contains the enzyme lipase, which begins the digestion process for the infant.

## Vitamins and Minerals

Vitamin and mineral needs are usually met if the infant is breastfed by a well-nourished mother or receives well-prepared infant formula. Infant formula is fortified with all essential vitamins and minerals according to guidelines established by the AAP and enforced by the FDA.

Vitamin $B_{12}$ is needed for the division of cells and normal folate metabolism. Recent research with vegan women showed that they produced milk containing only one-fourth to one-third as much vitamin $B_{12}$ as women consuming a mixed diet.[98] Another research study reported vitamin $B_{12}$ deficiencies in strict vegetarian breastfeeding mothers, which caused severe neurological deterioration in 4- to 8-month-old infants.[99] Mothers who included meat, fish, and dairy products in their diets produced milk that was adequate in vitamin $B_{12}$.[80] However, compared to meat, cow's milk alone is not a good source of $B_{12}$.

Vitamin D is important for calcium absorption and mineralization of bone. However, human breast milk contains more vitamin C and less vitamin D than cow's milk. The vitamin D precursor in breast milk can be converted to vitamin D in the infant's skin if the infant is exposed to sunlight. Therefore, vitamin D deficiency may be a concern for infants who are not exposed to sunlight.[80,94]

Infants need the same minerals as other human beings. The two-to-one calcium-to-phosphorus ratio of breast milk is ideal for calcium absorption, and both of these minerals, along with magnesium, support the rate of growth expected in a human infant. Calcium is needed for tooth development, muscle contraction, nerve irritability, blood coagulation, and heart muscle action. Infants can absorb approximately 67 percent of the calcium in breast milk, compared to 25 percent of the calcium in cow's milk.[92]

Another mineral that is important for the formation of hemoglobin and mental and psychomotor development is iron.[98,99] An infant's fetal iron stores are depleted 4 to 6 months after birth. Therefore, solid food additions at this time will help supply the iron the infant needs. Iron-fortified cereal, eggs, and later meat will achieve this task. Iron-fortified formula and foods were found to reduce the incidence of iron-deficiency anemia in children from homeless families enrolled in WIC.[100,101]

Breast milk contains less iron than cow's milk, but infants absorb about 49 percent of it compared to about 10 percent from cow's milk. Iron absorption from breast milk is better because it contains less protein and phosphorus and more lactose and vitamin C.[92] The bioavailability of zinc in breast milk is about 60 percent, compared to 43 to 50 percent in cow's milk and 27 to 32 percent in infant formulas.[48,102]

## ▶ Nutrition-Related Health Concerns During Infancy

Community nutritionists, parents, and other health-care professionals need to be observant about feeding practices that may cause health-related problems in infants. Some of the health-related problems are due to improper feeding practices and poor nutrient intakes. For example, mothers may replace human milk or formula with large amounts of fruit juice before 6 months of age; use goat's milk that is low in iron, folate, and vitamin C; and not provide a variety of foods to their infants. Other problems include, but are not limited to, feeding bottle tooth decay, iron-deficiency anemia, milk allergies, and failure to thrive.

### Feeding Bottle Tooth Decay

Tooth decay during infancy, also known as **dental caries**, is linked to putting infants to bed with bottles filled with milk, juice, or other carbohydrate-rich fluids that nourish decay-producing bacteria. The upper teeth are affected most because the tongue protects the lower teeth. The following will prevent feeding bottle tooth decay.[80,94]:

- Avoid giving a bottle filled with human milk, formula, or juice to quiet the infant or to encourage sleep.
- Encourage the infant to sleep by holding the baby snugly and creating a gentle, regular motion/rocking. (Other options are reading, or rubbing or patting the infant's back while holding him or her on the shoulder and chest.)
- Clean the infant's gums and teeth twice a day using a washcloth on the gums and a soft toothbrush with water on the teeth.
- Introduce a drinking cup at 6 months and provide juice in a cup instead of a bottle, limiting juice to 4 to 6 ounces per day.
- Use fluoridated water, approximately 0.8 to 1.0 mg/L parts per million (PPM).

### Iron-Deficiency Anemia

Iron deficiency in infants is not as common as in toddlers. Factors that may cause iron-deficiency anemia in infants are inadequate dietary iron intake, too much milk feeding (known as milk anemia), and not enough iron-fortified solid foods.[101,102] The onset of anemia is common in infants after their fourth month, when iron stores are depleted, their birth weight has increased, and they are synthesizing new red blood cells daily.[48]

The Pediatric Nutrition Surveillance System (PedNSS) reported that the highest prevalence of anemia in the United States was in children younger than 2 years; the prevalence decreased as the children grew older. The rate of anemia was high in infants ages 6 to 11 months (16.2 percent) and children ages 12 to 17 months (15.0 percent). The rate of anemia varied among racial and ethnic groups. African American children had the highest rate of anemia (19 percent). The overall prevalence of anemia in children in the United States decreased from 14 percent in 2010.[103]

The Healthy People 2010 objectives (19.12c and 19.13) are to reduce iron deficiency to less than 7 percent among females ages 12 to 49 years and to reduce anemia among low-income pregnant females in their third trimester. The progress data show a decrease of 13 percent in 2006.

## Milk Allergy

The risk for infants developing allergies doubles if a parent or sibling has allergies.[104] An infant may develop a food allergy to the protein in a cow milk–based formula over time. In a healthy infant, protein is broken down during digestion and allergy may result when small groups of two or three amino acids are absorbed in the small intestine. In some cases, the intestinal lining may allow larger chains of amino acids to be absorbed, triggering a reaction.[105]

The absorption of intact protein fragments is the basis for allergic reactions. When this happens with cow milk protein, the infant can be switched to a soy-based formula. In cases in which soy formula still produces an allergic reaction, the infant can be switched to a predigested protein formula. Approximately 6 to 8 percent of children younger than 4 years of age have allergies that started in infancy.[105] The most common allergic reactions are respiratory tract and skin symptoms, such as wheezing or skin rashes.[106]

## Failure to Thrive

**Failure to thrive (FTT)** is a term used when a decrease in or slow physical growth is observed over time using a national standard growth chart. Although the definitions of FTT vary, most practitioners diagnose FTT when a child's weight for age falls below the fifth percentile of the standard National Center for Health Statistics (NCHS) growth chart. Conversely, weight for height above the 95th percentile signifies a child who is overweight.[108] FTT is mainly used to describe conditions resulting from failure to obtain or use necessary calories.[107] FTT can occur in all socioeconomic strata, but it is more common in families living in poverty.[108]

Different classification systems have been developed to identify the reasons for FTT in children, such as organic (meaning a diagnosed medical illness is the basis), nonorganic (meaning not based on a medical diagnosis), or a mixed FTT. Nonorganic FTT is generally due to a variety of environmental and psychosocial factors. It is associated with interactions between the primary caregiver and the infant. Any disturbance in the relationship between the primary caregiver and the

infant can result in an inadequate provision of food. The following are some of the causes of nonorganic FTT[103]:

- Poor feeding or feeding-skills disorder
- Dysfunctional family interactions and difficult parent–child interactions
- Lack of preparation for parenting and lack of support (e.g., no friends, no extended family)

Organic FTT refers to growth failure due to an acute or chronic disorder known to interfere with normal nutrient intake, absorption, metabolism, or excretion or known to result in increased energy requirements to sustain and promote growth. The following are some examples of the causes of organic FTT[109]:

- Maternal malnutrition, alcohol use, smoking, medications, and infections during pregnancy
- Inborn error of metabolism

In mixed FTT, organic and nonorganic FTT overlap. The physician will determine each of the contributing factors to the child's abnormal growth. Mixed FTT is diagnosed in children who were born prematurely and who have evidence of disproportionate growth failure later in infancy and in those who have a deformity.[109]

The role of the dietitian is to assess the infant's growth and nutritional adequacy, establish a care plan, and provide follow-up as part of a team approach. The dietitian may work with other health specialists and work on medical or psychological aspects of treatment. One of the goals for the management of FTT is to increase the infant's growth rate. The median expected increase in weight per day for infants is summarized in **TABLE 8-13**. On average, infants gain 1 kg/month for the first 3 months, 0.5 kg/month from 3 to 6 months, 0.33 kg/month from 6 to 9 months, and 0.25 kg/month from 9 to 12 months.

Children with FTT will need 150 percent of their recommended daily caloric intake, based on their expected, not actual, weight.[109] In infants, this increased caloric intake may be accomplished by concentrating formula or adding rice cereal to pureed foods. WIC also provides

| **TABLE 8-13** Median Daily Weight Gain | | |
|---|---|---|
| **Age** | **Grams** | **Ounces** |
| 0-3 months | 26.0-31.0 | 0.9-1.09 |
| 3-6 months | 17.0-18.0 | 0.6-0.63 |
| 6-9 months | 12.0-13.0 | 0.42-0.46 |
| 9-12 months | 9.0 | 0.32 |

Data from: Bassali RW, Benjamin J. Failure to thrive. http://www.emedicine.com/PED /topic738.htm. Accessed September 27, 2005.

high-calorie milk drinks (e.g., PediaSure). It provides 30 calories per ounce, and one or two cans per day can be used.

# ▶ Methods of Feeding Infants

Breastfeeding is the preferred method for feeding infants and has advantages over other methods of feeding.[108] However, some mothers may prefer to use formula as opposed to breast milk when feeding their infants. Some formulas are prepared according to ethnic or religious practices. Community nutritionists and healthcare professionals need to monitor these formulas closely. Mothers who are on prescription or illegal drugs also may consider using formula to feed their infants,[110] as may mothers who are HIV positive. Research studies indicate that not all women have the same risk for transmitting HIV to their breastfed infants. The factors that may increase the risk for transmission include early mixed feedings, nipple lesions, and mastitis (inflammation of the breasts).[111,112] Guidelines for formula preparation can be found online at http://nutrition.jbpub.com/communitynutrition.

## Breastfeeding and Lactation

Human milk is the best choice for infants. It provides appropriate amounts of energy, nutrients, and **colostrum** that provide protection against infections, and it rarely causes allergic responses. The Academy of Nutrition and Dietetics has issued position statements in support of breastfeeding.[44] The La Leche League, an international nonprofit organization, provides encouragement to women who wish to breastfeed. **TABLE 8-14** presents the major components of human milk and their functions.

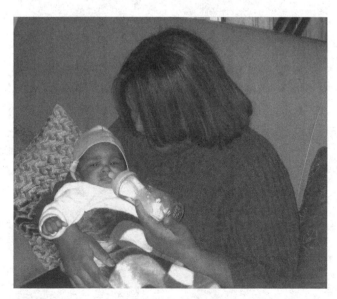

Mothers can use an electric pump to express breast milk. The mother should be instructed to wash her hands and breasts before handling the equipment or pumping. During feeding, the position of the baby and the bottle are both important

Some important changes must occur during the period of **lactogenesis** (transition from pregnancy to lactation) for milk volume to increase. These changes mainly occur from 2 or 3 to 8 days postpartum.[113] Lactogenesis is stimulated by a rapid drop of serum progesterone and maybe estrogen after the delivery of the placenta. It is also accompanied by a significant decrease in breast milk levels of sodium, chloride, and protein and an increase in lactose and milk lipids. The following hormones change during lactation[113-116]:

- A decrease in progesterone levels
- Release of prolactin from the anterior pituitary that stimulates lactogenesis and initiates milk secretion

In some situations, there can be a delay or impairment of lactogenesis on the third or fourth day postpartum. The reason for the delay in breast milk production is not clear in some cases, but it has been attributed to the following[114-116]:

- Cesarean birth
- Labor analgesia
- Obesity
- Premature delivery
- Insulin-dependent diabetes mellitus
- Placental retention (placental fragments)
- Stress

In the United States, the Healthy People 2010 objective for breastfeeding is to increase the number of mothers who breastfeed their babies in the early postpartum period to at least 75 percent. The progress report shows an increase of 74 percent. This Healthy People 2010 breastfeeding goal appears to be reached. However, considerable efforts have been made to achieve the 50 percent goal for breastfeeding up to 6 months and the new 25 percent goal for breastfeeding at 12 months.[117] Reports show that 56.3 percent of all infants are being breastfed at 6 months of age and 77.8 percent are being breastfed at 12 months.[118] The greatest benefits are associated with exclusive breastfeeding for at least 6 months and continued breastfeeding with complementary foods for at least 12 months.[119,120] In an endeavor to achieve these goals, federally supported breastfeeding promotion efforts have continued to expand in number and scope, including the national USDA and WIC social marketing campaign for breastfeeding.

## Barriers to Breastfeeding

Training new mothers in the hospital on how to initiate breastfeeding has the potential to boost breastfeeding, but the implementation of this practice is limited in some U.S. hospitals.[121] Delayed identification and treatment of lactation problems can lead to morbidity and excessive costs.[122] Several sociocultural factors also contribute to

**TABLE 8-14** Major Components of Human Milk and Their Functions

| Cells | Functions |
| --- | --- |
| Phagocytes (macrophages) | Engulf and absorb pathogens; release immunoglobulin A (IgA); polymorphonuclear (any of a group of white blood cells having granules in the cytoplasm) and mononuclear (white blood cells with a one-lobed nucleus). |
| Lymphocytes | T cells and B cells; essential for cell-mediated immunity; antiviral activity; memory T cells give long-term protection. |
| **Antiinflammatory Factors** | |
| Prostaglandins PGE1, PGE2 | Cytoprotective. |
| Cytokines/chemokines | Immunomodulating agents that bind to specific cellular receptors, activate the immune system, promote mammary growth, and move lymphocytes into breastmilk and across the neonatal bowel wall. Transforming growth factor-beta is the dominating cytokine in colostrum. |
| **Growth Factors** | |
| *Enzymes* | Facilitates infant digestion of polysaccharides. |
| Amylase | |
| Lipase | Hydrolyzes fat in infant intestines; bactericidal activity. |
| *Growth Factors and Hormones* | |
| Human growth factors | Polypeptides that stimulate proliferation of intestinal mucosa and epithelium; strengthen mucosal barrier to antigens. |
| Cortisol, insulin, thyroxine cholecystokinin (CCK) | Promote maturation of the neonate's intestines and intestinal host-defense process. Thyroxine protects against hypothyroidism; CCK enhances digestion. |
| Prolactin | Enhances development of B and T lymphocytes. |
| *Lipids (Fat)* | Major source of calories. |
| Long-chain polyunsaturated fatty acids (LC-PUFA) | Docosahexaenoic acid (DHA) and arachidonic acid (AA) are associated with higher visual acuity and cognitive ability; breast milk content depends on maternal diet. |
| Free fatty acids (FFA) | Antiinfective effects. |
| Triglycerides | Largest source of calories for infant; broken down to free fatty acids and glycerol by lipase; types of fat depend on maternal diet. |
| *Lactose* | Carbohydrate, major energy source; breaks down into galactose and glucose; enhances absorption of calcium, magnesium, and manganese. |
| Oligosaccharides | Microbial and viral ligands. |
| Glycoconjugates | Microbial and viral ligands. |

| Cells | Functions |
|---|---|
| *Minerals* | Regulate normal body functions; minimal influence by maternal diet. |
| *Protein* | |
| Whey | Contains lactoferrin, lysozyme, immunoglobulins, and alpha-lactalbumin. |
| Immunoglobulins (SIgA, IgM, IgG) | Immunity response to specific antigens in environment; SIgA pathways to mammary gland called GALT and BALT. |
| Lactoferrin | Antibacterial, especially against *E. coli*; iron carrier. |
| Lysozyme | Bactericidal and antiinflammatory; activity progressively increases starting 6 months after delivery. |
| Taurine | Abundant amino acid; associated with early brain maturation and retinal development. |
| Casein | Inhibits microbial adhesion to mucosal membranes. |
| *Vitamins A, C, E* | Antiinflammatory action; scavenge oxygen radicals. |
| *Water* | Constitutes 87.5% of human milk volume; provides adequate hydration to infant. |

lack of or short-term breastfeeding, including some of the barriers outlined in **TABLE 8-15**.

There are many ways to facilitate breastfeeding and, therefore, support infant health and the mother–infant bond. Providing home visits during the newborn period can compensate for short hospital stays if personnel with training in assessment and management of lactation perform these visits. Rental of an electric pump or purchase of other equipment (all of which are frequently not reimbursed by third-party payers) would be a valuable practice. Supportive work environments where mothers can have the infant present or have access to onsite or nearby facilities for time to pump and store milk would enhance the goal to increase the rate of breastfeeding.[123,125] **BOX 8-7** presents the advantages of breastfeeding and the benefits of breastfeeding for mothers.

## The Mother's Nutritional Needs During Lactation

The nutritional needs for a lactating mother are different from those of a pregnant woman. The best approach is to eat a balanced diet using the Dietary Guidelines for Americans. The diet should supply at least 1,800 kcal per day. Milk production requires approximately 800 kcal every day. Based on an average milk secretion of 750 to 800 mL/day in the first 6 months and 600 mL/day in the second 6 months, the additional daily energy requirements become 640 kcal and 510 kcal, respectively. The reason for recommending 500 kcal daily above prepregnancy levels is because the 4 to 6 lb (2 to 3 kg) of fat retained postpartum can provide the remaining energy needed for lactation. Weight loss of 1 to 4 pounds per month in the lactating mother is appropriate. Significant weight loss that occurs with severe dieting when an energy intake is less than 1,500 kcal/day greatly reduces milk output.[6,80,123]

## ▶ Management and Techniques for Successful Breastfeeding

Early mother–infant contact increases the duration of breastfeeding by as much as 50 percent, and nursing should be initiated immediately after delivery when possible. The guidelines for successful breastfeeding are presented in **BOX 8-8**. Monitoring and assessing infant

**TABLE 8-15** Barriers to Breastfeeding[123,124]

| Barriers to Breastfeeding | Possible Solutions |
|---|---|
| Loss of traditional knowledge and support for breastfeeding | ■ Reposition breastfeeding as a way for a family to establish a special relationship with their child from the very onset of the child's life. |
| Lack of generational breastfeeding experience | ■ Help mothers to breastfeed through mother-to-mother support.<br>■ Provide prenatal exposure to human milk.<br>■ Make home visits 2 weeks after discharge from the hospital.<br>■ Provide postpartum follow-up along with professional intervention.<br>■ Provide support from the pregnant woman's mother and healthcare professionals. |
| Teenage or single motherhood | ■ Communicate the importance of breastfeeding through family members and peers.<br>■ Provide prenatal exposure to human milk.<br>■ Provide home visits 2 weeks after discharge from the hospital.<br>■ Provide postpartum follow-up along with professional intervention. |
| Reliance on childcare outside the home | ■ Healthcare providers should assist mothers in identifying common misperceptions and help mothers work through them. |
| Relatively short-term maternity leave | ■ Companies should institute policies that promote breastfeeding. |
| Inflexible work hours when returning to work | ■ Healthcare professionals and mothers should use a variety of methods and a broad range of outlets, including legislative, policy, and organizational development, and the media to promote breastfeeding.<br>■ They should use grassroots advocacy, professional training and education, peer counselor programs, and direct marketing and advertising to promote breastfeeding. |
| Lack of paid breastfeeding or pumping breaks in the workplace | ■ Employers can contribute to the health of their employees and their families by establishing a policy of support for breastfeeding mothers.<br>■ Mothers can rent an electric pump.<br>■ Encourage mothers to use break times during the workday to express milk, which can be stored and taken home at the end of the day and used for feedings. |
| Prolonged separation from the infant | ■ Employers can provide childcare at the facility.<br>■ Managers should ensure it is possible for staff to take breaks as appropriate. |
| Advertising campaigns that promote early termination of breastfeeding in the first 2 weeks | ■ Distribute educational materials to reach mothers, friends, and relatives at home and in various environments in which mothers and their friends and relatives obtain infant care information. |
| Marketing or providing commercial products during hospital discharge that promote maternal–infant separation, undermine maternal confidence, and contribute to early mixed feedings | ■ Use media as well as grassroots advocacy with a congratulatory tone to stress the importance of breastfeeding.<br>■ Provide postpartum follow-up along with professional intervention. |

## BOX 8-7 Advantages of Breastfeeding for Infants and Mothers[36,77,82,88,92,104,123,126-130]

### Benefits for Infants

- Enhances protection against infectious disease early in life, including infectious diarrhea, lower respiratory tract disease, and middle ear infection
- Reduces overfeeding and decreases the incidence of obesity
- Promotes optimal development of the central nervous system
- Has a low sodium content and a low solute load
- Gathers minerals in breast milk that are bound to protein and are balanced to enhance bioavailability
- Is more economical
- Decreases tendencies toward obesity
- Avoids overfeeding as compared with formula feeding
- Lowers the incidence of constipation
- Provides immunological protection
- May protect against developing allergies later in life
- Avoids risk for allergies associated with cow's milk protein
- Reduces risk for foodborne illnesses
- Facilitates close contact that fosters the mother–child relationship
- Reduces the need for sterilized equipment and formula preparation
- Provides enzymes that aid digestion and absorption of nutrients
- Decreases insulin-dependent diabetes
- Provides generous amounts of essential fatty acids, especially docosahexaenoic acid, and is nutritionally superior to any alternative
- Contains the powerful antibacterial agent lactoferrin, which binds iron and keeps it from supporting the growth of harmful bacteria and fungi in the infant's intestinal tract

### Benefits for Mothers

- Lactation amenorrhea
- Can help regulate maternal weight or fat loss
- Protects against premenopausal breast cancer and ovarian cancer
- Results in more optimal blood glucose profiles in women with gestational diabetes
- Lowers the risk for ovarian cancer by inhibiting ovulation

## BOX 8-8 Guidelines for Successful Breastfeeding[101,120,161,162]

- Examine the breasts and nipples for any potential problems.
  - Explore the rooting reflex by placing light contact over the lips and cheeks with five fingertips.
  - Use a circular massage on the upper lip and anterior gum side for 5 minutes.
  - Continue massage toward the lateral gum side and inside the cheek for 3 minutes.
  - Place pressure on the suckling point (located in the central area of the hard palate behind the upper gum).
  - Apply tactile stimulus to the lower lip with little pressure.
- Inquire about the availability of prenatal breastfeeding classes.
- Seek breastfeeding support groups such as the La Leche League and local lactation consultants.
- Ensure appropriate positioning and latch-on to avoid breast soreness and/or engorgement.
- Schedule early follow-up visits at home or in a clinic setting.
- Nurse the baby at least 8 to 12 times in 24 hours (every 2 to 3 hours).
- Baby should have 4 to 6 wet diapers per day during days 2 to 4.
- Baby should have 6 to 8 wet diapers of light yellow urine per day after day 4.
- Baby should have 4 to 6 stools per day by the first week.
- Baby should sleep at least 2 hours after a feeding.
- Feedings should last at least 10 minutes per breast, but generally not more than 20 minutes per breast.
- The feeling of fullness in the breast signifies change from colostrum to milk.

growth is an important part of identifying potential lactation problems. Healthcare professionals should recognize the following signs and symptoms of insufficient milk[37]:

- Infant lethargy and/or irritability
- Jaundice
- Infrequent defecating or urinating
- Failure to gain weight
- Excessive weight loss (7 to 10 percent of birth weight)

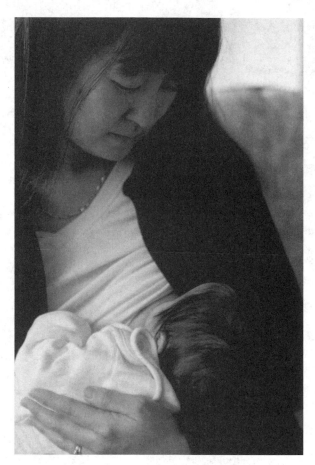

A mother's milk has the needed amounts of fat, sugar, water, vitamins, minerals, and protein for a baby's growth and development. Breastfeeding also helps a mother bond with her baby.

© Kari Weatherly/Photodisc/Getty Images

## ▶ Supplemental Nutrition Programs During Pregnancy, Infancy, and Lactation

In the United States, several resources are available to pregnant women. Some of the resources include programs such as the federally funded Commodity Supplemental Food Program (CSFP), WIC, the Supplemental Nutrition Assistance Program (SNAP), and other emergency food or financial assistance programs described in the following sections, as well as other state and local programs. Clients screened and found to be at nutritional risk can be referred to various federal and state assistance programs, many of which are described in the following sections.

An example of a successful state-sponsored program promoting prenatal care is BabyCal, a public awareness and education campaign carried out by the California Department of Health Services since 1991. The BabyCal outreach program used a statewide network of community-based support organizations (CBSOs), along with a focused media campaign involving pop music and television personalities, to reach low-income expectant mothers with messages stressing prenatal care, a healthy lifestyle during pregnancy, and the importance of infant immunization.[124]

In addition, the CBSOs used various other methods to carry out the BabyCal program. For instance, they conducted health fairs to reach the majority of participants and developed wallet-sized pocket calendars to help expectant mothers keep track of their prenatal appointments. The BabyCal campaign continually explored unique opportunities to support its CBSO network. For example, for BabyCal's 10th birthday campaign, it introduced a 60-minute video designed to help CBSOs educate pregnant women on the importance of prenatal care, healthy behaviors, and the availability of state programs that could help their clients pay for prenatal care services. The BabyCal program increased the rates of participation in prenatal care programs and over the past decade reduced statewide infant mortality by 15 percent.[124]

Another successful public health education and outreach to pregnant women uses current information technology to promote maternal and child health. It is an educational program of the National Healthy Mothers, Healthy Babies Coalition (HMHB) called text4baby. It provides pregnant women and new mothers with information they need to take care of their health and provide their babies the best possible start in life. Text-4baby is made possible through a broad, public–private partnership that includes government, corporations, academic institutions, professional associations, tribal agencies, and nonprofit organizations.[131] Women sign up for the service by texting BABY (or BEBE for Spanish) to receive free text messages each week, timed to their due date. They can stop the messages by texting STOP. Visit http://www.text4baby.org for more information.

### Commodity Supplemental Food Program

The Commodity Supplemental Food Program (CSFP) is a federal food assistance program that works to prevent malnutrition and improve the health of low-income pregnant and breastfeeding women, other new mothers up to 1 year postpartum, infants, and children up to age 6 by supplementing their diets with nutritious USDA commodity foods.[124] The population served by CSFP is similar to that of WIC, but CSFP also serves elderly people and provides food rather than the food vouchers that WIC participants receive. Eligible people may not participate in both programs at the same time.[124]

The USDA purchases food and makes it available to state agencies and Indian Tribal Organizations (ITOs). It also provides funds for administrative costs. State agencies that administer CSFPs are typically departments of health, social services, education, or agriculture. State agencies store the food and distribute it to public and nonprofit private local agencies for distribution to the recipients.[124]

Food packages include a variety of foods, such as infant formula and cereal; nonfat dry and evaporated milk; juice; farina; oats; ready-to-eat cereal; rice; pasta; egg mix; peanut butter; dry beans or peas; canned meat, poultry, or tuna; and canned fruits and vegetables. The most current list of foods is available at http://www.fns.usda.gov/fdd/programs/csfp.

## Special Supplemental Nutrition Program for Women, Infants, and Children

WIC provides food, nutrition counseling, and access to health services to low-income women, infants, and children.[132] It was established as a pilot program in 1972 and made permanent in 1974. The Food and Nutrition Service of the USDA administers WIC at the federal level.

The WIC program is funded as part of the Child Nutrition Program legislation to provide nutrition education and improve the nutritional status of pregnant and lactating women and children up to 5 years of age for low-income families. The new WIC food packages for breastfeeding mothers consist of two packages—one for exclusively breastfeeding mothers to help them establish a good milk supply and encourage new mothers to breastfeed and another package for formula-feeding mothers. WIC regulations require that income and nutritional-risk eligibility criteria be used to certify program participants. Although nutritional-risk criteria are established by each state agency, federal regulations recommend that the individual has medical-based (low hemoglobin levels) or dietary-based (poor diet) indicators of poor nutritional status.[133]

The program involves cash grants to state health departments and comparable agencies that make available supplemental foods and nutrition education through participating health clinics. It is intended to assist low-income persons who are at high risk medically. Studies have shown that WIC participants had lower medical costs for themselves and their babies, longer gestation periods, and higher birth weights. Lower infant mortality, improved children's diets, and decreased incidences of iron-deficiency anemia in children also were observed.[134,135]

Only 65 percent of people eligible to participate in WIC receive services because of lack of funding. WIC can collaborate with other agencies to provide nutrition education and improve the participants' diets. This chapter's Successful Community Strategies highlights the success stories of collaborative efforts. **TABLE 8-16** presents nutritional risk criteria for WIC. Visit http://www.nal.usda.gov/wicworks/ for more information on the new WIC food packages.

## WIC Farmers' Market Nutrition Program

The WIC Farmers' Market Nutrition Program (FMNP) provides vouchers redeemable for fresh fruits and vegetables at farmers' markets. The purpose of FMNP is to increase the awareness and use of farmers' markets to selected participants in the WIC program in addition to their regular WIC benefits. A study entitled Project FRESH examined the effects of the FMNP program on attitudes about buying, preparing, and eating fruits and vegetables; redemption of vouchers; and the number of fruit and vegetable servings consumed. Results showed that FMNP coupons had a direct effect on increasing fruit and vegetable consumption behavior. The maximum impact of the intervention was achieved through a combination of education and vouchers. This study demonstrated that incentives, such as vouchers, might encourage increased fruit and vegetable intake, especially in low-income populations.[138]

## Title V Maternal and Child Health Program

Title V of the Social Security Act provides federal support to strengthen the states' ability to promote, improve, and deliver maternal and child health (MCH) services and programs for children with special healthcare needs, mainly in rural areas and areas of severe economic distress.[139] When the Social Security Act was passed in 1935, the federal government, through Title V, pledged to support states' efforts to extend and improve health and welfare services for mothers and children. Although specific initiatives may vary among the states and jurisdictions using Title V funds, all programs must work to accomplish the activities listed in **BOX 8-9**.[140]

The Maternal and Child Health Bureau (MCHB) is a part of the Health Resources and Services Administration (HRSA) of the U.S. Department of Health and Human Services (DHHS), and it administers the Title V program. Some of the MCHB responsibilities include, but are not limited to, the following[140]:

- Coordinating the MCH Formula Grants to States program
- Promoting coordination at the federal level of the activities authorized under Titles V and XIX of the act, especially early and periodic screening, diagnosis, and treatment programs (EPSDT); related activities funded by the Departments of Agriculture

| TABLE 8-16 Nutritional Risk Criteria for Special Nutrition Program for Women, Infants, and Children[51,92,135-137] | |
| --- | --- |
| **Women** | **Infants** |
| **Nutritional Risks**<br><br>▪ Pregnant women and breastfeeding women determined to be at nutritional risk because of a nutrition-related medical condition (low hematocrit or hemoglobin). Also, underweight (BMI < 19 kg, low maternal weight gain < 0.45 kg/month), or overweight prenatal or postpartum weight gain<br>▪ Failure to meet the dietary guidelines or inappropriate nutrition practices (eating disorder, pica) Pregnant or breastfeeding women at nutritional risk because of an inadequate dietary pattern<br>▪ Alcohol, drug, or tobacco use<br>▪ Dietary deficiencies that impair or endanger health<br>▪ Nonbreastfeeding, postpartum women with any nutritional risk<br>▪ Individuals at nutritional risk only because they are homeless or migrants, and current participants who, without WIC foods, could continue to have medical and/or dietary problems<br>▪ Under the age of 18<br>▪ High parity and young age | ▪ Infants and children determined to be at nutritional risk because of a nutrition-related medical condition<br>▪ Infants up to 6 months of age whose mothers participated in WIC or could have participated and had a serious medical problem<br>▪ Infants and children at nutritional risk because of an inadequate dietary pattern<br>▪ Low-birth-weight or preterm infants<br>▪ Abnormal pattern of growth (short, underweight, overweight)<br>▪ Failure to thrive (low head circumference, underweight, etc.) |
| **Pregnancy Complications**<br><br>▪ Poor pregnancy outcomes (preterm delivery, low-birth-weight infant)<br>▪ Miscarriage or stillbirth<br>▪ Infant with congenital defect<br>▪ Gestational diabetes<br>▪ Neonatal death | |
| **Health Conditions**<br><br>▪ Cancer<br>▪ Depression<br>▪ Diabetes<br>▪ Eating disorders (bulimia, anorexia nervosa)<br>▪ Gastrointestinal disorders<br>▪ HIV/AIDS<br>▪ Infectious diseases<br>▪ Pregnancy-induced hypertension<br>▪ Renal diseases<br>▪ Thyroid disorders<br>▪ Urinary tract infections | ▪ Low hematocrit or hemoglobin (after 6 months of age)<br>▪ High blood lead levels<br>▪ Food allergies<br>▪ Fetal alcohol syndrome<br>▪ Inborn errors of metabolism (PKU, galactosemia, etc.)<br>▪ Otitis media |

and Education; and health block grants and categorical health programs, such as immunizations, administered by DHHS

▪ Administering the two types of discretionary grants: Special Projects of Regional and National Significance and Community Integrated Service Systems

Another federally funded program administered through the MCHB is the Healthy Start Program (HSP). This program began in 1991 to reduce the high rate of infant mortality, especially in U.S. minority groups. For example, the national infant mortality rates in 2006 were 13.4 per 1,000 live births for African Americans,

- Create services to decrease infant mortality and promote maternal, infant, and child health.
- Increase the number of children who are immunized against disease.
- Increase the number of children in low-income households who receive assessments and follow-up diagnostic and treatment services.
- Provide comprehensive perinatal care for women.
- Provide preventive and childcare services, including long-term care services for children with special healthcare needs and rehabilitation services for blind and disabled children under 16 years of age who are eligible for Supplemental Security Income.
- Facilitate the development of comprehensive, family-centered, community-based, culturally competent, coordinated systems of care for children with special healthcare needs.
- Provide nutrition assessment, dietary counseling, nutrition education, and referral to food assistance programs for infants, preschool, and school-age children.

11.1 for those of Hispanic and American Indian origin, and 9.3 for European Americans; the overall U.S. infant mortality rate was 6.0 per 1,000 live births. The high rate of infant mortality is due to limited availability of prenatal care.[143]

The HSP is designed to break down barriers to care by providing accessible, culturally competent, and, in some communities, mobile clinics to minority groups. The program addresses the clients' basic health as well as prenatal care needs and makes referrals for depression or substance abuse screenings. Through the HSP, women learn how to improve their overall health by not smoking or drinking before, during, and after pregnancy. HSP also works within communities by providing resources, such as job employment services, to assist families in finding employment. This program provides services to about 96 communities in 36 states, the District of Columbia, and Puerto Rico.[143]

## Community Health Center

The MCHB also administers the Community Health Center (CHC), which is designed to provide health services and related training to medically underserved areas. The CHC program was launched by the Office of Economic Opportunity in 1966 and was subsequently authorized by Section 330 of the Public Health Service Act. Priority for funding was given to medically underserved areas, particularly those with high infant mortality rates, older populations, and shortages of healthcare personnel. CHCs exist in areas where economic, geographic, or cultural barriers limit access to primary health care for a substantial portion of the population, and they tailor services to the needs of the community.[144]

The main health services include physicians' services, diagnosis, treatment, diagnostic x-rays, laboratory services, and emergency medical care. CHCs provide family-oriented primary preventive services, including prenatal and postpartum care, well-child care, children's eye and ear examinations, immunizations, preventive dental services, voluntary family planning services, health education, and nutrition assessments. They also provide links to welfare, Medicaid, substance abuse treatment, the WIC program, and related services. CHCs also provide pharmacy services as well as related services such as health education, transportation, translation, and prenatal services.[145]

## Supplemental Nutrition Assistance Program

Another program that provides assistance to low-income families is the Supplemental Nutrition Assistance Program (SNAP). SNAP was established as the Food Stamp Program in 1964 to supplement the food-buying power of low-income individuals and families. Monthly allotments of vouchers (Electronic Benefits Transfer card) are provided for approved food items in approved grocery stores. SNAP is an entitlement program, which means that clients who meet eligibility criteria are entitled to receive assistance. Eligibility and allotments are based on income, household size, assets, housing costs, work requirements, and other factors. To qualify for SNAP, households must have gross incomes below 130 percent of the official poverty level, and only net income is required for households with elderly people or individuals with disabilities.[146] See Chapter 4 for an overview of the SNAP.

## Personal Responsibility and Work Opportunities Reconciliation Act of 1996

The mid-1990s was a period of welfare reform. Many states had waivers of the rules for the cash welfare program, Aid to Families with Dependent Children (AFDC), before major welfare reform legislation was enacted in 1996. The Personal Responsibility and Work

Opportunities Reconciliation Act of 1996 (PRWORA) removed the entitlement of recipients to AFDC and replaced that with a new block grant to states called Temporary Assistance to Needy Families (TANF).[147]

Although the SNAP was reauthorized in the 1996 Farm Bill, major changes to the program were enacted through PRWORA. Some of the changes included, but were not limited to,[147] the following:

- Placing a time limit on SNAP receipts of 3 out of 36 months for able-bodied adults without dependents who are not working at least 20 hours a week or participating in a work program
- Reducing maximum allotments by setting them at 100 percent of the change in the Thrifty Food Plan (TFP), from 103 percent of the change in the TFP.

In May 2002, the Food Security and Rural Investment Act of 2002 was enacted, including reauthorization of the SNAP. Major changes to the program included the following[146]:

- Restoration of eligibility for SNAP to qualified aliens who have been in the United States at least 5 years
- Restoration of eligibility for immigrants receiving certain disability payments and for children, regardless of how long they have been in the country
- Adjusting the standard deduction to vary by household size and indexing each year for inflation
- Replacing enhanced funding for states with low error rates with a performance bonus system based on several different measures of performance
- Providing states with several options to simplify the program, including aligning the definition of income and/or resources to that used in TANF or Medicaid, adopting a simplified reporting system, and providing transitional benefits for clients leaving TANF

## Electronic Benefits Transfer

Households used to receive monthly allotments in the form of vouchers from state welfare or human services agencies that were redeemable for food at authorized grocery stores. However, since October 2002, benefits are issued to recipients in an electronic form known as the Electronic Benefits Transfer (EBT) card, which is similar to a bankcard. EBT allows a recipient to authorize transfer of their government benefits from a federal account to a retailer account to pay for products received. The EBT keeps an electronic record of all transactions and makes fraud easier to detect. EBT is

> **BOX 8-10** Food Stamp Nutrition Education Program Objectives[145,150]
>
> - Improved self-sufficiency of food stamp recipients
> - Decreased reliance on emergency food resources
> - Increased skills in food budgeting and meal planning
> - Improved diet for the entire family
> - Increased consumption of fruits and vegetables
> - Increased variety of food choices
> - Improved food preparation skills
> - Improved knowledge of safe food practices
> - Increased physical activity
> - Increased promotion of healthy lifestyles for youth as outlined in the *Dietary Guidelines for Americans*

currently being used in the majority of states to issue SNAP and other benefits.[148]

## The Supplemental Nutrition Assistance Program

The Supplemental Nutrition Assistance Program Education (SNAP-Ed) (formerly the Food Stamp Nutrition Education Program) started in 1986. Funding for the program is provided by the SNAP administrative budget. To qualify for the funds, participating states are required to provide 50 percent matching funds. The major goal is to improve the diet and nutrition-related skills of SNAP recipients and their families. **BOX 8-10** presents some of the SNAP-Ed objectives.[147]

## Nutrition Assistance Program in Puerto Rico, American Samoa, and the Commonwealth of the Northern Marianas Islands

The Nutrition Assistance Program (NAP) in Puerto Rico, American Samoa, and the Commonwealth of the Northern Marianas Islands provides food and nutrition assistance to low-income individuals through block grants to territory administrative agencies. The territories provide cash or checks to eligible participants. The NAP replaced the SNAP in Puerto Rico in 1982. The same program started in the Northern Marianas in 1982 and in American Samoa in 1994.[147,149]

## Food Distribution Program on Indian Reservations

The Food Distribution Program on Indian Reservations (FDPIR) began in the 1930s. It originally was known as the Needy Family Program and was the major type of food assistance program for all low-income individuals in the United States until the early 1970s when the SNAP was expanded.[149] The FDPIR provides monthly supplemental food packages to low-income households living on Indian reservations and to eligible American Indian households living in approved areas near reservations. The USDA commodities consist of canned meats and fish products; vegetables, fruits, and juices; dried beans; peanuts or peanut butter; milk, butter, and cheese; pasta, flour, or grains; adult cereals; corn syrup or honey; and vegetable oil and shortening. The participants may decide each month whether they will participate in SNAP or FDPIR. The majority of participants on reservations prefer the Food Distribution Program due to a lack of access to grocery stores.[149]

## The Emergency Food Assistance Program

The Emergency Food Assistance Program (TEFAP) provides commodity foods to emergency kitchens (often referred to as soup kitchens), homeless shelters, and similar organizations that serve meals to low-income individuals. Eligibility criteria are set between 130 and 150 percent of the poverty line for some states.[150] In many states, SNAP participants are automatically eligible for TEFAP. The types of foods the USDA purchases for TEFAP distribution vary depending on the preferences of each state and agricultural market conditions.

## Cooperative Extension Program and Expanded Food and Nutrition Education Program

The Cooperative Extension Program provides hands-on training in homes and community settings for the people of each community, usually through a state university. This program is funded under the USDA and operated in each U.S. state and territory. It has offices at the state land-grant universities and a network of local or regional offices. One component of the Cooperative Extension Program is the Expanded Food and Nutrition Education Program (EFNEP), which provides education tailored to low-income families.[151]

## Medicaid and Early and Periodic Screening, Diagnosis, and Treatment

The Early and Periodic Screening, Diagnosis, and Treatment (EPSDT) service is Medicaid's comprehensive and preventive child health program for individuals under the age of 21. It was established in 1969 by an amendment to Title XIX of the Social Security Act (Medicaid). The Deficit Reduction Act (PL 109-171) of 2005 (enacted February 2006) gave states the option to modify their approach to delivery of services to children enrolled in Medicaid. DRA gave states the option to restructure their approach to benefits under Medicaid without federal waiver and to extend Medicaid to underinsured, moderate-income children with serious disabilities.[152]

The EPSDT was defined by law as part of the Omnibus Budget Reconciliation Act of 1989 (OBRA 89) legislation and includes periodic screening, vision, dental, and hearing services. The EPSDT program consists of two mutually supportive operational components: 1) ensuring the availability and accessibility of required healthcare resources, and 2) helping Medicaid recipients and their parents or guardians effectively use these resources. These components enable Medicaid agencies to manage a comprehensive child health program of prevention and treatment and to seek out eligible clients and inform them of the benefits of prevention and the health services and assistance available. It also enables them to assess the child's health needs through initial and periodic examinations and evaluations and to ensure that the health problems found are diagnosed and treated before they become more complex and their treatment more expensive.[153] Children can be referred for nutrition intervention for growth retardation, iron-deficiency anemia, cardiovascular disease, obesity, and other nutrition-related conditions.[153] Nutrition counseling for these problems is reimbursable. Brochures from the state agency promote EPSDT services and inform clients about how to obtain health and nutrition information and services for children who need them. Following are elements to remember when working with clients[153]:

- *Early:* Identify problems early, starting at birth.
- *Periodic:* Check children's health at periodic, age-appropriate intervals.
- *Screening:* Conduct physical, mental, developmental, dental, hearing, vision, and other screening tests to detect potential problems.
- *Diagnosis:* Perform diagnostic tests to follow up when a risk is identified.
- *Treatment:* Treat the problems observed.

In addition, the OBRA of 1986 (PL 99-509) and 1987 (PL 100-203) gave states the option to expand Medicaid coverage and determine the income eligibility to provide health services to pregnant women, infants, and children up to age 5 with poor medical conditions. The new provisions of Medicaid now provide funding for nutrition assessment, counseling, and education.[154] Table 4-10 in Chapter 4 presents a list of federally funded food assistance programs.

## Successful Community Strategies

### WIC and EFNEP Collaborative Work[148]

The Cook County Expanded Food and Nutrition Education Program (EFNEP) in Chicago partnered with WIC. The purpose of this project was to provide nutrition education to WIC participants and increase clients' fruit and vegetable consumption. They accomplished this goal by partnering with the Cook County jail. The Cook County EFNEP provided seeds and gardening expertise to the prisoners. Then WIC bought the produce from the Chicago Farmer's Market. EFNEP then provided food demonstrations and recipes in the WIC Food Centers throughout the summer. The WIC participants were very receptive to the foods and were eager to try the foods on their own. This project also made a significant positive impact on the prisoners.

# Learning Portfolio

## Chapter Summary

- A mother brings to gestation her previous life experiences, diet, general health and fitness, lifelong dietary habits, and genetic heritage.

- Preconception nutritional status is more important than the mother's diet during the 9 months of gestation.

- Adequate vitamin and mineral intake at least 8 weeks before conception and during pregnancy can help prevent birth defects such as neural tube defects.

- Infant mortality rates can be used to monitor pregnancy outcomes in the population.

- Pregnant and breastfeeding mothers should not drink alcohol or ingest any substance that will harm the infant (tobacco, illegal drugs, etc.).

- Obese women have a greater risk for pregnancy complications, especially gestational diabetes, hypertensive disorders, cesarean deliveries, and postoperative morbidity.

- Pregnant women found to be at nutritional risk can be referred to a nutritionist and to the Special Supplemental Food Program for Women, Infants, and Children (WIC).

- Physical activity is important during pregnancy because research shows that being active can facilitate labor and reduce psychological stress.

- Infants have higher energy requirements than adults because of their rapid growth rate.

- Failure to thrive (FTT) may be queried when an infant's weight for age falls below the fifth percentile of the standard National Center for Health Statistics (NCHS) growth chart.

- Human milk contains all the essential amino acids and nutrients an infant needs.

- The greatest benefits of breastfeeding are associated with exclusive breastfeeding for at least 6 months and continued breastfeeding with complementary foods for at least 12 months.

- In the United States, the Centers for Disease Control and Prevention (CDC) advises women who are HIV positive not to breastfeed.

- Programs such as WIC, the CSFP, and the SNAP are available to low-income pregnant women.

## Critical Thinking Activities

- Examine health statistics and demographic data to identify the rate of infant mortality and maternal mortality in your geographic area. What resources and agencies are available in the area to support pregnant and lactating women? What services are available from federal, state, and local sources?

- Determine the eligibility criteria for women and infants' food assistance programs.

- Working with other students, make appointments with persons in charge of the WIC Farmers' Market Nutrition Program, social welfare agencies, and the Cooperative Extension Expanded Food and Nutrition Education Program to find out what each agency offers, how clients can access the services, who is eligible, how the agency receives funding, and what methods are used to evaluate the agency's ability to meet the needs of its target.

- Identify nutritionists in the community who work with pregnant and lactating women and other vulnerable groups. Invite these nutritionists to come to a class meeting to share their experiences. What constitutes a typical workday? What are the rewards and challenges of working with vulnerable populations? How do they deal with the frustrations and challenges of their work? What advice might they offer to students working with a vulnerable group? How are they involved in political advocacy related to vulnerable populations?

- Imagine a nutritionist working with a vulnerable population making a home visit to a family in an impoverished neighborhood. How have their life experiences and education prepared them (or not) for working in an impoverished neighborhood? What are their expectations? Write and discuss ideas with classmates.

- Discuss welfare reform with other students. How does the welfare system work? Who receives welfare? Who is eligible for benefits? What are the strengths and weaknesses of welfare reform in the United States? What are the financial and personal costs of welfare reform?

- Identify federal and state senators and representatives for your community. What is their position on the issue of welfare reform? How would they restructure the welfare system?

- As a group, design a nutrition education program to explain the importance of prenatal care visits to monitor the growth of the fetus and to prevent maternal complications such as anemia and spina bifida.

- Explain the effects of inadequate folate and iron intake and relate them to preconception care.

- Determine socioeconomic factors that influence eating practices such as income, ethnic food traditions, taboos, cravings, educational achievement, housing, and family situation of clients.

## CASE STUDY 8-1: Teenage Pregnancy and Its Complications

Amy is a 17-year-old who is at 24 weeks of gestation. She is attending high school and lives with the father of her baby. During her health checkup at the community center clinic, she complained of feeling tired most of the time. A blood sample was drawn and analyzed; her hemoglobin level was 8.5 mg/dl and hematocrit was 30 percent. The normal hemoglobin value is 12 to 16 g/dl and hematocrit 37 to 47 percent. Typically, many physiological and biochemical changes occur during pregnancy, but Amy's blood values were lower than what is usual. Amy indicated that she is still smoking three packs of cigarette a day because she is worried about gaining too much weight. She has only visited the community center clinic twice since she found out she was pregnant, and she has stopped taking her prenatal vitamins because one of her friends told her that the vitamins can cause constipation. She continues to wear the clothes she wore before the pregnancy even though the clothes are tight on her. The nurse at the clinic referred Amy to the local WIC program for more assessment. Additional assessment showed that Amy's weight for height (BMI) was less than 18.5, and she had spoon-shaped fingernails on two fingers. The dietitian assessed Amy's dietary intake using a 24-hour recall and the Nutritional Risk Score (see Table 8-8). Her 24-hour recall showed a lack of some of the essential nutrients such as protein, iron, folate, calories, and some vitamins. Amy's Nutritional Risk Score was less than 50. Her daily caloric intake was 1,000 kcal per day. She likes to drink espresso, at least 4 cups a day. Amy's present income is at 185 percent of the U.S. poverty guidelines. The WIC dietitian asked Amy if she wants to breastfeed her baby and if she could attend a workshop on breastfeeding.

### Questions

1. What are some of the Healthy People 2010 Maternal and Infant Health objectives? What are the objectives that have made the most progress that the WIC dietitian should know?
2. What are some of the physiological and biochemical changes that occur during a normal pregnancy?
3. What factors can affect the outcome of Amy's pregnancy? List some of the factors that Amy may be experiencing.
4. Amy's BMI was assessed at less than 18.5. What is the recommended range of weight gain for a woman of her weight and height? What is the typical weight distribution during pregnancy?
5. What is the role of the placenta during pregnancy?
6. What are some of the diet-related complications during pregnancy that Amy should know?
7. What are the guidelines for pregnant women to avoid contracting foodborne illnesses that Amy should know? Why does the U.S. Food and Drug Administration advise pregnant women to avoid consuming large fish?
8. Why is nutrition assessment so important during pregnancy? What would an assessment include?
9. What are some issues in adolescent pregnancy that influence nutritional well-being and need to be addressed in intervention strategies?
10. What are the requirements for energy and protein during infancy for Amy's baby? Why are carbohydrates and fat so important during infancy?
11. What vitamins and minerals are of main concern during infancy, and why should the WIC dietitian explain them to Amy?
12. List three actions and the associated alternative actions for introducing solid foods to infants that Amy might learn during the lactation workshop.

*(continues)*

## 🔍 CASE STUDY 8-1: Teenage Pregnancy and Its Complications (continued)

13. What are some of the nutrition-related health concerns during infancy? Briefly describe each of these health concerns.
14. The WIC dietitian informed Amy that her baby may experience failure to thrive if she did not correct her lifestyle. What are some of the causes of nonorganic and organic failure to thrive?
15. Why is human breast milk the best choice for Amy's baby? What are some reasons why women may decide not to breastfeed?
16. List three possible barriers to breastfeeding and the possible solutions to overcome these barriers.
17. What are some of the signs and symptoms of insufficient breast milk that healthcare professionals should recognize and that Amy must know if she decides to breastfeed?
18. What are some of the benefits of breastfeeding for infants? For Amy and other mothers?
19. What are some of the supplemental nutrition programs available for Amy during pregnancy, infancy, and lactation?
20. What is the Commodity Supplemental Food Program (CSFP)? What foods are included in the food packages provided by the CSFP?
21. List three nutritional risks for Amy and other women and their infants that would qualify them for WIC.
22. What are the activities covered by Title V funds that the dietitian should know?
23. The dietitian explained the Supplemental Nutrition Assistance Program Education Program (SNAP-Ed) to Amy. What are the objectives of SNAP-Ed?
24. What is colostrum, and why is it so beneficial to newborn infants?
25. What are three of the guidelines for successful breastfeeding?
26. Where could Amy be referred to for prenatal nutritional assessment and counseling?
27. What are the consequences of inadequate, absent, or delayed prenatal care?
28. Consuming large amounts of caffeine during pregnancy is discouraged because of its effect on some essential nutrients and on the fetus. What are the negative effects of excessive consumption of caffeine, which nutrients may be affected, and how many cups of coffee should a pregnant woman consume each day?
29. Amy is smoking three packs of cigarette a day. What are the consequences of cigarette smoking during pregnancy?
30. Explain to Amy why dieting during pregnancy is not recommended. What are the functions of calories during pregnancy? List the recommended amounts of calories during the second and third trimesters.
31. Amy's hemoglobin is very low due to inadequate iron intake. What are the consequences of low blood iron? List the foods that Amy should consume to increase her iron intake.
32. Work in small groups or individually to discuss the case study and practice using the Nutrition Care Process chart provided on the companion website. You can also add other nutrition and health-related conditions or assessments to the case study to make the case study more challenging and interesting.

## Think About It

**Answer:** Obese women have a greater risk for pregnancy complications, including gestational diabetes mellitus, hypertensive disorders, cesarean deliveries, postoperative morbidity, gestational hypertension, preeclampsia, fetal death, and possible birth defects. Infants of obese women also may be at greater risk for perinatal death and are twice as likely to be obese and to develop type 2 diabetes later in life.

Weight gain below the recommendations is associated with a risk for preterm delivery and low birth weight; those with weight gain above the suggested range have a higher risk for cesarean delivery and excessive postpartum weight retention. The food assistance programs Mary can recommend are the Supplemental Nutrition Assistance Program (SNAP), WIC Program, WIC Farmer's Market Maternal and Child Program, Community Health Center (CHC), Commodity Supplement Food Program (CSFP), and Medicaid and Early Periodic Screening Diagnosis and Treatment (EPSDT).

## Key Terms

**cesarean section:** Surgical childbirth in which the infant is delivered through an incision in the woman's abdomen and uterus.

**colostrum:** The first fluid secreted by the breast during late pregnancy and the first few days after birth. This thick fluid is rich in immune factors and protein.

**dental caries:** Tooth decay that results from formula or juice (and even human milk) bathing the teeth as the child sleeps with a bottle in his or her mouth.

**eclampsia:** Advanced pregnancy-induced hypertension (PIH) that is characterized by seizures.

**failure to thrive (FTT):** is when a child's weight for age falls below the fifth percentile of the standard National Center for Health Statistics (NCHS) growth chart.

**fetal alcohol syndrome:** The cluster of symptoms seen in an infant or a child whose mother consumed excessive alcohol during pregnancy.

**fetus:** The developing infant from 8 weeks after conception until birth.

**gestational diabetes mellitus:** Diabetes that appears during pregnancy.

**growth chart:** Charts that plot the weight, length, and head circumference of infants and children as they grow.

**head circumference:** Measurement of the largest part of an infant's head to determine brain growth.

**hyperemesis gravidarum:** Excessive vomiting that produces weight loss and dehydration during pregnancy.

**infancy:** The period between birth and 1 year of age.

**infant mortality rate:** The death of an infant under 1 year of age, expressed as a rate per 1,000 live births.

**insensible water losses:** The continual loss of body water by evaporation from the respiratory tract and diffusion through the skin, as well as a higher overall metabolic rate.

**ketone bodies:** The compounds, such as acetone and diacetic acid, formed when fat is metabolized incompletely.

**ketosis:** The physical state of the human body when ketone bodies are elevated in the blood and present in the urine; one example is diabetic ketoacidosis.

**lactogenesis:** The transition from pregnancy to lactation. The growth and proliferation of the ductal tree and further formation of lobules after birth is lactogenesis stage II (days 2 or 3 to 8 postpartum). During lactogenesis II, milk volume increases rapidly from 38 to 98 hours postpartum and then abruptly levels off.

**length:** The proper measurement method of infants and children not yet able to stand.

**low birth weight (LBW):** A birth weight less than 2.5 kg (5.5 lb) at birth; mostly due to preterm birth (born before 37 weeks of gestation).

**menarche:** The onset of menstruation (monthly bleeding); normally happens between 10 and 15 years of age.

**neural tube defect (NTD):** Developmental abnormality resulting in anencephaly (absence of a brain) or spina bifida (spinal-cord or spinal-fluid bulge through the back); related to folic acid deficiency.

**percentile:** Classification of a measurement of a unit into divisions of 100 units.

**phenylketonuria (PKU):** An inherited error in phenylalanine metabolism, most commonly caused by a deficiency of phenylalanine hydroxylase, which converts the amino acid phenylalanine to tyrosine.

**pica:** The practice of eating nonfood items such as dirt, laundry starch, or clay.

**placenta:** An organ that forms inside the uterus early in pregnancy. The placenta transfers oxygen and nutrients from the mother's blood to the fetus; fetal wastes are removed through the placenta, and it releases hormones that maintain the pregnancy.

**prenatal (antenatal):** Occurring before childbirth.

**small for gestational age (SGA):** Full-term newborns who weigh less than 2.5 kg (5.5 lb).

**trophoblast:** The outer layer of embryonic ectoderm that nourishes the embryo or develops into fetal membranes with nutritive functions.

# References

1. Cucó G, Fernández-Ballart J, Sala J, et al. Dietary patterns and associated lifestyles in preconception, pregnancy and postpartum. *Eur J Clin Nutr.* 2006;60(3):364-371.
2. Allen LH. Malnutrition and human function: a comparison of conclusions from the INCAP and nutrition CRSP studies. *J Nutr.* 1995;125(4):S1119-S1126.
3. US Dept of Health and Human Services. *National Health Promotion and Disease Prevention Objectives 2010.* Washington, DC: US Dept of Health and Human Services; 2000.
4. US Dept of Health and Human Services. *Healthy People 2010.* Conference edition in two volumes. Washington, DC: US Dept of Health and Human Services; 2000.
5. US Dept of Health and Human Services. *Healthy People 2020: Maternal, Infant, and Child Health.* https://www.healthypeople.gov/2020/topics-objectives/topic/maternal-infant-and-child-health. Accessed February 26, 2017.
6. William SR, Schlenker ED. *Essentials of Nutrition and Diet Therapy.* 9th ed. St. Louis, MO: Mosby; 2007.
7. Shils M, Olson JA. *Modern Nutrition in Health and Disease.* 11th ed. Baltimore MD: Lippincott Williams & Wilklins; 2012.
8. Huy AT. Biochemical tests in pregnancy. *Aust Prescr.* 2005;28:98-101.
9. Bruinse HW, Vandenberg H. Changes of some vitamin levels during and after normal pregnancy. *Eur J Obstet Gynecol Reprod Biol.* 1995;61(1):31-37.
10. Ackurt F, Wetherilt H, Loker M, Hacibekiroglu M. Biochemical assessment of nutritional status in pre-and post-natal Turkish women and outcome of pregnancy. *Euro J Clin Nutr.* 1995;49(8):613-622.
11. Brown AS, Fernhoff PM, Waisbren SE, Frazier DM, et al. Barriers to successful dietary control among pregnant women with phenylketonuria. *Genet Med.* 2002;4(2):84-89.

12. Centers for Disease Control and Prevention. Extending the successful prevention of mental retardation through newborn screening. 2002. https://www.cdc.gov/ncbddd/newbornscreening/. Accessed February 26, 2017.

13. Riskin-Mashiah S. Preconception counseling: for all. *Harefuah (Harefuah.).* 2004;143(7):530-547.

14. Dietrich M, Brown CJ, Block G. The effect of folate fortification of cereal-grain products on blood folate status, dietary folate intake, and dietary folate sources among adult non-supplement users in the United States. *J Am Coll Nutr.* 2005;24(4):266-274.

15. Botto LD, Lisi A, Robert-Gnansia E, Erickson JD et al. International retrospective cohort study of neural tube defects in relation to folic acid recommendations: are the recommendations working? *Obstet Gynecol Survey.* 2005;60(9):563-565.

16. Carter H, Petrini JR. Use of vitamins containing folic acid among women of childbearing age: United States, 2004. *Morb Mortal Wkly Rep MMWR.* 2004;53(36):847-850.

17. Norsworthy BB. Effects of once-a-week or daily folic acid supplementation on red blood cell folate concentrations in women. *Eur J Clin Nutr.* 2004;58(3):548-554.

18. Krishnaswamy K, Madhavan Nair K. Importance of folate in human nutrition. *Br J Nutr.* 2001;85(2 suppl):S115-S124.

19. Institute of Medicine, Food and Nutrition Board. *Dietary Reference Intakes for Thiamin, Riboflavin, Niacin, Vitamin B-6, Folate, Vitamin B-12, Pantothenic Acid, Biotin, and Choline.* Washington, DC: National Academies Press; 1998.

20. Anorlu RI, Oluwole AA, Abudu OO. Sociodemographic factors in anaemia in pregnancy at booking in Lagos, Nigeria. *J Obstet Gynaecol.* 2006;26(8):773-776.

21. Conrey EJ, Frongillo E, Dollahite JS, Griffin MR. Integrated program enhancements increased utilization of Farmers' Market Nutrition Program. *J Nutr.* 2003;133:1841-1844.

22. Luke B, Leurgans S. Maternal weight gains in ideal twins outcomes. *J Am Diet Assoc.* 1996;96(2):178.

23. Zhu BP. The effect of the interval between pregnancies on perinatal outcomes. *N Engl J Med.* 1999;340(8):589-594.

24. Shetty SS. Determining risk factors for candidemia among newborn infants from population-based surveillance: Baltimore, Maryland, 1998-2000. *Pediatr Infec Dis J.* 2005;24(7):601-604.

25. Sommers AS, Kenny GM, Dubay L. Implementation of mandatory Medicaid managed care in Missouri: impacts for pregnant women. *Am J Manag Care.* 2005;11(7):433-442.

26. Wen SW, Tan H, Yang Q, Walker M. Prediction of small for gestational age by logistic regression in twins. *Aust N Z J Obstet Gynaecol.* 2005;45(5):399-404.

27. Ness RB, Grisso JA, Hirschinger N, Markovic N, et al. Cocaine and tobacco use and the risk of spontaneous abortion. *N Engl J Med.* 1999;340(5):333-339.

28. Tillett J, Kostich L, VandeVusse L. Use of over-the-counter medications during pregnancy. *J Perinat Neonat Nurse.* 2003;17(1):3-18.

29. Kacew S. Fetal consequences and risks attributed to the use of prescribed and over-the-counter (OTC) preparations during pregnancy. *Int J Clin Pharmacol.* 1994;32(7):335-343.

30. Henry A, Crowther C. Patterns of medication use during and prior to pregnancy: the MAP study. *Aust N Z J Obstet Gynecol.* 2000;40(2):165-172.

31. Rubin J, Ferenez C, Loffredo C. The Baltimore-Washington Infant Study Use of prescription and non-prescription drugs in pregnancy. *J Clin Epidemiol.* 1993;46(6):581-589.

32. Rosa FW, Wilk AL, Kelsey FO. Teratogen update: vitamin A congeners. *Teratology.* 1986;33(3):355-364.

33. Ogunyemi DD. The impact of antenatal cocaine use on maternal characteristics and neonatal outcomes. *J Matern Fetal Neonatal Med.* 2004;15(4):253-259.

34. Shankaran SS. Association between patterns of maternal substance use and infant birth weight, length, and head circumference. *Pediatrics.* 2004;114(2):e226-e234.

35. Zuccato E, Chiabrando C, Castiglioni S, Calamari D, et al. Cocaine in surface waters: a new evidence-based tool to monitor community drug abuse. *Environ Health.* 2005;4:14-20.

36. Wardlaw G, Kessel M. *Perspectives in Nutrition.* 10th ed. New York, NY: McGraw Hill; 2016.

37. Berdanier CD. *Handbook of Nutrition and Food.* New York, NY: CRC Press; 2013.

38. Briggs GG, Freeman RK, Yaffe SJ. *Drugs in Pregnancy and Lactation.* Baltimore, MD: Williams & Williams; 1994.

39. Kaiser LL, Allen L. Position of the American Dietetic Association: nutrition and lifestyle for a healthy pregnancy outcome. *J Am Diet Assoc.* 2002;102(10):1479-1490.

40. Lundsberg LS, Backen MB, Saftlas AF. Low-to-moderate gestational alcohol use and intrauterine growth retardation, low birthweight and preterm delivery. *Ann Epidemiol.* 1997;7:498-508.

41. American Academy of Pediatrics. Parenting corner: breastfeeding Q&A. 2005. http://www.aap.org. Accessed February 24, 2016.

42. US Dept of Health and Human Services, Public Health Service. *Healthy People 2000 National Health Promotion and Disease Prevention Objectives.*

Washington, DC: US Government Printing Office; 1990.

43. Grosvenor M, Smolin L. *Nutrition: From Science to Life*. Philadelphia, PA: Harcourt College Publishers; 2016.

44. US Dept of Health and Human Services. *The Surgeon General's Report on Nutrition and Health*. PHS Publication No. 88-50210. Washington, DC: US Dept of Health and Human Services; 1988.

45. Crosby W. Pica. *JAMA*. 1976;235:2765.

46. Karanja N. Descriptive characteristics of the dietary patterns used in the Dietary Approaches to Stop Hypertension Trial: DASH Collaborative Research Group. *J Am Diet Assoc*. 1999;99(8):S19-S27.

47. US Dept of Health and Human Services. Your guide to lowering your blood pressure with DASH. https://catalog.nhlbi.nih.gov/catalog/product/Your-Guide-to-Lowering-Your-Blood-Pressure-with-DASH/06-4082. Accessed February 27, 2017.

48. Cataldo CB, DeBruyne LK, Whitney EN. *Nutrition and Diet Therapy*. 6th ed. Belmont, CA: Thomson Wadsworth; 2012.

49. Abrams B, Altman SL, Pickett KE. Pregnancy weight gain: still controversial. *Am J Clin Nutr*. 2000;71(suppl):S1233-S1241.

50. Suitor CW. *Maternal Weight Gain: A Report of an Expert Work Group*. Arlington, VA: National Center for Education in Maternal and Child Health; 1997.

51. Institute of Medicine. *Nutrition During Pregnancy and Lactation: An Implementation Guide*. Washington, DC: National Academies Press; 1992.

52. Schieve LA, Cogswell ME, Scanlon KS. An empiric evaluation of the Institute of Medicine's pregnancy weight gain guidelines by race. *Obstet Gynecol*. 1998;91:878-884.

53. Scholl TO, Hedinger ML, Schall JI. Gestational weight gain, pregnancy outcome and postpartum weight retention. *Obstet Gynecol*. 1995;86(3):423-427.

54. Villamor E, Cnattingius S. Interpregnancy weight change and risk of adverse pregnancy outcomes: a population-based study. *Lancet*. 2006;368(9542):1164-1170.

55. Centers for Disease Control and Prevention. Maternal and infant health research: pregnancy complications. http://www.cdc.gov/. Accessed February 26, 2016.

56. Borrelli FC, Capasso R, Aviello G, Pittler MH, et al. Effectiveness and safety of ginger in the treatment of pregnancy-induced nausea and vomiting. *Obstet Gynecol*. 2005;105(4):849-856.

57. Klebanoff MA, Levine RJ, DerSimonian R, Clemens JD, et al. Maternal serum paraxanthine, a caffeine metabolite, and the risk of spontaneous abortion. *N Engl J Med*. 1999;341:1639-1644.

58. Louik C, Hernandez-Diaz S, Werler MM, Mitchell A. Nausea and vomiting in pregnancy: maternal characteristics and risk factors. *Paediatr Perinatal Epidemiol*. 2006;20:270-278.

59. Prather CCM. Pregnancy-related constipation. *Curr Gastroenterol Rep*. 2004;6(5):402-404.

60. Casanova BF, Sammel MD, Macones GA. Development of a clinical prediction rule for iron deficiency anemia in pregnancy. *Am J Obstet Gynecol*. 2005;193(2):460-466.

61. Scholl T, Hediger ML, Bendich A, Schall JI, et al. Use of multivitamin/mineral prenatal supplements: influence on the outcome of pregnancy. *Am J Epidemiol*. 2000;146:134-141.

62. Allen LH. Biological mechanisms that might underlie iron's effects on fetal growth and preterm birth. *J Nutr*. 2001;131:S581-S589.

63. Allen HL. Anemia and iron deficiency: effects on pregnancy outcome. *Am J Clin Nutr*. 2000;71(5):S1280-S1284.

64. Williams DR. Racial/ethnic variations in women's health: the social embeddedness of health. *Am J Public Health*. 2002;92(4):588-597.

65. Lozoff B, Jimenez E, Smith JB. Double burden of iron deficiency in infancy and low socioeconomic status: a longitudinal analysis of cognitive test scores to age 19 years. *Arch Pediatr Adolesc Med*. 2006;1609(11):1108-1113.

66. Academy of Nutrition and Dietetics. Nutrition and women's health: position paper. 2016. http://www.eatright.org. Accessed July 12, 2016.

67. Belizán JM, Villar J, Gonzalez L. Calcium supplementation to prevent hypertensive disorders of pregnancy. *N Engl J Med*. 1991;325:1399-1405.

68. King H. Epidemiology of glucose intolerance and gestational diabetes in women of childbearing age. *Diabetes Care*. 1998;21(suppl 2):B9-B13.

69. Gellin B, Broome C, Bibb W, Weaver R, et al. The epidemiology of listeriosis in the United States: 1986—Listeriosis Study Group. *Am J Epidemiol*. 1991;133(4):392-401.

70. Voetsch AC, Angulo FJ, Jones TF, Moore MR, et al. Reduction in the incidence of invasive listeriosis in foodborne diseases active surveillance network sites 1996-2003. *Clin Infect Dis*. 2007;44(4):513-520.

71. Evans EC. The FDA recommendations on fish intake during pregnancy. *J Obstet Gynecol Neonatal Nurs*. 2002;31(6):715-720.

72. Raichel LL. Maternal obesity as a risk factor for complications in pregnancy, labor and pregnancy outcomes. *Harefuah*. 2005;144(2):107-111.

73. Bonapace FS, Fisher RS. Constipation and diarrhea in pregnancy. *Gastroenterol Clin North Am*. 1998;279(1):197-211.

74. Centers for Disease Control and Prevention. Multistate outbreak of listeriosis: United States. *Morb Mortal Wkly Rep MMWR*. 1998;47(50):1085-1086.

75. Food Safety and Inspection Service. Listeriosis and pregnancy: what is your risk? 2016. http://www.fsis.usda. Accessed September 27, 2016.

76. US Dept of Agriculture of Health Human Services. *Dietary Guidelines for Americans*. Washington, DC: US Government Printing Office; 2000.

77. Brabin BB. Anaemia prevention for reduction of mortality in mothers and children. *Trans R Soc Trop Med Hyg*. 2003;97(1):36-38.

78. Trissler RJT. The child within: a guide to nutrition counseling for pregnant teens. *J Am Diet Assoc*. 1999;99:516-520.

79. American Academy of Pediatrics. Committee on Adolescence Adolescent Pregnancy: current trends and issues. *Pediatrics*. 1999;103:516-520.

80. Worthington-Roberts B, Williams SR. *Nutrition Throughout the Life Cycle*. 4th ed. St. Louis, MO: Mosby; 2000.

81. Centers for Disease Control and Prevention. State-specific pregnancy and birth rates among teenagers: United States 1991-1992. *Morb Mortal Wkly Rep MMWR*. 1995;44:677-684.

82. Kirby D. *No Easy Answers: Research Findings on Programs to Reduce Teen Pregnancy*. Washington, DC: The National Campaign to Prevent Teen Pregnancy; 1997.

83. Clapp JF. The effect of continuing regular endurance exercise on the physiologic adaptations to pregnancy and pregnancy outcome. *Am J Sports Med*. 1996;24:S28-S29.

84. Bodnar L, Catov J, Zmuda J, Cooper ME, et al. Maternal serum 25-hydroxyvitamin D concentrations are associated with small-for-gestational age births in white women. *J Nutr*. 2010;140(5):999-1006.

85. National Center of health Statistics. New CDC report shows record low infant mortality rate. 2016. http://www.cdc.gov/nchs/pressroom/03facts/lowinfant.htm. Accessed February 28, 2016.

86. Maternal and Child Health Library. Knowledge path: infant mortality. https://nnlm.gov/sea/newsletter/2010/09/reviewers-needed-maternal-and-child-health-library-mortality-and-pregnancy-loss-resource-guides/. Accessed February 27, 2017.

87. Harvard Public Health Review. Bringing up baby better. 2002. http://www.hsph.harvard.edu/. Accessed February 25, 2011.

88. Goodell SL, Wakefield DB, Ferris AM. Rapid weight gain during the first year of life predicts obesity in 2-3 year olds from a low-income, minority population. *J Community Health*. 2009;34(5):370-375.

89. Trahms CM, Pipes P. *Nutrition in Infancy and Childhood*. 6th ed. New York, NY: WCB/McGraw-Hill; 1997.

90. Story M, Holt K. *Bright Futures in Practice: Nutrition Pocket Guide*. Washington, DC: Georgetown University: National Center for Education in Maternal and Child Health; 2002.

91. Worthington P. *Practical Aspects of Nutritional Support: An Advance Practice Guide*. Philadelphia, PA: Saunders; 2004.

92. Insel P, Ross D, McMahon K, Bernstein M. *Nutrition 2002 Update*. 5th ed. Sudbury, MA: Jones & Bartlett Learning; 2014.

93. American Academy of Pediatrics. Breastfeeding and the use of human milk. 2016. http://pediatrics.aappublications.org/content/early/2012/02/22/peds.2011-3552. Accessed February 27, 2017.

94. Kennedy E, Goldberg J. What are American children eating: implication for public policy. *Nutr Rev*. 1995;53:111-126.

95. Lutz C, Przytulski K. *Nutrition and Diet Therapy*. 5th ed. Philadelphia, PA: F.A. Davis; 2010.

96. Skinner JD, Carruth BR, Houck K, Moran J, et al. Transitions in infant feeding during the first year of life. *J Am Coll Nutr*. 1997;16(3):209-214.

97. Hamosh M. Digestion in the newborn. *Clin Perinatol*. 1996;23(2):191-209.

98. Hoffman DR, Birch EE, Castañeda YS, Fawsett SL, et al. Visual function in breast-fed term infants weaned to formula with or without long chain polyunsaturates at 4 to 6 months: a randomized clinical trial. *J Pediatr*. 2003;142(6):669-677.

99. Holst MC. Developmental and behavioral effects of iron deficiency anemia in infants. *Nutr Today*. 1998;33(1):27-36.

100. Hurtado EK, Hartl AH, Claussen A, Scott KG. Early childhood anemia and mild or moderate mental retardation. *Am J Clin Nutr*. 1999;69(1):115-119.

101. Partington S, Nitzke S, Csete J. The prevalence of anemia in a WIC: a comparison by homeless experience. *J Am Diet Assoc*. 2000;100:469-471.

102. Fomon SJ. Infant feeding in the 20th century: formula and beikost. *J Nutr*. 2001;131(2):409S-420S.

103. Soh P, Ferguson JE, McKenzie JE, Homs MY, et al. Iron deficiency and risk factors for lower iron stores in 6-24-month old New Zealanders. *Eur J Clin Nutr*. 2004;58(1):71-79.

104. Polhamus B, Dalenius K, Thompson D, Scanlon K, et al. *Pediatric Nutrition Surveillance 2003*. Atlanta, GA: US Dept of Health and Human Services, Centers for Disease Control and Prevention; 2004.

105. Garcia-Careaga M, Kerner JA. Gastrointestinal manifestations of food allergies in pediatric patients. *Nutr Clin Pract*. 2005;20(5):526-535.

106. Sicherer SH, Morrow EH, Sampson HA. Dose-response in double-blind, placebo-controlled oral food challenges in children with atopic dermatitis. *J Allergy Clin Immunol.* 2000;105:582-586.

107. Peroni DG, Piacentini GL, Bondini A, Rigotti E, et al. Prevalence and risk factors for atopic dermatitis in preschool children. *Br J Dermatol.* 2008;158(3):539-543.

108. Krugman SD. Failure to thrive. *Am Fam Physician.* 2003;68(5):879-884.

109. Bassali RW, Benjamin J. Failure to thrive. *eMedicine.* 2006. http://emedicine.medscape.com/article/985007-overview. Accessed February 16, 2017.

110. Laurence RM, Lawrence RA. Benefits, risks, and alternatives. *Curr Opin Obstet Gynecol.* 2000;12(6):519-524.

111. Dobson B, Murtaugh M. Position of the American Dietetic Association: breaking the barriers to breastfeeding. *J Am Diet Assoc.* 2001;101(10):11213-11220.

112. Embree JE, Njenga S, Datta P, Nagelkerke NJ, et al. Risk factors for postnatal mother-child transmission of HIV-1. *AIDS.* 2000;14(16):2535-2541.

113. Coutsoudis A, Pillay K, Kuhn L, Spooner E, et al. Method of feeding and transmission of HIV-1 from mothers to children by 15 months of age: Prospective cohort study from Durban, South Africa. *AIDS.* 2001;15(3):379-387.

114. Riordan J, Wambach K. *Breastfeeding and Human Lactation.* 4th ed. Sudbury, MA: Jones & Bartlett Learning; 2010.

115. Grajeda R, Perez-Escamilla R. Stress during labor and delivery is associated with delayed onset of lactation among urban Guatemalan women. *J Nutr.* 2002;132:3055-3060.

116. Hover K, Barbalinardo L, Pia Platia M. Delayed lactogenesis 2 secondary to gestational ovarian theca lutein cysts in two normal singleton pregnancies. *J Hum Lact.* 2002;18(3):264-268.

117. Sozmen M. Effects of early suckling of cesarean-born babies on lactation. *Biol Neonate.* 1992;62:67-68.

118. US Dept of Health and Human Services. *Healthy People 2010: Understanding and Improving Health.* 2nd ed. Washington, DC: Dept of Health and Human Services; 2000.

119. Ruowei L, Zhen Z, Mokdad A, Barker L, et al. Prevalence of breastfeeding in the United States: the 2001 National Immunization Survey. *Pediatrics.* 2003;111(5):1198-1201.

120. Raisler JA, Alexander C, O'Campo P. Breastfeeding: a dose-response relationship? *J Am Public Health.* 1999;89:25-30.

121. Kramer MS, Chalmers B, Hodnett ED, Sevkovsekaya Z, et al. Promotion of breastfeeding intervention trial (PROBIT): a randomized trial in the Republic of Belarus. *JAMA.* 2001;285(4):413-420.

122. World Health Organization. *Protecting Promoting and Supporting Breastfeeding: the Special Role of Maternity Services—A Joint WHO/UNICEF Statement.* Geneva, Switzerland: World Health Organization, United Nations International Childrens Fund; 1998.

123. Gielen AC, Faden RR, O'Campo P, Brown CH, et al. Maternal employment during the early period: effects on initiation and continuation of breastfeeding. *Pediatrics.* 1991;87:298-305.

124. Hills-Bonczyk SG, Avery MD, Savik K, Potter S, et al. Women's experiences with combining breastfeeding and employment. *J Nurse Midw.* 1993;38(5):257-266.

125. Cooper WO, Atherton HD, Kahana M, Kotagal UR. Increased incidence of severe breastfeeding malnutrition and hypermatremia in a metropolitan area. *Pediatrics.* 1995;96(5 Pt 1):957-960.

126. Mai X, Becker A, Liem J, Kozyrskyj A. Fast food consumption counters the protective effect of breastfeeding on asthma in children? *Clin Exp Allergy.* 2009;39(4):556-561.

127. Kleinman RE. *Pediatric Nutrition Handbook.* 4th ed. Elk Grove, IL: American Academy of Pediatrics; 1998.

128. Zavaleta N, Nombera J, Rojas R, Hambraeus L, et al. Iron and lactoferrin in milk of anemic mothers given iron supplements. *Nutr Res.* 1995;15(5):681-690.

129. US Dept of Health and Human Services. *Blueprint for Action on Breastfeeding.* Washington, DC: Office of Women's Health; 2000.

130. Tamborlane WV. *The Yale Guide to Children's Nutrition.* New Haven, CT: Yale Press; 1997.

131. California Department of Health Services. New corporate partners support BabyCal's efforts. Vol. VIII. Sacramento, CA: California Department of Health Services; 1999.

132. Text4baby. Educational program. http://www.text4baby.org/. Accessed February, 2011.

133. Boyle MA, Holben D. *Community Nutrition in Action: An Entrepreneurial Approach.* 4th ed. Belmont, CA: Thomson Wadsworth; 2013.

134. Kaufman M. *Nutrition in Promoting the Public's Health: Strategies, Principles, and Practice.* Sudbury, MA: Jones & Bartlett; 2009.

135. US Dept of Agriculture. Continuing survey of food intakes by individuals 1994-1996. Vol (CD-ROM) NITIS. Washington, DC: Agricultural Research Service; 2000.

136. Food and Nutrition Board. WIC nutrition risk criteria: a scientific assessment. In: *Committee*

*on Scientific Evaluation of WIC Nutrition Risk Criteria.* Washington, DC: National Academy Press; 1996.

137. US Dept of Agriculture Food and Nutrition Service. WIC program fact sheet. http://www.fns .usda.gov/. Accessed February 25, 2016.

138. Rose D, Habicht J-P, Devaney B. Household participation in the Food Stamp and WIC programs increases the nutrient intakes of preschool children. *J Nutr.* 1998;128:548-555.

139. Anderson JV, Bybee DI, Brown RM, McLean DF, et al. 5 a day fruit and vegetable intervention improves consumption in a low income population. *J Am Diet Assoc.* 2001;101(2):195-202.

140. US Dept of Health and Human Services. The report of the select panel for the promotion of child helath better health for our children: a national strategy analysis and recommendations for selected federal programs. Vol 2. Washington, DC: US Dept of Health and Human Service. PHS 79-55071; 1981.

141. US Dept of Health and Human Services. *The Report of the Select Panel for the Promotion of Child Health Better Health for Our Children: A National Strategy Analysis and Recommendations for Selected Federal Programs.* Vol 2. 79-55071. Washington, DC: US Dept of Health and Human Services, Public Health Service; 1981.

142. US Health Resources and Services Administration. Maternal and child health. http://bhpr.hrsa .gov/kidscareers/community_hc_program.htm. Accessed September 17, 2005.

143. US Health Resources and Services Administration. Understanding Title V of the Social Security Act. https://mchb.hrsa.gov/maternal-child-health-topics/maternal-and-womens-health. Accessed February 27, 2017.

144. US Dept of Health and Human Service. HHS Awards $80.5 million in healthy start grants to reduce infant mortality. http://www.hhs.gov/. Accessed February 25, 2011.

145. Bhutta ZA, Ali S, Cousens S, Ali TA, et al. Interventions to address maternal, newborn, and child survival: what difference can integrated primary health care strategies make? *Lancet.* 2008;372(9642):13-19.

146. US Health Resources and Services Administration. Community health centers. http://www.bhpr.hrsa .gov/. Accessed February 25, 2016.

147. US Dept of Agriculture, Economic Research Service. Supplemental Nutrition Assistance Program. http://www.fns.usda.gov/snap/. Accessed April 5, 2016.

148. US Dept of Health and Human Services, Administration for Children and Families. The Personal Responsibility and Work Opportunity Reconciliation Act of 1996. https://aspe.hhs.gov/report /personal-responsibility-and-work-opportunity -reconciliation-act-1996. Accessed February 25, 2016.

149. US Dept of Agriculture. Electronic Benefit Transfer (EBT). http://www.fns.usda.gov/. Accessed February 25, 2011.

150. Cooperative State Research Extension https:// articles.extension.org/sites/default/files/North%20 Carolina%20EFNEP%20Success%20Stories.pdf. Service. Expanded food and nutrition education program success stories: collaboration. Accessed February 25, 2017.

151. US Dept of Agriculture. The Emergency Food Assistance Program (TEFAP). https://www.fns .usda.gov/tefap/emergency-food-assistance-program -tefap. Accessed February 16, 2017.

152. US Dept of Agriculture. Cooperative State Research Education and Extension Office. htt:p//www.csrees .usda.gov/. Accessed March 4, 2016.

153. Rosenbaum S, Wise P. Crossing the Medicaid-private insurance divide: the case of EPSDT. *Health Affairs.* 2007;26(2):382-393.

154. Mahan KL, Escott-Stump S. *Krause's Food, Nutrition, and Diet Therapy.* 11th ed. St. Louis, MO: Mosby; 2012.

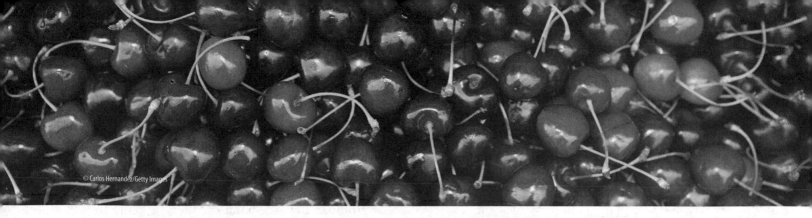

# CHAPTER 9

# Nutrition in Childhood and Adolescence

## CHAPTER OUTLINE

- Introduction
- Nutrition Status of Children and Adolescents in the United States
- Nutrition-Related Concerns During Childhood and Adolescence
- Malnutrition in Children
- Children and Adolescents with Special Healthcare Needs and Childhood Disability
- The Effect of Television on Children's Eating Habits
- Nutrition During Childhood and Adolescence
- Food and Nutrition Programs for Children and Adolescents
- Challenges to Implementing Quality School Nutrition Programs
- Promoting Successful Programs in Schools

## LEARNING OBJECTIVES

- Identify the nutritional needs of adolescents and school-age children.
- Discuss common nutrition problems during childhood and adolescence.
- List the diagnostic criteria for eating disorders in adolescents.
- Discuss the contributing factors to childhood overweight and obesity.
- Explain the causes of malnutrition in children globally and in the United States.
- Discuss the effect television has on children's eating habits.
- Outline different child nutrition programs.

## ▶ Introduction

Maintaining the proper physical, social, and cognitive development of children (ages 1 to 11) and adolescents is essential and depends upon adequate energy and nutrient intake. Children and adolescents who lack adequate energy and nutrient intake are at risk for a variety of nutrition-related health conditions, including growth retardation, malnutrition, iron-deficiency anemia, poor academic performance, protein–energy malnutrition, development of psychosocial difficulties, and an increased likelihood of developing chronic diseases such as metabolic syndrome, diabetes, heart disease, and osteoporosis during adulthood.[1] Children and adolescents who live below the national poverty level are more likely to experience nutrient deficiencies, food insecurity, and hunger.[2,3] In the United States, child nutrition programs subsidize meals served to children and adolescents in schools and other organizations that may help prevent malnutrition. The programs that make up the federal child nutrition programs are the Special Supplemental Nutrition Program for Women, Infants, and Children (WIC), National School Lunch Program (NSLP), School Breakfast Program (SBP), Summer Food Service Program (SFSP), and Special Milk Program (SMP). In addition, low-income families are eligible to enroll in the Supplemental Nutrition Assistance Program (SNAP). These programs will be discussed later in this chapter.

# ▶ Nutrition Status of Children and Adolescents in the United States

The diets of many children and adolescents in the United States are below the recommended dietary standards. A small number of U.S. children eat the recommended amounts of grains, fruits, vegetables, dairy products, and meat or meat alternatives from the MyPlate.[4] The majority of them consume calorie-dense snacks and meals, with added sugars and larger portion sizes, which increase the overall amount of caloric intake.[5-8] Children's total fat, saturated fat, and sodium intake generally are above recommended levels.[5,6] Children and adolescents also consume large amounts of beverages that are high in added sugars, such as soft drinks and fruit drinks.[9] These habits can lead to inadequate intakes of essential vitamins and minerals.

Overconsumption of calories and inactivity are major factors contributing to the increased rate of childhood overweight and obesity in the United States.[10] The prevalence of overweight and obesity in children ages 6 to 17 years has doubled in the past 30 years. Approximately 4.7 million children ages 6 to 17 years are seriously overweight or obese.[10,11] Overweight and obesity at any age increase the risk for type 2 **diabetes mellitus**, cardiovascular disease, and severe social and psychological problems.[11,12] Research shows that overweight and obese children with poor nutritional practices tend to have difficulty learning and concentrating and are more likely to be sick and miss school.[13] **TABLE 9-1** provides examples of fruits and vegetables that parents and caregivers can feed toddlers and preschoolers.

## Healthy People 2010

Two goals of Healthy People 2010 are to increase the proportion of adolescents who participate in daily school physical education to 50 percent and increase the proportion of adolescents who engage in moderate physical activity (> 30 minutes on at least 5 days of the previous 7 days) and vigorous physical activity that promotes cardiorespiratory fitness on more than 3 days per week for 20 minutes per occasion.[14] Report shows slight progress toward these objectives.[15] **TABLE 9-2** presents a progress review for the Healthy People 2010 objectives for children and adolescents.

## Growth and Physical Development and Assessment

After the first year of rapid growth, children's physical growth rate slows down during the preschool and school years until the pubertal **growth spurt** of adolescence.[16] By age 2, children quadruple their birth weight. They gain an average of 4.5 to 6.5 pounds (2 to 3 kg) per year between the ages of 2 and 5 years.[16] In addition, between these ages, children grow 2.5 to 3.5 inches (6 to 8 cm) in height per year.[17] The rate of growth during middle childhood is steady. On average, a 7-year-old child grows approximately 2 to 2.5 inches (5 to 6 cm) per year in stature and about 4.5 pounds (2 kg) per year in weight. By 10 years of age, the increase in weight is approximately 9 pounds (4 kg) per year.

A 1-year-old child has several teeth, and his or her digestive and metabolic systems are functioning at or near adult capability.[16,17] Also by 1 year of age, most children are walking or beginning to walk. With improved coordination over the next few years, their activity level increases noticeably.

The following are some eating behaviors of toddlers[18,19]:

- They can learn to feed themselves independently during the second year of life.
- They can manage to use a cup, with some spilling, at 15 months.
- Two-year-olds prefer foods that can be picked up with their fingers.
- Toddlers tend to be apprehensive of new foods and may refuse to eat them. (Continue to offer the new foods; it takes about 15 times before they will accept them.)
- They tend to play with food and refuse any help from the caregiver or mother.
- Young children are curious about new foods, but may be reluctant to try them.
- Childhood and adolescent eating behaviors are presented later in this chapter.

**TABLE 9-1** Food Guide for Toddlers and Preschoolers[4]

| Food Group | Servings Per Day | Foods | Toddler Amounts | Preschooler Amounts | Nutrients Supplied |
|---|---|---|---|---|---|
| Grains | 6 | Bread, tortilla pieces, waffle squares, noodles, rice, pasta, etc. | ¼–½ slice | ½ slice | Carbohydrates, iron, fiber, and thiamin |
| | | Hot cereal (oatmeal, grits) | ¼ cup | 1/3 cup | |
| | | Cold cereal (ready-to-eat cereal, any variety) | ¼ cup | 1/3 cup | |
| | | | ¼ cup | 1/3 cup | |
| Vegetables | 3–5 | Cooked vegetables (broccoli, peas, sweet potatoes, squash, mushrooms, green beans, winter squash, spinach, etc.) | 2 Tbsp | ¼ cup | Carbohydrates, magnesium, fiber, carotenoids, vitamin A, and phytochemicals |
| | | Raw vegetables (carrot sticks, tomatoes, etc.) | 2 Tbsp | ¼ cup | |
| Fruits | 2–4 | Fresh fruit (raisins, kiwi slices, berries, strawberries, melon, etc.) | 2 Tbsp | ¼ cup | Carbohydrates, vitamin C, potassium, fiber, and phytochemicals |
| | | Fruit juice (apple, pineapple, orange, etc.) | ¼ cup | ½ cup | |
| | | Canned fruit (any variety) | ¼ cup | ½ cup | |
| Milk and dairy products | 3–4 | Milk or yogurt | ½ cup | ¾ cup | Carbohydrates, protein, vitamin D, calcium, and phosphorus |
| | | Cheese (cheese cubes, cheese sticks) | 1 oz | 1½ oz | |
| Meat and poultry | 2–3 | Meat (beef cubes, turkey rollups) | 1 oz | 1½ oz | Protein, vitamin B, iron, zinc, and phytochemicals |
| | | Chicken | | | |
| | | Turkey | | | |
| | | Fish (tuna and salmon without bones) | 1 oz | 1½ oz | |
| | | Cooked beans | 2 Tbsp | ¼ cup | |
| | | Eggs | ½ an egg | 1 egg | |
| | | Peanut butter | 1 Tbsp | 2 Tbsp | |
| | | Nuts | | | |

U.S. Department of Agriculture

## Using Surveys to Monitor Nutrient Intake

The U.S. Department of Agriculture's (USDA's) Center for Nutrition Policy and Promotion (CNPP) developed the Healthy Eating Index (HEI) to evaluate and monitor the dietary status of the U.S. population. The HEI-2005 (see **TABLE 9-4**) represents different aspects of a healthful diet and provides an overall picture of the type and quality of foods people eat, their compliance with specific dietary recommendations, and the variety in their diets. The CNPP used the 2005 Dietary Guidelines for Americans based on the recommendation found in MyPlate, and the recommendations of the Committee on Diet and Health of the National Research Council to formulate the current HEI-2005. The USDA and CNPP revised the HEI so that it conforms to the 2005 Dietary Guidelines for Americans, maximizes variation in individual scores, and standardizes dietary scores.[20,21] The standards were created using a density approach that is expressed as the amount of food and nutrient intakes per 1,000 calories.

The total HEI-2005 score and standards are shown in Table 9-3. HEI-2005 consists of 12 components scores,

**TABLE 9-2** Healthy People 2010 Objectives Related to Children and Adolescents

| Healthy People 2010 Objectives Number | Healthy People 2010 Objective | Baseline (Year) | Progress Review (2002) | Healthy People 2010 Target |
|---|---|---|---|---|
| 19.2 | Decrease the occurrence of iron deficiency among children: a. 1–2 years b. 3–4 years | 9% (1988–1994) 4% (1988–1994) | 7% Not available | 7% Not available |
| 19.3 | Reduce the proportion of children and adolescents who are overweight or obese | 11% (1988–1994) | 16% | 5% |
| 19.4 | Reduce growth retardation among low-income children, 5 years and younger | 8% (1997) | 8% | 5% |
| 19.5 | Increase the proportion of persons age 2 years or older who consume at least three daily servings of fruit | 28% (1994–1996) | Little or no change | 75% |
| 19.6 | Increase the proportion of persons age 2 years or older who consume at least three daily servings of vegetables, with at least one-third being dark green or deep yellow vegetables | 3% | No change | 50% |
| 19.7 | Increase the proportion of persons age 2 years and older who consume at least six daily servings of grain products, with at least three being whole grains | 7% | Little or no change | 50% |
| 19.8 | Increase the proportion of persons age 2 years or older who consume less than 10% of calories from saturated fat | Females 2–11 years: 23% 12–19 years: 34% Males 2–11 years: 23%–25% 12–19 years: 27% (1994–1996) | No change | 75% |
| 19.9 | Increase the proportion of persons age 2 years or older who consume no more than 30% of calories from fat | 33% | No change | 75% |
| 19.11 | Increase the proportion of persons age 2 years or older who meet dietary recommendation for calcium | 46% | Data statistically unavailable | 75% |
| 22.6 | Increase the number of adolescents who engage in moderate physical activity for at least 30 minutes on 5 or more of the previous 7 days | 27% (1999) | 26% | 35% |
| 22.7 | Increase the proportion of the adolescents who engage in vigorous physical activity that promotes cardiorespiratory fitness 3 or more days per week for 20 or more minutes per occasion | 65% (1999) | 65% | 85% |
| 22.9 | Increase the number of adolescents who participate in daily school physical education | 29% (1999) | 32% | 50% |

Data from: National Center for Health Statistics. *Healthy People: Tracking the Nation's Health.* http://www.cdc.gov/nchs/about/otheract/hpdata2010/focusareas/fa16-mich.htm. Accessed August 9, 2016.

**TABLE 9-3** Healthy People 2020 Objectives Related to Children and Adolescents

| Healthy People 2020 Objectives Number | Healthy People 2020 Objective | Baseline (Year) | Progress Review (2020) | Healthy People 2020 Target |
|---|---|---|---|---|
| NWS–10 | Reduce the proportion of children and adolescents who are considered obese | | | |
| NWS–10.1 | Reduce the proportion of children aged 2–5 years who are considered obese | 9.4% (2013–2014) | N/A | 10.4%* |
| NWS–10.2 | Reduce the proportion of children ages 6–11 years who are considered obese | 17.4% (2013–2014) | N/A | 15.7%* |
| NWS–10.3 | Reduce the proportion of adolescents ages 12–19 years who are considered obese | 17.9% | N/A | 16.1%* |
| NWS–10.4 | Reduce the proportion of children and adolescents ages 2–19 years who are considered obese | 16.1% | N/A | 14.5%* |
| NWS–11 | (Developmental) Prevent inappropriate weight gain in youth and adults | | | |
| NWS–11.1 | (Developmental) Prevent inappropriate weight gain in children ages 2–5 years | N/A | N/A | N/A |
| NWS–11.2 | (Developmental) Prevent inappropriate weight gain in children ages 6–11 years | N/A | N/A | N/A |
| NWS–11.3 | (Developmental) Prevent inappropriate weight gain in adolescents ages 12–19 years | N/A | N/A | N/A |
| NWS–11.4 | (Developmental) Prevent inappropriate weight gain in children and adolescents ages 2–19 years | N/A | N/A | N/A |
| NWS–11.5 | (Developmental) Prevent inappropriate weight gain in adults ages 20 years and older | N/A | N/A | N/A |
| NWS–21.1 | Reduce iron deficiency among children ages 1–2 years | 15.9% of children ages 1–2 years were iron deficient in 2005-2008 | N/A | 14.3%* |
| NWS–21.2 | Reduce iron deficiency among children ages 3–4 years | 5.3% of children ages 3–4 years were iron deficient in 2005–2008 | N/A | 4.3% |
| NWS–21.3 | Reduce iron deficiency among females ages 12 to 49 years | 10.5% of females ages 12 to 49 years old were iron deficient in 2005–2008 | N/A | 9.4%* |

*Target-setting method: 10 percent improvement.

Data from: National Center for Health Statistics. *Healthy People Tracking the Nation's Health. Healthy People 2020.* https://www.healthypeople.gov/2020/topics-objectives/topic/nutrition-and-weight-status/objectives. Accessed August 9, 2016.

**TABLE 9-4** Healthy Eating Index—2005: Components and Standards for Scoring*

| Component | Maximum Points | Standard for Maximum Scoring | Standard for Minimum Score of Zero |
|---|---|---|---|
| Total fruit (includes 100% juice) | 5 | ≥ 0.8 cup equivalent per 1,000 kcal | No fruit |
| Whole fruit (not juice) | 5 | ≥ 0.4 cup equivalent per 1,000 kcal | No whole fruit |
| Total vegetables | 5 | ≥ 1.1 cup equivalent per 1,000 kcal | No vegetables |
| Dark green and orange vegetables and legumes† | 5 | ≥ 0.4 cup equivalent per 1,000 kcal | No dark green or orange vegetables or legumes |
| Total grains | 5 | ≥ 3.0 oz equivalent per 1,000 kcal | No grains |
| Whole grains | 5 | ≥ 1.5 oz equivalent per 1,000 kcal | No whole grains |
| Milk‡ | 10 | ≥ 1.3 cup equivalent per 1,000 kcal | No milk |
| Meat and beans | 10 | ≥ 2.5 oz equivalent per 1,000 kcal | No meat or beans |
| Oils§ | 10 | ≥ 12 g per 1,000 kcal | No oil |
| Saturated fat | 10 | ≤ 7% of energy⁵ | ≥ 15% of energy |
| Sodium | 10 | ≤ 0.7 g per 1,000 kcal | ≥ 2.0 g per 1,000 kcal |
| Calories from solid fats, alcoholic beverages, and added sugars | 20 | ≤ 20% of energy | ≥ 50% of energy |

*Intakes between the minimum and maximum levels are scored proportionately, except for saturated fat and sodium (see note 5).

†Legumes counted as vegetables only after Meat and Beans standard is met.

‡Includes all milk products, such as fluid milk, yogurt, and cheese, and soy beverages.

§Includes nonhydrogenated vegetable oils and oils in fish, nuts, and seeds.

⁵Saturated fat and sodium get a score of 8 for the intake levels that reflect the 2005 Dietary Guidelines, less than 10 percent of calories from saturated fat and 1.1 g of sodium/1,000 kcal, respectively.

Reproduced from: Guenther PM, Krebs-Smith SM, Reedy J, et al. USDA Center for Nutrition Policy and Promotion and National Cancer Institute. Available at: http://www.cnpp.usda.gov/HealthyEatingIndex.htm. Accessed October 21, 2016.

each representing a different aspect of diet quality with a minimum score of 0; the highest possible overall HEI-2005 score is 100. An HEI-2005 score over 80 is interpreted as a "good" diet, a score between 51 and 80 is interpreted as a diet that "needs improvement," and a score of less than 51 is interpreted as a "poor" diet.[21] Moderation is recommended for saturated fat (< 10 percent of total energy intake), sodium, and extra/discretionary calories for solid fat, including fat from milk and sugar.[22,23]

The data from the 2003 to 2004 National Health and Nutrition Examination Survey (NHANES) show that children ages 2 to 5 had the highest mean HEI-2005 score over children 6 to 11 and 12 to 17 years old in total fruits, whole fruits, milk, and extra calories. The overall HEI-2005 scores for children were 54.7 (6 to 17 years old) and 59.6 (2 to 5 years old) of a possible 100 points. The likely reasons for the poor-quality diet of older children are a diminished parental role in providing nutritious foods, peer pressure, and increased consumption of fast foods.[23] The consumption of dark green vegetables and legumes ranged from 0.5 to 0.6 of maximum points of 5. Whole grains score ranged between 0.6 and 0.9 of 5 points. The consumption of saturated fat, sodium, and extra calories was approximately 50 percent lower than the maximum scores for all age groups, suggesting that intake levels should be reduced.[21,22]

In the United States, national surveys of dietary intakes are used to determine the types and amounts of food people consume. Wilkinson et al.[23] compared nationally representative USDA surveys of dietary intakes of 6- to 11-year-old boys and girls using the Nationwide Food Consumption Survey (NFCS) 1977 to 1978, the Continuing Survey of Food Intakes by Individuals (CSFII) 1989 to 1991, and the CSFII 1994, 1996, and 1998 to assess whether the trends in children's food intake changed over time.[24-26] (The CSFII and NHANES merged into an integrated survey that acts as the primary source of nationally representative data on dietary intake of foods and nutrients and nutritional status.[27]) Results showed increases in intakes of soft drinks as well as decreases in intakes of total fluid milk due to decreases in whole milk intake. Higher intakes of crackers, popcorn, pretzels, corn chips, and potato chips and higher intakes of noncitrus juices, candy, and fruit drinks were observed. Results also showed lower intakes of yeast breads, rolls, green beans, corn, green peas, lima beans, beef, pork, and eggs.[23] These findings imply that these children were not consuming important nutrients such as vitamins and minerals that can promote growth and development. In addition, this trend of poor-quality diet may be one of the reasons for the high incidence of childhood obesity.

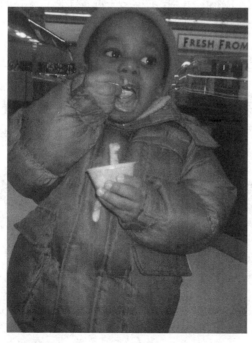

Children should consume a daily total of 3 cups of milk or the equivalent from other dairy products daily.

## ▶ Nutrition-Related Concerns During Childhood and Adolescence

Concern has been raised regarding poor dietary habits during childhood and adolescence. Appropriate food selection is essential because children of this age are still growing. Appropriate food selection also can reduce some of the negative consequences of inadequate food intake. Hence, it is important to monitor children's food and nutrient intakes to reduce nutrition-related health conditions, which include but are not limited to iron-deficiency anemia, lead poisoning, dental caries, overweight and obesity, and high blood cholesterol.

### Iron-Deficiency Anemia

Iron-deficiency anemia is a problem for all ages, but especially for children. Many iron-deficient children come from low-income families with poor diets.[28] Cultural traditions and lack of nutrition knowledge about iron requirements are also factors that contribute to iron deficiencies.[29] **Iron deficiency** is defined as absent bone marrow iron stores, an increase in hemoglobin concentration of less than 1 g/dl after treatment with iron, or other abnormal laboratory values, such as serum **ferritin** concentration.[30] Age- and sex-specific cutoff values for anemia are derived from NHANES III data. For children 1 to 2 years of age, the diagnosis of anemia would be made if the hemoglobin concentrations were less than 11 g/dl and hematocrit was less than 32.9 percent. For children ages 2 to 5 years, a hemoglobin value of 11.1 g/dl or a hematocrit of 33 percent signifies iron-deficiency anemia.[31]

One of the Healthy People 2010 objectives was to reduce iron deficiency in children ages 1 to 2 years from 9 percent to 5 percent and in children ages 3 to 4 years from 4 percent to 1 percent.[32] Healthy People 2020 objectives were to reduce iron deficiency by 10 percent. A 2010 progress report showed no progress in 1 to 2 and 3 to 4 year olds (see Table 9-2).40 Reaching this goal will require reducing or eliminating disparities in iron deficiency by race and family income level.

The prevalence of iron deficiency is higher in African American than in European American children (10 percent vs. 8 percent for children ages 1 to 2 years) and is highest in Mexican American children (17 percent of children ages 1 to 2 years).[33] Also, children of families with incomes less than 130 percent of the poverty threshold have higher incidences of iron deficiency than those with a higher income (12 percent vs. 7 percent).

Low blood iron levels affect a child's resistance to disease, attention span, behavior, and intellectual performance.[34,35] It is reported that excessive consumption of milk could contribute to low iron intake. Milk or soymilk intake should be limited to 3 to 4 cups per day or no more than 24 ounces; this will permit inclusion of iron-rich foods, such as lean meats, legumes, fish, poultry, and iron-enriched breads and cereals.[30] Larger intakes of milk or soymilk may replace foods that are high in iron.

Cultural and religious practices also may affect children's iron status. For example, it was reported that East Indian mothers living in Great Britain do not feed their children beef if they are Hindu; if they are Muslim, they do not feed children pork or meats that are not "halal" (permitted, or lawful, foods are called *halal*.) They often do not replace the nutrients in those items with equivalent foods, consequently causing anemia.[36] In contrast, it was reported that in Spain, preschool children showed better iron status when meat was included in their diets during their eighth month or earlier, compared to those who were given meat later.[37] There are no reports on the effect of kosher meat on iron status.

Iron-deficiency anemia is not common in school-age children. The NHANES III data from 1988 to 1994 and other studies have shown that more than 7 percent of older children were iron deficient, however. For adolescents, it was reported that iron deficiency was found in 2.8 to 3.5 percent of 11- to 14-year-old females, 4.1 percent of 11- to 14-year-old males, 6.0 to 7.2 percent of 15- to 19-year-old females, and 0.6 percent of 15- to 19-year-old males.[38,39] Dietary intake of iron ranges from 10.0 to 12.5 mg per day in females (ages 14 to 18 years old).[39] The Dietary Reference Intakes (DRIs) are 15 mg per day for girls and 11 mg per day for boys. Donovan et al.[39] reported that 32 percent of male and 83 percent of female adolescents consume less than the DRI for iron.[1,40]

## Lead Poisoning

Approximately 4.4 percent of children ages 1 to 5 years have high blood lead levels—higher than 10 µg/dl. Lead poisoning is common among children under age 6 and can cause learning disabilities and behavior problems, slow growth, brain damage, and central nervous system damage. Lead poisoning also can cause iron deficiency, and, in turn, iron deficiency can impair the body's ability to prevent lead absorption.[32,41] Satisfactory calcium intake may slow lead's absorption or interfere with its toxicity.

The U.S. Environmental Protection Agency's (EPA's) "Keep It Clean" public health campaigns to prevent lead poisoning have significantly reduced the amount of lead in the environment. Also, the U.S. ban on the use of leaded gasoline, leaded house paint, and lead-soldered food cans have helped reduce lead poisoning.[42] Other strategies for preventing lead poisoning include providing nutritious foods, screening children for lead poisoning, preventing children from eating nonfood items, avoiding water containing lead, and preventing children from putting dirty or old painted objects in their mouths. In addition, food providers must wash their hands before handling foods and require children to also wash their hands before eating.[14,17,43]

The prevalence of elevated blood lead levels above 10 µg/dl in U.S. children 1 to 5 years old has decreased.[44] Results show a decrease of 84 percent. Low-income children, especially African American children, are still at higher risk for lead poisoning than other U.S. children.[45] Among the different ethnic groups, the prevalence of lead poisoning decreased 84 percent in Mexican American children, 82 percent in African American, and 78 percent in European American. A study conducted in California identified Mexican-born children as being at a higher risk than Hispanic children born in the United States.[46] The Centers for Disease Control and Prevention (CDC) recommends universal lead screening for children living in neighborhoods where the risk for lead exposure is widespread, and the federal Medicaid program requires that all eligible children be screened for elevated blood lead levels. Children who live in housing built before 1950 are at high risk for lead poisoning because of the presence of lead-based paints.[47] Children who live in inner cities are also at risk for lead poisoning because of the lead in dirt. Also improper drinking water treatment that happened in the city of Flint Michigan in Detroit can expose children to high levels of lead.

## Successful Community Strategies

### Lead Poisoning Prevention in Hartford, Connecticut[40]

The Hartford Health Department, the Hartford Regional Lead Treatment Center, and the Hartford Lead Safe House established a Lead Poisoning Prevention and Education Program (LPPEP) in 1999. The program was a citywide effort to increase lead poisoning awareness and promote behaviors leading to lead poisoning prevention among the residents within the city of Hartford, Connecticut. They implemented a multifaceted public health campaign that involved several partnerships. The program was funded by the Centers for Disease Control and Prevention,

*(continues)*

the U.S. Department of Housing and Urban Development, the Connecticut Department of Public Health, and the U.S. Environmental Protection Agency. The campaign used 10 different strategies to carry out the intervention program, including an educational video that aired on public access television and was made available to 10 of the city's public libraries; drawings showing the hazards of lead poisoning that were chosen from a poster contest were displayed at the capitol building; and an educational table was displayed in front of a local Hartford hardware store for almost 1 year to reach patrons and pedestrians with messages about lead poisoning and lead-safe work practices. In addition, four educational notices highlighting lead poisoning prevention were placed for two consecutive months, from April 1 to June 30, 2000, in Connecticut's major newspaper and two smaller, local Hartford newspapers, to reach different segments of the population. One of the notices featured two African American boys encouraging readers to test their children and homes for lead. The notices included phone numbers for both the Hartford Health Department and the Connecticut Children's Medical Center. From April 2000 through April 2001, the Hartford Health Department posted an educational awareness message in English and in Spanish on 16 Hartford billboards. These messages featured a woman playing with a child; underneath was the phrase, "He got his eyes from grandma, his laugh from Daddy, and his lead poisoning from home." The billboards have continued to be posted throughout the city. In addition, the Hartford Health Department partnered with a local dairy to place lead awareness messages on almost 1 million milk cartons and 300,000 orange juice cartons that were distributed throughout Connecticut, Rhode Island, Westchester County in New York, and western Massachusetts. These notices featured drawings of children, along with the phrase "One good reason to prevent lead poisoning."

Additionally, the Hartford Health Department partnered with the Connecticut Transit Authority to place educational signs on the interiors of 120 city buses, on the exterior bus tails of 20 additional buses, and on the walls of five of the city's bus shelters. Plus, a series of 4- by 8-foot lead poisoning awareness signs were placed on the sides of Hartford's 13 municipal sanitation trucks. The signs posted messages in English and in Spanish about the hazards of lead poisoning and the importance of having children tested for lead. In addition, the city of Hartford collaborated with the U.S. Postal Service and the U.S. Department of Housing and Urban Development to implement, for the first time in the United States, postmarks aimed at the prevention of lead poisoning. This postmark was applied to almost every stamped, first-class card and letter mailed in Connecticut in October 2001. The postmark featured an illustration of a house accompanied by the phrase "Let's give every child a lead safe home."

At the end of the campaign, the Hartford Health Department conducted a survey to evaluate its effectiveness. Approximately 45 percent of the respondents said that they took specific steps to learn more about lead poisoning because of the campaigns just described. The survey also showed that:

- Approximately 73.3 percent of the respondents said that they asked their doctor about blood tests for lead poisoning.
- 21.3 percent said that they called a phone number to learn more about lead poisoning.
- 76 percent said that they changed the way they cooked or cleaned.
- 42.7 percent said that they changed the kinds of foods they fed their families.
- 41.3 percent said that they spoke to their landlord.
- 60 percent said that they took other steps to prevent lead poisoning.

Among those reporting that they took specific steps to learn more about how to prevent lead poisoning, approximately 51 percent specified that they took steps because of the newspaper notices. Consequently, the newspaper notices were the most effective campaign strategy in terms of self-reported lead poisoning prevention behavior.

## Dental Caries

**Dental caries** is a widespread problem for all age groups. Approximately one in five children ages 2 to 4 years has decay in their primary or permanent teeth.[48] Foods containing carbohydrates that stick to the surface of the teeth—for example, sticky candy such as caramel—can interact with the bacteria *Streptococcus mutans* and cause tooth decay.[49] The following suggestions may help reduce dental caries in children[17,31,50]:

- Brush the child's teeth to remove carbohydrates.
- Rinse the child's mouth with water.
- Use fluoridated water.
- Provide crunchy foods such as carrot sticks and apple slices for a snack. These are less likely to promote tooth decay than sticky candies or raisins.

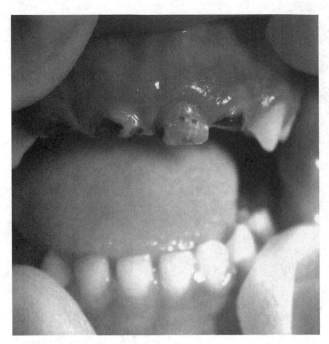

Tooth decay occurs when sugar in liquids is in contact with teeth for a prolonged time. Milk, formula, juice, Kool-Aid, and soft drinks contain sugar.

Courtesy of Dr. Hisham Yehia El Batawi.

## Overweight and Obesity

There has been a significant increase in the United States in the prevalence of overweight and obesity in children and adolescents. A body mass index (BMI) between the 85th and 95th percentiles for age and sex is considered at risk for overweight, and a BMI at or above the 95th percentile is considered overweight or obese.[51] According to the 2003 to 2004 NHANES data, approximately 18.8 percent of children 6 to 11 years old and 17.4 percent of adolescents 12 to 19 years are overweight. A research study conducted by Krebs et al.[50] showed that about 15.3 percent of 6- to 11-year-olds and 15.5 percent of 12- to 19-year-olds were at or above the 95th percentile for BMI on standard growth charts developed by the CDC. One of the Healthy People 2010 objectives is to reduce the prevalence of overweight from the baseline of 11 percent to 5 percent. However, the data show an increase of almost 45 percent from estimates of 11 percent obtained from NHANES III (1988 to 1994) and a threefold increase from the 1960s.[51]

Overweight and obesity occur at a higher rate in African American girls than Hispanic and European American girls. For example, the prevalence of overweight in girls ages 12 to 19 years for African Americans was 25.4 percent, for Mexican Americans was 14.1 percent, and for European Americans was 15.4 percent.[52] But for a boy of the same age group, there was a slight difference: for African Americans, 18.5 percent; for Mexican

Americans, 18.3 percent; and for European Americans, 19.1 percent. In addition, Hedley et al.[51] reported that 42.8 percent of Mexican American boys ages 6 to 19 years were at risk for overweight compared with 31 percent of African American boys and 29.2 percent of European American boys.[53] Among girls, 40.1 percent of African American girls were at risk for overweight compared to 36.6 percent of Mexican American girls and 27.0 percent of European American girls.[53] In addition, results from the 2007 to 2008 NHANES, using measured heights and weights, showed that about 16.9 percent of children and adolescents ages 2 to 19 years are obese.

The mechanism of obesity development is not well understood, but it is confirmed that obesity develops when energy intake exceeds energy expenditure. Many factors contribute to obesity in children and adolescents worldwide, including the amount of television viewing, an inactive and sedentary lifestyle, genetic factors, environmental factors, and cultural environment.[54,55] In a small number of cases, childhood obesity is due to medical causes such as hypothyroidism and growth hormone deficiency.[56] Other causes may be that low-income families lack safe places for physical activity and lack consistent access to healthful food choices, mainly fruits and vegetables.

The situations that encourage overweight or obesity evolved over a period of years; therefore, no single change will reverse the trend. Multicomponent, family-based, community-based, and school-based approaches, including diet, physical activity, and behavior modification for reducing overweight in children and adolescents, may be the best strategy.

Obesity is associated with major health problems in children and is an early risk factor for morbidity and mortality in adults.[57] Studies show that approximately one third of overweight preschool children, half of overweight school-age children, and three quarters of overweight teenagers grow up to be obese adults.[58]

## Medical Problems Related to Childhood Obesity

Obese children and adolescents commonly have problems that affect cardiovascular health (hypercholesterolemia, dyslipidemia, and hypertension),[57] the endocrine system (hyperinsulinism, insulin resistance, impaired glucose tolerance, type 2 diabetes mellitus, and menstrual irregularity),[59] and mental health (depression and low self-esteem).[60-62] Other major problems that can be caused by overweight and obesity include osteoporosis and some cancers (such as ovarian and breast cancer).[63] In addition, some children may develop sleep apnea and liver and gallbladder diseases.[64]

One health risk of notable concern is the prevalence of diagnosed diabetes coincident with increases in the prevalence of obesity and sedentary lifestyle.[65,66] Diabetes is a group of diseases marked by high levels of blood glucose due to defects in insulin production, insulin action, or both.[67] Type 1 diabetes is usually diagnosed in children and young adults, and was known as juvenile diabetes. Type 1 diabetes develops when the body's immune system destroys pancreatic beta cells, the only cells in the body that make the hormone insulin that regulates blood glucose. People with type 1 diabetes must have insulin administered by injection or a pump to help move glucose from the blood to the cells. Type 1 diabetes accounts for 5 to 10 percent of all diagnosed cases of diabetes.

Another kind of diabetes is type 2 diabetes. This is the most common form of diabetes and accounts for approximately 90 to 95 percent of all diagnosed cases. It usually begins as insulin resistance, a disorder in which the cells do not use insulin properly. As the need for insulin increases, the pancreas gradually loses its ability to produce it. Type 2 diabetes is associated with older age, obesity, a family history of diabetes, a history of gestational diabetes, impaired glucose metabolism, physical inactivity, and certain races/ethnicities. In the United States, African Americans, Hispanic Americans, American Indians, and some Asian Americans and native Hawaiians are at high risk for type 2 diabetes.[67] Clinically based reports and regional studies show that type 2 diabetes is increasing in children and adolescents.[67-71] Several factors are linked to type 2 diabetes. These children and adolescents are usually between 10 and 19 years old, obese, have a strong family history for type 2 diabetes, and have insulin resistance.

This trend of obesity and its relationship to diabetes is not restricted to only U.S. children. Among Japanese schoolchildren, the incidence of type 2 diabetes increased from 0.2 to 7.3 per 100,000 children per year between 1976 and 1995.[72,73] The increase was associated with changing dietary patterns and increasing rates of obesity among these children.[72] Similarly, Sinha et al.[72] reported the prevalence of impaired glucose tolerance in 25 percent of 55 obese children (4 to 10 years of age) and in 21 percent of 112 obese adolescents (11 to 18 years of age).[59] In addition, type 2 diabetes was observed in 4 percent of the 112 obese adolescents.[59]

The prevalence of childhood obesity indicates an urgent need for the development of effective strategies for primary, secondary, and tertiary prevention. Primary prevention may include family and/or school-based programs, regardless of the children's risk status. Secondary prevention may include routine assessments of eating and activity patterns that may include school-based or institution-based programs. The tertiary prevention efforts may include individual, family-based, and multiple-component–based (diet, physical activity, behavior, and parent training) programs.

## Dealing with Overweight and Obesity

Overweight and obesity are easier to prevent than to treat. Early intervention and prevention of obesity are valuable. (See Chapter 10 for more information on prevention of obesity in adults.) There is evidence that childhood eating and exercise habits can be modified more easily than adult habits.[74] Prevention of obesity needs to focus on parents' knowledge of nutrition. Parental education should include information about low-fat foods, good physical activities, and monitoring of television viewing. Wolf et al.[74] reported that adolescents spend an average of 22 to 25 hours per week watching television.[75] (More information about television viewing is presented later in this chapter.)

Reports from national surveys of parents showed the following[76]:

- Ninety-five percent thought physical education should be a part of school curriculum for all students grades K through 12 and regular, daily physical activity could help children do better academically.
- Approximately 85 percent thought parents and school officials should work together to decide what students should eat and drink at school and that they would support programs in schools to help fight childhood obesity.

Parents and family members play an important role in a successful weight loss or healthy lifestyle program. A 10-year follow-up study involving parents in a weight management program with their obese children showed that parental involvement led to a significant weight loss in obese children compared to obese children without parental involvement.[77]

Similarly, a British pilot study showed that school might be an appropriate setting for the promotion of healthy lifestyles in children. However, interventions require replication in other social settings, including the family setting. The researcher stated that successful efforts should be long-lasting, multifaceted, and sustainable; involve all school-age children; and be behaviorally focused.[78]

One program designed to encourage young children to be physically fit is VERB. The VERB campaign encouraged young people ages 9 to 13 years (tweens) to be physically active every day. This was a national, multicultural social marketing campaign coordinated by the CDC. The campaign used a combination of paid advertising, marketing strategies, and partnership efforts to reach the distinct audiences of tweens and adult role models. More information about VERB can be obtained from the CDC website (http://www.cdc.gov). The second Successful Community Strategies in this chapter presents a different successful obesity prevention program.

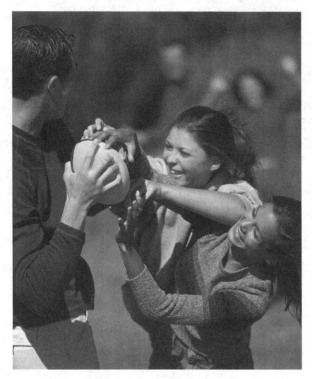

Physical activity is one of the answers for the prevention of childhood obesity.

© SW Productions/Photodisc/Getty Images.

## High Blood Cholesterol

**Atherosclerosis** is a progressive, complex disease that often begins in childhood and adolescence. It is related to high serum total cholesterol levels, consisting of low-density lipoprotein (LDL), very-low-density lipoprotein (VLDL), and high-density lipoprotein (HDL) levels. Children and adolescents with elevated serum cholesterol levels, mainly LDL cholesterol levels, often have family members with high incidence of coronary heart disease.[72]

Most parents do not know their children's cholesterol levels. The children fitting the following criteria are at risk[79]:

- If a parent or grandparent had coronary heart disease when age 55 years or younger.
- If a parent has a blood cholesterol level 240 mg/dl or above. (Approximately 90 percent of children with high cholesterol have a parent who also has high blood cholesterol.)
- If lipid abnormalities are in the family history.
- If a child has a medical condition that predisposes him or her to coronary heart disease, such as severe obesity, diabetes, elevated blood pressure, renal disease, or low thyroid activity.
- If family history is unknown.

Once a lipoprotein analysis report is obtained, it should be repeated so that an average LDL cholesterol level can be established. The average LDL cholesterol level determines the steps for risk assessment and treatment. **TABLE 9-5** lists the acceptable blood cholesterol profile for children as determined by the National Cholesterol Education Program's Expert Panel (NCEPEP) and major health organizations, including the American Heart Association (AHA) and the American Academy of Pediatrics (AAP).

It is encouraging to know that some children are making efforts to reduce fat intake. For instance, the results from the Bogalusa Heart Study showed a significant increase in the percentage of energy supplied by protein and carbohydrates and a significant decrease in the percentage of energy received from fat, mainly saturated and monounsaturated fat. The general dietary recommendations of the AHA for those age 2 years or older stress a diet that depends on fruits and vegetables, whole grains, low-fat and nonfat dairy products, beans, fish, and lean meat.[80,81]

Research also shows that children with high blood cholesterol levels can benefit from reducing the amount of fat, saturated fat, and cholesterol in their diets without

| TABLE 9-5 Cholesterol Levels in Children and Adolescents Ages 2-19 Years[78] | | | |
|---|---|---|---|
| **Cholesterol** | **Acceptable (mg/dl)** | **Borderline (mg/dl)*** | **High (mg/dl)†** |
| Total cholesterol | < 70 | 170–199 | ≥ 200 |
| LDL cholesterol | < 110 | 110–129 | ≥ 130 |

HDL levels should be ≥ 35 mg/dl and triglycerides should be ≤ 150 mg/dl.

*May require moderate changes to diet.
†May require changes in diet and possible drug treatment.

adversely affecting their normal development. In the Dietary Intervention Study in Children (DISC), children were asked to adopt a low-fat, low-cholesterol diet. The children maintained this diet for 7 years. The dietary modifications did not alter the children's growth, nutritional status, or sexual maturation throughout the 7-year study. In addition, the diet significantly helped decrease the children's blood levels of LDL for up to 3 years after they stopped following the diet.[82,83]

## Dieting Behavior and Abnormal Eating

Dieting and abnormal eating behaviors among adolescents, especially among girls, is very common. Studies indicate that overweight individuals are more likely to report engaging in dieting and other weight-control behaviors than nonoverweight individuals.[84,85] For instance, in a cross-sectional study, 17.5 percent of underweight girls (BMI < 15th percentile), 37.9 percent of average-weight girls (BMI 15th to 85th percentile), 49.3 percent of moderately overweight girls (BMI 85th to 95th percentile), and 52.1 percent of very overweight girls (BMI > 95th percentile) reported dieting behaviors.[86] Due to the nature of this study, it is not clear whether dieting led to higher BMI values or whether overweight status led to increased dieting behavior. However, Stice et al.[83] found that baseline dieting behaviors and dietary restraint were associated with the onset of obesity.[84]

Adolescents who diet are more likely to have poor body image and indulge in fasting, vomiting, taking diet pills, and binge eating.[84,87,88] It is estimated that 0.5 to 1 percent of the general population have **anorexia nervosa**, 2 percent have **bulimia nervosa**, and 2 percent have **binge eating** disorders.[89] In general, 95 percent of individuals diagnosed with clinical eating disorders are female.

## Screening or Diagnosis Tools for Eating Disorders

Clinical diagnosis of eating disorders is based on the psychological, behavioral, and physiological characteristics described by the *Diagnostic and Statistical Manual of Mental Disorders*, fourth edition (DSM-IV), criteria.[90,91] Some of the criteria for anorexia nervosa, bulimia nervosa, and binge eating disorders are presented in **BOX 9-1** and **FIGURE 9-1**. Researchers also have used self-figure drawing to assess eating disorders in 36 women with anorexia or bulimia and 40 women with no eating disorder, half of whom were overweight and half were normal weight. The participants were asked to draw themselves. The researchers found that women with anorexia or bulimia drew themselves with

---

**BOX 9-1** Some Criteria for Eating Disorders[92,93]

Anorexia nervosa

1. BMI of less than 17.5 kg/m$^2$ in adults
2. Intense fear of gaining weight
3. Disturbance in the way in which body size or weight is perceived
4. Amenorrhea if the individual is a postmenarchal female
5. Purposive avoidance of food and a steadfast and implacable attitude in pursuing a low body weight and then maintaining it
6. Active refusal to eat enough to maintain a normal weight and/or in determined, sustained efforts to prevent ingested food from being absorbed
7. Relentless pursuit of thinness

Bulimia nervosa

- Recurrent episodes of binge eating
- Recurrent purging behavior
- Excessive exercise or fasting
- Excessive concern about body weight or shape and absence of anorexia nervosa
- Self-evaluation unduly influenced by body shape and weight

Provisional criteria for binge eating

- Recurrent episodes of binge eating associated with at least three behavioral and attitudinal characteristics, such as:
  - Eating large amounts when not physically hungry
  - Feeling disgusted or guilty after overeating
  - Eating much more rapidly than normal
- Occurs, on average, at least 2 days per week for 6 months
- The regular use of purging, fasting, and excessive exercise

---

characteristics different from those of women without eating disorders. Results showed the following differences between the groups in four areas[92]:

- Women with anorexia or bulimia depicted themselves as having a larger neck, a disconnected neck, or no neck.
- Women with anorexia or bulimia emphasized their mouth more.
- Depictions of wider thighs were more common among participants with eating disorders.
- Women with anorexia or bulimia drew pictures without feet or with disconnected feet.

In addition, women with anorexia were more likely than those with bulimia to omit breasts from

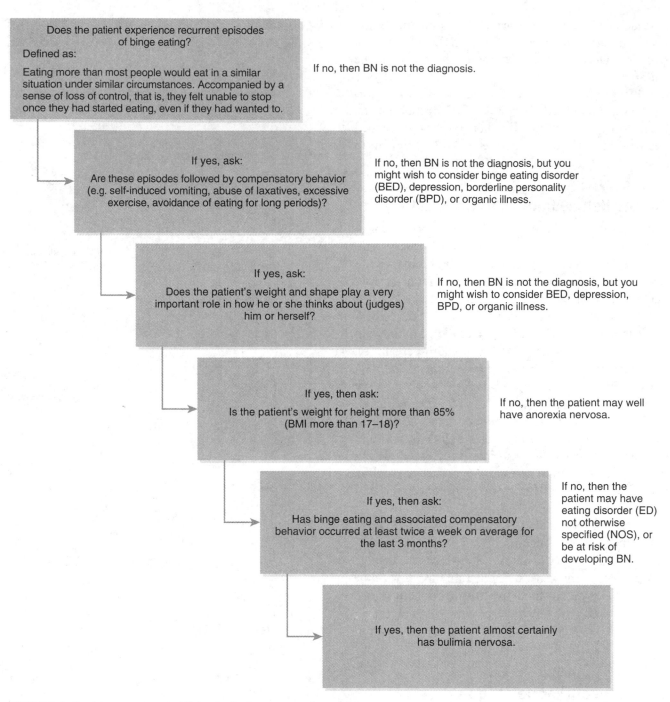

**FIGURE 9-1** Decision tree to establish a bulimia nervous diagnosis.

Modified from Cooper M, Todd G, Wells A. *Treating Bulimia Nervosa and Binge Eating: An Integrated Meta Cognitive and Cognitive Therapy Manual.* London and New York: Routledge Taylor & Francis Group; 2009:28. Reprinted with permission.

their drawings, to sketch less defined body lines, and to portray smaller figures in relation to the page size. The implication of these findings is that women with or prone to developing eating disorders, such as anorexia and bulimia, can be diagnosed with a simple and nonintrusive self-figure drawing assessment. Visit http://centerforchange.com/eating-disorder-characteristics/ for diagnostic features of anorexia nervosa and bulimia nervosa. https://www.nationaleatingdisorders.org /types-symptoms-eating-disorders and http://www .mayoclinic.org/diseases-conditions/eating-disorders /symptoms-causes/dxc-20182875 for types and symptoms of eating disorders.

## Helping to Prevent Eating Disorders

Michael Levine[92] developed 10 things that parents can do to help prevent eating disorders.[93] Community and public health nutritionists also can include this information as part of their nutrition education programs for parents. Nutritionists should ask parents to do the following:

- Consider their thoughts, attitudes, and behaviors toward their own body and the way they are shaped by the forces of weightism and sexism.
  - Parents need to educate their children about the genetic basis for the natural diversity of human body shapes and sizes and the nature and ugliness of prejudice.
  - Parents need to maintain positive attitudes and healthy behaviors.
- Examine their dreams and goals for their children and observe if they are overemphasizing beauty and body shape (mainly for girls).
- Discuss with their sons and daughters the dangers of trying to alter their body; emphasize the importance of eating at least three times per day and the value of moderate exercise for health.
- Avoid categorizing and labeling foods (e.g., good/bad or safe/dangerous). All foods can be eaten in moderation.
- Ask their children not to avoid activities (such as swimming, sunbathing, dancing, etc.) because they call attention to their weight and shape.
- Encourage their children to exercise for the joy of feeling their body move and grow stronger and not use it to compensate for calories, power, excitement, popularity, or perfection.
- Tell their children not to take people seriously when they comment on how slender or "well put together" they appear.
- Help their children appreciate and resist the ways television, magazines, and other media distort the true diversity of human body types and imply that a slender body means power, excitement, popularity, or perfection.
- Educate boys and girls about various forms of prejudice, including weightism, and help them understand their responsibilities for preventing them.
- Encourage their children to be active and to enjoy what their bodies can do and feel and not limit their caloric intake unless a physician prescribes it because of medical reasons.
- Promote their children's self-esteem and self-respect for all their intellectual, athletic, and social endeavors. Give boys and girls the same opportunities and encouragement; do not suggest that females are less important than males, for example, by exempting males from housework or childcare.

Eating disorders have many causes, and it is likely that several factors contribute to the development of the disorders in any given case. In some cases, sociocultural pressures may explain why eating disorders are high in economically privileged communities and countries; a cultural obsession with weight and thinness in women has been linked with increasing incidences of eating disorders during the past two decades.[91,94]

Nutritional factors and dieting behavior also may contribute to the development and course of eating disorders. The onset of bulimia nervosa usually follows a period of dieting to lose weight,[95,96] and a contributory link between dietary restraint and bulimia is strengthened by similar behavior among obese patients who binge eat following diet restriction and among normal subjects following a period of food deprivation.[97,98] Their abnormal eating patterns, as well as the physiological consequences of those patterns, perpetuate the disorder and contribute to its often difficult nature.

## ✎ Think About It

Diane, a university dietitian, provides nutrition education to college students. She is planning a program on eating disorders for the students. She posted fliers about the program in the residence halls and at the student center. Over 200 students responded to the invitation. She thought it would be beneficial to screen participants for eating disorders during the nutrition education program. How can she determine who is at risk for eating disorder? Why is the level of eating disorders high in economically privileged communities?

## Successful Community Strategies

### Pathways: An Obesity Prevention Program for American Indian Schoolchildren[98]

Pathways was a culturally appropriate obesity prevention program for third-, fourth-, and fifth-grade American Indian schoolchildren. The purpose of the program was to increase individual attributes such as children's knowledge about physical activity and food selections; their values about health, physical activity, and nutrition; and their sense of personal control over their choices.

*(continues)*

## Successful Community Strategies (continued)

An intervention committee composed of universities, American Indian nations, schools, and families (working groups) coordinated the development of the Pathways intervention program. The committee modified the intervention based on feedback from the review process and from a highly organized process of evaluation that included feedback from students, teachers, school administrators, families, and food service workers. Approval for the study was obtained from each academic institution's review board. Similar approval was obtained from each tribe. The content and approach of the Pathways intervention combined constructs from social learning theory and cultural concepts that included American Indian customs and practices. Therefore, the intervention team drew on the indigenous beliefs and values of each participating American Indian nation to create a program that supported healthier lifestyles and reflected the nations' traditional cultures. The program also equipped children with experience in self-monitoring and goal setting to effect changes in their existing habits.

The Pathways intervention targeted four areas: 1) classroom curriculum, 2) physical education, 3) family education, and 4) school food service. Formative assessment was conducted in each of the participating communities to identify the main risk factors for obesity specific to the study populations; design and evaluate culturally appropriate interventions based on people's beliefs, perceptions, and behaviors; and engage members of each tribe in the development and implementation of the program. Data were collected from school staff members (teachers, food service workers, and administrators), third- to fifth-grade students and their caregivers, and other community members using in-depth interviews, semi-structured interviews, focus groups, and direct observation.

Teacher response to the 12 lessons of the third-grade curriculum showed a trend toward increased satisfaction with the lessons overall, with the students' enjoyment of the lessons, and with the students' attainment of knowledge and skills as the weeks advanced. Classroom observation by Pathways staff members complemented these responses, showing that the children participated actively in and enjoyed the lessons (particularly the story circle and music) and clearly retained some of the primary concepts.

## ▶ Malnutrition in Children

Malnutrition and hunger are responsible for nearly half of the deaths of preschool children throughout the world. Deficiencies in vitamin A, zinc, iron, and protein also result in illness, stunted growth, limited development, and in the case of vitamin A, possibly permanent blindness.[99,100]

Malnutrition is caused by continual consumption of foods that provide less or more than the nutrients or energy required to support the everyday needs of the human body. Malnutrition includes **undernutrition**, which means the body is not receiving enough nutrients, and **overnutrition**, which includes excessive consumption of any particular nutrient.[100,101]

Undernutrition is a significant cause of malnutrition in developing countries, and poverty is its main cause. Poor families often do not have the economic, social, or environmental resources to purchase or produce enough food. Poor soil conditions also contribute to a family's inability to grow enough food to prevent malnutrition and its complications. In addition, low wages, underemployment, and food prices beyond the reach of families contribute to undernutrition in the urban poor.

Children, mainly infants and those under 5 years of age, are at increased risk for undernutrition due to the greater need for energy and nutrients during periods of rapid growth and development. Protein-energy

malnutrition (PEM) occurs throughout the life cycle, but is more common during infancy and childhood and in the elderly. PEM is classified into two parts: primary and secondary. Primary PEM, presented in **BOX 9-2**, refers to a deficit of available food. This may be due to biological, sociological, ecological, and economic conditions. Secondary causes of PEM, presented in **BOX 9-3**, may have biological or social causes. Biological conditions may

### BOX 9-2 Primary Causes of Protein-Energy Malnutrition[99]

Biological
- Maternal malnutrition prior to or during pregnancy and lactation
- Genetic factors

Sociological
- Poverty
- Limited or selective unavailability of food

Ecological
- Disasters leading to famine
- Profound social inequalities either at the individual level (discrimination, refugees, prisoners) or at the community or country level
- War

**BOX 9-3** Secondary Causes of Protein-Energy Malnutrition[99]

Biological conditions that may interfere with food intake and utilization

- Congenital anomalies (e.g., cleft lip)
- Gastrointestinal problems that may cause malabsorption of nutrients (e.g., tropical sprue)
- Genetic factors (e.g., phenylketonuria [PKU])

Biological conditions that may increase the need for energy and other nutrients

- AIDS
- All infectious diseases accompanied with fever
- Other diseases that increase catabolism (e.g., tuberculosis)

Social causes

- Lack of education
- Inadequate weaning practices
- Child abuse
- Alcoholism and other drug addictions

interfere with food intake or utilization or may increase the need for energy and other nutrients. In most cases, PEM is caused by a combination of both, but the concept of two parts may be useful for targeting interventions.[101]

## The Prevalence and Effect of Malnutrition in Children

In the United States, approximately 15.3 million children live in families with incomes below the federal poverty level. About 20 percent of children under 6 years old and approximately 20.7 percent of children 6 years or older live in poor families.[102] About 24.4 percent of households with children under 6 years old were food-insecure, and more than 46 percent of these households experienced hunger in 2009.[103,104] In 2014, 46 million U.S. households obtained food from food pantries.[105]

The World Health Organization (WHO) Program of Nutrition compiled the most recent estimates about the distribution of PEM worldwide; the report is available online at http://www.worldhunger.org. The database covered 95 percent of the total population of children younger than 5 years of age who lived in about 200 countries, as was reported in nationally representative surveys available in 2013. According to the data:

- About 161 million children under 5 years old were stunted (low height for age).[105]
- About 99 million children were underweight (low weight for age) and 10 percent were severely underweight.

- The largest percentage of children diagnosed with PEM was from Asia, at 70 percent.
- Africa had 26 percent of children diagnosed with PEM.
- Latin America and the Caribbean showed 4 percent stunted growth.
- About 17 million children died of malnutrition worldwide in 2013.[100,104,105]

Globally, there is an adequate food supply and the technical expertise necessary to address the problems and complications of malnutrition. All that is lacking is the political cooperation to address this devastating situation.[100]

In the United States, federal programs such as the WIC Program, NSLP, SBP, Summer Feeding Program, and SMP provide a safety net for children. The WIC program is designed to follow children through their fifth birthday. It provides vouchers for milk, eggs, cereal, juice, cheese, and either peanut butter or dried beans. However, the WIC program does not reach all the children in need. Many parents do not understand that WIC is still available after a child is weaned from formula, do not have transportation to get to a WIC grocery site, or are homeless.

## ▶ Children and Adolescents with Special Healthcare Needs and Childhood Disability

The prevalence of **childhood disability** is increasing—approximately 7 to 18 percent of children and adolescents from birth to 18 years in the United States have a chronic physical, behavioral, developmental, or emotional condition. These conditions limit their activities and/or require special care.[106] The health and health-related needs of children with disabilities are very broad, and it is not possible to adequately cover all aspects in this chapter.

There are various causes of developmental disabilities, and special healthcare needs are comprehensive. Children may have physical impairments, developmental delays, or chronic medical conditions caused by or associated with the following factors[107,108]:

- Genetic conditions (e.g., diabetes, sickle cell anemia)
- Congenital infections
- Inborn errors of metabolism (e.g., phenylketonuria, lactose intolerance, **galactosemia**)
- Prematurity
- Neural tube defects
- Maternal substance abuse
- Environmental toxins (e.g., lead, mercury)

Children and adolescents with special healthcare needs are at risk for nutrition-related health problems. It is estimated that up to 40 to 50 percent of children and adolescents with special healthcare needs have nutrition-related risk factors or health problems that require the attention of a registered dietitian, nutritionist, or healthcare professional.[109,110] Some of the nutrition risk factors include, but are not limited to, those that are physical, biochemical, psychological, or environmental in nature. Physical conditions such as a cleft lip or palate or a disease process such as galactosemia may limit an individual's ability to feed, digest, or absorb food. Drug–nutrient interactions may alter digestion, absorption, or the bioavailability of nutrients from the diet. Also, psychological factors may contribute to an individual's ability to accept and cope with a disability or treatment plan.[110] For example, depression or stress may alter an individual's appetite and motivation to follow a specified diet plan. Environmental factors such as family and social support, finances, and other factors will have a significant impact on the children's access to nutritious foods and support for following certain dietary regimens. One or a combination of these factors may put a child or an adolescent with special needs at nutritional risk.[111] Common nutrition problems for children and adolescents with special healthcare needs may include the following[109,110,112,113]:

- Altered energy and nutrient needs
- Delayed or stunted linear growth
- Underweight
- Overweight or obesity
- Feeding delays or oral–motor dysfunction
- Drug–nutrient interactions
- Appetite disturbances
- Unusual food habits (e.g., rumination, voluntary regurgitation of food, pica, disordered eating)
- Dental and gum disease

It is important to perform a comprehensive assessment of the problems. The assessment process should include anthropometric data, biochemical and laboratory data, clinical findings, medical history, a dietary history or food frequency questionnaire, and feeding skills assessment (chewing ability, etc.).[113] The assessment and care plan processes require a multidisciplinary team approach that allows individuals from different disciplines to address the problems that may have an impact on nutrition and other needs. The multidisciplinary team members can include physicians, nurses, dietitians, dentists, community resource personnel, and social workers.[112] The child and caregiver(s) should be the main members of the team who identify problems and set priorities to be addressed in the treatment plan.

After the assessment process is completed and a treatment plan is established, the best strategy for incorporating nutrition goals and objectives outside the home is to collaborate with the school system. In local communities, public schools use the Child and Adult Care Food Program to provide resources to children and adolescents with special needs. Public schools also administer the NSLP and SBPs. Federal government regulations allow modified school meals for students with disabilities or chronic medical problems needing special diets at no extra cost. Food substitutions and modified meals required for a medical or special dietary need are provided for individuals identified by the school system as having a disability.[110] The provision of comprehensive nutrition services to 3 to 5 year olds with disability was mandated by Congress in 1986 (Education of the Handicapped Act Amendments PL99-457).[114] In this provision, nutritionists are recognized as the health professionals qualified to provide developmental services to children with special healthcare needs.[114]

The Special Olympics program is a nongovernmental program that promotes health, nutrition, and physical fitness for disabled children and adolescents. The program provides year-round sports training and athletic competition in a variety of community-based Olympic-type sports for children. The activities include nutrition, physical fitness, and the sharing of gifts, skills, and friendship. To receive the nutrition benefits, the child must have a diet prescription from a physician. The prescription must include the following information[110,112]:

- A statement identifying the disability and how the disability affects the adolescent's diet
- A statement identifying the major life activity affected by the disability
- A specific list of dietary changes, modifications, or substitutions required for the diet

The goals set by Healthy People 2010 for the nation's disabled children and adolescents were to achieve more physical activity, better nutrition, weight control, and improved access to healthcare and preventive services and mental health services.

## ▶ The Effect of Television on Children's Eating Habits

It appears that television advertisements influence children's dietary habits. Children watch an average of 3 hours of advertisements per week and 19,000 to 22,000 commercials over a 1-year period.[115] It is reported that children from families with high television use consume an average of 6 percent more of their total daily energy intake from meats; 5 percent more from pizza, salty snacks, and soda; and nearly 5 percent less of their energy intake from fruits, vegetables, and juices than children from families with low television use.[115] Research shows that nutrient content of advertised foods exceeded the recommended amounts for fat, saturated fat, and sodium, and failed to provide the recommended amount of fiber and certain vitamins and minerals.[31,116] Children from families with a high level of television viewing derived fewer of their total calories from carbohydrates and consumed twice as much caffeine as children from families with a low level of television viewing.[117]

Television and the Internet are the favorite advertising media of the food industry,[118] and it is reported that children are exposed to too much television advertising, playing digital games, and using computers, leading to a sedentary lifestyle.[119,120] Research studies examined food advertising during children's Saturday morning television programming and found that over half (56 percent) of all advertisements were for food. The foods promoted were high in fat or sugar, and many were low in nutritional value. Thus, the diet presented on Saturday morning television is in direct contrast to what is recommended for healthful eating for children.[116,120] There is also a growing trend toward food commercialism and marketing in schools. Channel One, the daily news program that broadcasts to millions of students in grades 6 to 12 in thousands of schools, has 2 minutes of each daily 12-minute program devoted to paid commercials for products that include candy bars, snack chips, and soft drinks.[120]

One of the Healthy People 2010 and 2020 objectives is to increase the proportion of children who view television 2 or fewer hours per day from 60 percent to 75 percent. A progress report shows an increase of 67 percent. **BOX 9-4** presents the highlights of adolescent snacking patterns based on 2005 to 2006 NHANES data, and **BOX 9-5** presents the Youth Risk Behavior Surveillance System (YRBS) and School Health Policies and Practice Study (SHPPS).

**BOX 9-4** Food Surveys Research Group Highlights Adolescent Snacking Patterns Based on 2005 to 2006 NHANES Data

The percentage of adolescents (12 to 19 years old) snacking increased from 61 percent in 1977 to 1978 to 83 percent in 2005 to 2006, and the mean snacking frequency increased significantly from 1.0 to 1.7 snacks in a day. The percentage of adolescents who consumed three or more snacks per day increased from 9 percent to 23 percent during the same period. Snacks provided 23 percent of daily calories, 31 percent of total sugars, and lesser proportions of most vitamins and minerals. Snacking provided 11 to 38 percent of daily intakes from MyPlate's grains, fruits, vegetable, milk, meat/beans, and oils groups; 27 percent of discretionary calories; 34 percent of added sugars; and 20 percent of solid fats.

Reproduced from: U.S. Department of Agriculture, Agricultural Research Service. Available at: http://www.cdc.gov/nchs/data/nhanes/nhanes_05_06/jan05intprocman.pdf. Accessed October 22, 2016.

**BOX 9-5** The Youth Risk Behavior Surveillance System and School Health Policies and Practices Study

The combined results from the 2009 national Youth Risk Behavior Surveillance System (YRBS) and School Health Policies and Practices Study (SHPPS) Obesity Epidemic in the U.S. Survey indicates the following among U.S. high school students:

Obesity

1. Based on reference data, 12 percent were above the 95th percentile for BMI by age and sex.

Unhealthy Dietary Behaviors

2. 78 percent ate fruits and vegetables fewer than five time per day during the 7 days before the survey; 66 percent ate fruit and drank 100 percent fruit juices fewer than two times per day during the 7 days before the survey.
3. 86 percent ate vegetables fewer than three times per day during the 7 days before the survey.
4. 29 percent drank a can, bottle, or glass of soda or pop at least one time per day during the 7 days before the survey.

Physical Inactivity

1. 23 percent did not participate in at least 60 minutes of physical activity on any day during the 7 days before the survey.
2. 82 percent were physically active at least 60 minutes per day on fewer than 7 days during the 7 days before the survey.

*(continues)*

3. 44 percent did not attend physical education (PE) classes in an average week when they were in school.
4. 67 percent did not attend PE classes daily when they were in school.
5. 33 percent watched television 3 or more hours per day on an average school day.
6. 25 percent used computers 3 or more hours per day on an average school day.

The School Health Policies and Programs Study 2006 indicated that among U.S. high schools:

Health Education

1. 69 percent required students to receive instruction on health topics as part of a specific course.
2. 53 percent taught 14 nutrition and dietary behavior topics in a required health education course.
3. 38 percent taught 13 physical activity topics in a required health education course.

PE and Physical Activity

1. 95 percent required students to take PE; among these schools, 59 percent did not allow students to be exempted from taking a required PE course for certain reasons.

## Special Milk Program

The Special Milk Program (SMP), established in 1955 by the USDA, provides reimbursement for milk served to children. It is available to schools and childcare institutions that are not eligible for other federal child nutrition service programs. Children whose families are eligible for free school lunches or breakfasts are also eligible for free milk through this program.[121,122]

In 2009, nearly 4,272 schools and residential childcare institutions participated, along with 704 summer camps and 630 nonresidential childcare institutions. The SMP also may provide milk to children in half-day prekindergarten and kindergarten programs in which children do not have access to the school meal programs.

Schools or institutions may choose pasteurized fluid types of unflavored or flavored whole milk, low-fat milk, skim milk, and cultured buttermilk that meet state and local standards. All milk should contain vitamins A and D at levels specified by the U.S. Food and Drug Administration. The federal reimbursement for each half-pint of milk sold to children in school year 2010 to 2011 was 17.75 cents.[123] For children who receive free milk, the USDA reimburses schools the net purchase price of the milk.

Because of the expansions made in the NSLP, there has been a substantial decrease in the SMP since the 1960s. In fiscal year 2009, the SMP cost $14.0 million. By comparison, the program cost $101.2 million in 1970, $145.2 million in 1980, and $19.1 million in 1990.[123]

## ► Nutrition During Childhood and Adolescence

Adequate nutrition is very important during the school-age years. Although clinical signs of malnutrition are not common in children in North America, some children receive diets that are inadequate in quantity or quality. Nutrients most likely to be low or deficient are calcium, iron, zinc, vitamin $B_6$, and vitamin A.[124,125] Similarly, national survey data show that children continue to consume foods high in sugar and sodium and insufficient amounts of fruits and vegetables.[126] Children living in poor families are more likely to follow diets low in calories; vitamins A, C, E, and $B_6$; folate; iron; zinc; thiamin; and magnesium.[127] Community nutritionists can encourage parents and caregivers to provide adequate foods using the recommendation presented in **TABLE 9-6**.

## Growth and Development

The normal events of puberty and the simultaneous growth spurt are the primary influences on nutritional requirements during adolescence. During puberty, height and weight increase, many organ systems enlarge, and body composition is altered due to increased lean body mass and changes in the quantity and distribution of fat. The timing of the growth spurt is influenced by genetic as well as environmental factors. Children who weigh more than average for their height tend to mature early and vice versa.[15]

Normally, growth spurts begin between ages 10.5 and 11 for girls and peak at about 12 years of age. Boys'

| **TABLE 9-6** The Recommended Daily Calorie Intake | | |
|---|---|---|
| **Age Category (Years)** | **Not Active** | **Active** |
| Children 2-3 | 1,000 | 1,400 |
| Females 4-8 | 1,200 | 1,800 |
| Females 9-13 | 1,600 | 2,200 |
| Females 13-18 | 1,800 | 2,400 |
| Females 19-30 | 2,000 | 2,400 |
| Males 4-8 | 1,400 | 2,200 |
| Males 9-13 | 1,800 | 2,600 |
| Males 14-18 | 2,200 | 3,200 |
| Males 19-30 | 2,400 | 3,000 |

Reproduced from: USDA. MyPlate Sample Menus. Available at: http://www.choosemyplate.gov/tipsresources/menus.html. Accessed October 6, 2016.

growth spurts start between 12.5 and 13 and peak at about age 14. This spurt lasts about 2 years.[17] The most rapid linear growth spurt for an average American boy occurs between 12 and 15 years of age. For the average American girl, the spurt occurs about 2 years earlier, between 10 and 13 years of age. The growth spurt during adolescence contributes about 15 percent of final adult height and about 50 percent of adult weight. During adolescence, boys tend to gain more weight than girls and boys experience greater increases in lean body mass. Girls accumulate more body fat, specifically around the hips and buttocks, upper arms, breasts, and upper back.

Growth charts are tools used for monitoring the growth of a child.[128] These charts, which are pertinent to the school-age child, include weight for age, stature for age, and BMI for age for boys and girls.

## Adolescent Eating Behaviors

The eating habits of adolescents are not static; they fluctuate throughout adolescence. Adolescents may use foods to establish individuality and express their identity. Experimentation may lead to certain eating behaviors such as skipping meals, and the rate of meal skipping may increase as they mature.[127] Breakfast is

the most frequently skipped meal; only 29 percent of adolescent females eat breakfast daily.[129,130] Adequate nutrition, especially eating breakfast, has been associated with improved academic performance and reduced tardiness and absences.[11] Lunch is another meal that about 25 percent of adolescents skip.[11,129] Reasons for their changes in eating habits include spending less time with family and more time with their peer group.[129] They eat more meals and snacks away from home, including many fast foods high in fat and calories.[131] The average teenager eats at fast-food restaurants twice a week. Fast-food visits account for 31 percent of all food eaten away from home and make up 83 percent of their visits to restaurants. [132,133]

The results of the HEI showed that in general, children ages 11 through 18 had poorer quality diets compared to younger children (2 to 3 years old). The possible reasons for the poor diet may be that parents are less attentive to the diets of this age group (11 through 18) and that children from low-income families are more likely to have a poorer diet. In addition, studies show that as children become more independent, they make inadequate dietary choices such as consuming more fast foods and salty snacks.[132,133] The average HEI scores for females ages 11 to 18 was 61.5 and for males of the same age was 60.4. As mentioned earlier in the chapter, an HEI score over 80 implies that the person has a good diet; a score between 51 and 80 means the diet needs improvement.

## ▶ Food and Nutrition Programs for Children and Adolescents

Child nutrition programs contribute significantly to the food and nutrient intake of school-age children. The purpose of these programs is to provide nutritious meals to all children. These programs also can reinforce nutrition education in the classroom. Child nutrition programs include the NSLP, SBP, SFSP, and SMP (see also Chapter 4). In addition, President Obama signed the Healthy, Hunger-Free Kids Act of 2010 into law. This law contains elements crucial to First Lady Michelle Obama's "Let's Move" anti–childhood obesity campaign. The Healthy, Hunger-Free Kids Act of 2010 is intended to allow children throughout the country to have access to good-quality meals in school cafeterias. Also, this bill will allow the USDA to be more effective and aggressive in responding to obesity and hunger challenges.[134]

## Think About It

Fedelia is a nutritionist in a community composed mostly of young families with children with mixed income—both high- and low-income status. She needs to prepare a nutrition education program for mothers about nutrient needs during childhood. She wants to focus on those nutrients that have been found to be deficient during childhood. Which nutrients are likely to be low or deficient during childhood? Are children living in poor families more likely to be deficient in nutrients? If so, which ones? What are some of the nutrition-related concerns during childhood that Fedelia needs to consider? What are some of the food assistance programs that can help the poor families obtain nutritious foods?

## National School Lunch Program

The National School Lunch Program (NSLP) provides nutritious lunches and the opportunity for professionals to practice skills learned in nutrition education classes. This program also offers after-school snacks at sites that meet eligibility requirements.

School food programs for children started in the early 1900s when free, compulsory, and universal education was established.[121] Philanthropic organizations, local school districts, and private individuals made the first efforts to establish free lunches in schools. With increasing federal involvement, primarily in the form of donations from the accumulation of surplus foods, states gradually expanded the number of food programs.[121] In 1946, legislation was passed establishing the NSLP under the direction of the USDA. Today, federal cash reimbursements and donated foods from the Commodity Supplemental Food Program are provided to schools that serve a lunch meeting specified nutritional requirements (see **TABLE 9-7**). Modifications in 1971 established the provision that children from families with incomes at or below 130 percent of the poverty level are eligible for a free lunch, and children in families with incomes between 130 percent and 185 percent below the poverty level are eligible for a reduced price lunch.[135] **TABLE 9-8** shows the eligibility standards for the federal child nutrition programs.

A small reimbursement also is provided to the school for all lunches, but children from families with incomes above 185 percent of the poverty level pay the established price (see Table 9-8). Most of the support that the USDA provides to schools in the NSLP comes in the form of a cash reimbursement for each meal served.

**TABLE 9-7** Acceptable National School Lunch Program Meals

| Food Items | Type A* | Type B* |
|---|---|---|
| Milk, whole | ½ pint | 2 pints |
| Protein-rich foods consisting of any of the following or a combination thereof: | | |
| Fresh or processed meat and poultry | 2 oz | 1 oz |
| Cheese, cooked or canned fish | | |
| Dry peas, or beans, or soybeans, cooked | ½ cup | ¼ cup |
| Peanut butter | 4 Tbsp | 2 Tbsp |
| Eggs | 1 | ½ |
| Raw, cooked, or canned vegetables, fruits, or both | ¾ cup | ½ cup |
| Bread, muffins, or hot bread made of whole grain cereal or enriched flour | 1 portion | 1 portion |
| Butter or fortified margarine | 2 tsp | 1 tsp |

*The Type A lunch was designed to meet one third to half of the minimum daily nutritional requirements of a child 10 to 12 years of age. The Type B pattern was devised to provide a supplementary lunch in schools in which adequate facilities for the preparation of a Type A lunch could not be provided.
Reproduced from: U.S. Department of Agriculture, Food and Nutrition Services. School Meal Programs Income Eligibility Guidelines. Available at: http://www.fns.usda.gov/cnd. Accessed April 24, 2016.

In 1994, the Food and Nutrition Service (formerly Food and Consumer Service) launched the School Meals Initiative for Healthy Children. The purpose of this initiative was twofold: 1) to educate children about the importance of making healthy food choices and 2) to provide support for school food service professionals to offer healthy school meals that meet the Dietary Guidelines for Americans. The recommendation included that no more than 30 percent of an individual's calories come from fat and less than 10 percent from saturated fat. Regulations also established a standard for school lunches to provide one third of the Recommended Dietary Allowances for protein, vitamin A, vitamin C,

**TABLE 9-8** Annual Income Eligibility Guidelines for the Federal Child Nutrition Programs: Effective from July 1, 2016 – June 30, 2017

| Household Size | Federal Poverty Guidelines Annual | Reduced Price Meals – 185% | | | | | Free Meals – 130% | | | | |
|---|---|---|---|---|---|---|---|---|---|---|---|
| | | Annual | Monthly | Twice per Month | Every Two Weeks | Weekly | Annual | Monthly | Twice per Month | Every Two Weeks | Weekly |
| **48 Contiguous States, District of Columbia, Guam, and Territories** | | | | | | | | | | | |
| 1 | 11,880 | 21,978 | 1,832 | 916 | 846 | 423 | 15,444 | 1,287 | 644 | 594 | 297 |
| 2 | 16,020 | 29,637 | 2,470 | 1,235 | 1,140 | 570 | 20,826 | 1,736 | 868 | 801 | 401 |
| 3 | 20,160 | 37,296 | 3,108 | 1,554 | 1,435 | 718 | 26,208 | 2,184 | 1,092 | 1,008 | 504 |
| 4 | 24,300 | 44,955 | 3,747 | 1,874 | 1,730 | 885 | 31,590 | 2,633 | 1,317 | 1,215 | 608 |
| 5 | 28,440 | 52,614 | 4,385 | 2,193 | 2,024 | 1,012 | 36,972 | 3,081 | 1,541 | 1,422 | 711 |
| 6 | 32,580 | 60,273 | 5,023 | 2,512 | 2,319 | 1,160 | 42,354 | 3,530 | 1,765 | 1,629 | 815 |
| 7 | 38,730 | 67,951 | 5,663 | 2,832 | 2,614 | 1,307 | 47,749 | 3,980 | 1,990 | 1,837 | 919 |
| 8 | 40,890 | 75,647 | 6,304 | 3,152 | 2,910 | 1,455 | 53,157 | 4,430 | 2,215 | 2,045 | 1,023 |
| For Each Additional Family Member add: | 4,150 | 7,696 | 642 | 321 | 296 | 146 | 5,408 | 451 | 226 | 208 | 104 |
| **Alaska** | | | | | | | | | | | |
| 1 | 14,840 | 27,454 | 2,288 | 1,144 | 1,056 | 528 | 19,292 | 1,608 | 804 | 742 | 371 |
| 2 | 20,020 | 37,037 | 3,087 | 1,544 | 1,425 | 713 | 26,028 | 2,169 | 1,085 | 1,001 | 501 |
| 3 | 25,200 | 46,620 | 3,885 | 1,943 | 1,794 | 897 | 32,760 | 2,730 | 1,365 | 1,260 | 630 |
| 4 | 30,380 | 56,203 | 4,684 | 2,342 | 2,162 | 1,081 | 39,494 | 3,292 | 1,646 | 1,519 | 760 |
| 5 | 35,360 | 65,786 | 5,483 | 2,742 | 2,531 | 1,266 | 46,228 | 3,853 | 1,927 | 1,778 | 889 |
| 6 | 40,740 | 75,389 | 6,281 | 3,141 | 2,899 | 1,450 | 52,962 | 4,414 | 2,207 | 2,037 | 1,019 |
| 7 | 45,920 | 84,952 | 7,080 | 3,540 | 3,268 | 1,634 | 59,696 | 4,975 | 2,488 | 2,296 | 1,148 |
| 8 | 51,120 | 94,572 | 7,881 | 3,941 | 3,638 | 1,819 | 66,458 | 5,538 | 2,789 | 2,556 | 1,278 |
| For Each Additional Family Member add: | 5,200 | 9,620 | 602 | 401 | 370 | 185 | 6,760 | 564 | 282 | 260 | 130 |
| **Hawaii** | | | | | | | | | | | |
| 1 | 13,670 | 25,290 | 2,108 | 1,054 | 973 | 487 | 17,771 | 1,481 | 741 | 684 | 342 |
| 2 | 18,430 | 34,096 | 2,842 | 1,421 | 1,312 | 656 | 23,959 | 1,997 | 999 | 922 | 461 |
| 3 | 23,190 | 42,902 | 3,576 | 1,788 | 1,651 | 826 | 30,147 | 2,513 | 1,257 | 1,160 | 580 |
| 4 | 27,950 | 51,708 | 4,309 | 2,155 | 1,989 | 995 | 36,335 | 3,028 | 1,514 | 1,398 | 699 |
| 5 | 32,710 | 60,514 | 5,043 | 2,522 | 2,326 | 1,164 | 42,523 | 3,544 | 1,772 | 1,636 | 818 |
| 6 | 37,470 | 69,320 | 5,777 | 2,869 | 2,667 | 1,334 | 48,711 | 4,060 | 2,030 | 1,874 | 937 |
| 7 | 42,230 | 78,126 | 6,511 | 3,256 | 3,005 | 1,503 | 54,899 | 4,575 | 2,288 | 2,112 | 1,056 |
| 8 | 47,010 | 86,969 | 7,248 | 3,624 | 3,345 | 1,673 | 61,113 | 5,093 | 2,547 | 2,351 | 1,176 |
| For Each Additional Family Member add: | 4,700 | 8,843 | 737 | 369 | 341 | 171 | 6,214 | 518 | 259 | 239 | 120 |

Modified from: U.S. Department of Agriculture, Food and Nutrition Services. School Meal Programs Income Eligibility Guidelines. Available at: http://www.fns.usda.gov/cnd/governance/notices/iegs/IEGs11-12.pdf. Accessed August 04, 2016.

iron, calcium, and calories. School lunches must meet federal nutrition requirements, but local school food authorities make decisions about what specific foods to serve and how they are prepared. The initiative was implemented in schools throughout the United States at the beginning of the 1996 to 1997 school year.[136]

In fiscal year 2009, more than 31.3 million children received their lunch through the NSLP each day. Since the modern program began, more than 219 billion lunches have been served.[137] However, not all children participate in the NSLP program or the SBP.[137]

## School Breakfast Program

The School Breakfast Program (SBP) began as a pilot project in 1966 and was made permanent in 1975. Eligibility criteria are the same as for the NSLP. The SBP was implemented for many reasons, some of which are the obvious nutrition-related ones. However, studies have shown that children who participate in the SBP also have higher standardized achievement test scores than eligible nonparticipants.[121]

Children often skip breakfast because of busy schedules, long bus rides, and lack of resources.[138] Meal standards and children's access to healthy foods improve the health status and academic performance of students. School breakfasts must provide one fourth of the Recommended Daily Allowances (RDAs) for calories, protein, calcium, iron, vitamin A, and vitamin C for the applicable age or grade groups.[139,140] In the fiscal year 2009, an average of 9.1 million children participated in the SBP every day.[141]

## Summer Food Service Program

Millions of U.S. children depend on free and reduced-price school meals for 9 months of the year, but many communities do not offer a summer program; therefore, a large number of children do not eat breakfast during summer months, consequently contributing to overall poor eating habits.[142]

The Summer Food Service Program (SFSP) was established in 1975 after a pilot program in 1968. The program provides free nutritious meals to low-income children during school vacations. It is offered in areas, for example, community centers or at activity programs, such as day camps, in which at least half of the children are from households with incomes below 185 percent of the poverty level.

The program provides one or two meals per day except on special conditions (for example, very low income situations), when three meals are provided daily. All meals are served free to eligible participants, and the USDA reimburses the sites for the meals served.[143]

## Team Nutrition Program

In 1995, the USDA started its School Meals Initiative for Healthy Children, called Team Nutrition, to "improve the health and education of children through better nutrition."[144] The initiative's major objectives are 1) to provide meals that are consistent with the Dietary Guidelines for Americans and other current scientific recommendations for children at school, and 2) to improve child health and nutrition by developing creative public–private partnerships through the media, schools, businesses, families, and the community. Partnership with the private sector also enhances the nutrition education efforts. For instance, a subsidiary of the Walt Disney Company used two movie characters to help promote nutrition. Scholastic, Inc., an educational publisher, developed teaching kits for use in schools. The Cooperative State Research, Education, and Extension Services (CSREES) implemented community nutrition action kits. Training and technical assistance were provided to develop new recipes for use in the updated school meals program by changing the specification for foods offered in school meals and by funding training grants to assist states in developing a sustainable training infrastructure for local school districts.[145] The Healthy School Meals Resource System is an information system for food service professionals available in print form, on a computer disk, and on the Internet at http://www.fns.usda.gov.

Team Nutrition uses an extensive nationwide network of public and private organizations to develop and disseminate products, including private sector companies, nonprofit organizations, and advocacy groups. The purpose of the relationships is to leverage resources, expand the reach of messages, and build a broad base of support.

**TABLE 9-9** Current Basic Cash Reimbursement Rates (July 1, 2014 to June 30, 2015)[*,131]

| Current Basic Cash Reimbursement Rates (July 1, 2011 to June 30, 2012)[*,131] | | | |
|---|---|---|---|
| Free lunches: | $2.93 | Free snacks: | $0.80 |
| Reduced-price lunches: | $2.53 | Reduced-price snacks: | $0.40 |
| Paid lunches: | $0.28 | Paid snacks: | $0.07 |

*Higher reimbursement rates are in effect for Alaska and Hawaii and for some schools with high percentages of low-income children.

The success of Team Nutrition depends on effective partnerships among federal, state, and local agencies that administer child nutrition programs. Team Nutrition schools are the focal point for this initiative; however, the roles and responsibilities presented in **TABLE 9-10** are critical at each level.[144]

## Head Start Program

The Head Start Program is a comprehensive child health development program for children between the ages of 3 and 5 years from families that meet the federal poverty guidelines. The Head Start Act of 1965 established this program, which provides all enrolled children with a broad array of services, including education, health services (medical, nutritional, dental, and mental health), social services, parent involvement activities, and special services to children with disabilities.[146] Visit http://www.acf.hhs.gov/programs/ohs for the most current information about Head Start.

## National Youth Sports Program

The National Youth Sports Program (NYSP) is a federal program designed to assist low-income children ages 10 to 16 in a summer program. The main goal of the program is to motivate low-income children to learn self-respect through a program of sports instruction and competition.

In 1968, representatives of the National Collegiate Athletic Association (NCAA) and the President's Council on Physical Fitness piloted the NYSP concept during the summer at two university athletic facilities. On March 17, 1969, the White House announced that the federal government was committing $3 million to establish a sports program for economically disadvantaged young children. The federal grant has increased significantly since then, and funding appropriations are renewed on a yearly basis. An annual grant is provided to a national, nonprofit organization to operate the NYSP.

The NYSP provides a comprehensive developmental and instructional sports program for approximately 78,148 low-income children. The program includes supervised sports instruction in at least four sports, using the campus facilities of colleges and universities. The enrichment part of the program provides the children with information about career and educational opportunities, study habits, drug and alcohol abuse, and nutrition.[147]

**TABLE 9-10** The Roles and Responsibilities of Federal, State, and Local Agencies in Team Nutrition

| FNS and the USDA | State Agencies | School Districts and Other School Food Authorities | Schools |
|---|---|---|---|
| • Establish policies.<br>• Develop materials that meet needs identified by the FNS and its state and local partners.<br>• Disseminate materials in ways that meet state and local needs.<br>• Develop partnerships with other federal agencies and national organizations.<br>• Promote Team Nutrition messages through the national media. | • Make recommendations to FNS regarding Team Nutrition materials and dissemination methods.<br>• Provide training and technical assistance to strengthen current Team Nutrition schools.<br>• Recruit new Team Nutrition schools.<br>• Develop partnerships with other state agencies and organizations.<br>• Promote Team Nutrition messages through the state media. | • Recruit Team Nutrition schools.<br>• Receive Team Nutrition materials from FNS, distribute to schools, and provide training for their use.<br>• Develop partnerships with other school district departments and community organizations.<br>• Coordinate Team Nutrition activities among schools, especially community events.<br>• Provide support as needed by Team Nutrition schools. | • Offer a variety of healthy menu choices.<br>• Provide behavior-based nutrition education in pre-K through grade 12.<br>• Establish policies and provide resources that ensure a school environment supportive of healthy eating and physical activity.<br>• Involve parents and communities in Team Nutrition activities that reinforce team nutrition messages.<br>• Establish partnerships among teachers, food service staff, school administrators, parents, community leaders, and the media. |

In addition, each participant receives a free complete medical examination prior to participation in NYSP. Any physical problems identified receive adequate follow-up treatment. Every participant is covered by an accident-medical insurance policy, and liability insurance is provided for sponsoring institutions. In addition, a minimum of one USDA-approved meal is provided on a daily basis and funded by the USDA.

## ▶ Challenges to Implementing Quality School Nutrition Programs

Research shows that students who participate in school meal programs have improved academic performance and healthier eating habits.[148] However, less than 60 percent of students choose the NSLP or SBP.[149] School meals face a variety of challenges[149]:

- Students' preferences for fast foods, soft drinks, and salty snacks
- Mixed messages sent by school personnel
- School food preparation and serving space limitations
- Inadequate meal periods
- Lack of education standards for school food service directors

Studies have shown that school meal programs improve children's academic, behavioral, emotional, and social functioning.[11,150,151] Children participating in the NSLP are more likely than nonparticipants to consume more vegetables, milk and milk products, and meat and meat substitutes and fewer soft drinks and/ or fruit drinks.[152] Consequently, they consume higher amounts of calcium, riboflavin, phosphorus, magnesium, zinc, thiamin, and vitamins $B_6$ and $B_{12}$ than do nonparticipants. The contribution of school meals to total daily intake of vitamins and minerals ranges from 45 percent of the RDA for iron to 77 percent of the RDA for calcium. School lunches provide approximately 35 percent of total energy intake. Thirty-three percent of the energy is from fat and 12 percent from saturated fatty acids. School lunches contribute one third of the total sodium intake and 8 percent of total sucrose intake. For some 10-year-old children, approximately 50 to 60 percent of total daily intake of energy, protein, cholesterol, carbohydrate, and sodium are from school meals.[153,154]

In many schools, the continued success of child nutrition programs is in trouble. The environment in these schools discourages students from eating meals provided by the NSLP and SBP and encourages food choices and eating habits that are not consistent with the Dietary Guidelines for Americans.[154,155]

The sale of foods in snack bars, school stores, and vending machines competes with school meals for students' appetites, time, and money.[155] **Competitive foods** are any foods sold in competition with USDA school meals and are considered as "foods of minimal nutritional value (FMNVs)" and "all other foods offered for individual sale."[155] FMNVs provide less than 5 percent of the DRI of each of the following eight nutrients per serving: protein, niacin, riboflavin, thiamin, calcium, iron, and vitamins A and C. FMNVs include soft drinks, nonfruit water ices, chewing gum, candies, jellies and gums (gum drops, jelly beans, and jellied and fruit-flavored slices), marshmallow candies, fondant (candy, soft mints), licorice, spun candy (cotton candy), and candy-coated popcorn. These foods may not be sold in the food service area during the serving period by law.[155]

Many foods that are served in competition with the NSLP and SBP are made available as a result of school administrators finding loopholes in competitive food regulations. For example:

1. Government regulations restrict the sale of FMNV only during actual meal times and only in food service areas where meals are prepared and/or served. They do not prohibit competitive foods from being sold on school campuses all day in locations other than where school meals are being served.
2. The USDA's definition of FMNV does not include many high-fat, high-sodium snack items such as cookies, doughnuts, potato chips, tortilla chips, and cheese puffs.
3. Other foods offered for individual sale in food service areas (e.g., cookies, potato chips, and muffins) are allowed if the income from the sale of such foods benefits the food service, school, or school student organizations. This creates an opportunity for schools to compete with their own NSLP and SBP for revenue, contributing to decreases in student participation in these programs.
4. The sale of competitive foods is also not prohibited in elementary schools, a place where most students are not mature enough to make wise food choices.[155] There is the potential for overconsumption of food when competitive foods are purchased in addition to school meals or in large quantities. This could lead to the risk for overweight or obesity.

To exacerbate these problems, many school districts negotiate exclusive pouring rights and marketing contracts with major beverage companies to promote their beverage and food products. Many of these contracts provide lucrative packages worth millions of dollars and make provisions to increase the percentage of profits schools receive when refreshment stand and vending sales volumes increase. School budgets are continually squeezed, so administrators find pouring rights contracts desirable and often do not consider the nutritional well-being of students.[155] For many schools, competitive foods, especially soft drinks, represent additional income that can be spent for discretionary purposes not necessarily related to food service.

As school populations grow and budgets shrink, schools give higher priority to building classrooms than to expanding food service facilities, which that are often inadequate for preparing and serving appealing meals to students. In some schools, inadequate cafeteria capacity requires lunch periods to begin as early as 10:00 AM and end as late as 1:30 PM. Due to inadequate dining facilities and less time to eat, many students rely on less nutritious foods that are available in vending machines, snack bars, and school stores.[156,157]

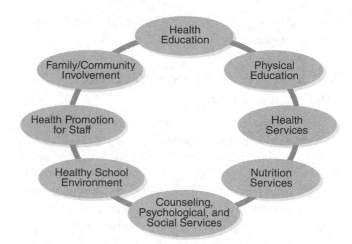

**FIGURE 9-2** Eight components of a coordinated school health program.

Reproduced from: Centers for Disease Control and Prevention, Division of Adolescent and School Health. Available at: http://www.cdc.gov/healthyyouth/CSHP/index.htm.

## ▶ Promoting Successful Programs in Schools

Inconsistent funding and severe reduction in funding from year to year, mainly in nutrition education, have decreased the effectiveness of nutrition education for children. An effective way to support nutrition-related action that encourages healthful eating and helps reduce childhood overweight and obesity is through implementation of a coordinated school health program (CSHP).[138] A CSHP combines health education, disease prevention, health promotion, and access to health and social services in an integrated, comprehensive manner.[158] **FIGURE 9-2** presents the eight components of a CSHP. Community nutritionists working as CSHP team members can provide leadership and coordination for issues related to many of the components of the school health program.[159]

The CDC provided guidelines that summarize the most effective strategies for promoting healthy eating among school-age children within the CSHP.[159] The guidelines are available at http://www.cdc.gov.

As Figure 9-2 shows, nutrition services is one of the eight components of a coordinated CSHP. The other components are discussed in the following sections.

### Comprehensive School Health Education

Health education provides pre-K through grade 12 classroom instruction to increase health knowledge, support positive health attitudes, and develop skills necessary for the adoption of a healthful lifestyle. Dietetics professionals

can work with school health educators to incorporate health education curricula, nutrition education, and opportunities to practice healthful eating behaviors.

### Physical Education

Physical education provides planned and sequential instruction that promotes physical activity designed to develop basic movement skills, sports skills, and physical fitness and to enhance physical, mental, social, and emotional abilities. Dietetics professionals can be advocates for pre-K through grade 12 education that promotes lifelong physical activity and focuses on components of health-related fitness.

### School Health Services

These are services coordinated by a certified school nurse that provide preventive services, education, emergency care, referral, and management of acute and chronic health conditions. Dietetics professionals can assist individuals in these services by developing policies for weight management and obesity programs and can provide nutrition education programs in conjunction with classroom teachers.

### School Nutrition Services

School nutrition services integrate nutritious, affordable, and appealing meals; nutrition education; and an environment that promotes healthful eating behaviors. Food service directors, as well as dietetics professionals and parents of school-age children, can advocate for policies to 1) provide more nutritious food offerings, 2) limit or remove competitive food sales and FMNV from school fundraisers, and 3) establish a list of nutritious foods allowed in vending machines, at school parties, and as classroom rewards.

## School Counseling, Psychological, and Social Services

Psychological, counseling, and social assistance can be integrated into school environment activities that focus on the cognitive, emotional, behavioral, and social needs of individuals, groups, and families to prevent and address problems and facilitate health and learning. Individual and group discussions regarding body image, physical changes, and weight management also can be provided. Dietetics professionals can provide encouragement and support to families who want to practice healthful eating behaviors.

## Healthy School Environment

Attention to the school environment means addressing the physical, emotional, and social climates of a school to provide a safe and supportive environment to enhance health and learning. Policies should be developed to support healthful eating environments related to vending machines, competitive foods, fundraisers, and classroom rewards and party treats. Dietetics professionals can help promote healthful eating environments by serving on nutrition-related school committees and advocating for policies that place precedence on nutrition and learning.

## School-Site Health Promotion for Staff

Staff health promotion includes assessment of education and fitness activities for school faculty and staff that are designed to maintain and improve students' health and well-being. Faculty and staff should be provided with opportunities to participate in workshops and classes for healthful eating and physical activity. Dietetics professionals can offer nutrition-related workshops and classes to school faculty and staff.

## Family and Community Involvement in School Health

Family and community involvement consists of developing partnerships among schools, families, community groups, and individuals to share and maximize resources and expertise in addressing the healthful development of children, adolescents, and families. Dietetics professionals can partner with schools and community organizations to establish nutrition, food preparation, weight management, and exercise programs for students, faculty, staff, and families.[158] This chapter's third Successful Community Strategies presents a program created by the Aptos Middle School in San Francisco, California.

## Successful Community Strategies

### The Aptos Middle School (San Francisco, California) Pilot Program[160]

During a pilot project for the San Francisco Unified School District (SFUSD), Aptos Middle School made significant changes in its vending and à la carte food service programs. The purpose of the project was to make more healthful foods and beverages available to students and establish nutrition standards for competitive foods. Approximately 860 to 900 racially diverse students were enrolled in Aptos Middle School during the 2002 to 2003 school year. About 36.5 percent of students were eligible for free and reduced-price school meals. The new principal, a new physical education program, and a group of parents, teachers, and volunteers initiated the change in the food service program. The San Francisco superintendent of schools supported this pilot project, which helped make it successful as a district-wide change.

With strong support from the administration, a nutrition committee composed of parents and teachers was formed to lead the changes. This group met electronically (via e-mail) to share concerns and data and to attain a consensus on appropriate changes for Aptos Middle School. The committee conducted a student survey to discover what foods students wanted the school to provide as à la carte choices. The students' preferences closely matched the parents' ideas of "more fresh foods." The most popular choices were submarine sandwiches, California rolls (sushi), soup, pasta, and smoothies.

The committee collaborated with a creative cafeteria supervisor and investigated products and ingredients that would offer students healthful versions of the foods they wanted to purchase.

This process presented both opportunities and challenges. In several cases, food suppliers and manufacturers were willing to adapt their products to adhere to the nutrition committee's standards (e.g., sushi). However, it has not been possible, at least so far, to find smoothie options with appropriate ingredients at an acceptable price.

*(continues)*

## Successful Community Strategies

Changes instituted included:

- All soft drinks were removed from the vending machines located in the physical education department and replaced with bottled water.
- Fruit options for students were expanded beyond apples, oranges, and bananas to include such fruits as kiwifruit, grapes, strawberries, and melons; jicama, raw broccoli, spinach, and romaine lettuce were available for salads.
- Soft drinks were removed from the à la carte line in the cafeteria and replaced with water, milk, and 100-percent juice (no more than 12 ounces per serving).
- FMNV and high-fat foods, such as French fries and nachos, were removed from cafeteria meals.
- During the 2002 to 2003 school years, high-fat/high-sugar foods were also removed from the à la carte line and replaced with fresh, healthier options and more appropriate portion sizes.
- The new food options included turkey sandwiches, sushi, homemade soup, salads, and baked chicken with rice.
- All vending machines, fundraising sales, and any other food sold outside cafeterias had to adhere to the standards by January 2004.

Results showed that students were buying more units of water than they used to buy soft drinks. Because the larger water bottle is sold at a higher price, vending machine revenues in the physical education department increased. Net revenues increased because food costs were lower for the healthier items. The Aptos cafeteria ended the 2002 to 2003 year with a surplus of $6,000. The administrators and teachers reported better student behavior after lunch, fewer afternoon visits to the counseling office, less litter in the school yard, and more students sitting down to eat. Aptos Middle School also reported higher scores on standardized tests. The "Healthy Food, Healthy Kids" policy at Aptos won an award from the State of California, and the changes made at Aptos were implemented throughout the San Francisco Unified School District for the school year 2003 to 2004. The district-wide trend appears to be a move away from à la carte purchases and toward the National School Lunch Program.

# Learning Portfolio

## Chapter Summary

- The nutrients most likely to be low or deficient in school-age children are calcium, iron, vitamins $B_6$ and A, and zinc.
- It is estimated that approximately 4.4 percent of children ages 1 to 5 years have blood lead levels higher than 10 mg/dl.
- Protein-energy malnutrition (PEM) is classified into two parts: primary and secondary. Primary PEM refers to a deficit of available food; secondary causes of PEM may be biological or social.
- Approximately 40 to 50 percent of children and adolescents with special healthcare needs have nutrition-related risk factors or health problems that require the attention of a registered dietitian, nutritionist, or healthcare professional. Dietitians are recognized as health professionals qualified to provide developmental services to children with special needs.
- Children from families with high television use consume an average of 6 percent more of their total daily energy intake from meats; 5 percent more from pizza, salty snacks, and soda; and nearly 5 percent less from fruits, vegetables, and juices than children from families with low television use.
- Experimentation and idealism during adolescence may lead to certain eating behaviors such as skipping meals. The rate of meal skipping increases as children mature. Breakfast is the most skipped meal; only 29 percent of adolescent females eat breakfast daily. Lunch is another meal that adolescents tend to skip.
- Eating disorders have many causes, and it is likely that several factors contribute to the development of the disorder in any given case. Nutritional factors and dieting behavior may be contributing factors to the development and course of eating disorders.
- Children from families with incomes at or below 130 percent of the poverty level are eligible for a free lunch, and children in families with incomes between 130 percent and 185 percent below the poverty level are eligible for a reduced price lunch.

## Critical Thinking Activities

- In groups of four or five, review the national health objectives in Healthy People 2010 for physical activity and weight control for children and adolescents. Pick an objective from each section, and brainstorm possible community programs a community or public health nutritionist could initiate to reach that objective.

- Visit a high school in the community and evaluate the school lunch meals, including the availability of foods of minimal nutritional value.
- A family with four children (ages 3, 7, 9, and 12) earns $17,000 per year. Using the Annual Income Eligibility Guidelines, determine the different types of food assistance programs from which they are eligible to receive benefits.

- Conduct a 24-hour recall on two WIC participants (preferably 4- to 5-year-old children) or on two school-age children to determine nutrient intake.
- Identify what federal and state assistance programs may be needed.
- Provide a list containing foods that are high in essential nutrients (vitamins, minerals, and protein).
- Determine/calculate the children's daily caloric and nutrient needs.
- Devise a list of foods with high iron content.

# 🔍 CASE STUDY 9-1: Special Supplemental Nutrition Program for Women, Infants, and Children (WIC) and Children's Health

Sandra is a single mother with three children: Sara is 2 years old, Alice is 6, and James is 13. To support her family, Sandra has a full-time job with an annual income of $18,000, and lives below the poverty line for a family of four. Recently, Sandra expressed to her friend Lisa that she is concerned about Alice and James's and her own weight gain. She explained that an elderly neighbor, Mary, takes care of the children after school and she likes to bake cookies for the children. Since the children have not made friends in their neighborhood, their main leisure activities are watching television and playing video games. Though time constraints lead Sandra to rely more on take-out and fast-food meals, she recently started attending an aerobics class with a friend and is interested in developing healthier eating habits.

Sara is under 5 years old, so Lisa suggested that Sandra enroll her in the Special Supplemental Nutrition Program for Women, Infants, and Children (WIC) and use the opportunity to speak to the WIC nutritionist about her concerns for the other children. Sandra scheduled an appointment with the WIC nutritionist, and nutritional assessments were conducted using such methods as 24-hour recall and anthropometric measurements. The evaluations revealed that Sara receives an inadequate dietary intake of essential nutrients such as calcium (400 mg/day) and iron (5 mg/day). The public health nurse assessments showed that the three children were anemic due to lack of adequate iron intake and the 6- and 13-year-olds were overweight because their BMIs were between the 85th and 95th percentiles on the CDC and National Center for Health Statistics growth chart.

Sandra was encouraged to:

- Enroll her children in the after-school program at the YWCA near their neighborhood that includes different types of physical activities. The program also provides after-school transportation assistance.
- Enroll in the WIC Farmers' Market program to obtain more fresh fruits and vegetables.
- Enroll in the Supplemental Nutrition Assistance Program and National School Lunch Program.
- Shop for foods once a week using MyPlate as a guide and purchase low-fat foods.
- Start weekend activities such as swimming instead of watching television or playing video games.
- Schedule a 3-month follow-up visit to see the WIC nutritionist.

## Questions

1. Sandra should be aware of the costs of overweight and obesity during childhood and adolescence. What are the consequences of overweight and obesity?
2. What are some of the foods that Sandra, other parents, and caregivers can feed toddlers and preschoolers? How many servings of foods per day should be given for each food group, and what are the nutrients supplied from each food group?
3. List and give a description of three of the Healthy People 2010 objectives related to children and adolescents, including the progress toward these three objectives.
4. Sandra wants to know how toddlers commonly behave while eating. What are some of the eating behaviors of toddlers?

*(continues)*

# 🔍 CASE STUDY 9-1: Special Supplemental Nutrition Program for Women, Infants, and Children (WIC) and Children's Health *(continued)*

5. The nutritionist wants to talk to Sandra about the Healthy Eating Index. What is the Healthy Eating Index? What are the components of the Healthy Eating Index?
6. There are some concerns about Sandra's children's food habits. Discuss some of the nutrition-related concerns during childhood and adolescence.
7. What criteria place Sandra's children and other children at risk for high blood cholesterol? What are the recommended cholesterol levels for children and adolescents ages 2 to 19 years?
8. The nutritionist explained eating disorders to Sandra because she was concerned about them. What are the three most prevalent disordered eating patterns? Briefly describe each.
9. Although Sandra's children do not have special healthcare needs, what are some common nutrition problems for children and adolescents with special healthcare needs?
10. Sandra's children are deficient in some important nutrients. Which nutrients are most commonly deficient or low in school-age children?
11. What are some additional food and nutrition assistance programs for Sandra's children and for other children, including adolescents with similar situations?
12. Sandra's children are in the school system. What are some of the challenges schools face when implementing successful nutrition programs?
13. Work in small groups or individually to discuss the case study and practice using the Nutrition Care Process chart provided on the companion website. You also can add other nutrition and health-related conditions or assessments to the case study to make the case study more challenging and interesting.

## Think About It

**Answer 1:** Nutrients that are likely to be low or deficient during childhood are calcium, iron, vitamin $B_6$, and vitamin A. Children living in poor families are likely to be deficient in calories; vitamins A, C, E, and folate; iron; zinc; thiamin; and magnesium.

Some of the nutrition-related concerns during childhood that Fedelia needs to consider are iron-deficiency anemia, dental caries, lead poisoning, overweight, and obesity. Food assistance programs such as the NSLP, SBP, SMP, and SFSP have been successful in reducing malnutrition in children.

**Answer 2:** She can use the *Diagnostic and Statistical Manual of Mental Disorders* or the information in Box 9-1, Table 9-7, and Figure 9-1 as screening tools. In addition, she can ask the participants to draw themselves on an 8½- by 11-inch piece of paper. Their drawings will help her determine their risk for eating disorder and the type of eating disorder.

Eating disorders have many causes, and it is likely that several factors contribute to the development of the disorders in any given case. In some cases, sociocultural pressures may be the reason why eating disorders are high in economically privileged communities and countries; a cultural obsession with weight and thinness in women and, possibly, dieting behaviors may contribute to eating disorders.

## Key Terms

**adolescence:** The period of life between 12 and 19 years of age.

**anorexia nervosa:** An eating disorder characterized by extreme weight loss, poor body image, and irrational fears of weight gain and obesity.

**atherosclerosis:** A progressive, complex disease that often begins in childhood and adolescence and is related to high serum total cholesterol levels.

**binge eating:** A disorder characterized by consuming large quantities of food in a very short period until the individual is uncomfortably full, which normally is not followed by vomiting or the use of laxatives. The individual typically feels out of control during a binge episode, followed by feelings of guilt and shame. People must experience eating binges twice a week on average for over 6 months to qualify for this diagnosis.

**bulimia nervosa:** An eating disorder characterized by recurrent episodes of rapid, uncontrolled eating of large amounts of food in a short period. Purging often follows episodes of binge eating.

**childhood disability:** Children and adolescents who have or are at increased risk for a chronic physical, developmental, behavioral, or emotional condition and who require health and related services.

**competitive foods:** Any foods sold in competition with U.S. Department of Agriculture school meals and that are considered as foods of minimal nutritional value (FMNV) available at concession stands, vending machines, and fundraisers that are in direct competition with the Child Nutrition Program during meal services anywhere on campus.

**dental caries:** Tooth decay.

**diabetes mellitus:** A disease caused by insufficient insulin secretion by the pancreas or insulin resistance by body tissues causing high blood glucose level.

**ferritin:** A complex of iron and apoferritin that is a major storage form of iron.

**galactosemia:** Lack of the enzyme needed to metabolize galactose.

**growth spurt:** A period of peak growth rate that begins at about ages 10 to 13 years in girls and 12 to 15 years in boys.

**iron deficiency:** Absent bone marrow iron stores, an increase in hemoglobin concentration of less than 1.0 g/dl after treatment with iron, or other abnormal laboratory values, such as serum ferritin concentration.

**Overnutrition:** Excessive consumption of any specific nutrient.

**undernutrition:** A health condition caused by a deficiency of one or more nutrients.

# References

1. Halterman JS, Kaczorowski JM, Aligne CA, Auinger P, et al. Iron deficiency and cognitive achievement among school-aged children and adolescents in the United States. *Pediatrics.* 2001;107:1381-1386.

2. Grantham-McGregor S. Can the provision of breakfast benefit school performance? *Food Nutr Bull.* 2005;26(2):S144-158.

3. Cook JT, Frank DA, Berkowitz C, Black MM, et.al. Food insecurity is associated with adverse health outcomes among human infants and toddlers. *J Nutr.* 2004;134:1432-1438.

4. Services USDA. Center for Nutrition Policy and Promotion *MyPyramid 2005.* www.mypyramid.gov/. Accessed February 28, 2011.

5. Gleason P, Suitor C. Changes in Children's Diets: Report (CN-01-CD2) to US Department of Agriculture, Food and Nutrition Service. Data taken from the 1994–96 and 1994–96 Continuing Survey of Food Intakes by Individuals (CSFII). 1989–91 to 1994–96 (2001).

6. Gleason P, Suitor C. Children's Diets in the Mid-1990s: Dietary Intake and Its Relationship With School Meal Participation (2001) Report (CN-01-CD) to US Department of Agriculture, Food and Nutrition Service. Data taken from the 1994–96 Continuing Survey of Food Intakes by Individuals (CSFII).

7. Nestle M. Increasing portion sizes in American diets: More calories, more obesity. *J Am Diet Assoc.* 2003;103:41-47.

8. Smiciklas-Wright H, Mitchell DC, Mickle SJ, Goldman JD, et al. Foods commonly eaten in the United States, 1989–1991 and 1994–1996: Are portion sizes changing? *J Am Diet Assoc.* 2003;103:39-40.

9. Rampersaud GC, Bailey LB, Kauwell GP. National survey beverage consumption data for children and adolescents indicate the need to encourage a shift toward more nutritive beverages. *J Am Diet Assoc.* 2003;103:97-100.

10. U.S. Department of Health and Human Services. The Surgeon General's call to action to prevent and decrease overweight and obesity. 2001. http://www.cdc.gov/nccdphp/dnpa/obesity/consequences.htm.

11. Troiano R, Flegal KM, Kuczmarski RJ, Campbell SM, et al. Overweight prevalence and trends for children and adolescents. *Arch Pediatr Adolesc Med.* 1995;149:1085–1091.

12. Franks P, Hanson H, Knowler H. Childhood obesity, other cardiovascular risk factors, and premature death. *N Engl J Med.* 2010;362:485-493.

13. American School Food Service Association. Impact of hunger and malnutrition on student achievement. *School Food Serv Res Rev.* 1989;13:17-21.

14. U.S. Department of Health and Human Services. *Healthy People 2010 Understanding and Improving Health.* 2nd ed. Washington, DC: Department of Health and Human Services; 2000. https://www.amazon.com/Healthy-People-2010-Understanding-Improving/dp/0160505283. Accessed March 10, 2017.

15. Nation Center for Health Statistics. Healthy People 2010: Progress Review Focus Area 16 Maternal Infant and Child Health. www.cdc.gov. Accessed March 7, 2011.

16. Berdanier CD. *Handbook of Nutrition and Food.* New York, NY: CRC Press; 2013.

17. Story M, Holt, K. *Bright Futures in Practice: Nutrition-Pocket Guide.* Arlington, VA: National Center for Education in Maternal and Child Health; 2002.

18. Insel P, Elaine Turner and Don Ross. *2002 Update Nutrition.* Sudbury, MA: Jones and Bartlett; 2002.

19. Frank G. *Community Nutrition: Applying Epidemiology to Contemporary Practice.* Rockville, MD: Aspen; 2007.

20. Kennedy ET, Ohls J, Carlson S, Fleming K. The healthy eating index: design and applicationl. *J Am Diet Assoc.* 1995;95(10):1103-1108.

21. Basiotis PP, Carlson A, Gerrior SA, Juan W, et al. The Healthy Eating Index, 1999-2000: Charting

dietary patterns of Americans. *Fam Econ Nutr Rev.* 2004;16(1):1-11.

22. Basiotis P, Carlson A, Gerrior S, Juan W, et al. The Healthy Eating Index: 1999-2000. CNPP-12. 2000. Accessed March 3, 2011.

23. Wilkinson EC, Mickle SJ, Joseph D. Trends in food and nutrient intakes by children in the United States. *Fam Econ Nutr Rev.* 2002;14(2):56-68.

24. U.S. Department of Agriculture. Food Intakes: Individuals in 48 States, Year 1977-78. U.S. Department of Agriculture, Human Nutrition Information Service, Nationwide Food Consumption Survey 1977-78, Rep. I-1; NTIS No. PB91-103523; 1983.

25. U.S. Department of Agriculture. Continuing survey of food intakes by individuals 1994-1996. Vol [CD-ROM] NITIS. Washington, DC: Agricultural Research Service; 2000.

26. Woteki RR, Briefel CJ, Klein PF, Jacques PM, et al. Nutrition Monitoring: Summary of a Statement from an American Society for Nutritional Sciences Working Group. *J Nutr.* 2002;132:3782-3783.

27. Bentley ME, Griffiths PL. The burden of anemia among women in India. *Eur J Clin Nutr.* 2003;57(1):52-60.

28. Thane CCW. Risk factors for low iron intake and poor iron status in a national sample of British young people aged 4-18 years. *Public Health Nutr.* 2003;6(5):485-496.

29. Center for Disease Control and Prevention. Recommendation to prevent and control iron deficiency in the United States. 1998;47 RR-03:1-36. Accessed April 3.

30. Brown JE, Sugarman I, Krinke UB, Murtaugh MA, et al. *Nutrition Through Life Cycle.* Belmont, CA: Wadsworth Thomson; 2002.

31. U.S. Department of Health and Human Services. Healthy People 2010, 2nd ed. With Understanding and Improving Health and Objectives for Improving Health. Vol 2. Washington, DC: U.S. Government Printing Office; 2000.

32. Centers for Disease Control and Prevention, National Center for Health Statistics. *National Center for Health Statistics-at-a-Glance.* Hyattsville, MD: CDC; 2002.

33. Kennedy E, Powell R. Changing eating patterns of American children: a view from 1996. *J Amer Coll Nutr.* 1997;16:524-529.

34. Pollitt E. Iron deficiencies and educational deficiency. *Nutr Rev.* 1997;55:133-141.

35. Riley E, McGee, C. Fetal alcohol spectrum disorders: an overview with emphasis on changes in brian and behavior. *Exp Bio Med.* 2005;230:357-365.

36. Requejo AM. The age at which meat in first include in the diet affects the incidence of iron deficiency and ferropenic anaemia in a group of pre-school children from Madrid. *Int J Vitam Nutr Res.* 1999;69:127-131.

37. Hine R. Folic acid contemporary clinical perspective. *Perspect Appl Nutr.* 1993;1:3-14.

38. Maloni J, Faan, D. Reducing the risk for preterm birth: evidence and implications for neonatal nurses. *Ad Neonatal Care.* 2004;4(3):166-174.

39. Donovan UM, Gibson, RS. Iron and zinc status of young women aged 14 to 19 years consuming vegetarian and omnivorous diets. *J Am Coll Nutr.* 1995;14:463-472.

40. McLaughlin TJ, Humphries O, Nguyen T, Maljanian R, et al. Getting the lead out in Hartford, Connecticut: a multifaceted lead-poisoning awareness campaign. *Environ Health Perspect.* 2004;112(1):1-5.

41. Markowitz M, Rosen JF, Clemente I. Clinicaian follow-up of children screened for lead poisoning. *Am J Public Health.* 1999;89.1088.

42. Wardlaw GM, Kessel M. *Perspecives in Nutrition.* 5th ed. New York, NY: McGraw-Hill; 2002.

43. Matte TD. Reducing blood lead levels. *JAMA.* 1999;281:2340-2342.

44. Ryan D, Levy B, Levy BS, Pollack S, et al. Protecting children form lead poisoning and building healthy communities. *Am J Public Health.* 1999; 89:822-824.

45. Snyder DC. Development of a population-specific risk assessment to predic elevated blood lead levels in Santa Clara County, California. *Pediatrics.* 1995;96:643-646.

46. Center for Disease Control and Prevention. Center for Disease Control and Prevention. Screening young children for lead poisoning; guidance for state and local public health officials; 1997. http:www.cdc.gov/nceh/programs/lead/guide/1997/guide97.htm.

47. Casamassimo P. *Bright Futures in Practice: Oral Health.* Arlington, VA: National Center for Education in Maternal and Child Health; 1996.

48. Mushak P,Crocetti A. Lead and nutrition: Biologic interactions of lead with nutrients. *Nutrition Today.* 1996;31:12-17.

49. Lutz P. *Nutrition and Diet Therapy.* 5th ed. Philadelphia, PA: F.A. Davis Company; 2010.

50. Krebs NF, Jacobson MS; American Academy of Pediatrics Committee on Nutrition. Prevention of pediatric overweight and obesity. *Pediatrics.* 2003;112:424-430.

51. Hedley AA, Ogden CL, Johnson CL, Carroll MD, et al. Prevalence of overweight and obesity among US children, adolescents, and adults, 1999-2002. *JAMA.* 2004;29(23):2847-2850.

52. Center Disease Control and Prevention. Overweight and Obesity: An Overview. www.cdc.gov/. Accessed March 10, 2011.

53. Phillips SM, Bandini LG, Compton DV, Naumova EN, et al. A longitudinal comparison of body composition by total body water and bioelectrical impedance in adolescent girls. *J Nutr.* 2003;133:1419-1425.

54. Hill JO, Peters JC. Environmental contributions to the obesity epidemic. *Science.* 1998;280:1371-1374.

55. Link K, Moell C, Garwicz S, Cavallin-Stahl E, et al. Growth hormone deficiency predicts cardiovascular risk in young adults treated for acute lymphoblastic leukemia in childhood. *J Clin Endocrinol Metab.* 2004;89:5003-5012.

56. Freedman DS, Dietz WH, Srinivasan SR, Berenson GS. The relation of overweight to cardiovascular risk factors among children and adolescents: The Bogalusa Heart Study. *Pediatrics.* 1999;103: 1175-1182.

57. Saelens BE, Sallis JF, Wilfley DE, Patric K, et al. Behavioral weight control for overweight adolescents initiated in primary care. *Obes Res.* 2002;10:22-32.

58. Guo SS, Chumlea WC. Tracking of body mass index in children in relation to overweight in adulthood. *Am J Clin Nutr.* 1999;70 Suppl:145S-148S.

59. Strauss RS. Childhood obesity and self-esteem. *Pediatr.* 2000;105(1):e15-e20.

60. Center Disease Control Prevention/National Center for Health Statistics. Prevalence of overweight and obesity among adults: United States, 1999-2002. 2005. http://epsl.asu.edu/ceru/Documents/NCHS_obesity.pdf. Accessed March 10, 2017.

61. Davison KK, Birch LL. Weight status, parent reaction, and self-concept in five-year-old girls. *Pediatrics.* 2001;107:46-53.

62. Nutrition and Your Health. *Dietary Guidelines for Americans.* Washington, DC: Departments of Agriculture and Health and Human Services; Home and Garden Bulletin No. 32.;2000.

63. Dietz WH. Health consequences of obesity in youth: childhood predictors of adult disease. *Pediatrics.* 1998;101(3 Pt 2):518-525.

64. Flegal KM, Carroll MD, Ogden CL, Johnson CL. Prevalence and trends in obesity among US Adults, 1999-2000. *JAMA.* 2002;288:1723-1727.

65. Mokdad A, Ford E, Bowman B. Prevalence of obesity, diabetes, and obesity-related health risk factors. *JAMA.* 2003;289:187-193.

66. Center Disease Control and Prevention. National diabetes fact sheet: general information and national estimates on diabetes in the United States. Atlanta, GA: U.S. Department of Health and Human Services; 2005. https://www.cdc.gov/diabetes/library/factsheets.html. Accessed March 10, 2017

67. Aye T, Levitsky LL. Type 2 diabetes: an epidemic disease in childhood. *Curr Opin Pediatr.* 2003;15(4):411-415.

68. Sung R, Tong P, Yu CW, Lau PW, et al. High prevalence of insulin resistance and metabolic syndrome in overweight/obese preadolescent Hong Kong Chines children aged 9-12 years. *Diabetes Care.* 2003;26:250-251.

69. Steinberger J, Daniels SR. Obesity, insulin resistance, diabetes, and cardiovascular risk in children. *Circulation.* 2003;107:1448-1456.

70. Prevention CDC. A. Diabetes Project. www.cdc.gov. Accessed March 6, 2011.

71. Kida K, Ito T, Yang SW, Tanpaichitr V. Effects of western diet on risk factors of chronic diseases in Asia. In: Bendich A, Deckelbaum RJ, eds. *Preventive Nutrition: the Comprehensive Guide for Health Professionals.* 2nd ed. Totowa, NJ: Humana Press; 2001:435-446.

72. Sinha R, Fisch G, Teague B. Prevalence of impaired glucose tolerance among children and adolescents with marked obesity. *N Engl J Med.* 2002;346:802-810.

73. Dwyer JT, Stone EJ, Yang M. Prevalence of marked overweight and obesity in a multiethnic pediatric population: Findings from the Child and Adolescent Trial for Cardiovascular Health (CATCH) Study. *J Am Diet Assoc.* 2000;100:1149-1156.

74. Wolf M, Cohen, KR, Rosenfeld JG. School-based interventions for obesity: Current approaches and future prospects. *Psychol Schools.* 1985;22:187-200.

75. Center Disease Control and Prevention. Healthy Schools Healthy Youth! www.cdc.gov. Accessed March 7, 2017.

76. National Association for Sport & Physical Education. Parents believe physical activity key to preventing childhood obesity. 2003.https://pgpedia.com/n/national-association-sport-and-physical-education. Accessed March 7, 2017.

77. Warren JM, Henry CJ, Lightowler HJ, Bradshaw SM, et al. Evaluation of a pilot school programme aimed at the prevention of obesity in children. *Health Promot Int.* 2003;18(4):287-296.

78. American Academy of Pediatrics. Cholesterol in Childhood. 2005; http://aappolicy.aappublications.org/. Accessed March 7, 2011.

79. Kavey RE, Daniels SR, Lauer RM, Atkins DL, et al. American Heart Association. American Heart Association guidelines for primary prevention of atherosclerotic cardiovascular disease beginning in childhood. *Circulation.* 2003;107:1562–1566.

80. Association AH. Dietary recommendations for children and adolescents: A guide for practitioners: consensus statement from the American Heart Association. *Circulation.* 2005;112:2061-2075.

81. National Heart, Lung, and Blood Institute. New NHLBI sponsored study shows programs can teach children to eat healthier. https://www.nhlbi.nih.gov/news/press-releases/2005/new-nhlbi-sponsored-study-shows-programs-can-teach-children-to-eat-healthier. Accessed March 7, 2017.

82. Obarzanek E, Kimm S, Barton B, Van Horn L, et al. Long-term safety and efficacy of cholesterol-lowering diet in children with elevated low-density lipoprotein cholesterol: seven-year results of the Dietary Intervention Study in Children (DISC). *Pediatrics.* 2001;107:256-264.

83. Stice E, Cameron RP, Killen JD, Hayward C, et al. Naturalistic weight-reduction efforts prospectively predict growth in relative weight and onset of obesity among female adolescents. *J Consult Clin Psychol.* 1999;67:967-974.

84. Mackey E, La Greca A. Adolescents' eating exercise and weight control behaviors: does peer crowd affiliation play a role? *J Pediatr Psychol.* 2007;32(1):13-23.

85. Freedman D, Dietz W, Srinivasan S, Berenson G. The relation of childhood BMI to adult adiposity: the Bogalusa Heart Study *Pediatrics.* 2005;115(1):22-27.

86. Neumark-Sztainer D, Story M, Falkner NH, Behuring T, et al. Sociodemographic and personal characteristics of adolescents engaged in weight loss and weight/muscle gain behaviors. Who is doing what? *Prevent Med.* 1999;28:4-5.

87. Moore D. Body image and eating behavior in adolescents,. *J Am Coll Nutr.* 1993;12:505-510.

88. Polivy J, Herman CP. Dieting and binging. A causal analysis. *Am Psychol.* 1985;193-201:193-201.

89. Schweiger U, Fichter M. Eating disorders: Clinical presentation, classification and aetiological models. *Bailliere's Clin Psych.* 1997;3:199-216.

90. Coulston A, Rock C, Monsen E. *Nutrition in the Prevention and Treatment of Disease.* New York, NY: Academic Press; 2001.

91. Guez J, Lev-Wiesel R, Valetsky S, Kruszewski D, et al. Self-figure drawings in women with anorexia; bulimia; overweight; and normal weight: a possible tool for assessment *Arts Psychother.* 2010;37(5):400-406.

92. Levine M. Ten things parents can do to help prevent eating disorder. www.nationaleatingdisorder.org Accessed March 2, 2011.

93. American Psychiatric Association. Diagnostic and Statistical Manual of Mental Disorders. 4th ed. Washington, DC: American Psychiatric Association; 1994.

94. Hsu L. Epidemiology of the eating disorders. *Psych Clin N Am.* 1996;19:681-700.

95. Haiman C, Devlin MJ. Binge eating before the onset of dieting: a distinct subgroup of bulimia nervosa. *Int J Eat Disord.* 1999;25:151-157.

96. Kirkley BG. Bulimia: Clinical characteristics, development, and ethiology. *J Am Diet Assoc.* 1986;86:472-486.

97. Lilenfeld LR, Kaye WH, Strober M. Genetics and family studies of anorexia nervosa and bulimia nervosa. *Bailliere's Clin Psych.* 1997;3:177-197.

98. Davis SM, Going D, Nicolette H, Teufel I, et al. Pathways: a culturally appropriate obesity-prevention program for American Indian schoolchildren. *Am J Clin Nutr.* 1999;69(4):796S-802S.

99. Katz SH, Weaver WW. *Encyclopedia of Food and Culture.* New York, NY: Scribner; 2003.

100. American Dietetic Association. Position of the American Dietetic Association: dietary guidance for healthy children aged 2 to 11 years. *J Am Diet Assoc.* 1999;99:93-101.

101. Fass S, Hancy K. Who are American's poor children. 2005. http://www.nccp.org/. Accessed March 7, 2011.

102. Nord M, Andrews M, Carlson S. *Household Food Security in the United States, 2004 (ERR-11).* Alexandria, VA: US Department of Agriculture, Economic Research Services; 2005.

103. America's Second Harvest. Hunger study: Key findings. 2016. http://www.shfblv.org/edu_hstats.php. Accessed March 7, 2017.

104. World Hunger Education Service. World Hunger Facts 2006. http://www.worldhunger.org/. Accessed March 7, 2011.

105. World Hunger Education Service. World Hunger Facts 2016. http://www.worldhunger.org/2015-world-hunger-and-poverty-facts-and-statistics. Accessed March 10, 2017.

106. Newacheck PW, Halfon N. Prevalence and impact of disabling chronic conditions in childhood. *Am J Public Health.* 1998;88(4):610-617.

107. Stang J, Story M. Guidelines for Adolescent Nutrition Services. 2005. http://www.epi.umn.edu/let/pubs/adol_book.shtm. Accessed March 7, 2011.

108. Hine RJ, Cloud HH, Carithers T, et al. Early nutrition intervention services for children with special health care needs. *J Am Diet Assoc.* 1989;89(11):1636-1639.

109. Willis JH. Adolescent Nutrition with Special Health Needs. *Guidelines for Adolescent Nutrition Services.* http://www.epi.umn.edu/let/pubs/adol_book.shtm. Accessed March 7, 2017.

110. Stallings V, Zemel B, Davies J, Cronk C, et al. Energy expenditure of children and adolescent with severe disabilities: a cerebral palsy model. *Am J Clin Nutr.* 1996;64(4):627-634.

111. Horsley JW. Children and adolescents with special health care needs. In: Story M, Holt K, Sofka D, eds. *Bright Futures in Practice: Nutrition.* Arlington, VA: National Center for Education in Maternal and Child Health; 2002:145-152.

112. Baer MT, Harris AB. Pediatric nutrition assessment: identifying children at risk. *J Am Diet Assoc.* 1997;97(Suppl 2):S107-115.

113. Boyle MA, Holben D. *Community Nutrition in Action: An Entrepreneurial Approach.* 4th ed. Belmont, CA: Thomson Wadsworth; 2013.

114. Robert Wood Johnson Foundation. Making the Grade: State and Local Partnerships to Establish School-Based Health Centers. Washington, DC: George Washington University; 2000.

115. Coon K, Goldberg J, Rogers B, Tucker K. Relationship between use of television during meals and children's food consumption paterns. *Pediatrics.* 2001;107(1):E1-E9.

116. Gallo AE. Food advertising in the United States. In "America's Eating Habits: Changes and Consequences" (E. Frazao, Ed.) Washington, DC: U.S. Department of Agriculture; 1999:173-180.

117. Kotz K, Story M. Food advertisement during children's Saturday morning television programming: Are they consistent with dietary recommendations? *J Am Diet Assoc.* 1994;94:1296-1300.

118. Consumers Union Education Services. *Captive Kids: Commercial Pressures on Kids at School Consumers Union of United States.* Yonkers, NY: Consumers Union Education Services; 1990.

119. Alaimo K, McDowell MA, Briefel RR. *Dietary Intake of Vitamins, Minerals, and Fiber of Persons Ages 2 months and over in the United States.* Hyattsville, MD: National Center for Health Statistics. Third National Health and Nutrition Examination Survey, Phase 1, 1988-91;1994.

120. Kennedy E, Goldberg, J. What are American children eating: implication for public policy. *Nutr Rev.* 1995;53:111.

121. United States Department of Agriculture. Food and Nutrition Service. Healthy Meals Resources System. www.fns.usda.gov/. Accessed March 7, 2011.

122. U.S. Department of Agriculture/Economic Research Service. Food Assistance Programs. 2000. https://www.ers.usda.gov/topics/food-nutrition-assistance/. Accessed March 10, 2017

123. Willis JT. Those lazy, hazy, crazy days of summer. *Nurs Times.* 1997;93:24-26.

124. Cook JT, Martin LS. *Differences in Nutrient Adequacy Among Poor and Non-poor Children.* Medford, MA: Tufts University School of Nutrition Center on Hunger; 1995.

125. Center for Disease Control and Prevention National Center on Health Statistics. National Center or Health Statistics. CDC growth charts: United States. https://www.cdc.gov/growthcharts/cdc_charts.htm. Accessed March 10, 2017.

126. Wilkinson C, Mickle S, Goldman J. Trends in food and nutrient intakes by adolescents in the United States. *Fam Econ Nutr Rev.* 2003;15(2):15-27.

127. Boynton-Jarrett R. Impact of television viewing patterns on fruit and vegetable consumption among adolescents. *Pediatrics.* 2003;112(6):1321.

128. Frisch RE, McArthur JW. Menstrual cycles: fatness as a determinant of minimum weight for height necessary for their maintenance or onset. *Science.* 1974;185:949-951.

129. Meyers AF, Sampson AE, Weitzman M, Rogers BL, et al. School breakfast program and school performance. *Am J Dis Child.* 1989;143:1234–1239.

130. Lin B, Guthrie J, Blaylock JR. *The diets of America's children: influences of dining out, household characteristics, and nutrition knowledge.* US Department of Agriculture Economic Report; 1996:746.

131. Siega-Ruz A, Carson T, Popkin B. Three squares or mostly snacks-what do teens really eat? A xociodemographic study of meal patterns. *J Adolesc Health.* 1998;22:29-36.

132. Agriculture USDDo. President Obama Signs Healthy, Hunger-Free Kids Act of 2010 Into Law. www.usda.gov. Accessed March 2, 2011.

133. Olver L. The Food Timeline: American Public School Lunch History. www.foodtimeline.org. Accessed March 7, 2011.

134. United States Department of Agriculture Food and Nutrition Service. Nutrition Assistance Programs. https://www.ers.usda.gov/topics/food-nutrition-assistance/. Accessed March 7, 2017.

135. U.S. Department Department of Agriculture Food and Nutrition Service. National School Lunch Program. https://www.ers.usda.gov/topics/food-nutrition-assistance/child-nutrition-programs/national-school-lunch-program.aspx. Accessed March 7, 2017.

136. Briggs M, Safaii D, Beall DL. Position of the American Associton: Nutrition services: an essential component of comprehensive health programs. *J Am Diet Assoc.* 2003;103:505-514.

137. Aschner JL. New therapies for pulmonary hypertension in neonates and children. *Pediatric Pulmonolo.* 2004;26(Supplement):132-135.

138. National Research Council. *Recommended Dietary Allowances.* Washington, DC: National Academy Press; 1989.

139. U.S. Department Department of Agriculture Food and Nutrition Service. School Breakfast. https://www.ers.usda.gov/topics/food-nutrition-assistance/child-nutrition-programs/school-breakfast-program.aspx. Accessed March 7, 2017.

140. Mahan KL, Escott-Stump S. *Krause's Food , Nutrition, and Diet Therapy.* 11th ed; 2012.

141. U.S. Department Department of Agriculture Food and Nutrition Service. Special Milk Program. https://www.ers.usda.gov/webdocs/publications/fanrr194/30216_fanrr19-4_002.pdf. Accessed March 7, 2017.

142. U.S. Department Department of Agriculture. Healthy Schools. http://teamnutrition.usda.gov. Accessed March 10, 2017.

143. U.S. Department of Agriculture. *Team nutrition:program summary.* Washington, DC: USDA; 1995. https://www.fns.usda.gov/tn/team-nutrition. Accessed March 10, 2017.

144. Administration for Children and Families. Head Start Fact Sheet. https://www.nhsa.org/facts. Accessed March 7, 2017.

145. National Youth Sports Program. The Office of Community Services, Division of Community Demonstration Programs (DCDP/DISC) administers this program. https://www.acf.hhs.gov/. Accessed March 7, 2017.

146. Powell CA, Walker SP, Chang SM, Grantham-McGregor SM. Nutrition and education: A randomized trial of the effects of breakfast in rural primary school children. *Am J Clin Nutr.* 1998;68:873-879.

147. Gross SM, Cinelli, B. Coordinated school health program and dietetics professionls: partners in promoting healthful eating. *J.Am Diet Assoc.* 2004;104(5):793-798.

148. Pollitt E. Does breakfast make a difference in school? *J Am Diet Assoc.* 1995;95:1134–1139.

149. Black S. Nutrition and learning. *Am School Board J.* 2000;187:49-51.

150. United States Department of Agriculture. Food and Nutrition Service. *Children's Diets in the Mid-1990s: Dietary Intake and Its Relationship with School Meal Participation.* Office of Analysis. Nutrition and Evaluation, Washington, DC;2001.

151. Farris RP, Nicklas TA, Webber LS, Berenson GS. Nutrient contribution of the school lunch program: implications for healthy people 2000. *J Sch Health.* 1992;62:180-184.

152. Nutrition and Your Health. *Dietary Guidelines for Americans. the optimal choice (131).* 5th ed. Washington, DC: US Departments of Agriculture and Health and Human Services; Home and Garden Bulletin No. 232;2000.

153. US Department of Agriculture Food and Nutrition Service. Foods Sold in Competition with USDA Meal Programs. https://www.fns.usda.gov/tags/competitive-foods. Accessed March 7, 2017.

154. U.S. Department Department of Agriculture. National School Lunch Program and School Breakfast Program nutriton objectives for school meals. Vol 59. Fed Reg1994:3021-3025.

155. Bergman EA, Buergel NS, Joseph E, Sanchez A. Time spent by school children to eat lunch. *J Am Diet Assoc.* 2000;100:697-698.

156. Center Disease Control and Prevention. Success story: make more healtful foods and veverages available. https://www.cdc.gov/obesity/strategies/food-serv-guide.html. Accessed March 7, 2017.

157. Nader PR, Sellers DE, Johnson CC, Perry CL, et al. The effect of adult participation in a school-based family intervention to improve children's diet and physical activity: The Child and Adolescent Trial for Cardiovascular Health. *Prev Med.* 1996;25:455-464.

158. Duker M, Slade, R. *Anorexia Nervosa and Bulimia: How to Help.* 2nd ed. Buckingham, PA: Open University Press; 2003.

159. National Center for Chronic Disease Prevention and Health Promotion. Coordinated School Health Program. https://www.cdc.gov/healthyschools/wscc/index.htm. Accessed March 10, 2017.

160. Centers for Disease Control and Prevention. *Guidelines for School Health Programs to Promote Lifelong Healthy Eating.* US Dept of Health and Human Services. MMWR;1996. 45(RR-9): 1-41.

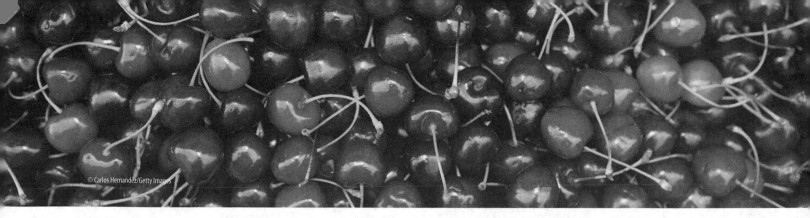

© Carlos Hernandez/Getty Images

# CHAPTER 10

# Adulthood: Special Health Issues

## LEARNING OBJECTIVES

- Discuss the significance of cardiovascular disease as it relates to morbidity and mortality.
- State the risk factors for cardiovascular disease.
- Discuss different factors that increase or decrease cardiovascular disease.
- Discuss the influence of different types of fat on heart disease.
- List the guidelines for reducing heart disease risk.
- Discuss the prevalence of obesity.
- Discuss the causes of obesity.
- Define obesity and overweight.
- Discuss the medical and social costs of obesity.
- Describe the dietary, behavioral, and physical activity modifications for the management of obesity.
- List major food sources or food components and how they protect the body and reduce the risk for cancer.
- List the ways in which foods are implicated in the development of cancer.
- Discuss the nutrients and other factors important in building bone density.
- Describe normal bone development.

# ▶ Introduction

A **chronic condition** is an occurrence of a disease that cannot be cured and that extends over a period of time. It has been recognized that chronic illness is an important issue in the health of older adults.[1] The cause of chronic diseases is associated with several factors, not just a single origin. It is often related to factors in lifestyle, genetics, and/or environment and in some situations is totally unknown.

An important part of public health is risk factor identification, which can lead to risk reduction through specific interventions aimed at reducing morbidity and mortality related to chronic illness. Risk factors can be classified as modifiable or nonmodifiable. For instance, data from 2007 show that 1 in every 18 deaths in the United States was due to stroke. On average, every 40 seconds, someone in the United States has a stroke. However, from 1997 to 2007, the stroke death rate decreased by 44.8 percent and 36.5 percent in 2014.[2] Modifiable risk factors for stroke include high blood cholesterol, hypertension, cigarette smoking, and obesity. The nonmodifiable risk factors are heredity, race, age, and gender.[3,4] Although each chronic disease must be considered individually, the risk factors of dietary practices are significant in several common chronic diseases, including heart disease, stroke, cancer, **obesity**, and **osteoporosis**, all of which will be discussed in this chapter. Diet is a primary intervention in the prevention of nutrition-related chronic health conditions.

The high prevalence of chronic conditions is one of the challenges of health promotion among older adults. It is assumed that the wear and tear that occurs with aging is inevitable and "normal," but that is not necessarily true in all cases because some individuals can age successfully by slowing the number and rate of aging changes through positive lifestyle choices and still have chronic conditions such as hypertension and osteoporosis. In the United States and other countries, people are living healthy, productive lives through their 70s, 80s, 90s, and beyond. Generally, health deteriorates with aging through an accumulation of chronic disorders and disabilities. According to the Centers for Disease Control and Prevention (CDC), chronic conditions significantly limit daily activity for 39 percent of persons over 65 years of age and account for about 36 percent of their healthcare costs.[5]

Community and public health nutritionists are involved in health promotion and disease prevention activities that require taking scientific research information and applying it to the community and to population-based health practices. They are poised to be the primary information resource regarding the relationships among diet, health, and disease prevention.

# ▶ Healthy People 2010 and 2020

One of the goals of Healthy People 2010 and 2020 was to prevent and control chronic diseases such as heart disease, obesity, cancer, and osteoporosis. The Healthy People 2010 progress report on weight status of adults showed that the proportion of adults ages 20 years or older who were at a healthy weight (body mass index [BMI] between 18.5 and 25.0) decreased from 42 percent in 1988 to 1994 to 34 percent in 1999 to 2000 and at 31 percent from 2005 to 2008 and 29.5 between 2009 to 2012. The target is 60 percent and 33.9 for the 2020 objectives. Data also showed that the age-adjusted proportion of adults age 20 years or older who were obese (i.e., BMI of 30.0 or more) increased from 23 percent in the survey period 1988 to 1994 to 31 percent in 1999 to 2000 and is currently 37.7 percent (2013 to 2014). The 2010 target for adult obesity, based on measured weights and heights, was 15 percent.[6]

As shown in **TABLE 10-1**, the Healthy People 2010 objectives to reduce the overall cancer and heart disease death rate showed little or no change. In regard to the objectives for fruits and vegetables, the age-adjusted average number of daily servings of fruit consumed showed little change, from 1.6 servings each day in 1994 to 1996 to 1.5 in 1999 to 2000; currently 0.56 percent (2009 to 2012) of people eat more than two servings of fruit each day. Two to four servings are recommended. In addition, vegetable consumption showed little change: an average of 3.4 daily servings in 1994 to 1996 compared with 3.3 in 1999 to 2000. Three to five servings are recommended; at least one third of the servings should be from dark green or orange vegetables. Data showed that from 2003 to 2004, four percent of adults 20 years of age or older ate dark green and orange vegetables, and 0.77 cup equivalents per 1,000 calories (2009 to 2012 for 2 years of age and older and 22 percent consumed fried potatoes. In 1999 to 2000, the proportion of all grain products consumed that were whole grain was 13 percent for adults. The target for whole grain products was 0.6 ounces equivalents per 1,000 calories. However, between 2009 and 2012, it was 0.44 ounce equivalents per 1,000 calories for 2 years of age and older. See Table10-1 and **TABLE 10-2** for more information on the 2010 progress report and the 2020 objectives.

These findings are not encouraging in regard to decreasing the incidence of chronic health conditions (obesity, heart disease, cancer, etc.) in older adults. Due to the results of the most recent review of Healthy People 2010 objectives, several strategies have been recommended to advance the progress toward achieving the objectives in relation to promoting healthy weight and food choices. (See **BOX 10-1**.)

**TABLE 10-1**  Healthy People 2010 Objectives for Adults

| Healthy People 2010 Objectives Number | Healthy People 2010 Objectives | Baseline (Year) | Progress Review (2002) | 2010 Target |
|---|---|---|---|---|
| 3.1 | Reduce the overall cancer death rate (age adjusted per 100,000 standard population). | 200.8 deaths (1999) 201.0 deaths (2000) 193.3 deaths (2002) | 190.1 deaths (2003) | 158.6 |
| 5.3 | Reduce the overall rate of diabetes per 1,000 population. | 40 cases (1997) 41 cases (1998-1999) 45 cases (2000) | N/A | 25 cases |
| 7.5 | Increase the proportion of worksites with 50 or more employees that offer a comprehensive employee health promotion program to their employees. | 34% | N/A | 75% |
| 12.1 | Reduce coronary heart disease deaths (age adjusted per 100,000 standard populations). | 204 (1999) 196 (2000) | N/A | 166 |
| 12.14 | Reduce the proportion of adults (age 20 years or over) with high total blood cholesterol levels ($\geq$ 240 mg/dl). | 21.0% (1988-1994) 18.3% (2000) | N/A | 17% |
| 19.1 | Increase the proportion of adults' ages 20 years or over who are at a healthy weight (BMI 18.5-25). | 42% (1988-1994) 34% (1999-2000) | N/A | 60% |
| 19.2 | Reduce the proportion of adults who are obese. | 23% (1988-1994) 31% (1999-2000) | N/A | 15% |
| 19.5 | Increase the proportion of persons age 2 years or older who consume more than two daily servings of fruit. | 28% (1994-1996) | N/A | 75% |
| 19.6 | Increase the proportion of persons age 2 years or older who consume more than three daily servings of vegetables, with at least one-third being dark green or deep yellow vegetables. | 3% (1994-1996) | N/A | 50% |
| 19.7 | Increase the proportion of persons age 2 years or older who consume at least six daily servings of grain products, with more than three being whole grains. | 7% (1994-1996) | N/A | 50% |
| 19.8 | Increase the proportion of persons age 2 years or older who consume less than 10% of calories from saturated fat. | 36% (1994-1996) | N/A | 75% |

*(continues)*

**TABLE 10-1** Healthy People 2010 Objectives for Adults *(continued)*

| Healthy People 2010 Objectives Number | Healthy People 2010 Objectives | Baseline (Year) | Progress Review (2002) | 2010 Target |
|---|---|---|---|---|
| 19.9 | Increase the proportion of persons age 2 years or older who consume no more than 30% of calories from total fat. | 33% (1994-1996) | N/A | 75% |
| 19.10 | Increase the proportion of persons ages 2 years or older who consume 2,400 milligrams or less of sodium daily. | 21% (1988-1994) | N/A | 65% |
| 19.11 | Increase the proportion of persons ages 2 years or older who meet dietary recommendations for calcium. | 45% (1988-1994) | N/A | 75% |
| 19.17 | Increase the proportion of physician office visits made by patients with a diagnosis of cardiovascular disease, diabetes, or hyperlipidemia that include counseling or education related to diet and nutrition. | 42% (1997)<br>38% (1998)<br>36% (1999)<br>40% (2000) | N/A | 75% |
| 19.18 | Increase food security among U.S. households and in so doing reduce hunger. | 88% (1995)<br>90% (1999)<br>89% (2001) | 89% | 94% |
| 22.2 | Increase the proportion of adults who engage regularly, preferably daily, in moderate physical activity for at least 30 minutes per day. | 32% (1997) | 33% (2003) | 50% |

Reproduced from: National Center for Health Statistics, Department of Health and Human Services. Healthy People 2010 Progress Review. Hyattsville, MD: Public Health Service, Healthy People 2010; 2004. Available at: http://www.cdc.gov/nchs/hphome.htm. Accessed August 9 2016.

**TABLE 10-2** Healthy People 2020 Objectives for Adults

| Healthy People 2020 Objectives Number | Healthy People 2020 Objectives | Baseline (Year) | Progress Review | 2020 Target |
|---|---|---|---|---|
| HDS-2 | Reduce coronary heart disease deaths. | 129.2 coronary heart disease deaths per 100,000 population occurred in 2007 (age adjusted to the year 2000 standard population). | 102.6 (2013) | 103.4 deaths* per 100,000 population |
| HDS-7 | Reduce the proportion of adults with high total blood cholesterol levels. | 15.0 percent of adults ages 20 years and older had total blood cholesterol levels of 240 mg/dl or greater in 2005-2008 (age adjusted to the year 2000 standard population). | 12.9 (2009-2012) | 13.5 percent* |

| Healthy People 2020 Objectives Number | Healthy People 2020 Objectives | Baseline (Year) | Progress Review | 2020 Target |
|---|---|---|---|---|
| HDS-8 | Reduce the mean total blood cholesterol levels among adults. | 197.7 mg/dL was the mean total blood cholesterol level for adults ages 20 years and older in 2005-2008 (age adjusted to the year 2000 standard population). | 195.3 (2009-2012) | 177.9 mg/dL (mean)* |
| C-1 | Reduce the overall cancer death rate. | 179.3 cancer deaths per 100,000 population occurred in 2007 (age adjusted to the year 2000 standard population). | 163.2 (2013) | 161.4 deaths* per 100,000 population |
| C-16 | Increase the proportion of adults who receive a colorectal cancer screening based on the most recent guidelines. | 52.1 percent of adults ages 50 to 75 years received a colorectal cancer screening based on the most recent guidelines in 2008 (age adjusted to the year 2000 standard population). | 58.2 (2013) | 70.5% |
| D-1 | Reduce the annual number of new cases of diagnosed diabetes in the population. | 8.0 new cases of diabetes per 1,000 population aged 18 to 84 years occurred in the past 12 months, as reported in 2006 to 2008 (age adjusted to the year 2000 standard population). | 6.7 (2012-2014) | 7.2 new cases* per 1,000 population aged 18 to 84 years |
| NWS-4 | (Developmental) Increase the proportion of Americans who have access to a food retail outlet that sells a variety of foods encouraged by the Dietary Guidelines for Americans. | TBD | TBD[†] | TBD[†] |
| NWS-6.1 | Increase the proportion of physician office visits made by patients with a diagnosis of cardiovascular disease, diabetes, or hyperlipidemia that include counseling or education related to diet or nutrition. | 20.8% of physician office visits by adult patients with a diagnosis of cardiovascular disease, diabetes, or hyperlipidemia included counseling or education related to diet or nutrition in 2007 (age adjusted to the year 2000 standard population). | N/A | 22.9%* |

*(continues)*

| TABLE 10-2 Healthy People 2020 Objectives for Adults | | | | *(continued)* |
|---|---|---|---|---|
| **Healthy People 2020 Objectives Number** | **Healthy People 2020 Objectives** | **Baseline (Year)** | **Progress Review** | **2020 Target** |
| NWS-7 | (Developmental) Increase the proportion of worksites that offer nutrition or weight management classes or counseling. | TBD | TBD[†] | TBD[†] |
| NWS-8 | Increase the proportion of adults who are at a healthy weight. | 30.8% of persons ages 20 years and older were at a healthy weight in 2005-2008 (age adjusted to the year 2000 standard population). | 29.5% (2009-2012) | 33.9%[*] |
| NWS-13 | Reduce household food insecurity and in doing so reduce hunger. | 14.6 % of households were food insecure in 2008. | 14.3% (2013) | 6.0%[*,‡] |
| NWS-14 | Increase the contribution of fruits to the diets of the population ages 2 years and older. | 0.53 cup equivalent of fruits per 1,000 calories was the mean daily intake by persons ages 2 years and older in 2005 to 2008 (age adjusted to the year 2000 standard population). | N/A | 0.93 cup equivalent per 1,000 calories |
| NWS-15.1 | Increase the contribution of total vegetables to the diets of the population ages 2 years and older. | 0.76 cup equivalent of total vegetables per 1,000 calories was the mean daily intake by persons ages 2 years and older in 2005-2008 (age adjusted to the year 2000 standard population). | N/A | 1.16 cup equivalent per 1,000 calories |
| NWS-15.2 | Increase the contribution of dark green vegetables, red and orange vegetables, and beans and peas to the diets of the population ages 2 years and older. | 0.29 cup equivalent of dark green vegetables, red and orange vegetables, and beans and peas per 1,000 calories was the mean daily intake by persons ages 2 years and older in 2005-2008 (age adjusted to the year 2000 standard population). | N/A | 0.53 cup equivalent per 1,000 calories |
| NWS-16 | Increase the contribution of whole grains to the diets of the population ages 2 years and older. | 0.34 ounce equivalent of whole grains per 1,000 calories was the mean daily intake by persons ages 2 years and older in 2005-2008 (age adjusted to the year 2000 standard population). | N/A | 0.66 ounce equivalent per 1,000 calories |

| Healthy People 2020 Objectives Number | Healthy People 2020 Objectives | Baseline (Year) | Progress Review | 2020 Target |
|---|---|---|---|---|
| NWS-17.1 | Reduce consumption of calories from solid fats. | 16.6 percent was the mean percentage of total daily calorie intake from solid fats for the population ages 2 years and older in 2005-2008 (age adjusted to the year 2000 standard population). | N/A | 14.2% |
| NWS-17.2 | Reduce consumption of calories from added sugars. | 15.1 percent was the mean percentage of total daily calorie intake from added sugars for the population aged 2 years and older in 2005-2008 (age adjusted to the year 2000 standard population). | N/A | 9.7% |
| NWS-18 | Reduce consumption of saturated fat in the population ages 2 years and older. | 11.3 percent was the mean percentage of total daily calorie intake provided by saturated fat for the population ages 2 years and older in 2005-2008 (age adjusted to the year 2000 standard population). | N/A | 9.9% |
| WS-19 | Reduce consumption of sodium in the population ages 2 years and older. | 3,658 milligrams of sodium from foods, dietary supplements, antacids, drinking water, and salt use at the table was the mean total daily intake by persons ages 2 years and older in 2009-2012 (age adjusted to the year 2000 standard population). | N/A | 2,300 milligrams |
| NWS-20 | Increase consumption of calcium in the population ages 2 years and older. | 1,099 milligrams of calcium from foods, dietary supplements, antacids, and drinking water was the mean total daily intake by persons ages 2 years and older in 2005-2008 (age adjusted to the year 2000 standard population). | N/A | 2,300 milligrams |
| PA-1 | Reduce the proportion of adults who engage in no leisure-time physical activity. | 36.2% of adults engaged in no leisure-time physical activity in 2008 (age adjusted to the year 2000 standard population). | 30.0% (2014) | 32.6%* |
| AOCBC-10 | Reduce the proportion of adults with osteoporosis. | 5.9% of adults ages 50 years and older had osteoporosis in 2005-2008 (age adjusted to the year 2000 standard population). | N/A | 5.3%* |

*(continues)*

| | | | | |
|---|---|---|---|---|
| **TABLE 10-2** Healthy People 2020 Objectives for Adults | | | | *(continued)* |
| **Healthy People 2020 Objectives Number** | **Healthy People 2020 Objectives** | **Baseline (Year)** | **Progress Review** | **2020 Target** |
| AOCBC-11 | Reduce hip fractures among older adults. | 823.5 hospitalizations for hip fractures per 100,000 females ages 65 years and older occurred in 2007 (age adjusted to the year 2000 standard population). | 778.2 (2010) | 741.2* hospitalizations per 100,000 population |
| OA-11 | Reduce the rate of emergency department (ED) visits due to falls among older adults. | 5,235.1 ED visits per 100,000 due to falls occurred among older adults in 2007 (age adjusted to the year 2000 standard population). | 6893.5 (2011) | 4,711.6 ED* visits per 100,000 due to falls among older adults |
| OA-7.6 | Increase the proportion of registered dieticians with geriatric certification. | 0.30 percent of registered dieticians had geriatric certification in 2009. | 0.60% (2013) | 0.33%* |

*Target-setting method: 10 percent improvement.
†To be determined
‡Retention of Healthy People 2010 target.
Reproduced from: National Center for Health Statistics, Department of Health and Human Services. Healthy People 2020. Public Health Service, Healthy People 2010; 2004. Available at: https://www.healthypeople.gov/2020/topics-objectives Accessed August 10, 2016.

| | |
|---|---|
| **BOX 10-1** Recommended Strategies for Achieving Healthy People 2010 and 2020 Objectives for Weight and Food Choice[6] | |

- Promote partnerships with community planners to design neighborhoods that encourage and support increased opportunities for physical activity in appropriate and safe locations.
- Educate the public about the health benefits of being physically active at any size and the possible added benefit of thereby attaining modest weight reduction.
- Educate the public on how to use the Nutrition Facts Panel on food products and on how to select appropriate portion sizes for healthful diets, including clarification of the difference between "serving size" and "portion size."
- Urge medical schools to incorporate training on the prevention and treatment of obesity into their curricula. In a parallel effort, work with medical associations and healthcare organizations on developing means for educating healthcare professionals already in practice.
- Offer incentives for worksites to provide safe, convenient, and affordable venues for employees to engage in physical activity.

- Promote food policy councils as a way to improve the food environment at state and local levels.
- Improve local food systems that will increase fruit and vegetable consumption.
- Improve access to retail stores that sell high-quality fruits and vegetables or increase the availability of high-quality fruits and vegetables at retail stores in underserved communities.
- Start or expand farm-to-institution programs in schools, hospitals, workplaces, and other institutions.
- Start or expand farmers' markets in all settings.
- Ensure access to fruits and vegetables in workplace cafeterias and other food service venues.
- Support and promote community and home gardens.
- Include fruits and vegetables in emergency food programs.

Source: Centers for Disease Control and Prevention. Strategies to Prevent Obesity and Other Chronic Diseases: The CDC Guide to Strategies to Increase the Consumption of Fruits and Vegetables. Atlanta: U.S. Department of Health and Human Services; 2011. http://www.cdc.gov/obesity/downloads/FandV_2011_WEB_TAG508.pdf Accessed July 20, 2016.

# ▶ Cardiovascular Disease

Cardiovascular disease (CVD) is one of the chronic health conditions affecting millions of people around the world. The cardiovascular system includes the heart, blood vessels, and blood-forming organs. Some common diseases of the heart and blood vessels can be influenced by diet and behavioral changes through primary and secondary prevention. CVDs are the leading cause of death in the United States and most of the industrialized countries.[7] CVDs killed over 17.3 million individuals globally in 2015 and 635,000 in the United States (2014), more than the next six leading causes of death combined.[8,9] Men have a greater risk for heart disease and are at risk at an earlier age than women, but this gap closes with age.

One aspect of CVD is **atherosclerosis**. This hardening of the arteries occurs when fibrous plaques, which are composed mainly of cholesterol, build up in the arteries, especially at branch points. The first sign of atherosclerosis is soft fatty streaks visible along the walls of the arteries. This disease process interferes with the pumping of blood through the artery in two ways: 1) the deposits gradually narrow the opening, and 2) the fibrosis makes it increasingly harder for the artery to constrict or dilate in response to the tissues' need for oxygenated blood.

Coronary heart disease (CHD) is the most common form of CVD. It usually involves atherosclerosis and hypertension and causes one third of all deaths in both men and women. Despite the dramatic decline in mortality over the past 25 years, it remains the most common cause of death in the United States. CHD costs the United States about $215.6 billion per year in medical treatment and lost wages.[2]

Many long-term studies, including the Framingham Study, the Honolulu Heart Study, and the Chicago Gas and Electric Company Study, have provided unique data concerning the role of genetic and environmental factors in increasing the risk for developing atherosclerotic cardiovascular disease (ASCVD).[10-12] The occurrence of CVD cannot be predicted with certainty; however, many attributes and behaviors are believed to interact to produce the illness. These break down into unmodifiable risk factors and modifiable risk factors.

## Unmodifiable Risk Factors

Certain risk factors that are not under the control of the individual, such as age, gender, ethnicity, and family history, can be predictive of atherosclerosis and hypertension in some people. Although these factors cannot be controlled, nutritionists, public health professionals, physicians, and other health educators need to increase awareness of heart disease in people in at-risk groups.

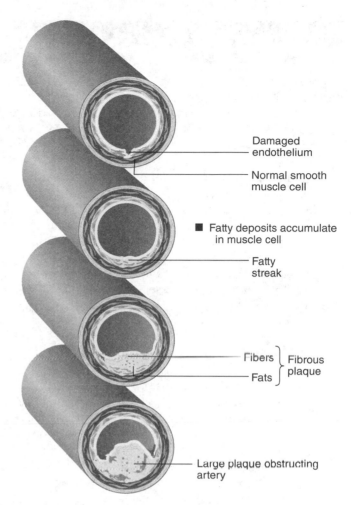

Damaged endothelium

Normal smooth muscle cell

■ Fatty deposits accumulate in muscle cell

Fatty streak

Fibers ⎫ Fibrous
Fats ⎭ plaque

Large plaque obstructing artery

This mold of an artery demonstrates dramatically how plaque build-up can restrict blood flow.

A family history of premature CHD in a parent or sibling increases a person's risk for the disease (see **CASE STUDY 10-1**). Premature CHD is defined as occurring in a male under the age of 50 or a female under age 60.[13] Individuals who suffer the highest risk for premature CVD have a rare genetic defect that substantially blocks the clearance of chylomicrons and triglycerides from the blood, reduces low-density lipoprotein (LDL) uptake by the liver, limits synthesis of high-density lipoprotein (HDL), or enhances blood clotting.[14] Other medical conditions, such as certain forms of liver and kidney disease, low concentrations of thyroid hormone, and use of certain medications to treat hypertension, can increase LDL and increase the risk for heart disease.[14]

## Modifiable Risk Factors

Unlike age, gender, ethnicity, and family history, some risk factors for CVD can be modified. The major modifiable risk factors for CVD are hypertension, obesity, cigarette smoking, **hypercholesterolemia**,

## 🔍 CASE STUDY 10-1: Risks Factors for Cardiovascular Disease

A 28-year-old gold-medal-winning ice skater, Sergei Grinkov, died suddenly of a heart attack as he was ice-skating. After a thorough evaluation, it was established that he died of a protein abnormality in his blood that causes more blood clot formation than normal. Sergei had normal blood lipid levels (total cholesterol 195 mg/dl, HDL of 45 mg/dl and normal blood triglycerides and LDL). Sergei's major risk factor was that his father died of heart disease at the age of 52.[126] It is reported that approximately 25 percent of people living in the United States have this protein abnormality.[126] The only risk factor is a family history of heart-related death under age 60. Therefore, it is important for all adult Americans to ask their physician to evaluate their cardiovascular disease risks.

Chinonye, a community nutritionist, was employed to identify individuals who may have this trait in the community she serves. She wrote a grant proposal and obtained funds from the AHA; she called the program "Know Your Risks for a Heart Attack." She collected data from 5,000 participants and found that some of the clients had several chronic conditions. She also found that 30 percent of individuals surveyed had high blood pressure, high blood cholesterol, high LDL, low HDL, high triglyceride levels, and obesity. Dietary analysis showed low fiber, fruit, and vegetable intakes. She proposed to use the social marketing framework for this program in the community. Social marketing has an impact on the practice of dietetics by boosting clients' awareness of health issues and helps move clients toward behavioral change. See Chapter 17 for more information on social marketing.

### Questions

1. What is the definition of a chronic condition? What are some of the factors related to chronic conditions?
2. What are three of the Healthy People 2010 objectives that Chinonye may relate to the clients?
3. What are some of the unmodifiable and modifiable risk factors of cardiovascular disease?
4. What are some of the successful strategies for the treatment of modifiable dyslipidemia?
5. What are the desirable levels for adult blood cholesterol and triglycerides? What are the borderline and high levels?
6. What are the major dietary components that can have an effect on total cholesterol and LDL cholesterol?
7. What are the strategies for primary prevention of hypertension?
8. What are the NCEP guidelines for reducing the risk for heart disease that Chinonye can use for her nutrition education?
9. Work in small groups or individually to discuss the case study and practice using the Nutrition Care Process chart provided on the companion website. You also can add other nutrition and health-related conditions or assessments to the case study to make the case study more challenging and interesting.

and diabetes.[15] **BOX 10-2** presents strategies for treating modifiable dyslipidemia, which is excess levels of blood lipids such as cholesterol, LDLs, and triglycerides.

## Hypertension

**Hypertension** is one of the major risk factors for CHD. There is a direct link between every increase of blood pressure above normal levels and cardiovascular complications.[19] A decrease in systolic pressure by 2 millimeters of mercury (mm Hg) is estimated to have the potential to reduce annual mortality from stroke by 6 percent and from CHD by 4 percent.[19]

Approximately 32 percent of U.S. adults have hypertension, a major risk factor for CHD, stroke, and premature death.[20] It is more common in people of African descent.[21] The cause of hypertension is unknown, except that in about 5 percent of cases, it is secondary to an underlying pathophysiological correctable condition.

Data suggest that dietary factors such as salt, sugar, alcohol, and body weight are important to regulate blood pressure. Other nonpharmacological recommendations include increasing potassium intake and aerobic exercise and quitting smoking.[22] These factors are all recommended as part of the first-line therapy for **low-risk individuals**, defined as those without diabetes or CVD and with a systolic blood pressure less than 160 mm Hg and diastolic blood pressure less than 100 mm Hg and as part of a combination therapy program for high-risk individuals.[22,23] The new guideline for the prevention and management of hypertension is to consider initiating therapy with two agents if blood pressure is more than 20/10 mm Hg above the goal. One of the agents used should be a thiazide-type diuretic. The guideline also states that the most effective therapy prescribed by even the most careful clinician will control hypertension only if individuals are motivated.[23] Magnesium, calcium, fiber, fat, protein, and certain carbohydrates have been

Research studies from human clinical and epidemiological trials show that dyslipidemia is one of the most important modifiable risk factors for CHD. Dyslipidemia is characterized by increased fasting concentrations of total cholesterol, LDL cholesterol (LDL-C), and triglycerides, in addition to decreased concentrations of HDL cholesterol (HDL-C).

The treatment for dyslipidemia has been mostly with pharmacological therapy. But, because of safety concerns about the use of pharmaceutical agents, the demand for alternative nonpharmacological therapies has increased.

The National Cholesterol Education Program (NCEP) Adult Treatment Panel III (ATP III) recommends lifestyle therapies, which include a combination of diet and exercise modifications in place of drug treatment for individuals who are in the intermediate range of CHD risk. This review examined the effectiveness of cholesterol lowering of the two NCEP-recommended combination therapies:

1. Low-saturated-fat diets combined with exercise
2. Nutritional supplementation (e.g., fish oil, oat bran, or plant sterol supplementation) combined with exercise

Results showed that low-saturated-fat diets combined with exercise:

- Lowered total cholesterol by 7% to 18%
- Lowered LDL cholesterol by 7% to 15%
- Lowered triglyceride concentrations by 4% to 18%
- Increased HDL-C levels by 5% to 14%

Alternatively, nutritional supplements combined with exercise:

- Decreased total cholesterol by 8% to 26%
- Decreased LDL-C levels by 8% to 30%
- Decreased triglyceride concentrations by 12% to 39%
- Increased HDL-C levels by 2% to 8%

These findings suggest that community nutritionists should provide nutrition education that uses combination lifestyle therapies because they are more effective strategies for improving cholesterol levels in those diagnosed with dyslipidemia in their community. Also, including a low-saturated-fat diet as part of the combination will increase HDL-C levels.

hypothesized to affect blood pressure, although information linking these dietary factors to blood pressure reduction is not consistent.

One objective of Healthy People 2010 was to reduce the proportion of adults with high blood pressure from 28 percent to 14 percent. However, the prevalence of hypertension between 2005 and 2008 increased from 25 percent to 30 percent among individuals ages 18 years and older. Research in 1972 showing the importance of blood pressure to health led to the introduction of the first large-scale public outreach and education campaign to reduce high blood pressure by the National Heart, Lung, and Blood Institute (NHLBI).[24] Its promotion of the detection, treatment, and control of high blood pressure has been credited with influencing the dramatic increase in the public's understanding of hypertension and its role in heart attacks and strokes, as well as a related reduction in deaths. The percentage of people who were able to control their high blood pressure through lifestyle changes and through antihypertensive drug therapy increased from about 16 percent in 1971 to 1972 to approximately 65 percent in 1988 to 1994.[25,26] Approximately 90 percent of all adults now have their blood pressure measured at least once every 2 years.[27] The 2020 objectives on hypertension are presented on Table 10-2.

The Dietary Approaches to Stop Hypertension (DASH) trial, the DASH-Sodium trial, and the Optimal Macro-Nutrient Intake to Prevent Heart Disease (OmniHeart) study evaluated the effects of diets with different macronutrient profiles on established CVD risk factors (blood pressure and blood lipids) in the setting of stable weight. The DASH and DASH-Sodium trials showed that a carbohydrate-rich diet that emphasized fruits, vegetables, low-fat dairy products, and reduced saturated fat, total fat, and cholesterol significantly lowered blood pressure and LDL cholesterol. The OmniHeart trial showed that partial replacement of carbohydrates with either protein (about half from plant sources) or unsaturated fat (mostly monounsaturated fat) also reduced blood pressure, LDL cholesterol, and CHD risk. Results from these trials showed the importance of macronutrients as a determinant of CVD risk.[28] Community nutritionists can use these results to promote heart-healthy diets that provide enough flexibility to increase individuals' ability to consume them.

What proven actions are possible for reducing hypertension and avoiding its complications?[29]

- Reduce weight, as little as 10 pounds (4.5 kg) will reduce blood pressure and/or prevent hypertension in a large proportion of overweight persons, but it is important to maintain a normal body weight (not become underweight).
- Use the DASH eating plan. (Add more fruits, vegetables, nuts/beans/seeds, and low-fat dairy products, and consume moderate amounts of lean

meat/fish/poultry with a reduced content of dietary cholesterol as well as saturated and total fat for the whole diet.) The DASH plan is rich in potassium and calcium content (see **TABLES 10-3** and **10-4**).

■ Reduce dietary sodium intake to no more than 2.4 g of sodium per day. Do not add salt to foods at the table. In cooking, use only 1 teaspoon of salt (contains 2,000 mg of sodium).

**TABLE 10-3** Daily Nutrient Goals Used in the DASH Studies (for a 2,000-Calorie Eating Plan)

| Nutrient | Daily Goal |
|---|---|
| Total fat | 27% of calories |
| Saturated fat | 6% of calories |
| Protein | 18% of calories |
| Carbohydrate | 55% of calories |
| Cholesterol | 150 mg |
| Sodium | 2,300 mg* |
| Potassium | 4,700 mg |
| Calcium | 1,250 mg |
| Magnesium | 500 mg |
| Fiber | 30 g |

*1,500 mg sodium was a lower goal tested and found to be even better for lowering blood pressure. It was particularly effective for middle-aged and older individuals, African Americans, and those who already had high blood pressure.

g, grams; mg, milligrams

Reproduced from: U.S. Department of Health and Human Services, National Heart Lung and Blood Institute. Diseases and conditions index. What is the DASH eating plan? Available at: http://www.nhlbi.nih.gov/ health/public/heart/hbp/dash/how_plan.html. Accessed October 9, 2016.

**TABLE 10-4** The DASH Diet Plan

| Type of Food | Number of Servings for 1,600- to 3,100-Calorie Diets | Servings on a 2,000-Calorie Diet |
|---|---|---|
| **Grains and grain products**<br>■ Whole-wheat flour, bulgur, cracked wheat<br>■ Oatmeal, whole cornmeal, brown rice, whole grain foods<br>■ Whole wheat pasta, whole wheat sandwich buns and rolls, whole wheat tortillas | 6–12 | 7–8 |
| **Fruits**<br>■ Apples, apricots, avocados, bananas<br>■ Strawberries, blueberries, raspberries<br>■ Grapefruit, grapes, kiwi fruit, lemons, limes, mangoes<br>■ Cantaloupe, honeydew, watermelon<br>■ Oranges, tangerines, peaches, pears, papaya, pineapple, plums, prunes, raisins | 4–6 | 4–5 |

| Type of Food | Number of Servings for 1,600- to 3,100-Calorie Diets | Servings on a 2,000-Calorie Diet |
|---|---|---|
| **Vegetables**<br>■ *Dark green vegetables* Bok choy, broccoli, collard greens, dark green leafy lettuce, kale, mustard greens, spinach, turnip greens, watercress<br>■ *Orange vegetables* Squash, butternut squash, carrot, pumpkin, sweet potatoes<br>■ *Other vegetables* Artichokes, asparagus, bean sprouts, beets, Brussels sprouts, cabbage, cauliflower, celery, cucumbers, eggplant, green or red peppers, mushrooms, okra, onions, tomatoes, zucchini<br>■ *Dry beans and peas* Black beans, black-eyed peas, garbanzo beans (chickpeas), kidney beans, lentils, lima beans (mature), navy beans, pinto beans, soybeans<br>■ *Starchy vegetables* Corn, potatoes, green peas, lima beans (green) | 4–6 | 4–5 |
| **Low-fat or nonfat dairy foods**<br>■ Milk, including all fluid milk, lactose-reduced milks, and lactose-free milks<br>■ Yogurt, ice cream, cheese, cottage cheese | 2–4 | 2–3 |
| **Lean meats, fish, poultry** | 1.5–2.5 | 2 or less |
| **Nuts, seeds, and legumes**<br>■ Almonds, cashews, hazelnuts, peanuts, peanut butter, pecans, pistachios, pumpkin seeds, sesame seeds, sunflower seeds, walnuts | 3-6 per week | 4-5 per week |
| **Fats and sweets**<br>■ Canola oil, corn oil, cottonseed oil, olive oil, safflower oil, soybean oil, sunflower oil<br>■ Some oils are used mainly as flavorings, such as walnut oil and sesame oil. A number of foods are naturally high in oils, such as nuts, olives, and some fish.<br>■ Sweets: jelly or jam, jelly beans, lemonade | 2–4 | Limited |

Reproduced from: U.S. Department of Health and Human Services, National Heart Lung and Blood Institute. Your Guide to Lowering Your Blood Pressure With DASH. How Do I Make the DASH? Available at: http://www.nhlbi.nih.gov/health/public/heart/hbp/dash/how_make_dash.html. Accessed October 9, 2016.

■ Engage in regular aerobic physical activity such as brisk walking, dancing, and the like at least 30 minutes per day most days of the week.

■ Reduce the amount of alcohol intake to no more than 1 oz (30 ml) of ethanol, the equivalent of two drinks per day in most men and no more than 0.5 oz of ethanol (one drink) per day in women and lighter weight persons. A drink is 12 oz of beer, 5 oz of wine, or 1.5 oz of 80-proof liquor. Alternatively, abstain from drinking alcohol.

■ Quit smoking.

Community-based programs may be an important strategy for primary prevention of hypertension. The Joint National Committee on Detection, Evaluation and Treatment of High Blood Pressure suggests that communities consider the items presented in **BOX 10-3**).

## Other Modifiable Risk Factors

Other major modifiable risk factors include tobacco and cigarette smoking, hypercholesterolemia, and obesity. Smoking stresses the cardiovascular system by depriving the heart of oxygen and raising the blood pressure. It also damages platelets, making blood clot formation more likely. Toxins in tobacco smoke damage the blood vessels, setting the stage for plaque formation. People who smoke cigars and pipes have an increased risk for

## Successful Community Strategies

### New York: Campaign Increases Awareness Among State Residents

In New York, a Healthy Heart Program was conducted using campaigns. The purpose of the program was to increase awareness about the symptoms of stroke. The program was conducted in four counties: Albany, Rensselaer, Saratoga, and Schenectady.

Information about symptoms of stroke was advertised by television, radio, and public transit.
Results showed:

- 18 percent increase in the number of people who arrived at hospital emergency departments in less than 2 hours after experiencing the first symptoms of a stroke.
- 13 percent increase in the number of people arriving at hospitals by ambulance.

### BOX 10-3 Strategy for Primary Prevention of Hypertension[22,27]

- Detection, education, and referral for other cardiovascular risk factors
- Various strategies to improve adherence:
  - Public, client, and professional education activities
  - Culturally sensitive approaches
  - Informative food labeling
  - Heart-healthy menus in restaurants
  - Safe trails for walking and biking
- Multiple channels for outreach:
  - Healthcare settings
  - Schools
  - Worksites
  - Churches and community centers
  - Supermarkets and pharmacies
- Media promotion
- Second-order prevention efforts directed toward individuals with "normal" risk factor levels who need education and support to maintain preventive behavior (e.g., weight control, physical activity, and good nutrition)

CHD, but the risk is not as high as that for people who smoke cigarettes.

It is reported that the segment of the public who has had their blood cholesterol checked increased from 67.6 percent in 1991 to 73.1 percent in 2003. The recommended frequency for checking blood cholesterol is every 5 years for healthy people.[30] The government's and healthcare practitioners' concern is that mass screenings increase healthcare costs through repetitive testing of known cases.[31]

Disorders of lipoprotein metabolism can lead to alterations in plasma cholesterol and triglyceride levels; these disorders are usually associated with an increased risk for CVD. A total blood cholesterol level of over 200 mg/dl, especially when it is at or over 240 mg/dl together with LDL cholesterol over 130 to 159 mg/dl, is associated with CVD. The higher the LDL, the greater the risk for CVD; therefore, the primary target of cholesterol-lowering management is the LDL cholesterol. In contrast, the higher a person's HDL levels, the lower is the risk for CHD. Individuals with high serum cholesterol concentrations are at lower risk if they also show higher levels of HDL cholesterol; conversely, individuals with low HDL cholesterol concentrations ($< 40$ mg/dl) are at a higher risk regardless of their total cholesterol concentrations. A high HDL level ($\geq 60$ mg/dl) counteracts one other risk factor in totaling a person's risk.[32] **TABLE 10-5** presents the range of adult blood cholesterol and triglyceride levels.

Although the liver produces cholesterol, diet also influences serum cholesterol levels. Only foods of animal origin contain cholesterol. Limiting foods containing animal products can reduce the risk for CVD. For people with elevated LDL cholesterol, pre-existing CVD (including a past heart attack or stroke), or diabetes, the recommended diet reduces saturated fat to 7 percent of daily calories and reduces cholesterol to less than 200 milligrams per day. Compared to the diet for healthy people, the diet for high-risk groups provides less lean meat, skinless poultry, fish, and eggs and strictly limits high-fat meats, especially organ meats (liver, brain, and kidney). Dietitians can help plan a person's diet to ensure that saturated fats and cholesterol are reduced without sacrificing the nutritional quality of the diet.[33]

It has been reported that polyunsaturated fatty acids, monounsaturated fatty acids, and, to a lesser extent, soluble fiber lower LDL cholesterol. However, fat from all sources should not exceed 30 percent of the total calories.

Fish oils, rich in omega-3 polyunsaturated fatty acids, improve blood lipids (primarily by lowering

| TABLE 10-5 Adult Blood Cholesterol and Triglyceride Levels | | | |
|---|---|---|---|
| **Lipids (mg/dl)** | **Desirable** | **Borderline** | **High** |
| Total cholesterol | < 200 | 200–239 | ≥ 240 |
| LDL cholesterol | < 100 | 130–159 | ≥ 160 |
| Triglycerides | < 150 | 150–199 | ≥ 200–499 |
| Body mass index | 18.5–24.9 | 25–29.9 | ≥ 30 |

Reproduced from: National Cholesterol Education Program. Third Report of the Expert Panel on Detection, Evaluation, and Treatment of High Blood Cholesterol in Adults (Adult Treatment Panel III). NIH Publication No. 02-5215. September 2002. Available at: http://www.nhlbi.nih.gov/guidelines/cholesterol/atp3full.pdf. Accessed April 11, 2016.

triglycerides), prevent blood clots, and reduce the risk for sudden death associated with CHD.[34] For these reasons, the dietary guidelines recommend at least two servings of fish per week. Plant sources of omega-3 fatty acids, such as flaxseed and flaxseed oil, canola oil, soybean oil, and nuts, also may be beneficial.[35]

In addition, high intakes of dietary sugars worldwide are causing an epidemic of obesity, CVD, and metabolic abnormalities (e.g., diabetes). Data show that the main sources of the added sugars are soft drinks and other sugar-sweetened beverages in the amount of about 22.2 teaspoons per day (355 calories per day). To address this problem, the American Heart Association (AHA) recommends a reduction in the intake of added sugars. Depending on the caloric level, recommendations for added sugars vary from 5 teaspoons per day (or 80 calories) for a daily energy expenditure of 1,800 calories for an average adult woman to 9 teaspoons per day (or 144 calories) for a daily energy expenditure of 2,200 calories for an average adult man. For reference, one 12-ounce can of cola contains 8 teaspoons of added sugar, for 130 calories.[36]

In comparison to a number of other CVD risk factors, the prevalence of obesity has increased over the past several decades, which has had a negative impact in reducing CVD morbidity and mortality. Some of the increased risk for CVD observed in individuals with diabetes is attributed to the concurrent presence of other risk factors such as hypertension and obesity. In addition, the amount and type of fatty acids ingested and the dietary cholesterol level as well as the caloric content and macronutrient composition of the diet can influence the composition, concentration, and metabolism of plasma lipoproteins. **TABLE 10-6** presents the major dietary components or conditions and their effect on total cholesterol and LDL cholesterol. Lifestyle interventions

that combine counseling for dietary management, weight reduction, and increased physical activity are essential in the management of diabetes and CHD.

Prevention of CVD depends on minimizing a person's risk factors (hypertension, overweight/obesity, sodium intake, irregular exercise, etc.) and moderating alcohol consumption.[54] Community nutritionists can use such strategies as cessation of tobacco use and cigarette smoking, decreased saturated fat intake, and control of diabetes mellitus for modifying the risk factors for CHD.

## The National Cholesterol Education Program

Healthy People 2010 set a goal of reducing total blood cholesterol among adults from an average of 206 mg/dl to 199 mg/dl, as well as reducing the percentage of adults with high blood cholesterol from 21 percent to 17 percent; current reports show a decrease of 15 percent, exceeding the 2010 target. The 2020 objectives target is to reduce mean total blood cholesterol level among adults to 177.9 mg/dl. The Third Report of the National Cholesterol Education Program (NCEP) Expert Panel on Detection, Evaluation, and Treatment of High Blood Cholesterol in Adults provided further evidence of the importance of diet in treating CVD.[55] The NCEP recommended several different strategies for identifying and managing individuals and communities at risk for heart disease. The strategies include either primary prevention for healthy individuals in the community or secondary prevention for those already screened and are at risk for heart disease. **BOX 10-4** and **TABLE 10-7** present the approaches for reducing the risk for heart disease and managing hypercholesterolemia in the community.

**TABLE 10-6** The Major Dietary Components or Conditions and Their Effect on Total Cholesterol and LDL Cholesterol

| Component | Effect |
|---|---|
| **Polyunsaturated Fatty Acids** | |
| Omega-6 fatty acids (corn oil, cottonseed oil, soybean oil, sunflower oil, etc.)<br>Omega-3 fatty acids (eicosapentaenoic acid [EPA] and docosahexaenoic acid [DHA]—ocean fish, king mackerel, salmon, sardines, albacore tuna, fish oil capsules, flaxseed, etc.) | Lower total cholesterol and LDL cholesterol levels.[37]<br>Lower blood pressure, total cholesterol, LDL, and triglyceride levels and are antithrombotic (interfere with blood clotting).[38]<br>High intake prolongs bleeding time, impairs immune function, and increases the potential intake of environmental toxins. At a high intake level of 30-40 ml of cod liver oil per day, there is a risk for vitamin A and vitamin D toxicity.[39] |
| **Monounsaturated Fatty Acids** | |
| Oleic acid (olive oil, rapeseed oil, etc.) | Lowers total and LDL cholesterol without lowering HDL.[40] |
| **Cholesterol** | |
| Animal products<br>Meats<br>Egg yolks<br>Shellfish | Raise total cholesterol and LDL cholesterol levels.<br>Most individuals compensate for different exogenous cholesterol levels and show no serum cholesterol change. Other individuals are sensitive to changes in cholesterol intake.[41] |
| **Saturated Fatty Acids** | |
| Lauric acid (coconut, palm kernel oil)<br>Myristic acid (coconut)<br>Palmitic acid (palm oil, beef)<br>Stearic acid (cocoa butter, beef) | Increases plasma total cholesterol.<br>Increases plasma total cholesterol (four to six times more hypercholesterolemic than palmitic and lauric acid).<br>Increases plasma total cholesterol.<br>Neutral—has no effect on blood lipoproteins due to its desaturation to oleic acid shortly after absorption and its high incorporation into phosphatidylcholine.[42] |
| **Trans Fatty Acids** | |
| Animal foods<br>Hydrogenated vegetable oil<br>Margarines (stick margarines have more trans-fat than tub margarine, baked goods, etc.) | Increase LDL cholesterol to about the same extent as saturated fatty acids and also can reduce HDL cholesterol concentrations.[43] |
| **Carbohydrates** | |
| Soluble fiber (pectins, gums, mucilages, legumes, oats, fruits, etc.)<br>High simple sugar (table sugar, candy, fructose, etc.) | Lower serum cholesterol and LDL cholesterol.<br>Lower risk for heart disease.<br>Increase plasma triglycerides.[44] |

| Component | Effect |
|---|---|
| **The Mediterranean Diet** | |
| High fiber<br>Fruits<br>Vegetables<br>Complex carbohydrates<br>Grains | Lowers incidence of coronary heart disease and possibly cancer.[45] |
| **Protein** | |
| Soy protein<br>Animal protein | The mechanism is not clear, but the assumption is that soy protein stimulates LDL receptors' activities, which are chronically reduced in hypercholesterolemia.[46]<br>Arginine is high in plant protein and seems to lower blood cholesterol, whereas lysine and methionine, amino acids that are higher in animal proteins, seem to raise plasma cholesterol levels.[47]<br>High levels of the amino acid homocysteine may contribute to heart disease by promoting atherosclerosis, excessive blood clotting, or blood vessel rigidity.[48]<br>Folic acid and vitamins $B_6$ and $B_{12}$ are all important in the metabolism of homocysteine by reducing its level. Scientists believe that a diet rich in these vitamins helps prevent blood vessel damage from homocysteine.[49] |
| **Moderate Alcohol Intake** | |
| Red or white wine<br>Beer<br>Distilled liquor | Has a protective factor.[50]<br>In addition to alcohol, wine contains phytochemicals that also may protect against cardiovascular disease.[51]<br>These substances may act as antioxidants, reducing LDL oxidation and blood clot formation, and may alter prostaglandin metabolism.<br>Wine also contains resveratrol, an antifungal compound in grape skins that increases HDL cholesterol and inhibits LDL oxidation.[49] |
| **Regular Aerobic Physical Activity** | |
| | Lowers LDL, raises HDL, lowers blood pressure, speeds weight loss and loss of body fat, improves blood glucose control in people with type 2 diabetes, and reduces emotional stress.[52] |
| **Coffee and Garlic** | |
| | Evidence relating coffee to increases and garlic consumption to decreases in serum total cholesterol, LDL cholesterol levels, or CHD has been inconsistent.[53] |

## BOX 10-4 The NCEP Guidelines for Reducing the Risk for Heart Disease[55,56]

- Recommend a cholesterol test every 5 years for all adults over age 20.
- Define low HDL as being less than 40 mg/dl compared to an earlier value of 35 mg/dl.
- Intensify the use of nutrition, physical activity, and weight control in the treatment of elevated blood cholesterol.
- Identify metabolic risk factors, collectively known as "metabolic syndrome" risk factors, linked to insulin resistance, which often occur together and dramatically increase the risk for heart attacks.
- Assess diet and lifestyle behaviors and use behavioral strategies to enhance adherence.
- Treat elevated triglycerides aggressively. Table 10-2 earlier in the chapter shows triglyceride levels

and levels of total and LDL cholesterol considered desirable, borderline high, and high according to the new guidelines.
- Treat high cholesterol more aggressively in people with diabetes.

Since its inception in 1985, the NCEP has made population-wide dietary recommendations. The following are the latest recommendations:

- Choose foods low in saturated fat.
- Choose foods low in total fat.
- Choose foods high in starch and fiber.
- Choose foods low in cholesterol.
- Be more physically active.
- Maintain a healthy weight, and lose weight if you are overweight.

## TABLE 10-7 The NCEP Two-Step Approach to Managing Hypercholesterolemia

| Nutrient | Step 1 Diet | Step 2 Diet | Therapeutic Lifestyle Changes |
|---|---|---|---|
| Total fat | < 30% of total calories | < 30% of total calories | 25%–35% of total calories |
| Saturated fatty acids* | < 8%–10% of total calories | < 7% of total calories | < 7% of total calories |
| Polyunsaturated fatty acids | Up to 10% of total calories | Up to 10% of total calories | Up to 10% of total calories |
| Monounsaturated fatty acids | 10%–15% of total calories | 10%–15% of total calories | Up to 20% of total calories |
| Carbohydrates† | 50%–60% of total calories | 50%–60% of total calories | 50%–60% of total calories |
| Protein | 10%–29% of total calories | 10%–20% of total calories | Approximately 15% of total calories |
| Cholesterol | < 300 mg/day | < 200 mg/day | < 200 mg/day |
| Fiber | 20–35 g/day | 20–35 g/day | 20–30 g/day |
| Total calories‡ | To achieve and maintain desirable | To achieve and maintain desirable | To balance energy intake and expenditure and to maintain desirable body weight/prevent weight gain |

*Trans-fatty acids are an LDL-raising fat that should be kept at a low intake.

†Carbohydrates should be derived predominantly from foods rich in complex carbohydrates, including grains (especially whole grains), fruits, and vegetables.

‡Daily energy expenditure should include at least moderate physical activity, contributing approximately 200 kcal per day.

Reproduced from: National Institutes of Health. National Heart, Lung, and Blood Institute, National Cholesterol Education Program. Expert Panel on Detection, Evaluation, and Treatment of High Blood Cholesterol in Adults (Adult Treatment Panel III). And National Institutes of Health, National Heart, Lung, and Blood Institute. NIH Publication No. 02-5215. September 2002. Available at: http://www.nhlbi.nih.gov/guidelines/cholesterol/atp3full.pdf. Accessed May 21, 2016.

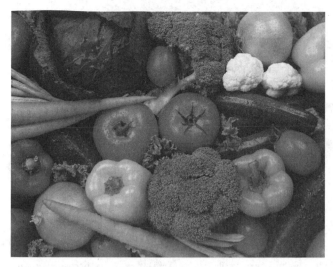

Consuming a variety of fruits and vegetables can reduce the risk for heart disease.

© Mitch Hrdlicka/Photodisc/Getty Images

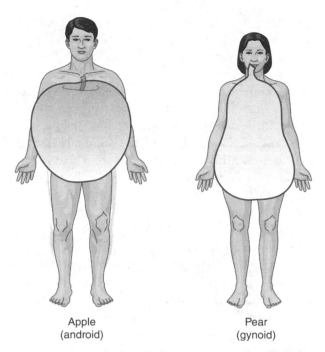

Apple (android)　　　Pear (gynoid)

Excessive body fat in the abdomen is associated with increased risk for morbidity.

## ▶ Obesity

Obesity is a persistent disease, and it is one of the most chronic health conditions in the world. It is reported that more than 1 billion adults worldwide are estimated as **overweight** and about 300 million of them are clinically obese.[34] In the United States, more than half of the population is either overweight or obese, and this condition affects all ages, genders, and ethnic groups.[57,58]

Obesity increases the risk for high blood pressure, high blood cholesterol, type 2 diabetes, insulin resistance, CHD, and many other physical ailments.[59] Several studies have demonstrated that increases in obesity also increase the number of lives lost to obesity,[60-62] as well as disease burdens of obesity. It is clear that obesity has become a leading public health problem in the United States. The first principle of the 2001 Surgeon General's Call to Action is to "promote the recognition of overweight and obesity as a major public health problem."[63]

### ☑ Think About It

After listening to a lecture about cardiovascular disease, Oliver asked, "What can I do to reduce my risk for heart disease?"

### Defining Obesity and Overweight

Obesity is caused by the accumulation of excess body fat. Although some methods to measure body fat do exist, they are expensive and unrealistic for general use. Body weight has traditionally been used to measure excess body fat. In recent years, however, the body mass index (BMI) has become the recommended method for screening and monitoring the population's body fat and for defining both overweight and obesity in a clinical setting.[42] BMI is determined by weight in kilograms divided by height in meters squared (BMI = $kg/m^2$). For adults, a BMI of 25.0 to 29.9 is classified as overweight and a BMI of 30.0 or more is classified as obese. See Chapter 2 for more about BMI calculation.

Although BMI is the most used criterion for obesity, there are limitations to this method. The measure may be incorrect for individuals with large muscle mass (e.g., body builders, weight lifters) or those with low muscle mass (e.g., the elderly). The location of body fat (fat distribution) is also important because fat distributed around the abdomen ("apple" shape or **android obesity**), found mainly in men, is linked to high blood lipids, glucose intolerance and insulin resistance, and high blood pressure. It also increases the risk for heart disease and diabetes mellitus. Fat that is distributed around the hips and thighs ("pear shape" or **gynoid obesity**) is common in women. Excess body fat at both locations has detrimental consequences for both men and women. A waist circumference of larger than 40 inches in men or larger than 35 inches in women is a sign of increased risk for CVD.[64]

### Epidemiology of Obesity and Overweight

Obesity and diabetes have reached epidemic proportions in the United States. According to 2005 to 2006 data from the CDC, 33.3 percent of men and 35.3 percent of women are obese (BMI > 30 kg/m$^2$), and those with a BMI of 40 or higher are at an increased risk for diabetes.[64,65] In 2015, 34.9 percent of U.S. adults were obese. In 2009, six states had obesity prevalence rates of 30 percent or more; 32 states, including those six, had rates of approximately 25 percent; and only one state, Colorado, had less than 20 percent.[64,66] The results from the National Health and Nutrition Examination Survey reported that between 2007 and 2008, 34.2 percent of U.S. adults were overweight (BMI > 27 kg/m$^2$), 33.8 percent were obese, and 5.7 percent were extremely obese.

The Healthy People 2010 target for adult obesity, based on measured weights and heights, was 15 percent among racial and ethnic groups for whom data were available. The trend toward obesity is high for adult African American females ages 49.6 between 2007 and 2008 and for adult Mexican American females, 35.9 of whom were obese in 2007 to 2008. Approximately 33 percent of Caucasian American women of the same age were obese. However, among men, the prevalence of obesity did not differ significantly by race or ethnic group. The report showed that 37.3 percent of African American men, 35.9 percent of Mexican American men, and 31.9 percent of Caucasian American men were obese.

## Medical and Social Costs of Obesity

Overweight and obesity and their associated health problems have substantial economic consequences for the U.S. healthcare system.[66] The increasing prevalence of overweight and obesity is associated with both direct and indirect costs. Direct healthcare costs refer to preventive, diagnostic, and treatment services related to overweight and obesity (e.g., physician's office visits, hospital visits, and nursing home care). Indirect costs refer to the value of wages people lost when they were unable to work because of illness or disability, as well as the value of future earnings lost by premature death. In 2003 to 2004, $431 billion was attributed to the direct and indirect costs of obesity.[67] Most of the costs associated with obesity were due to type 2 diabetes, CHD, and hypertension. Data show that U.S. medical expenses in 2003 related to obesity were as high as $75 billion.[68] Medicaid and Medicare paid about half of these costs.[69]

At the state level, estimates of annual Medicare costs due to obesity ranged from $87 million (Wyoming) to $7.7 billion (California), and Medicaid costs due to obesity ranged from $23 million (Wyoming) to $3.5 billion (New York). (The state differences in obesity expenditures were due to differences in the size of each state's population.)[69,70] These state-estimated data are limited to direct medical costs of obesity, not indirect costs (e.g., absenteeism and decreased productivity).[66] Overall, persons who are obese spent $1,429 (42 percent) more for medical care in 2006 than did normal-weight people.[71]

Overweight and obese individuals are at increased risk for many diseases and health conditions, including the following[66]:

- Hypertension
- Dyslipidemia (e.g., high total cholesterol or high levels of triglycerides)
- Type 2 diabetes
- Coronary heart disease
- Stroke
- Gallbladder disease
- Osteoarthritis
- Sleep apnea and respiratory problems
- Some cancers (endometrial, breast, prostate, rectum, uterus, cervical, and colon)
- Complications during pregnancy
- Complications during surgical procedures
- Depression

Society's emphasis on body weight may contribute to the emotional suffering of obese people. Emphasis on physical appearance, especially for women, makes overweight people feel unattractive.[72] Obese people regularly encounter prejudice or discrimination in the workplace, at school, and in social situations. Feelings of rejection, shame, or depression are common in obese individuals.[73] One research study suggested that improved self-image may be an avenue to promoting weight control in women.[74]

## Determinants of Obesity

Weight gain occurs due to an imbalance of energy intake and expenditure. Initially, when energy intake exceeds output, fat cells increase in size. When fat cells can no longer expand, they can increase in number. The size of the fat cells can decrease with weight loss, but the number of cells does not decrease. The reasons for the imbalance between energy intake and expenditure vary based on an individual's genes, emotional state, age, gender, psychological makeup, and environmental factors.[75]

### Genes

Scientists have identified some genes that cause obesity when they are damaged, but the actual mechanism that predisposes an individual to obesity is not clear. However, it is clear that when both parents are obese (body weight 100 percent above normal), the likelihood that their children will be obese is high (80 percent); however, when neither parent is obese, the chance that their children will be obese is low (less than 10 percent). Conversely, about 25 to 30 percent of obese persons have normal-weight parents.[76] The relationship between genetics and environment is not clear. It is estimated that genes alone account for about 50 to 90 percent of the variation in the amount of body fat stored.[77] However, having an obese relative does not guarantee that an individual will be obese.

## Emotions

Some people overeat because of depression, hopelessness, anger, boredom, and many other reasons besides hunger.[78] This does not indicate that overweight and obese people have more emotional problems than other people, but that their feelings seem to influence their eating habits, causing them to overeat. In these cases, as with other emotional issues, psychological intervention may be helpful.[79]

## Environmental Factors

The most important environmental factor is lifestyle. Individuals' eating habits and activity level may be learned from the people around them. Overeating and sedentary habits (inactivity) are the most important risk factors for obesity. The term **obesogenic environment** is defined as "the sum of influences that the surroundings, opportunities, or conditions of life have on promoting obesity in individuals or populations."[80,81] The environment is broader than just the physical environment; it includes costs, laws, policies, social and cultural attitudes, and values.

## Gender

Men typically have more muscle mass than women. Individuals with more muscle mass tend to have a higher **basal metabolic rate (BMR)**. Other factors that influence BMR include age, genetics, temperature, hormones, growth, and physical activity. Thus, women are more likely than men to gain weight with the same amount of calorie intake. In addition, women often gain weight after pregnancy and at menopause. During pregnancy, women store more body fat to be used for lactation. Menopause causes a decrease in estrogen level, causing increased body fat storage. In addition, both men and women tend to lose muscle mass and gain more body fat as they age. Their metabolism also slows slightly, which lowers their caloric needs.[82]

## Certain Medical Conditions and Medications

Although these situations are less common causes of obesity than overeating and inactivity, community nutritionists should be aware that individuals with the following conditions may gain excess body fat[81]:

- Hypothyroidism
- Cushing syndrome
- Depression
- Prader-Willi syndrome
- Polycystic ovarian syndrome

Also, certain medications (e.g., steroids, antidepressants, birth control pills, etc.) can cause an increase in body fat.

In addition to the causes listed, obesity is associated with other factors such as poverty; portion sizes; types of food consumed (high-fat foods, fast foods, soft drinks, and potato chips, and fewer complex carbohydrates); agricultural and technological innovations, which cause a decrease in food prices; and a sedentary lifestyle.[83,84]

## Obesity Prevention and Treatment Intervention

Extensive scientific research in the area of obesity has contributed significantly to the prevention and treatment of overweight and obesity. Obesity is now viewed as a complex disorder with several contributing factors, including genetic, sociocultural, environmental, and behavioral. Hence, the recommendations for weight management emphasize moderation and a balanced diet, behavior change, and moderate to vigorous physical activity for improving fitness. This section discusses different strategies for weight management.

### Lifestyle Modification

The bases of most obesity management programs are diet modification and physical activity. These modifications are inexpensive, and if the lifestyle changes can be maintained, they have the potential for long-term effectiveness.[85] In addition to creating changes in diet and physical activity, the lifestyle modification component of obesity interventions usually includes some form of behavioral modification to increase the long-term effectiveness of the program.

In 1994, the National Weight Control Registry, an ongoing observational study, was established to assess factors associated with sustained weight loss.[85] The requirement for this observational study was that participants must have maintained at least 30 pounds of weight loss for at least 1 year. Initial results indicated that more than 3,000 participants (80 percent women, 97 percent Caucasian Americans, with a mean age of 45 years) reported an average weight loss of 66 pounds and that the average duration of weight loss was 5.5 years. Approximately 90 percent of the participants reported previous unsuccessful attempts at weight loss. In this report, 89 percent of the participants reported modifying both diet and exercise to achieve their initial weight loss. The most common methods used were restricting certain types of foods (88 percent), limiting quantities

(44 percent), and counting calories (44 percent). Overall, 40 percent of the women and 63 percent of the men reported losing weight on their own, while the remainder used a commercial weight loss program to achieve their weight loss. The most common weight loss strategies used for those who modified their dietary intake were 1) eating a low-fat, low-calorie diet; 2) frequent self-monitoring; and 3) engaging in regular physical activity.[86]

## Dietary Modification

The interest in dieting is high because the prevalence of overweight and obesity is very high. Approximately 70 percent of U.S. adults are trying to lose weight or maintain their weight, and almost all report modifying their diet in some way to achieve their goals.[87] The common component of dietary modification for weight loss is reduced caloric intake. The recommendation is to encourage a slow rate of weight loss through an energy deficit (energy output minus energy intake). Small changes in reducing calorie intake by 200 to 300 kilocalories each day is more successful in long-term weight control than a drastic diet of only 1,000 to 1,200 total kilocalories per day. An individual can reduce kilocalorie intake by eliminating one can of soda each day, which is about 150 kilocalories; also, eating half a serving of fries instead of a whole serving would save another 100 kilocalories.[64] Making such changes as replacing whole milk with skim milk and including more fruits and vegetables also will reduce the total kilocalorie intake.

## Physical Activity Modification

In general, physical activity is used for the management of obesity. However, studies using only physical activity for weight loss show a small reduction in body weight.[88] Weight losses in the range of 0.09 to 0.1 kg/week have been reported when exercise is used alone compared to a no-treatment control group.[89,90]

Although its impact on weight loss may be minimal, physical activity has a critical role in the long-term maintenance of weight loss. One correlation study showed a strong association between self-reported exercise at follow-up and maintenance of a weight loss program.[91]

## Behavior Modification

The most effective weight reduction programs use group **behavior modification**. Behavior modification programs are usually conducted on a weekly basis in university or hospital clinics and have produced average reductions of 8 to 10 percent of body weight over 16 to 26 weeks.[92] The main behavioral modification components utilized in the management of obesity include self-monitoring, **stimulus control**, and relapse prevention strategies (see **CASE STUDY 10-2**). Self-monitoring includes the

---

## 🔍 CASE STUDY 10-2: How Effective Is Your Weight Loss Program

A group of women in the community have been trying to lose weight, but when they feel stressed, they binge. They are having trouble staying on a food plan and exercising regularly and are becoming discouraged. Cindy, a registered dietitian, listened to their doubts and lack of confidence. She gave them positive feedback, telling them, "I know it's frustrating trying to lose weight, but you're doing a good job. You've already lost some weight. I have confidence you can stick to your goals and lose the weight you want to lose." She assured the women that if they worked hard they would lose weight. The group seemed inspired to work harder at their weight loss plan because Cindy listened to their frustration, motivated them by reinforcing their self-esteem, and recognized that they were doing a good job. Cindy did further investigation and found that they were enrolled in a very-low-calorie (800 calories/day) weight loss program. The program also encouraged minimal physical activity and promised quick weight loss of 6 to 7 pounds per week. Cindy asked the women to keep records of the types of physical activities and the amount of time they spent on them for 1 week. She also provided them the MyPlate graphic and asked them to keep a 3-day dietary record. Analysis of the 3-day dietary record revealed low calories, calcium, iron, protein, vitamin D, and vitamin A intake. Cindy explained to the women that consuming adequate calories, including fruits and vegetables in their diets, reducing alcohol intake, and participating in physical activity would not only help them lose weight, but also help them reduce the incidence of cancer, heart disease, osteoporosis, obesity, and hypertension.

### Questions
1. What are the diseases and health conditions associated with overweight and obesity?
2. What is the difference between android obesity and gynoid obesity that Cindy must know?
3. What are some of the determinants of obesity?
4. What are obesogenic environments that Cindy must know so she can educate her clients about obesity adequately?

## ⌕ *CASE STUDY 10-2: How Effective Is Your Weight Loss Program* *(continued)*

5. What are some of the techniques that Cindy can use for obesity prevention, treatment, and intervention?
6. What is the definition of behavior modification? Cindy asked her clients to monitor their behaviors and eating habits. What does self-monitoring include?
7. What are two of the nine initiatives of the World Heart Federation (WHF) obesity strategies that Cindy can apply to her weight loss program?
8. What is the relationship among high fat intake, cooking methods, alcohol consumption, and cancer that these women should know?
9. Cindy explained the difference between intrinsic and extrinsic factors of bone mass to the women. What are the intrinsic and extrinsic factors that determine normal bone mass? What are some of the lifestyle factors that help maintain normal bone mass?
10. Work in small groups or individually to discuss the case study and practice using the Nutrition Care Process chart provided on the companion website. You also can add other nutrition and health-related conditions or assessments to the case study to make the case study more challenging and interesting.

systematic recording of food intake, exercise activities, and/or weight change. The use of stimulus control involves the identification and modification of environmental cues associated with overeating and sedentary activity and is widely accepted as clinically effective.[90] The available scientific literature on obesity suggests that consistent self-monitoring, particularly of food intake, is associated with improved outcome,[93] even during high-risk periods such as holidays.

When clients decide to participate in a weight loss program, finding a program that meets their needs becomes important. Some clients choose to participate in programs that include spirituality as a central component. Fitzgibbon et al.[94] conducted a faith-based weight loss intervention study that compared a culturally tailored, faith-based weight loss program to a culturally tailored weight loss intervention with no active faith component.[94] The results were not statistically significant, but suggested that the addition of the faith component improved results.[94] Two weight loss programs based on spirituality are the Thin Within Program, which was founded in 1975 and publicizes itself as a spiritually based, 12-week program that teaches participants to listen to their body's natural internal hunger/fullness signals, and the Weight Down Workshop, founded in 1986 by a registered dietitian, that takes a similar approach to weight loss.[95] In 2004, it was estimated that nearly 30,000 Weight Down Workshop groups were in existence nationwide, with many offered through churches. Reports indicate that for some women, spirituality was an important aspect of adhering to program principles.[96]

Hearts N' Parks is a national, community-based program designed to increase physical activity and reduce the incidence of obesity and other chronic health conditions. It was developed and supported by the NHLBI of the National Institutes of Health and the National Recreation and Park Association. The purpose of the program, which was created in 1999, is to reduce the growing trend of obesity and the risk for CHD in the United States. The program encourages all age groups in the United States to aspire for a healthy weight, follow a heart-healthy eating plan, and engage in regular physical activity. The American Dietetic Association is also working with Hearts N' Parks communities to provide expertise on heart-healthy nutrition.[97] About 50 Hearts N' Parks sites ("magnet centers") exist in 11 states.

The magnet centers carry out special "FunFit" events in July, including many activities tied to local Fourth of July celebrations. For instance, approximately 40,000 people attended a July 4 event in Athens, Georgia where a special Hearts N' Parks tent with games, prizes, and health and wellness information were displayed. On July 5, residents of Roswell, New Mexico, measured their body fat and learned how to grill low-fat foods in conjunction with the city's annual Alien Chase. Over 100,000 people attended a July 6 concert and fireworks event in South Bend, Indiana, that featured Hearts N' Parks displays and nutrition and fitness quizzes.

The Hearts N' Parks model supports the U.S. Department of Health and Human Services' Steps to a Healthier US initiative, based on President Bush's Healthier US initiative. These initiatives promote healthy lifestyles and behaviors aimed at achieving and maintaining good health for individuals of all ages. They also encourage public–private partnerships to support community-driven programs on healthy lifestyles that contribute directly to the prevention or treatment of one of three main health problems: obesity, diabetes, and asthma.

In 2002, data collected from the magnet centers included information on 68 programs that varied in size and duration. A pretest and posttest were administered and collected by 36 Hearts N' Parks sites during their first year as a magnet center. Programs for adults lasted an average of 12 weeks, attracting mainly seniors and women.

Results showed that adult participants significantly improved their scores in all areas of knowledge, attitude, and behavior. They increased their knowledge of heart-healthy nutrition by 9 percent. Scores increased from 6 to 7 percent in knowledge of overweight/obesity risks, physical activity, causes of high blood pressure, and ways to control cholesterol levels. Results also showed healthier attitudes toward overweight/obesity, heart-healthy eating habits, and physical activity and improvements on how frequently participants chose nutritious foods, based on self-reports. Adult participants reported adding, on average, 2 hours of moderate physical activity per week (from 8 hours to 10 hours), such as bicycling, walking, and golfing, after participating in the Hearts N' Parks program. In addition, they reduced the time spent in sedentary activities by an average of 8 hours per week, down to 33 hours.

Older adults (60 years or older) showed greater overall improvement than younger adults. Seniors' pretest knowledge scores were lower than younger adults' scores, but posttest knowledge scores were comparable. Seniors also significantly increased time spent weekly in physical activity on average, from slightly fewer than 6 hours to more than 8.5 hours, and significantly lowered the amount of time each week in sedentary tasks by 10 hours.[98]

# Public Health Policy for Addressing Global Obesity

In 2006, the Trust for America's Health (TFAH) reported that national and state policies were inadequate for obesity control and reduction. Some important findings from a study it conducted included the following[99]:

- The federal government faces organizational issues, including a lack of designated leadership, a bureaucratic tangle of involved agencies, and a need to learn to balance the competing interests of industry and public health.
- Obesity and obesity-related disease rates are increasing throughout the nation. Adult obesity exceeds 20 percent in 41 states and Washington, D.C. Alabama ranked as the heaviest state with 28.4 percent obesity; Colorado ranked as the least obese at 16 percent.
- Most of the states were on track to fail the national Healthy People 2010 goal of reducing the proportion

of adults who are obese to 15 percent or lower by the year 2010.[100]

Similarly, the Society for Nutrition Education (SNE) designed a public policy position paper (Improved Nutrition and Physical Activity IMPACT]) to address the obesity epidemic in the United States. SNE supports local communities to promote good nutrition and increased levels of physical activity among their citizens through community interventions, school-based activities, and healthcare delivery programs. In addition, SNE supports establishing grants for training health professionals and health science students to identify those at risk for obesity and provide health services for prevention and treatment of these conditions. SNE also supports collecting and analyzing data as part of NHANES and other data sources that can monitor and control obesity.[101]

At the international level, a proactive involvement with food, physical activities, and industries is critical to reduce the risks associated with the global obesity epidemic. This requires collective action, including the development of international strategies, together with supportive government policies. The World Heart Federation (WHF) is an international organization whose goal is to improve life through prevention and control of heart disease and stroke, with a focus on low- and middle-income countries. It is one of the international nongovernmental organizations (NGOs) for the World Health Organization's (WHO's) Global Strategy on Diet, Physical Activity and Health. Through its national members, the WHF supports the development of food labeling programs. The following are nine initiatives of the WHF's obesity strategies[102]:

- Supporting WHO's strategy on diet, physical activity, and health
- Calling for an international alliance with other global NGOs (IOTF, UICC, International Diabetes Federation, International Council of Nurses, etc.) against an environment may encourage the development of obesity. The World Heart Federation proposes a specific internet network to strengthen international action against obesity and to share positive experiences.
- Increasing awareness of the obesity epidemic and the benefits of healthy diets and physical activity among the population and policy makers through active support of the media.
- Making people aware that childhood obesity is a critical risk factor for later ill health.
- Replacing advertisements for candy, snacks, fast foods and soft drinks on television aimed at children and shown at times and on programs commonly watched

by children with advertisements promoting healthy lifestyles. Make fruits and vegetables readily available.

- Stressing among families and teachers the importance of traditional food and enhancing the value of healthy cooking skills.
- Creating public/private partnerships so as to improve content labeling on all foods, to decrease portion size, to reduce salt and sugar levels, to encourage fat substitution, and to implement education programs on nutrition to help people achieve energy balance.

- Promoting increased physical activity by any sustainable form of exercise.
- Advocating to governments through World Heart Federation members:
  - To provide incentives to communities to develop areas for physical activity such as bicycle paths, jogging trails, and sports areas (swimming pools, tennis courts, ball fields, etc.).
  - To change school based curricula to increase physical activity. To use legislation when voluntary action is insufficient.

# Successful Community Strategies

## The Burden of Obesity in Washington[103]

The CDC's Division of Nutrition, Physical Activity, and Obesity (DNPAO) funded 25 states to address the problems of obesity and other chronic diseases through statewide efforts with multiple partners. The program's primary focus was to create policy and environmental changes to increase physical activity, consumption of fruits and vegetables, and breastfeeding and to decrease television viewing, consumption of sugar-sweetened beverages, and consumption of high-energy-dense foods (high calorie/low nutrient foods). Washington received funding for this program in 2001.

In Washington, Behavioral Risk Factor Surveillance System data showed that 36 percent of adults were overweight and 26 percent were obese. Problems were also seen in factors related to obesity and other chronic diseases.

- Eighteen percent of Washington adults reported no leisure time physical activity in the past month.
- Only 26 percent of adults ate fruits and vegetables five or more times a day.

The problem was not limited to adults. Data from Washington's 2006 Healthy Youth Survey showed that 11 percent of 10th graders were obese and 14 percent were overweight. Fewer than half of youth surveyed ate at least five fruits and vegetables each day: 30 percent of 8th graders, 25 percent of 10th graders, and 22 percent of 12th graders.

One successful project in Washington was Healthy Communities, which assembled 12 communities to make significant changes in policy and the community environment to support community members with easy access to healthy foods and physical activity opportunities.

The project resulted in many policy and environmental changes: nonmotorized transportation plans and better access to healthy foods through community gardens, parks, open space, and recreational facilities. The project encouraged mixed-use development and a connected grid of streets, so that homes, businesses, schools, and stores are accessible to pedestrians and bicyclists. The Department of Health, with the Washington State Department of Transportation, and Community, Trade, and Economic Development, helped communities develop partnerships with transportation, planning, public health, and parks professionals. These partnerships promoted policies and plans that permitted citizens to be physically active in their daily lives.

To improve access to healthy foods for people in Washington, the Department of Health supported many projects and partnerships, including the following:

- Energize Your Meetings, a guide to serving healthy foods during meetings and events for worksites
- A healthy vending initiative called Fit Pick, in which healthy items in vending machines are labeled as such
- Participating in the Access to Healthy Foods Coalition, a nonprofit organization that serves as a connecting point among communities working to improve the nutritional environment
- Coordinating the Fruits and Veggies—More Matters program for the state.

Washington had a great success with rule and policy changes at the state and local levels. For example, the state legislature passed a bill requiring communities to include environmental health impacts to support physical activity in their growth management plans. The Seattle Board of Health now requires chain restaurants to include nutritional information on their menus. Also, results of the Healthy Communities project showed that many cities and communities have implemented pedestrian and bicycle transportation planning, designated funds to develop and maintain the trails and path systems, and implemented Safe Routes to School programs.

Source: Centers for Disease Control and Prevention. The burden of obesity in Washington. Available at: www.cdc.gov/obesity. Accessed October 23, 2016.

# ▶ Cancer

Cancer, a disease of the body's cells, is one of the most devastating chronic health conditions in the United States and worldwide. It is the second most common fatal disease in the United States. Its development involves damage to cells' DNA; this damage occurs over a long period and grows at the expense of the healthy cells. The characteristics common to all types of cancer are uncontrolled growth and the ability to spread to distant sites (to **metastasize**).

Individuals who are alive and without recurrence of cancer 5 years after diagnosis are considered cured. This is termed the **5-year survival rate**. Survival rates vary significantly depending on the site where the cancer occurred. Overall, the survival rate for some types of cancer is approximately 52 percent for Caucasian Americans and 38 percent for African Americans.[104] Regardless of ethnicity, the 5-year survival rate for poor Americans is estimated to be 10 to 15 percent lower than for middle-class and affluent Americans.[105] This chapter discusses cancer prevention and dietary factors implicated in the development of cancer.

## Links Between Cancer and Diet

The causes of cancer are complex and often not understood. Certain cancers occur in great numbers in some countries. It has been estimated that 35 percent of the cancer mortality in the U.S. population is attributable to diet and about 80 percent to environmental factors.[106] For example, stomach and esophageal cancers are common where nitrates and nitrites are prevalent in food and water or where cured and pickled foods are popular. Some of the countries where this occurs are the United States, China, Japan, and Iceland.

Studies of migration between cultures demonstrate the strong effect of environmental factors. These studies reveal that the pattern of occurrence of many types of cancer changes when people move to a new country. For example, in Japan there is more stomach cancer and less prostate, colon, and breast cancer than in the United States. In second-generation Japanese immigrants to the United States, however, the rates and types of cancers are similar to those of other Americans.[86] Similar outcomes for prostate cancer are reported in Polish men.[106] The changes coincide with differences in environmental exposure, lifestyle, and diet.

## Dietary Components and Cancer

It is hard to review the role of dietary components in cancer development without also considering the other factors that might add to the development of cancer. It is estimated that 35 percent of cancers may be related to diet, including 40 percent of those in men and 60 percent of those in women, notwithstanding the fact that women consume a more varied diet and less alcohol than men.[83] Cooking methods also may be linked to cancer, and some nutrients are associated with cancer when they are consumed in large quantities. The nutrients that may cause cancer include fat and calories; other factors such as alcohol also may cause cancer. **TABLE 10-8** presents dietary components and their effect on cancer.

---

**TABLE 10-8** Dietary Components and Their Effect on Cancer[107-110]

| Dietary Components | Effect |
|---|---|
| Fats<br>Animal<br>**Linoleic acid** (polyunsaturated fat)<br>Omega-3 fatty acids<br>Monounsaturated fatty acids | Higher incidences of breast, colon, prostate, and pancreatic cancers.<br>A high level promotes cancer rather than initiates it.<br>Have a protective effect against the development of cancer.<br>Have a neutral effect. |
| Cooking methods | High-temperature cooking of meat, such as frying, broiling, and grilling, produces **carcinogens** such as heterocyclic amines (HCAs), polycyclic aromatic hydrocarbons, and nitrosamines (PAHs) in animals. These substances can damage the DNA and cause mutations, which may result in cancer of the stomach and esophagus.[110]<br>Low-temperature, high-moisture cooking, such as stewing and pot-roasting, does not produce the same level of carcinogens. |
| Alcohol | High consumption causes oropharyngeal, laryngeal, esophageal, breast,[111] and colorectal cancer. |

A research study on the relationship between cancer and calcium and dairy products reported that higher consumption of milk/dairy products reduced the risk for colon cancer and that high calcium intake reduced the risk for colorectal cancer.[112] In another study, an estimated minimum increase of serum 25(OH)D level to 40 to 60 µg/ml (100 to 50 µmol/L) throughout the year would prevent about 58,000 new cases of breast cancer and 49,000 new cases of colorectal cancer each year and three fourths of deaths from these diseases in the United States and Canada. This is based on observational studies combined with a randomized trial. In addition, the proposed intakes may reduce case-fatality rates of patients who have breast, colorectal, or prostate cancer by half.[111,113]

## Protective Effects of Certain Food Components Against Cancer

One of the Healthy People 2010 objectives was to reduce both new cases and the current rate of cancer in the United States. This can be accomplished by eating a moderately low-fat diet and increasing the consumption of fruits, vegetables, and whole grains. These foods contain vitamins, minerals, and other substances that are beneficial to one's health, such as phytochemicals. This section discusses some of the dietary components that can protect people from the risk for cancer.

### Fiber

Strong evidence shows that fiber has physiological effects on the gastrointestinal tract that may prevent the occurrence of chronic diseases. Dietary fiber refers to plant materials that are not easily digested by enzymes in the human gut. Water-soluble fibers include pectin, gums, and mucilages. Insoluble fibers include cellulose and other hemicelluloses.

Early studies suggested that fiber intake was related to the low incidence of colorectal cancer in Africans consuming high-fiber diets.[114] In the United States, populations with a higher per capita intake of fiber usually have a lower incidence of colorectal cancer compared with those with a lower intake. However, epidemiological studies on the relationship between dietary fiber and colorectal cancer are inconclusive. A recent prospective study using the Nurses' Health Study cohort found no association between fiber intake and the risk for colorectal cancer.[115] Two clinical trials have shown that increasing total fiber intake did not influence the risk for recurrent colorectal **adenomas**,[116,117] which are cancers that arise from glandular tissues. Fiber also plays a protective role in preventing breast and ovarian cancer.[118]

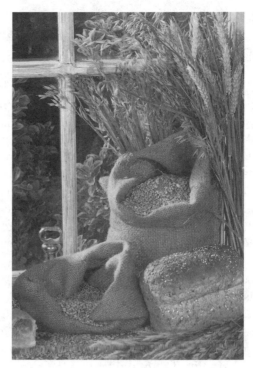

Instead of using white flour, substitute with different types of whole grains in your regular recipes for cookies, muffins, quick breads, and pancakes.
© AbleStock

The anticarcinogenic effects previously attributed to fiber may be due to the effects of the nonfiber constituents of fruits and vegetables, such as **antioxidants**, vitamins, and minerals. In addition, high fiber intake is mostly associated with lower caloric intake, which may also decrease the risk for cancer.[119,120]

Adequate dietary fiber intake is encouraged because of its role in maintaining normal bowel function and its possible role in disease prevention. The recommended amount of dietary fiber ranges from 25 to 30 g/day or 10 to 13 g/1,000 kcal.[121] Mean dietary fiber intake in the United States is about 14 to 15 g/day.[94] Because some of the benefits of high-fiber foods may be due to other components in fiber-rich diets, high-fiber foods, rather than isolated fiber, are recommended. The recommendation is to consume whole fruits and whole grains instead of fruit juices and refined grains.

Certain fibers exist in higher concentrations in specific foods. For example, insoluble fiber such as pectin is found in fruits and vegetables, especially apples, oranges, strawberries, and carrots. Gums are found in oat bran, barley, and legumes. Whole-wheat flour, wheat bran, and vegetables are good sources of celluloses, and hemicellulose is found in wheat bran, whole bran, and whole grains.

### Antioxidants

Free radicals are short-lived, highly reactive chemicals often derived from oxygen-containing compounds, which can have detrimental effects on cells, especially cellular DNA and cell membranes. The body has an antioxidant defense system that prevents free radical damage.[64] This includes antioxidant nutrients, which can directly scavenge free radicals and deactivate them. Alpha-tocopherol (vitamin E), ascorbic acid (vitamin C), beta-carotene (carotenoid, a provitamin A), and flavonoids are antioxidants that have been shown to be active in the prevention of cancer in vitro. Vitamins C and E and green tea can prevent the formation of **carcinogenic** nitrosamines and nitrosamides.[122] A 5-year trial of beta-carotene, vitamin E, and selenium showed that consumption of higher levels of these nutrients resulted in the incidence of stomach cancer being reduced by 20 percent and total mortality by 10 percent among residents of Linxian County, China, who have one of the world's highest rates of esophageal and gastric cancer.[123]

The consumption of tomatoes and tomato sauce has been reported to reduce the incidence of prostate and gastrointestinal cancers. Lycopene, found in tomatoes, is the most efficient antioxidant of the carotenoids. A high intake of raw tomatoes, more than seven servings per week, was significantly related to decreased risk for gastrointestinal cancers compared to an intake of less than two servings per week.[35,124] Tomatoes have other components besides lycopene, such as vitamin C, that may contribute to these findings. Because the cancer-reducing effect may be influenced by other nutrients or a combination of nutrients, eating a variety of whole foods, not individual micronutrients, is the appropriate formula for decreasing the risk for cancer.

Fruits and vegetables are low in calories and good sources of fiber, vitamins, minerals, and other bioactive substances (**phytochemicals**). (See **TABLE 10-9**.) Several epidemiological studies have examined the relationship between fruit and vegetable intake and the occurrence of cancer. Populations with the lowest intake of fruits and vegetables have double the rate of most cancers, such as genitourinary, gastrointestinal, and pulmonary malignancies as well as stomach, pancreatic, oral cavity, esophageal, colorectal, and bladder cancer.[35] Raw vegetables were shown to provide protective effects in 87 percent of studies. Specifically, vegetables from the allium family (e.g., onions, garlic), carrots, green vegetables, cruciferous vegetables (e.g., broccoli, cauliflower), and tomatoes were shown to be protective in 70 to 80 percent of the studies. Total fruits

**TABLE 10-9** Possible Anticarcinogens in Vegetables and Fruits[14,107,125]

| Nutrients and Substances | Food Sources |
|---|---|
| Carotenoids | Carrots, peppers, parsley, greens, spinach |
| Ascorbate (vitamin C) | Oranges, strawberries, green peppers, tomatoes |
| Tocopherols (vitamin E) | Wheat germ, safflower oil, sunflower seeds |
| Selenium | Lean ground beef, crab, turkey, dark meat |
| Folate | Fortified grain products |
| Dietary fiber | All plants, fruits, and vegetables |
| Allium compounds | Onions, garlic |
| Isoflavones | Soybeans |
| Flavonoids | Grapefruit, citrus |
| Protease inhibitors | Seeds, legumes, potatoes, sweet corn |
| Anthocyanidins | Grapes, cherries, raspberries. |
| Lignans | Grains, flaxseed |
| Ellagic acid | Raspberries, spinach, strawberries, blueberries, cranberries |
| Phytochemicals/indoles | Broccoli, Brussels sprouts, cabbage, kale |

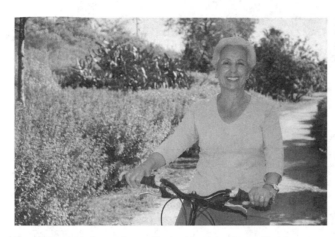

Engaging in leisure time physical activity is the first step toward developing a pattern of regular physical activity.

© Carme Balcells/ShutterStock, Inc.

and citrus fruits were shown to be protective in about 65 percent of the studies.[35] The majority of case-control studies indicate that high versus low consumption of vegetables and fruits reduces the risk for cancer by about half. For example, the risk for stomach cancer decreased by about 60 percent as vegetable intake increased from 100 g/day to 350 g/day and more than 50 percent as fruit intake increased from 50 g/day to 300 g/day.

## Physical Activity, Exercise, and Cancer

Several studies, including the Nurses' Health Study, show a direct relationship between physical activity and colon cancer.[107,126] Individuals with high levels of activity throughout their lives were found to have the lowest risk, whereas those who reported high levels of activity only in later life were associated with a weaker protective effect of physical activity.[126,127]

These studies also reported that mild to moderate physical activity and exercise significantly reduced colon cancer and adenoma risk.[127,128] The American Cancer Society guidelines are consistent with guidelines from the AHA and the American Diabetes Association for the prevention of CHD and diabetes, as well as for general health promotion, as defined by the U.S. Department of Health and Human Services' 2005 *Dietary Guidelines for Americans*. The dietary guidelines are[129,130]:

- Reduce fat intake to 30 percent or less of calories.
- Increase fiber intake to 20 to 30 g/day, with an upper limit of 35 g/day.
- Include a variety of vegetables and fruits in the daily diet.
- Avoid obesity.
- Consume alcoholic beverages in moderation, if at all.
- Minimize consumption of salt-cured, salt-pickled, or smoked foods and high-fat meats, particularly those from animal sources.
- Be physically active.
- Achieve and maintain a healthy weight.
- Be moderately active for 30 minutes or more on most days of the week.

Community and public health nutritionists may find that primary and secondary prevention of all cancers involves a more aggressive approach toward eating behavior. (See **CASE STUDY 10-3**.) Equally, understanding the screening and detection approaches recommended for several major cancers, even if there is no known dietary link, prepares nutritionists with the skills to communicate more effectively with their clients.[104] **BOX 10-5** presents a dietary research approach to prevention of cancer, and **BOX 10-6** describes a successful strategy for increasing the antioxidant content of pizza crust.

## ⌕ CASE STUDY 10-3: Nutrition Education and Cancer Prevention

Chimma, a registered dietitian and a public health nutritionist in an urban-based wellness program, plans to begin a cancer prevention program that includes nutrition education and smoking cessation classes. Her goal is to provide nutrition programs that address some of the Healthy People 2010 objectives. She wants to increase the proportion of persons age 2 years or older who:

- Consume at least two daily servings of fruits, from 28 to 75 percent.
- Consume at least three daily servings of vegetables, with at least one third being dark green or deep yellow vegetables, from 3 to 50 percent.
- Consume at least six daily servings of grain products, with at least three being whole grains, from 7 to 50 percent.
- Consume less than 10 percent of calories from saturated fat, from 36 to 75 percent.
- Consume no more than 30 percent of total calories from fat, from 33 to 75 percent.
- Participate in at least 30 minutes of daily physical activity.

Chimma attended and completed the Freedom from Smoking course from the American Lung Association and studied hypnosis and behavior modification during her master's degree program in Public Health Nutrition at the University of Minnesota. Chimma's first project will be a needs assessment of the clients attending her program and in the surrounding community in order to determine an ideal time for the classes and the best type of cost-effective nutrition assessment, and

*(continues)*

## 🔍 *CASE STUDY 10-3: Nutrition Education and Cancer Prevention* (continued)

to understand the nutritional knowledge of the community. The assessment showed that current health problems include heart disease, hypertension, obesity, and lung cancer; further analysis showed low iron intake, inadequate intake of fruits and vegetables, high calorie intake, and lack of physical activity. Chimma explained to the community that achieving the listed objectives will help reduce the likelihood of cancer, heart disease, osteoporosis, obesity, and hypertension.

### Questions

1. What are the recommended strategies for achieving the Healthy People 2010 objectives for weight and food choice?
2. List and briefly describe three of the Healthy People 2010 objectives.
3. What is atherosclerosis? What are the two components of coronary heart disease (CHD)?
4. What is the relationship between physical activity and cancer?
5. What are the effects of vegetarianism on colon cancer?
6. What are the Dietary Guidelines for Americans that directly relate to cancer prevention?
7. What are phytochemicals? What are antioxidants that the community needs to know about?
8. What is the definition of carcinogenic? What is a carcinogen?
9. What are some food components that have protective effects against cancer? What are some possible anticarcinogens in vegetables and fruits?
10. Work in small groups or individually to discuss the case study and practice using the Nutrition Care Process chart provided on the companion website. You also can add other nutrition and health-related conditions or assessments to the case study to make the case study more challenging and interesting.

### BOX 10-5   Dietary Research Approach Strategy for the Prevention of Cancer

#### Dietary Fiber and Colorectal Cancer Risk[131,132]

Le Marchand et al.[132] conducted a population-based case-control study among different ethnic groups in Hawaii using personal interviews. (See Chapter 3 for more information on case-control research design.) Between 1987 and 1991, 698 males and 494 females were diagnosed with adenocarcinoma of the colon or rectum, compared to 1,192 population controls matched by age, sex, and ethnicity. They found a protective association in both sexes with fiber intake from vegetable sources (but not from fruits, except bananas, and cereals). Intakes of carotenoids, light green and yellow-orange vegetables, broccoli, corn, carrots, garlic, and legumes (including soy products) reduced the risk, even after adjustments were made for vegetable fiber. The data supported a protective role of fiber from vegetables against colorectal cancer independent of its water solubility property and the effects of other phytochemicals.

Aligning with these findings, the National Cancer Institute (NCI) designed its Fruits and Veggies—More Matters program to increase per capita fruit and vegetable consumption. The NCI's 5-a-Day program promotes a simple nutrition message that physicians, nurses, community and public health nutritionists, and other healthcare professionals can reinforce to their clients. The basic goal is to promote eating five or more servings of fruits and vegetables every day for better health.

### BOX 10-6   Increasing the Antioxidant Content of Pizza Dough[133,134]

Whole grains contain higher levels of fiber and more types of vitamins and minerals, such as folate, vitamin E, and selenium, than refined flour products. These antioxidants have been shown to reduce the risk for some forms of cancer, including prostate and colon cancers. Dr. Liangli Lucy Yu and other nutritionists at the department of nutrition and food science at the University of Maryland conducted a research study to enhance the antioxidant content of pizza dough by incorporating whole wheat flour. The nutritionists increased the antioxidant content by increasing the fermentation process and baking conditions; it is recognized that chemical reactions induced by yeast during the fermentation process release antioxidants that gather in the dough. The researchers extended the time the dough was allowed to rise (48 hours) and baked the dough for a longer time (7 to 14 minutes), which increased the antioxidant content of the crust by 60 percent. Also, results showed that the higher the baking temperature (from 400° to 550° Fahrenheit), the more antioxidants accumulated, increasing the antioxidant content in the crust by 82 percent.

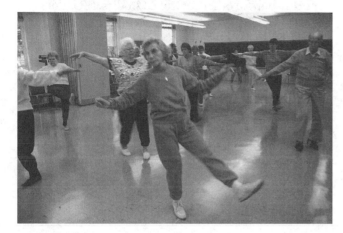

Vigorous physical activity is recommended for improved cardiorespiratory fitness.

Courtesy of Bill Branson/National Cancer Institute

# ▶ Osteoporosis

Osteoporosis is porous bone due to reduction in bone mass. According to NHANES III, 13 to 18 percent of women, or 4 to 6 million, have osteoporosis, and 37 to 50 percent, or 13 to 17 million, have reduced bone mineral density (BMD). For men, 1 to 2 million have osteoporosis and 28 to 47 percent (8 to 13 million) have reduced BMD. Of women 65 or older, 29.3 percent have osteoporosis.[56,103,135-137] Therefore, preventive strategies to retard bone loss and prevent osteoporosis are very important.

## Normal Bone Development

Both intrinsic and extrinsic factors determine normal bone mass. Intrinsic factors include genetics, family history, and ethnicity. Extrinsic factors include diet, hormonal milieu, specific illness, and exercise. Each of these factors is discussed in detail in this section.

Genetic factors account for 60 to 80 percent of the variance seen in bone mineral density.[108] Daughters of postmenopausal women with a family history of osteoporosis were found to have a lower than normal BMD,[138,139] and both elderly men and women have an increased risk

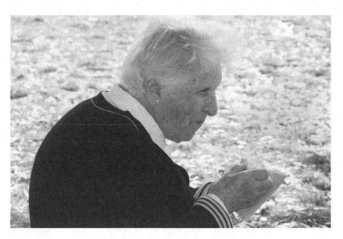

Osteoporosis makes the vertebrae susceptible to compression fractures from minor trauma. The elderly (especially women) should be concerned about potential fractures if they experience height loss, a limited ability to twist and bend the back, and/or a deformity that develops in the spine.

© frantab/Shutterstock

for osteoporosis when other family members have been affected.[140]

Gender and ethnicity are important factors in consideration of bone density. Males have a higher bone mass, including peak bone mass, at all ages.[141] Men also have a slower reduction of sex steroids with aging, resulting in less dramatic reduction in BMD. Osteoporosis and fractures are lowest among African Americans compared with other races/ethnicities, and bone mass is higher in African Americans compared to Hispanics, Caucasian Americans, and Asians Americans.[141]

Calcium intake seems to increase and maintain bone mass. The recommended daily intake for men and women age 51 years or older is 1,200 mg elemental calcium.[140] Dairy products are the most important sources of dietary calcium, providing approximately 75 percent of the calcium in a typical North American diet.[142] Epidemiological data suggest that osteoporosis is more prevalent in regions where dairy intake is low and that milk consumption in childhood and adolescence is directly correlated with postmenopausal BMD.[143] (Calcium requirements increase during periods of rapid growth.) It has been reported that calcium alone may not be sufficient for optimal bone accretion, however. In one study, women consuming more than 1,000 mg of calcium daily exhibited no significant gains in BMD if they did not concomitantly increase their activity patterns.[114] Research evaluating the effects of calcium supplementation on BMD have yielded varying results; controlled supplementation trials in healthy children and adolescents, including twin studies, suggest that calcium supplementation improves bone density.[144,145]

Vitamin D is an important complement to calcium because it facilitates absorption of calcium from the diet. In addition to being absorbed through the intestines, vitamin D is synthesized endogenously in the skin under the influence of ultraviolet sunlight. Risk factors for vitamin D deficiency include inadequate diet, deficient sunlight exposure, low body weight and BMI, the use of anticonvulsants, and malabsorption.[145] In addition, it is important to observe that a study reported the incidence of hypovitaminosis D in African American and Caucasian American women. Hypovitaminosis D also was found in African American women who consumed the adequate intake of vitamin D from supplements of 200 IU per day.[146]

Regular moderate exercise seems to have a beneficial effect on BMD. Studies have suggested that a positive correlation exists between BMD and both body weight and BMI. Low body weight from various conditions has been recognized as an independent risk factor for fractures.[147,148] Several studies have shown that impact (weight-bearing) exercise may have a positive effect on both bone size and mineralization, and a twin study showed that the twin with the longer duration of weight-bearing exercise showed an increased femoral neck BMD.[149,150]

It has been suggested that estrogen helps preserve bone mass in young women with anorexia nervosa by impairing osteoclast-mediated bone resorption. Oral contraceptive use by these young women in a retrospective cross-sectional study was shown to be associated with a higher BMD.[151] In a small pilot study of women with anorexia nervosa and hypothalamic amenorrhea, estrogen replacement therapy (ERT) increased BMD.[152] Unfortunately, in other controlled studies, ERT alone has not been shown to consistently reverse the bone loss in young women with anorexia nervosa, with the possible exception of the most severely underweight patients ($< 70$ percent of ideal body weight).[153] Despite the fact that its effects on bone accretion have been disappointing, ERT, combined with psychological support, is a therapy usually used to maintain skeletal health in patients with anorexia.[154] The following Successful Community Strategies presents a successful osteoporosis education program.

# Successful Community Strategies

## The University of Nebraska's Osteoporosis Education[105]

A team of healthcare professionals consisting of registered dietitians, faculty, and Extension specialists collaborated and designed a community-based health education program. They also formed partnerships and coalitions with individuals, communities, organizations, government agencies, and businesses to educate people about the prevention of osteoporosis.

The program was publicized by placing advertisements in the local newspaper and displaying posters in local businesses. The educational session emphasized prevention, risk factors, diagnosis, and treatment of osteoporosis. The program also had a question and answer session. The participants were able to ask physicians and nutrition professionals questions about osteoporosis. Local health professionals presented the educational session, with local physicians being the primary presenters. Pre-event and post-event data were obtained from the participants using written questionnaires. The following general issues were incorporated into the educational session: knowledge of osteoporosis, the need for an optimal calcium intake and bioavailability; food sources of calcium; parents as role models; issues affecting consumption, such as weight concerns; lactose intolerance; vitamin D inadequacy; dietary factors aiding calcium retention; weight-bearing exercise; prevention and treatment of osteoporosis; bone density scans; and avoidance of smoking and excessive alcohol intake.

Results showed that 82 percent of respondents knew a great deal about osteoporosis after the sessions, as opposed to only 24 percent before the sessions. After the sessions, 86 percent of those who had a bone density scan prior to the sessions indicated they had a great deal of knowledge about osteoporosis compared with only 21 percent before the educational sessions. In addition, 55 percent of those who had never had a bone density scan indicated that they had a great deal of knowledge about osteoporosis compared to 27 percent before the sessions.

About 20 percent of the respondents reported "always" taking calcium supplements after the sessions. Thirty-two percent indicated "always" eating a calcium-rich diet prior to the program, whereas 41 percent did following the sessions. Thirty-four percent "always" did weight-bearing exercises at least three times weekly before the sessions, compared to 40 percent after the sessions.

There were requests for additional nutrition and health education sessions due to the success of the educational program. The team approach in presenting the educational sessions and answering/discussing participants' questions contributed to the success of the program.

# Learning Portfolio

## Chapter Summary

- A low-fat diet accompanied by a high intake of complex carbohydrates may prevent heart disease and cancer.
- In some people, certain risk factors such as age, genetics, gender, and ethnicity can be predictive of atherosclerosis and hypertension.
- Smoking has a significant influence on the risk for acquiring cardiovascular disease.
- A diet containing soybeans may be an effective dietary tool to treat hypercholesterolemia.
- The National High Blood Pressure Education Program (NHBPEP) was the first large-scale public outreach and education campaign to reduce high blood pressure. Its promotion of the detection, treatment, and control of high blood pressure has been credited with influencing the dramatic increase in the public's understanding of hypertension and its role in heart attacks and strokes.
- The diet and lifestyle strategies discussed in this chapter to reduce cardiovascular disease risk are appropriate for primary prevention (where a heart attack has not yet taken place, but there are risk factors).
- There are links between obesity and an increased risk for high blood pressure, high blood cholesterol, type 2 diabetes, insulin resistance, and coronary heart disease.
- BMI is determined by weight in kilograms divided by height in meters squared (BMI = kg/m$^2$).
- The basis of a weight loss program is diet, behavior, and physical activity modification.
- Cancer is a disease of the body's cells and is one of the most common chronic health issues.
- About 35 percent of the cancer mortality in the U.S. population is due to diet and about 80 percent to environmental factors.
- Many cancers may be related to obesity and excessive caloric intake.
- Low-temperature, high-moisture cooking methods, such as stewing and pot-roasting, do not produce carcinogens.
- High-temperature cooking of meat, for example, frying, broiling, and grilling, may produce carcinogens.
- Excessive alcohol consumption is associated with an increased risk for laryngeal and esophageal cancers.
- Research shows that populations with a higher per capita intake of fiber have a lower incidence of colorectal cancer.
- Fruits and vegetables are good sources of fiber, vitamins, minerals, and other bioactive substances such as phytochemicals. Studies show that populations with the lowest intake of fruits and vegetables have double the rate of most cancers.
- Individuals with high levels of activity throughout their lives were found to have the lowest risk for some cancers.
- Genetic factors account for about 60 to 80 percent of the variance seen in bone mineral density.
- Vitamin D is an important complement to calcium because it facilitates absorption of calcium from the diet.
- Regular moderate exercise seems to have a beneficial effect on bone mineral density.
- Estrogen helps preserve bone mass in young women with anorexia nervosa by impairing osteoclast-mediated bone resorption.

## Critical Thinking Activities

Community and public health nutritionists need to be aware of other healthcare professionals (nurses, physicians, health educators) who are also marketing to the same targeted community audience, for example, those needing information about heart disease, obesity, cancer, and osteoporosis prevention. Programs can overlap and negative reactions occur if a competitive/collaborative market analysis is not conducted prior to initiating any prevention or intervention programs in the community.

- Identify a nutrition and health education program that the community needs.
  - Identify the current providers of heart disease, cancer, osteoporosis, and obesity prevention programs for your community or target audience.
  - Determine your strengths and weaknesses in competing with other healthcare professionals (e.g., nurses, doctors, etc.) who are providing similar education programs.
  - Determine how you can collaborate with the current service providers in the community (e.g., AHA to develop a Heart Healthy program).
  - Outline the distinctive characteristic of your program that sets it apart from other healthcare disease prevention programs in your community.
- Divide into groups and indicate how you can publicize classes for smoking cessation using various media methods.
- Decide how to provide clients with a way to change their dietary habits.

- Identify funding sources for the smoking cessation program (see http://go.jblearning.com/nnakwe2 for examples of funding agencies).
- Identify different types of screening methods for obesity (discussed in Chapter 2) to use in the weight loss program.
- Provide a list of different heart disease risk factors.
- Provide examples of other ways of making the public aware of the impact of heart disease.

## Think About It

**Answer 1:**

Choose foods low in saturated fat.

Choose foods low in total fat.

Choose foods high in starch and fiber.

Choose foods low in cholesterol.

Be more physically active.

Maintain a healthy weight, and lose weight if you are overweight.

**Answer 2:** She should add more fruits, vegetables, nuts/beans/seeds, and low-fat dairy products to her diet and eat moderate amounts of lean meat/fish/poultry, with a reduced content of dietary cholesterol as well as saturated and total fat for the whole diet. She should also reduce her dietary sodium intake to no more than 2.4 g of sodium daily.

## Key Terms

**5-year survival rate:** The number of individuals who are alive and without recurrence of cancer 5 years after diagnosis.

**adenomas:** Cancers that arise from glandular tissues.

**android obesity:** Excess storage of fat, mainly in the abdominal area.

**antioxidants:** Vitamins C and E and beta-carotene, which neutralize free radicals and other reactive chemicals and terminate harmful chemical reactions.

**atherosclerosis:** A common form of arteriosclerosis in which plaque forms within the intima of medium and large arteries; a group of diseases characterized by thickening and loss of elasticity of arterial walls.

**basal metabolic rate (BMR):** The minimum amount of energy that an awake, fasted, resting body needs to maintain itself; often used interchangeably with resting metabolic rate (RMR). BMR measurements are performed in a warm room in the morning before the individual rises, and at least 12 hours after the last food intake and activity.

**behavior modification:** A process used to gradually and permanently change habitual behaviors.

**carcinogen:** An agent that can cause cancer.

**carcinogenic:** Producing cancer; a substance that can produce or enhance the development of cancer.

**chronic condition:** An occurrence of a disease that cannot be cured and extends over a period of time.

**gynoid obesity:** Excess storage of fat, mainly in the buttocks and thigh. Also called gynecoid obesity.

**hypercholesterolemia:** Elevated cholesterol level in the blood.

**hypertension:** A condition in which blood pressure remains persistently elevated.

**linoleic acid:** An essential omega-6 fatty acid that contains 18 carbon atoms and 2 carbon–carbon double bonds (18:2).

**low-risk individual:** An individual without diabetes or cardiovascular disease and with systolic blood pressure less than 160 mm Hg and diastolic blood pressure less than 100 mm Hg.

**metastasize:** To spread cancer by the movement of cancer cells from one part of the body to another.

**obesity:** A condition characterized by excess body fat. It is defined as a body mass index of 30 kg/m² or greater or a body weight that is 20 percent or more above the healthy body weight standard.

**obesogenic environments:** The sum of influences that the surroundings, opportunities, or conditions of life have on promoting obesity in individuals or populations.

**osteoporosis:** Porous bone due to reduction in bone mass.

**overweight:** A body mass index of 25 to 29.9 kg/m² or a body weight 10 to 19 percent above the healthy body weight standard.

**phytochemicals:** Nonnutrient compounds found in plant-derived foods that produce biological activity in the body.

**stimulus control:** Altering the environment to minimize the stimuli for eating; for example, removing foods from sight and storing them in kitchen cabinets.

## References

1.    Agency for Health Care Research and Quality. Chronic disease in adults. http://www.ahrq.gov/. Accessed March 17 2017.
2.    Véronique LR, Turner MB, Alan S, Donald M, et al. Heart disease and stroke statistics: 2011 update—a report from the American Heart Association. *Circulation.* 2011;123:e18-e209.
3.    Morrison C, Bare L, Chambless L, Ellis S, et al. Prediction of coronary heart disease risk using

a genetic risk score: the atherosclerosis risk in communities study. *Am J Epidemiol.* 2007;166:28-35.

4.   Position of the American Dietetic Association. The role of dietetics professionals in health promotion and disease prevention. *J Am Diet Assoc.* 2002;102(11):1680-1687.

5.   Centers for Disease Control and Prevention. *Healthy Aging: Preserving Function and Improving Quality of Life Among Older Americans at a Glance.* 2008. http://www.cdc.gov/. Accessed March 17, 2017.

6.   US Dept of Health and Human Services. *Healthy People 2010 Understanding and Improving Health* (2nd ed.). Washington, DC: US Dept of Health and Human Services; 2000.

7.   Vatten LL. Adiposity and physical activity as predictors of cardiovascular mortality. *Eur J Cardiovasc Prev Rehab.* 2006;13(6):909-915.

8.   Thom T, Haase N, Rosamond W, Howard VJ. Heart disease and stroke statistics: 2006 update—a report from the American Heart Association Statistics Committee and Stroke Statistics Subcommittee. AHA statistical update. *Circulation.* http://www.circulationaha.org. Accessed March 17, 2017.

9.   American Heart and Stroke Association. Heart disease and stroke statistics   at a  glance. https://www.heart.org/idc/groups/ahamah-public/@wcm/@sop/@smd/documents/downloadable/ucm_470704.pdf. Accessed March 17, 2017.

10.   Council NR. *Diet and Health Implications for Reducing Chronic Disease Risk.* Washington, DC: National Academies Press; 1989:12.

11.   Keavney B. Genetic epidemiological studies of coronary heart disease [Review]. *Int J Epidemiol.* 2002;31:1730-1738.

12.   Simon J, Rosolova H. Family history and independent risk factors for coronary heart disease: it is time to be practical. *Eur Heart J.* 2002;23(21):1637-1638.

13.   Radomyska BB. [Screening programme for hyperlipidemia in children and adolescents: prophylactic aspects of atherosclerosis]. *Med Wieku Rozwoj.* 2001;5(1):27-34.

14.   Wardlaw G, Kessel M. *Perspectives in Nutrition.* 10th ed. New York, NY: McGraw Hill; 2016.

15.   Hubert H, Eaker E, Garrison R, Castelli W. Life-style correlates of risk factor change in young adults: an eight-year study of coronary heart disease risk factors in the Framingham offspring. *Am J Epidemiol.* 2008;125(5):812-831.

16.   Ferdinand KC. The importance of aggressive lipid management in patients at risk: evidence from recent clinical trials. *Clin Cardiol.* 2004;27:12-15.

17.   Meagher EA. Addressing cardiovascular disease in women: focus on dyslipidemia. *J Am Board Fam Pract.* 2004;17:424-437.

18.   Varady KA, Jones PJ. Combination diet and exercise interventions for the treatment of dyslipidemia: an effective preliminary strategy to lower cholesterol levels. *J Nutr.* 2005;135(8):1829-1835.

19.   Atilla KK. Prehypertension and risk of cardiovascular disease. *Expert Rev of Cardiovasc Ther.* 2006;4(1):111-117.

20.   Wolf-Maier K, Cooper RS, Banegas JR, Giampaoli S, et al. Hypertension more prevalent in Europe than U.S. and Canada. *JAMA.* 2003;289(18):2363-2369.

21.   Clark RR. Interactive but not direct effects of perceived racism and trait anger predict resting systolic and diastolic blood pressure in black adolescents. *Health Psychol.* 2006;25(5):580-585.

22.   Edward JR. The Seventh Report of the Joint National Committee on Prevention, Detection, Evaluation, and Treatment of High Blood Pressure *JAMA.* 2003;289:2560-2572.

23.   Magill MK, Gunning K, Saffel SS, Gay C. New developments in the management of hupertension. *Am Fam Physician.* 2003;68:853-858.

24.   Burt VL. Prevalence of hypertension in the US adult population: results from the Third National Health and Nutrition Examination Survey 1988-91. *Hypertension.* 1995;25:305-313.

25.   National Center for Health Statistics. *Health: United States—2003 With Chartbook on Trends in the Health of Americans.* Hyattsville, MD: Centers for Disease Control and Prevention; 2006.

26.   Jones D, Hall J. Seventh report of the Joint National Committeee on Prevention, Detection, Evaluation and Treatment of High Blood Pressure and evidence from new hypertension trials. *Hypertension.* 2004;43(1):1-3.

27.   National Center for Health Statistics. *Health: United States 2007—With Chartbook on Trends in the Health of Americans.* Hyattsville, MD: National Center for Health Statistics; 2006. http://www.cdc.gov/nchs/hus.htm. Accessed March 8, 2011.

28.   Miller ER, Erlinger TP, Appel LJ. The effects of macronutrients on blood pressure and lipids: an overview of the DASH and OmniHeart trials. *Curr Atheroscler Rep.* 2006;8(6):460-465.

29.   US Dept of Health and Human Services, National Institutes of Health, National Heart, Lung, and Blood Institute. The seventh report of the Joint National Committee on Prevention, Detection, Evaluation, and Treatment of High Blood Pressure. http://www.nhlbi.nih.gov/. Accessed March 17, 2017.

30. Centers for Disease Control and Prevention, US Dept of Health and Human Services. Trends in cholesterol screening and awarness of high blood cholesterol: United States—1991-2003. *Morb Mortal Wkly Rep MMWR.* 2005;54(35):865-870.

31. Finkelstein EE, Troped PJ, Will JC, Palombo R. Cost-effectiveness of a cardiovascular disease risk reduction program aimed at financially vulnerable women: the Massachusetts WISEWOMAN project. *J Womens Health Gend Based Med.* 2002;11(6):519-526.

32. American Heart Association. About cholesterol. http://www.americanheart.org/. Accessed March 17, 2017.

33. Allman-Farinelli MA, Gomes K, Favaloro EJ, Petocz P. A diet rich in high-oleic-acid sunflower oil favorably alters low-density lipoprotein cholesterol, triglycerides, and factor VII coagulant activity. *J Am Diet Assoc.* 2005;105(7):1071-1079.

34. Oh RR. The fish in secondary prevention of heart disease (FISH) survey: primary care physicians and omega 3 fatty acid prescribing behaviors. *J Am Board of Fam Med.* 2006;19(5):459-467.

35. Kris-Etherton PM, Hecker KD, Bonanome A. Bioactive compounds in foods: their role in the prevention of cardiovascular disease and cancer. *Am J Med.* 2002;113(suppl 9B):71s-88s.

36. Johnson RK, Lawrence JA, Brands M, Howard BV, et al. Dietary sugars intake and cardiovascular health: a scientific statement from the American Heart Assoc. *Circulation.* 2009;120(11):1011-1020.

37. Vijaimohan K, Jainu M, Sabitha K, Subramaniyam S, et al. Beneficial effects of alpha linolenic acid rich flaxseed oil on growth performance and hepatic cholesterol metabolism in high fat diet fed rats. *Life Sci.* 2006;79(5):448-454.

38. Denke MM. Dietary fats, fatty acids, and their effects on lipoproteins. *Curr Atheroscler Rep.* 2006;8(6):466-471.

39. Bourre JJ. An important source of omega-3 fatty acids, vitamins D and E, carotenoids, iodine and selenium: a new natural multi-enriched egg. *J Nutr Health Aging.* 2006;10(5):371-376.

40. Appel LL. Effects of protein, monounsaturated fat, and carbohydrate intake on blood pressure and serum lipids: results of the OmniHeart randomized trial. *JAMA.* 2005;294(19):2455-2464.

41. Herron KL, Vega-Lopez S, Conde K. Pre-menopausal women, classified as hypo- or hyper-responders, do not alter their LDL/HDL Ratio following a high dietary cholesterol challenge. *J Am Coll Nutr.* 2002;21(3):250-258.

42. Haub MM. Beef and soy-based food supplements differentially affect serum lipoprotein-lipid profiles because of changes in carbohydrate intake and novel. *Metab Clin Exp.* 2005;54(6):769-774.

43. Pedersen JJ. Palm oil versus hydrogenated soybean oil: effects on serum lipids and plasma haemostatic variables. *Asia Pacific J Clin Nutr.* 2005;14(4):348-357.

44. Weggemans R, Zock PL, Ordovas J, Pedro-Botet J, et al. Apoprotein E genotype and the response of serum cholesterol to dietary fat, cholesterol and cafesto. *Atherosclerosis* 2001;154(3):547-555.

45. Nagyova AA. Effects of dietary extra virgin olive oil on serum lipid resistance to oxidation and fatty acid composition in elderly lipidemic patients. *Bratisl Lék Listy.* 2003;104(7-8):218-221.

46. Reynolds KK. A meta-analysis of the effect of soy protein supplementation on serum lipids. *Am J Cardiol.* 2006;98(5):633-640.

47. Smulyan H. Nitrates, arterial function, wave reflections and coronary heart disease. *Adv Cardiol.* 2007;44:302-314.

48. Herrmann WW. Significance of hyperhomocysteinemia. *Clin Lab.* 2006;52(7-8):367-374.

49. Clarke RR. Effects of B-vitamins on plasma homocysteine concentrations and on risk of cardiovascular disease and dementia. *Curr Opin Clin Nutr Metab Care.* 2007;10(1):32-39.

50. Genovefa D, Kolovou D, Salpea KK. Alcohol use, vascular disease, and lipid-lowering drugs. *J Pharmacol Exp Therapeut.* 2006;318(1):1-7.

51. Oak MH. Antiangiogenic properties of natural polyphenols from red wine and green tea. *J Nutr Biochem.* 2005;16(1):1-8.

52. Booth FW. Waging war on modern chronic diseases: primary prevention through exercise biology. *J Appl Physiol.* 2000;88(2):774-787.

53. Tattelman E. Health effects of garlic. *Am Fam Physician.* 2005;72(1):103-106.

54. Reeves MJ, Rafferty AP. Healthy lifestyle characteristics among adults in the United States 2000. *Arch Intern Med.* 2005;165(8):854-857.

55. National Cholesterol Education Program. Executive summary of the third report of the National Cholesterol Education Program (NCEP) Expert Panel on Detection, Evaluation and Treatment of High Blood Cholesterol in Adults (Adult Treatment Panel II). *JAMA.* 2001;285(19):2486-2498.

56. Van Horn L. A summary of the science supporting the new national cholesterol education program dietary recommendations: what dietitians should know. *J Am Diet Assoc.* 2001;101(10):1148-1154.

57. Ogden CL, Carroll MD, Curtin LR, Lamb MM, et al. Prevalence of high body mass index in U.S.

children and adolescents 2007-2008. *JAMA.* 2010;303(3):242-249.

58. Ogden CL, Carrol MD, Curtin LR, McDowell MA, et al. Prevalence of overweight and obesity in the United States, 1999-2004. *JAMA.* 2006;295(13):1549-1555.

59. US Dept of Health and Human Services. *The Surgeon General's Call to Action to Prevent and Decrease Overweight and Obesity.* 2001. https://www.ncbi.nlm.nih.gov/books/NBK44206/. Accessed March 15, 2017.

60. Mokdad A, Ford E, Bowman B. Prevalence of obesity, diabetes, and obesity-related health risk factors. *JAMA.* 2003;289:187-193.

61. Fontaine K, Redden D, Wang C, Westfall A, et al. Years of life lost due to obesity. *JAMA.* 2003;289:187-193.

62. Peters A, Barendregt J, Willenkens F, Mackenbach J, et al. Obesity in adulthood and its consequences for life expectancy: a life-table analysis. *Ann Intern Med.* 2003;138(1):24-32.

63. Wang G, Dietz WH. Economic burden of obesity in youths aged 6 to 17 years: 1979–1999. *Pediatrics.* 2002;109(5):e81-e86.

64. Inscl PT, Ross D, McMahon K, Bernstein M. *Nutrition: 2002 Update.* 5th ed. Sudbury, MA: Jones & Bartlett; 2014.

65. Nation Center for Health Statistics. New CDC study finds no increase in obesity among adults but levels still high. https://www.extension.umd.edu/healthyliving/adult-nutrition/new-cdc-study-finds-no-increase-obesity-among-adults-levels-still-high. Accessed March 17, 2017.

66. Mokdad AH, Ford ES, Bowman BA. The continuing increase of diabetes in the US. *Diabetes Care.* 2001;24(8):412-417.

67. Wang Y, Beydoun M. The obesity epidemic in the United States gender, age, socioeconomic, racial/ethnic, and geographic characteristics: a systematic review and meta-regression analysis. *Epidemiol Rev.* 2007;29(1):6-28.

68. Moreno LA, Blay MG, Rodríguez G, Blay VA, et al. A screening performances of the International Obesity Task Force body mass index cut-off values in adolescents. *J Am Coll Nutr.* 2006;25(5): 403-408.

69. Centers for Disease Control and Prevention. Quick facts: economic and health burden of chronic disease. http://www.cdc.gov/. Accessed March 17, 2017.

70. Finkelstein EA, Fiebelkorn IC, Wang G. State-level estimates of annual medical expenditures attributable to obesity. *Obes Res.* 2004;12(1): 18-24.

71. Centers for Disease Control and Prevention. Study estimates medical cost of obesity may be as high as $147 billion annually new community recommendations show ways to reduce burden. http://www.cdc.gov/. Accessed March 17, 2017.

72. Forrest K, Stuhldreher W. Patterns and correlates of body image dissatisfaction and distortion among college students. *Am J Health Stud.* 2007;22(1): 18-25.

73. Sjoberg RL, Nilsson KW, Leppert J. Obesity, shame, and depression in schoolaged children: a population-based study. *Pediatrics.* 2005;116(3):e389-e392.

74. O'Dea JA, Abraham S. Knowledge, beliefs, attitudes, and behaviors related to weight control, eating disorders, and body image in Australian trainee home economics and physical education teachers. *J Nutr Educ.* 2001;33(6):332-340.

75. Centers for Disease Control and Prevention. Overweight and obesity: an overview. http://www.cdc.gov/. Accessed March 17, 2017.

76. Wright C, Parker L, Lamont D, Craft A. Implications of childhood obesity for adult health: findings from thousand families cohort study. *BMJ.* 2001;323(7324):1280-1284.

77. Barsh GS, Faroogi S, O'Rahilly S. Genetics of body-weight regulation. *Nature.* 2000;404(6778):644-651.

78. Wellman N, Friedberg B. Causes and consequences of adult obesity: health, social and economic impacts in the United States. *Asia Pacific J Clin Nutr.* 2002;11(suppl 8):S705-S709.

79. Swinburn B, Egger G, Raza F. Dissecting obesogenic environments: the development and application of a framework for identifying and prioritizing environmental interventions for obesity. *Prev Med.* 1999;29(6 Pt 1):563-570.

80. Chang CJ, Wu C, Yao WJ, Yang YC, et al. Relationships of age, menopause and central obesity on cardiovascular disease risk factors in Chinese women. *Int J Obes.* 2000;24(12):1699-1704.

81. Adler G, Dipp S. Cushing syndrome. WebMed. http://www.emedicine.com/med/topic485.htm. Accessed March 10, 2016.

82. Wyatt SB, Winters KP, Dubbert PM, Dubbert, P. Overweight and obesity: prevalence consequences and causes of a growing public health problem. *Am J Med Sci.* 2006;331(4):166-174.

83. Finkelstein E, Ruhm CJ, Kosa KM. Economic causes and consequences of obesity. *Ann Rev Public Health.* 2005;26:239-257.

84. US Dept of Agriculture, Cooperative State Research, Education, and Extension Service. Obesity and healthy weight: obesity white paper. http://www.usda.gov/. Accessed March 17, 2017.

85. McAuley KK. Long-term effects of popular dietary approaches on weight loss and features of insulin resistance. *Int J Obes*. 2006;30(2):342-349.

86. Appel LJ. Lifestyle modification: is it achievable and durable? The argument for. *J Clin Hypertens*. 2004;6(10):578-581.

87. Linde JA, Erickson DJ, Jeffery RW, Pronk NP, et al. The relationship between prevalence and duration of weight loss strategies and weight loss among overweight managed care organization members enrolled in a weight loss trial. *Int J Behav Nutr Phys Act*. 2006;17:3.

88. Klohe-Lehman DD. Nutrition knowledge is associated with greater weight loss in obese and overweight low-income mothers. *J Am Diet Assoc*. 2006;106(1):65-75.

89. Greenwald A. Current nutritional treatments of obesity. *Adv Psychosom Med*. 2006;27:24-41.

90. Melin I. Conservative treatment of obesity in an academic obesity unit: long-term outcome and drop-out. *Eat Weight Disord*. 2006;11(1):22-30.

91. Bish CC. Health-related quality of life and weight loss among overweight and obese U.S. adults, 2001 to 2002. *Obesity*. 2006;14(11):2042-2053.

92. Suastika KK. Update in the management of obesity. *Acta Med Indones*. 2006;38(4):231-237.

93. Germann JN, Kirschenbaum DS, Rich BH. Child and parental self-monitoring as determinants of success in the treatment of morbid obesity in low-income minority children. *J Pediatr Psychol*. 2007;32(1):111-121.

94. Fitzgibbon L, Stolley MR, Ganschow P. Results of a faith-based weight loss intervention for black women. *J Natl Med Assoc*. 2005;97(10):1393-1402

95. Thin Within. http://www.thinwithin.org/. Accessed March 17, 2017.

96. Reicks M, Mills J, Henry H. Qualitative study of spirituality in weight loss program: contribution to self-efficacy and locus of control. *J Nutr Educ Behav*. 2004;36(1):13-19.

97. National Institute of Health. Hearts N' Parks Program continues to help participants of all ages adopt Hearty-Healthy behaviors. http://www.nhlbi.nih.gov/. Accessed March 17, 2017.

98. National Institute of Health; National Heart, Lung, and Blood Institute. Reducing nationalwide obesity starts in neighborhoods: Hearts N' Parks Progrtam brings science, skills to 50 communities. https://www.nhlbi.nih.gov/news/press-releases/2003/reducing-nationwide-obesity-stars-in-neighborhoods. Accessed March 17, 2017.

99. Trust for Americans Health. F as in fat: how obesity policies are failing in America. 2006. http://healthyamericans.org/. Accessed March 11, 2016.

100. Segal L. New report finds 41 states have obesity levels over 20 percent, state and federal obesity policies are failing. http://healthyamericans.org/. Accessed March 11, 2016.

101. Orr R, Thompson P, McCullum C. Impact position paper. *SNE J Nutr Educ Behav*. 2004;36(4):169-171.

102. World Heart Federation. A statement on obesity from the World Heart Federation. 2004. http://www.worldheart.org/. Accessed March 17, 2017.

103. Centers for Disease Control and Prevention. The burden of obesity in Washington. http://www.cdc.gov/obesity. Accessed March 17, 2017.

104. Reisfield GG. Survival in cancer patients undergoing in-hospital cardiopulmonary resuscitation: a meta-analysis. *Resuscitation*. 2006;71(2):152-160.

105. Spurlock WW. Cancer fatalism and breast cancer screening in African American women. *ABNF J*. 2006;17(1):38-43.

106. Mahan KL, Escott-Stump S. *Krause's Food, Nutrition, and Diet Therapy*. 11th ed. St. Louis, MO: Mosby; 2012.

107. Kushi LH, Byers T. American Cancer Society guidelines on nutrition and physical activity for cancer. *CA Cancer J Clin* 2006;56:254-281.

108. Rodriguez C, Freedland SJ, Deka A, Jacobs EJ, et al. Body mass index, weight change, and risk of prostate cancer in the Cancer Prevention Study II Nutrition Cohort. *Cancer Epidemiol Biomarkers Prev*. 2007;16(1):63-69.

109. Hiom SS. Public awareness regarding UV risks and vitamin D: the challenges for UK skin cancer prevention campaigns. *Progr Biophys Mol Biol*. 2006;92(1):161-166.

110. Calle EE, Rodriguez C, Walker-Thurmond K, Michael J. Overweight, obesity, and mortality from cancer in a prospectively studied cohort of U.S. adults. *N Engl J Med*. 2003;348(17):1625-1638.

111. Hines SL, Jorn H, Thompson KM. Breast cancer survivors and vitamin D: a review. *Nutrition* 2010;26(3):255-262.

112. Huncharek M, Muscat J. Colorectal cancer risk and dietary intake of calcium, vitamin D, and dairy products: a meta-analysis of 26,335 cases from 60 observational studies. *Nutr Cancer*. 2009;61(1):47-69.

113. Cedric FG, Edward D, Sharif B, Frank C. Vitamin D for cancer prevention: global perspective. *Ann Epidemiol*. 2009;19(7):468-483.

114. Navarro SS. Risk factors for thyroid cancer: a prospective cohort study. *Int J Cancer*. 2005;116(3):433-438.

115. Park Y, Hunter DJ, Spiegelman D, Bergkvist L. Dietary fiber intake and risk of colorectal cancer: a pooled analysis of prospective cohort studies. *JAMA*. 2005;294(22):2849-2857.

116. Schatzkin A, Lanza E, Corie D, Lance P, et al. Lack of effect of a lowfat, high-fiber diet on the recurrence of colorectal adenomas. *N Engl J Med*. 2000;342(16):1149-1155.

117. Alberts DS, Martinez ME, Roe DJ. Lack of effect of a high-fiber cereal supplement on the recurrence of colorectal adenomas. *N Engl J Med*. 2000;342(16):1156-1162.

118. Shin A, Li H, Shu XO, Yang G, et al. Dietary intake of calcium, fiber and other micronutrients in relation to colorectal cancer risk: results from the Shanghai Women's Health Study. *Int J Cancer*. 2006;119(12):2938-2942.

119. Boffetta P, Pagona L, Naska A, Benetou V. Fruit and vegetable intake and overall cancer risk in the European Prospective Investigation into Cancer and Nutrition (EPIC). *JNCI*. 2010;102(8): 529-537.

120. Park SY, Clooney RV, Wilkens LR, Murphy SP, et al. Plasma 25-hydroxyvitamin D and prostate cancer risk: the multiethnic cohort. *Eur Cancer*. 2010;46(5):932-936

121. American Dietetic Association and Dietitians of Canada. Position of the American Dietetic Association and Dietitians of Canada: vegetarian diets. *J Am Diet Assoc*. 2003;103(6):748-765.

122. Adhami VM, Ahmad N, Mukhtar H. Molecular targets for green tea in prostate cancer prevention. *J. Nutr*. 2003;133(7 suppl):2417S-2424S.

123. Blot WJ, Li JY, Taylor PR, Guo W, et al. Nutrition intervention trials in Linxian, China: supplementation with specific vitamin/mineral combinations, cancer incidence, and disease-specific mortality in the general population. *J Natl Cancer Inst*. 1993;83:1483–1492.

124. Wang S. Tomato and soy polyphenols reduce insulin-like growth factor-I-stimulated rat prostate cancer cell proliferation and apoptotic resistance in vitro via inhibition of intracellular signaling pathways involving tyrosine kinase. *J Nutr*. 2003;133(7):2367-2376.

125. Kanadaswami C, Lee LT, Hwang JJ, Huang YT. The antitumor activities of flavonoids. *In Vivo*. 2005;19(5):895-909.

126. World Cancer Research Fund, American Institute for Cancer Research. *Food, Nutrition and the Prevention of Cancer: A Global Perspective*. Washington, DC: World Cancer Research Fund, American Institute for Cancer Research; 1997.

127. Ahmed FE. Effect of diet, life style, and other environmental chemopreventive factors on colorectal cancer development, and assessment of the risks. *J Environ Sci Health C Environ Carcinog Ecotoxicol Rev*. 2004;22(2):91-147.

128. US Dept of Health and Human Services. *Dietary Guidelines for Americans*. 6th ed. Washington, DC: US Government Printing Office; 2005.

129. US Dept of Agriculture and US Dept of Health Human Services. *Dietary Guidelines for Americans*. Washington, DC: US Government Printing Office; 2000:232.

130. Lichtenstein AH, Appel LJ, Brands M, Carnethon M, et al. Diet and lifestyle recommendations revision 2006: a scientific statement from the American Heart Association Nutrition Committee. *Circulation* 2006;114:82-96.

131. Centers for Disease Control and Prevention. *5 A Day Almost Everyone Needs to Eat More Fruits and Vegetables*. http://www.cdc.gov/. Accessed March 17, 2017.

132. Le Marchand L, Hankin JH, Wilkens LR. Dietary fiber and colorectal cancer risk. *Epdemiology*. 1997;8(6):658-665.

133. US Dept of Agriculture, Cooperative State Research, Education, and Extension Service. Pizza: the cancer fighting food. http://www.csrees.usda.gov/. Accessed March 17, 2017.

134. Borek C. Dietary antioxidants and human cancer. *Integr Cancer Ther*. 2004;3(4):333-341.

135. Driskell JA, Pohlman DH, Naslund MM. Value of an educational program on osteoporosis. *J Extn*. 2003;41(5).

136. Araujo B, Travison T, Harris S, Holick M, et al. Race/ethnic differences in bone mineral density in men. *Osteo Inter*. 2007;18(7):943-953.

137. Looker A. Prevalence of low femoral bone density in older U.S. adults from NHANES III. *J Bone Miner Res*. 1997;12(11):1761-1768.

138. Steelman J, Zeitler P. Osteoporosis in pediatrics. *Pediatr Rev*. 2001;22:56-65.

139. Magaña JJ, Gómez R, Cisneros B, Casas L, et al. Association of the CT gene (CA) polymorphism with BMD in osteoporotic Mexican women. *Clin Genet*. 2006;70(5):402-408.

140. Morita A. Genetic factors of osteoporosis and fracture and the application of genetic information to the preventive medicine. *Clin Calcium*. 2005;15(8):1364-1371.

141. Centers for Disease Control and Prevention. Hip fractures among older adults. http://www.cdc.gov/. Accessed March 11, 2016.

142. Borges JLC, Brandão CMA. Low bone mass in children and adolescents. *Arq Bras Endocrinol Metabol*. 2006;50(4):775-782.

143. Brown J. Proposals for prevention and management of steroid-induced osteoporosis in children and adolescents. *J Paediatr Child Health*. 2005;41(11): 553-557.

144. Pongchaiyakul C, Nguyen TV, Kosulwat V, Rojroongwasinkul N. Effects of physical activity and dietary calcium intake on bone mineral density and osteoporosis risk in a rural Thai population. *Osteoporos Int.* 2004;15(10):807-813.

145. Faibish D, Ott SM, Boskey AL. Mineral changes in osteoporosis: a review. *Clin Orthop Relat Res* 2006;443:28-38.

146. Nicklas T. Calcium intake trends and health consequences from childhood through adulthood. *J Am Coll Nutr.* 2003;22(5):340-356.

147. Nesby-O'Dell S, Scanlon K, Cogswell M, Gillespie C, et al. Hypovitaminosis D prevalence and determinants among African American and white women of reproductive age: third National Health and Nutrition Examination Survey, 1988–1994. *Am J Clin Nutr.* 2002;76(1):187-192.

148. Blum M, Harris SS, Must A. Weight and body mass index at menarche are associated with premenopausal bone mass. *Osteoporosis Int.* 2001;12:588-591.

149. Elgan C, Fridlund B. Bone mineral density in relation to body mass index among young women: a prospective cohort study. *Int J Nurs Stud.* 2006;43(6):663-672.

150. Rideout CC. Self-reported lifetime physical activity and areal bone mineral density in healthy postmenopausal women: the importance of teenage activity. *Calcif Tissue Int.* 2006;79(4):214-222.

151. Lewiecki EE. Redefining osteoporosis treatment: who to treat and how long to treat. *Arq Bras Endocrinol Metabol.* 2006;50(4):694-704.

152. Liu SL, Lebrun CM. Effect of oral contraceptives and hormone replacement therapy on bone mineral density in premenopausal and perimenopausal women: a systematic review. *Br J Sports Med.* 2006;40:11-24.

153. Golden H, Lanzkowski N, Schebendach L, Mard J, et al. Hormone replacement therapy (hRT) and bone mineral density in anorexia nervosa a 3-year prospective observational study. *J Pediatr Adolesc Gynecol.* 2002;15(3):135-143.

154. Klibanski A, Biller BM, Schoenfeld DA, Herzog DB, et al. The effects of estrogen administration on trabecular bone loss in young women with anorexia nervosa. *J Clin Endocrinol Metab.* 1995;80(3):898-904.

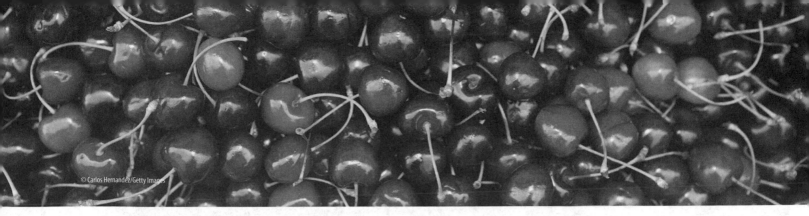
© Carlos Hernández/Getty Images

# CHAPTER 11

# Promoting Health and Preventing Disease in Older Persons

## CHAPTER OUTLINE

- Introduction
- Nutrition, Longevity, and Demographics of Older Persons
- Leading Causes of Death and Disability in Older Persons
- Theories of Aging
- Lifestyle and Socioeconomic Factors That May Influence the Aging Process
- Physiological Changes That Can Affect Nutritional Status
- Nutrition Screening for Older Persons
- Anorexia in the Elderly
- Water Requirements
- Alzheimer's Disease
- Multivitamin and Mineral Supplements
- Nutrition Assessment
- Nutrition Services That Promote Independent Living
- Home Healthcare Services

## LEARNING OBJECTIVES

- Define old age and discuss the demographic shift of the U.S. population.
- Identify the normal physiological changes of aging that can affect nutritional status.
- Discuss the lifestyle and socioeconomic factors that may influence the aging process.
- Describe the Nutrition Screening Initiative.
- List the government nutrition programs for older persons.

# ▶ Introduction

Aging is a biological, psychological, and social process that most individuals will experience. Although the biological and physical changes that occur during the aging process are unavoidable, the rate and manner at which these changes occur vary among individuals. It is encouraging to know that the older population in the United States is increasing. This is due to advances in modern medicine and technology, which contributed to the increase in longevity. Similarly, several characteristics of older persons influence their health and well-being. Some of the characteristics of aging discussed in this chapter include nutrition, lifestyle, and socioeconomic factors.

# ▶ Nutrition, Longevity, and Demographics of Older Persons

The average **life expectancy** at birth has increased from 47 years in 1900 to 78.8 years in 2014. In 2014, the life expectancy in the United States was 76.5 years for Caucasian American men and 72 years for African American men. The same report also showed that the life expectancy for Caucasian American women was 81.1 years and for African American women was 78.1 years. Life expectancy for Hispanic men was 79.2 and 84 for the women.[1] For all Americans, most deaths occur after age 65.[2] The 65 years and older age group is expected to constitute an increasingly larger share of the U.S. population.

The maximum age to which humans can live (life span) is about 100 to 120 years,[1] but most people do not live this long. The goal to increase life expectancy and the number of years of healthy life is known as compression of morbidity. **Compression of morbidity** can be achieved by slowing the biological changes that accrue over time and delaying the diseases of aging enough to reach the limits of life span before any symptoms emerge.[1-4] **FIGURE 11-1** presents life expectancy by race and sex. From 2000 to 2007, life expectancy at age 65 increased by 6 percent. In 2015, the population 65 years or older was 46 million, an increase of 6.4 million from 2009.[4]

Nutrition plays an important role in **successful aging**. Research suggests that a diet based on rice, fish, vegetable proteins, fruits, vegetables, and some meat contributes to **longevity**.

Adequate food intake is necessary for successful aging. The consequence of inadequate food intake is malnutrition, which can lead to nutrition-related health conditions (osteoporosis, anemia, cancer, etc.), increased disability, decreased resistance to infection,

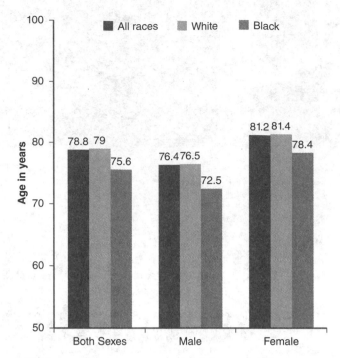

**FIGURE 11-1** Life expectancy at birth, by race and sex: United States, 2014.

Reproduced from: Center for Disease Control and Prevention. National Center for Health Statistics, National Vital Statistics System. Available at: https://www.cdc.gov/nchs/data/hus/2015/fig18.pdf. Accessed September 06, 2016.

and extended hospital stays among elderly persons.[5,6] Therefore, nutrition is one important component of ensuring that the added years at the end of the lifecycle are healthful and productive. However, almost 9 percent of older adults live below poverty level. The poorest of the older adults have inadequate income for their food and nutrition requirements. The majority of their income is spent on housing, transportation, medication, and other essential commodities.[7] The decrease in their earnings has the potential of making them vulnerable to malnutrition. Research shows that those experiencing food insecurity have lower intakes of micronutrients and energy, more health problems, and functional limitations.[7] In addition, almost 9 percent of all older Americans are food insecure and 3.9 percent are very low food secure.[8] This indicates that approximately 14 million older adults are at risk for hunger and about 24 million have hunger due to financial constraints. The most difficult aspect of this situation is that older adults with incomes above 130 percent of poverty guidelines are ineligible for some of the food and nutrition assistance programs.[9]

According to a study using the Healthy Eating Index-2005 (HEI-2005), 83 percent of older adults do not consume a good-quality diet, and those who are poor have lower scores than do higher income older adults.[8] The following are the segments of older adults most at risk for hunger[10,11,12]:

- 60 years or older
- Living at or below poverty level
- High school dropouts
- African Americans
- Hispanic Americans
- Divorced or separated
- Living with a grandchild
- Renters
- Living alone
- Living in low-quality housing

Dietetics professionals are distinctly qualified to provide a wide variety of appropriate, culturally sensitive nutrition programs for older persons. In the United States, nutrition programs such as the Elderly Nutrition Program, Meals on Wheels, Child and Adult Care Food Program, Senior Farmers Market Nutrition Program, soup kitchens, food pantries, subsidize meals or others discussed later in this chapter provide food assistance to older persons that may help prevent malnutrition. You will find an overview of some of these programs in Chapter 4. In addition, the U.S. Department of Agriculture (USDA) Food and Nutrition Service (FNS) developed an intervention called Eat Smart, Live Strong to help program providers and communities improve the health of an increasing number of low-income older adults 60 to 74 years old. The intervention is based on the Dietary Guidelines for Americans and MyPlate. The two main goals of Eat Smart, Live Strong are to increase fruit and vegetable consumption to 3 ½-cup servings per day and participate in at least 30 minutes of physical activity most days of the week. Visit http://www.choosemyplate.gov for more information.

As the aged population grows larger, there is an increased awareness that successful aging is not trying to stay young, but rather trying to discover the rewards of a life fully lived to the end.[11] Although many dimensions of successful aging have been recognized, the four features of successful aging identified by Fisher[13] are outlined here:

1. Interactions with others
2. Autonomy and sense of purpose
3. Personal growth
4. Self-acceptance

A positive attitude is the first step toward enhancing quality of life, whether it is an individual's attitude about his or her own aging or the attitude toward older persons in the community. It has been reported that fear and negative attitudes are prevalent among many persons nearing retirement age, mainly among men.[14] This fear of growing old may affect an individual's ability to experience an enhanced quality of life at old age. In addition, many retirement education campaigns focus on financial security

without considering nutrition, fitness, fun, volunteerism, community resources, caregiving, or living environments.

Kerschner[15] developed a philosophy of productive aging in the late 1980s, which viewed older adults as representing the following[13,16]:

- An opportunity rather than a crisis
- A solution rather than a problem
- An asset rather than a burden
- A resource rather than a drain on resources
- A group that can make social, economic, and cultural contributions rather than one that merely constitutes an expanding portion of the population

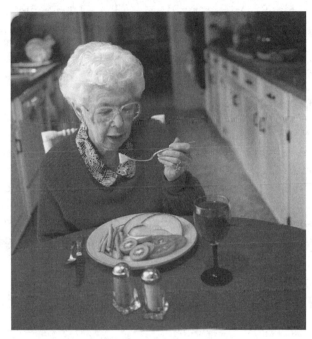

In older persons, appetite is a decisive factor of food intake.
© Photodisc

## ▶ Leading Causes of Death and Disability in Older Persons

Studies show that when older people are asked how they feel about their health, only 10 percent say their health is fair or poor, whereas 90 percent consider their health to be good, very good, or excellent.[13,15] Chronic health conditions did not change their perception about how they felt about their health. In contrast to older adults' perceptions, public health professionals objectively monitor health by measuring leading causes of death (mortality) and leading diagnoses of health conditions (morbidity). Heart disease and cancer are the leading causes of death for all persons age 65 or older and in all ethnic groups. Other chronic health conditions, such as cerebrovascular diseases (stroke) and chronic lower respiratory tract diseases also affect older persons significantly.[17,18] The following are the top causes of death for adults over the age of 65 starting with the leading cause[4]:

- Heart disease
- Cancer
- Chronic obstructive pulmonary disease (COPD)
- Cerebrovascular disease (stroke)
- Alzheimer's disease
- Diabetes
- Pneumonia and influenza
- Accidents

**FIGURE 11-2** presents the age-adjusted death rates by race and Hispanic origin, and **FIGURE 11-3** presents the percentage distribution of five leading causes of death by age group.

## National Goals: Healthy People 2010 and 2020

The primary goal of the U.S. Department of Health and Human Services' (DHHS's) Healthy People 2010 initiative is to help individuals of all ages increase life expectancy and improve their quality of life. The 2020 goal is to improve the health, function, and quality of life of older adults. Therefore, Healthy People 2010 and 2020 include many objectives related to aging. A few examples of the objectives set to promote healthy lifestyles for older adults include access to quality healthcare services; reduction of rates of chronic diseases such as arthritis, cancer, diabetes, kidney disease, and osteoporosis; reduction in hospitalization rates for heart disease and stroke; increased immunizations for influenza and pneumococcal disease; and increased physical activity and fitness for older adults; increase the proportion of registered dietitians with geriatric certification; and reduce the proportion of adults who engage in no leisure-time physical activity.[17,19] Little progress has been made toward these objectives, however. Tables 10-1 and 10-2 in Chapter 10 provide information on the Healthy People 2010 and 2020 progress report.

## ▶ Theories of Aging

Aging is a process that involves the entire body. Individuals age at different rates, but the processes that control the rate at which people age, and how aging affects the development of chronic diseases, are not well understood.[20,21] Although the degenerative changes that come with aging are poorly understood, several theories have been proposed to explain the aging process. One theory is that the aging process depends on genetic, environmental, and lifestyle factors.[21] This

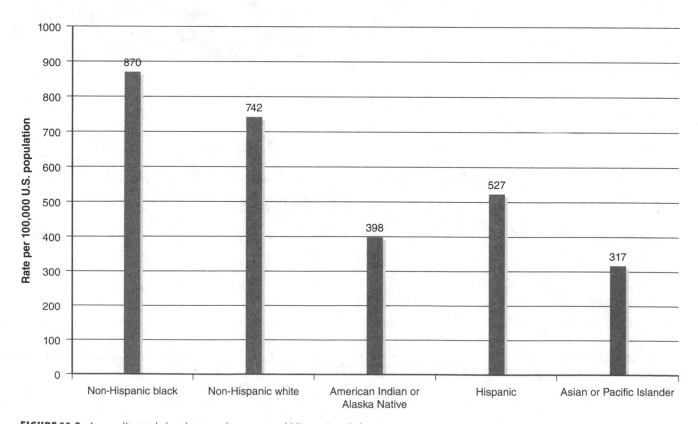

**FIGURE 11-2** Age-adjusted death rates, by race and Hispanic origin.

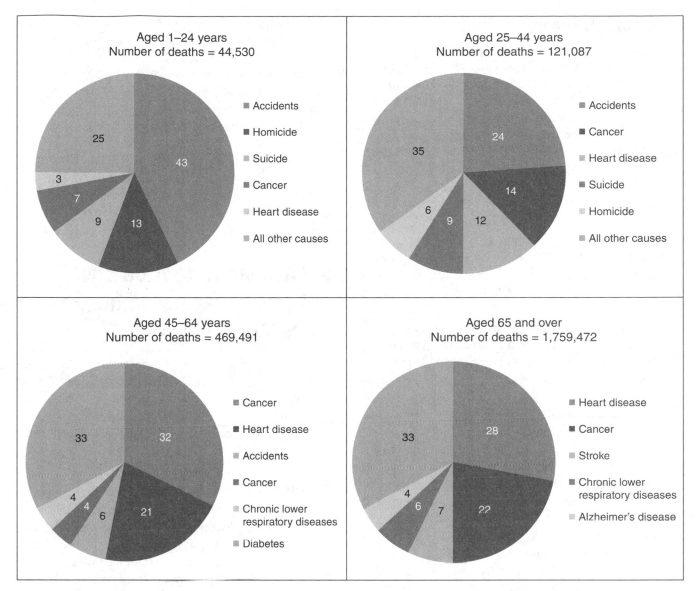

**FIGURE 11-3** Percent distribution of five leading causes of death, by age group: preliminary, 2007.

Reproduced from: Center for Disease Control and Prevention. National Center for Health Statistics, National Vital Statistics System. FastStats. Available at http://www.cdc.gov/nchs/fastats/. Accessed March 29, 2011.

theory recognizes that every individual has a unique genetic makeup and environment, which interact with each other to control the aging process. Another theory of aging is the free radical theory. **Free radicals** are short-lived, very reactive chemicals often derived from oxygen compounds that damage cells, especially cellular DNA and cell membranes, that may speed up the aging process. However, only the third theory, the nutritional model, which involves severe caloric restriction, has been successful in prolonging life in mammalian species.[22]

## Genetic, Environment, and Lifestyle Theory

The rates at which changes occur with aging depend on heredity. Genes determine the competence with which cells are maintained and repaired. Fundamental biological processes involved in aging are mostly determined by genetics.[23] However, environmental factors such as pollution, poor living conditions, and personal lifestyle habits related to diet, smoking, alcohol abuse, or level of physical activity influence expression of the genetic code by intensifying certain traits. For instance, an individual's height and weight are determined genetically, but diet and other environmental exposures can modify this effect. People with a family history of high levels of low-density lipoprotein cholesterol (i.e., bad cholesterol) and eventually death from cardiovascular disease can deter the effects of their genetic programming by losing weight, consuming diets low in saturated fat, performing regular physical activity, and abstaining from tobacco use.[24] Individuals with a family history of type 2 diabetes can reduce their risk for developing the disease with a proper diet, physical activity, and maintenance of normal weight.

## Free Radicals Theory

Free radicals are unstable oxygen compounds formed normally during metabolism. These can damage cells by initiating reactions that break down cell membranes and modify the normal metabolic processes that protect people from disease.[25] Exposure to oxidizing agents such as environmental pollutants, ozone, smoking, and solar radiation also can damage the cells.[26] Free radicals cause oxidative damage to proteins, lipids, carbohydrates, and DNA and also may indirectly destroy cells by producing toxic products. For instance, spots that appear on the skin with age are caused by the oxidation of lipids, which produces a pigment called lipofuscin, or age pigment.[1,27] The cell damage due to free radicals has been implicated in the development of several chronic diseases, such as cardiovascular disease and cancer, common among older persons.[27-29]

Unstable oxygen compounds can be neutralized when they combine with an antioxidant.[30] The antioxidants prevent them from interfering with normal cell functions. The body can produce antioxidant enzymes (e.g., catalases, glutathione, peroxidase, reductases, and superoxide dismutase).[26] In addition, some antioxidants can be obtained from the diet. Dietary antioxidants include selenium, vitamins C and E, and other phytochemicals, which are plant substances such as beta-carotene, lycopene, flavonoids, lutein, zeaxanthin, resveratrol, and isoflavones that contribute to normal metabolism. For instance, flavonoids found in grapes, apples, broccoli, and onions act as antioxidants. In contrast, it is not effective to consume cellular enzymes designed to break down the damaging compounds, such as superoxide dismutase, because ingested enzymes are broken down during digestion before they can act in the body. Despite this, some health food stores sell superoxide dismutase.[25]

## Caloric Restriction Theory

The one nutritional model that has been successful in prolonging life in mice, rats, and other rodents involves severe dietary restriction of energy.[31] The original study in this area demonstrated that dietary restriction in rats increased longevity, but led to diminished sexual maturation and fertility, lower bone strength, and lower bone calcium and phosphorus contents.[31,32] Studies involving less severe dietary restrictions (a 50 to 60 percent lower energy intake than animals allowed to eat as needed) showed increased longevity in rats, mice, and hamsters without developmental abnormalities. Furthermore, the age-related physiological changes were also delayed. Although the animals in these studies were leaner than the control animals, the results do not point to reduction of body fat as the mechanism by which food restriction extends length of life.[31-34] Research on a moderately reduced

energy and protein diet in growing pigs showed a significant increase in intramuscular lipids.[31-34] In obese humans, the accumulation of intramuscular lipids is associated with insulin resistance and the subsequent development of type 2 diabetes mellitus, which is one of the chronic diseases that affect older persons.[35,36]

The most appropriate caloric restriction approach is to add more fruits and vegetables to a diet to decrease chronic disease risk and subsequently reduce the aging process. Eating nutrient-dense foods and avoiding obesity enhance prospects for longevity. Therefore, there seems to be a relationship among genetics, environment, nutrition, and lifestyle in the process of aging.

# ▶ Lifestyle and Socioeconomic Factors That May Influence the Aging Process

A variety of social and economic factors affect aging and can affect the nutritional status of individuals. These factors can interrelate and decrease an individual's ability to socialize, eat, and acquire and enjoy food. The socioeconomic changes affecting the nutritional status of the elderly are presented in **BOX 11-1**.

## Alcohol Use

Alcohol consumption increases the risk for malnutrition in older persons. Alcohol is high in calories and provides few nutrients. Too much alcohol intake damages the brain, heart, liver, and other organs.[37] It impairs judgment and balance, thereby increasing the frequency of falls. Too much intake also makes it harder to eat and take medications appropriately.[37] Older persons should limit alcohol consumption to no more than one drink (4 to 5 ounces of wine, 12 ounces of beer, or a 1.5-ounce shot of 80-proof liquor) per day for women and two drinks per day for men.[38]

---

**BOX 11-1** Socioeconomic Changes Affecting the Nutritional Status of the Elderly

- Reduced income with retirement
- Insufficient funds for purchase of food
- Skipping meals
- Increased medical expenses
- Inability to drive to doctor's appointments or to the grocery store
- Inadequate food storage facilities
- Diminished self-esteem
- Social isolation

Data from: Williams SR. Essentials of Nutrition and Diet Therapy. 8th ed. Davis, CA: Mosby; 2003.

**TABLE 11-1** Risk Factors for Drug–Nutrient Interactions[37,40]

| Factors | Examples of Health Conditions |
| --- | --- |
| Restrictive diets | Diabetes and other chronic health conditions |
| Existing malnutrition | Protein-energy malnutrition |
| Drastic changes in eating patterns | Eating disorders |
| Chronic disease with long-term drug treatment | Cancer, HIV, etc. |
| Alcohol abuse | Alcoholism |
| Need for multiple-drug regimens | Heart disease, hypertension, and other chronic health conditions |
| Extremes in age: young children and the elderly | Underweight and/or frail |
| Use of a high-potency vitamin or mineral supplement | Quackery and chronic use of medication |

The incidence of alcoholism among the elderly is approximately 13 percent for men, 2 percent for women, and 6 percent for both sexes.[39] Late-onset alcoholism occurs mainly in women with high socioeconomic status after stressful life events such as the death of a spouse or retirement.[40,41] It is also important to note that 75 percent of adults 65 years of age or older who misuse alcohol are also taking prescription drugs.[42] Even small amounts of alcohol can react negatively with various medications that many older persons routinely take.

Some of the symptoms of alcoholism in older persons include trembling hands, sleep problems, memory loss, and unsteady gait; these can be easily overlooked simply because they are similar to symptoms of old age.[43] Older adults become intoxicated on a smaller amount of alcohol than younger persons because older persons metabolize alcohol more slowly.[43] In addition to having adverse effects on the liver, drinking large amounts of alcohol increases the risk for hemorrhagic stroke and may exacerbate hypertension in older adults.[25]

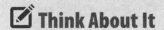 **Think About It**

How might drugs affect an elderly individual's nutritional status?

## Increased Use of Medications and Aging

Persons at highest risk for drug–nutrient interactions (DNIs) are those who 1) take many drugs, including alcohol; 2) require long-term drug therapy; or 3) have poor or marginal nutrition status.[42] These and other risk-increasing factors are listed in **TABLE 11-1**. Older persons are likely to take medications because health problems increase with age. Almost half of older Americans take multiple medications daily (**polypharmacy**).[44,45] The information on DNI is continually updated as new products enter the market or additional, sometimes conflicting, reports appear in the literature.[46]

Twenty-three percent of women and 19 percent of men over 65 years of age take five or more prescription medications per week.[47] Several situations contribute to the increased risk for DNI among the elderly[36,48]:

- They are more likely to take more medications for longer periods to manage chronic diseases.
- Their medications are more likely to be toxic.
- Their responses to medications vary significantly.
- Their bodies have less capability to handle medications effectively.
- They are more likely to be nutritionally deficient.
- They are more likely to make mistakes in self-care because of illness, mental confusion, or lack of medication information.

The use of over-the-counter and prescription medications can affect nutritional status and contribute to malnutrition. Medications commonly used by older individuals include aspirin, laxatives, diuretics, antacids, anticoagulants (blood thinner), anticonvulsants, heart medications, and pain medications.[36]

Drugs can affect nutritional status by changing food intake patterns. Medications may interfere with an individual's ability to gather and prepare meals. Drug-induced alterations in mental status, blood pressure, urinary continence, coordination, or gait may affect nutritional status by diminishing interest in food and the ability to carry out activities involved in meal preparation.[36,44,45,47-49]

Drugs may have a primary effect on diminishing or increasing appetite or may cause an unwanted side effect; for example, drugs that alter taste perception also can cause gastrointestinal discomfort and decrease food intake. The incidence of nausea and vomiting can be common with many medications and, if severe (e.g., with chemotherapy), may result in weight loss and nutrient deficiencies. **TABLE 11-2** presents common medications that the elderly use and food and nutrient interactions.[48]

## Dependent Living

Many older individuals continue to live in a family setting; however, the number and proportion of older U.S. adults living alone have increased significantly in the past three decades, and there is concern that these individuals may have poor dietary quality.[53] Malnutrition can be a problem among older adults regardless of where they live. It is reported that older individuals living independently have reduced intakes of energy and protein.[54,55] Also, older adults who live alone are vulnerable to poverty and social isolation, which affect the quality of food intake and could lead to malnutrition.[53] Alternatively, dependent-living older adults (e.g., those in nursing homes) may have medical conditions that increase nutrient requirements and interfere with food intake and/or nutrient absorption, causing malnutrition. In addition, persons with less education and those who smoke, drink excessive amounts of alcoholic beverages, do not exercise, and have low energy intake are at greater risk for malnutrition. Community nutritionists should consider all of these characteristics when designing programs to improve dietary quality among older persons.[53]

**TABLE 11-2** Common Medications and Food and Nutrient Interactions[50-52]

| Common Medications Used by Older Adults | Effects of Nutrient/Food Interaction | Recommendations |
|---|---|---|
| Laxative/mineral oil | Steatorrhea, rickets, and dehydration. Electrolyte, vitamin (fat-soluble), and mineral deficiency due to a decrease in the absorption of many vitamins and minerals, electrolytes, and calcium. | Provide fluid and electrolytes. Provide foods that are high in vitamins and minerals (fruits, vegetables, dairy products). |
| Aluminum hydroxide (contained in some antacids) | Phosphorus deficiency leading to osteomalacia and muscle weakness due to the inhibition of phosphorus absorption from food over a long period. | Avoid late evening meals and snacks and avoid lying down, sleeping, or swimming soon after meals to guard against reflux. Follow the Dietary Guidelines for Americans. |
| Anticonvulsants | Megaloblastic anemia due to a decrease in folate absorption. | Increase folic acid in the diet to alleviate anemia. Include green leafy vegetables, citrus fruits, animal products, and grain products fortified with folate (enriched breads, flours, cornmeals, rice, etc.). |
| Cholesterol-lowering medications (e.g., cholestyramine/colestipol) | Vitamins A, D, E, and K deficiency due to the removal of bile acids over a long period that can decrease absorption of fat-soluble vitamins, calcium, cobalamin, and folate. | Increase vitamin D and calcium intake; also increase vitamin $B_{12}$ and folate intake. Include animal products, dairy products, fruits, and vegetables. |
| Antibiotics | Vitamin K deficiency due to destruction of the bacteria that produce vitamin K in the intestine. Foods: dietary calcium can bind to tetracycline and reduce its absorption. | Avoid taking tetracycline with dairy products, antacids, and vitamins containing iron because they interfere with the medication's effectiveness. Follow the Dietary Guidelines for Americans. |

| Common Medications Used by Older Adults | Effects of Nutrient/Food Interaction | Recommendations |
|---|---|---|
| Diuretics (e.g., hydrochlorothiazide) | Potassium deficiency causing dehydration and impairment of the heart and other muscle due to increase in the loss of potassium and fluids. Increased urinary loss of sodium, chloride, magnesium, zinc, and riboflavin ($B_2$). | When taking triamterene, limit the intake of bananas, oranges, and green leafy vegetables or salt substitutes that contain potassium. Follow the Dietary Guidelines for Americans. |
| Large amounts of aspirin | Anemia iron deficiency due to stomach bleeding over a long period and a decrease in vitamin C and folate utilization. | Increase folate and vitamin D intake. Avoid taking omega-3 fatty acids in fish oil capsules, which can cause hypervitaminosis A and D if taken in large doses. |
| Alcohol (ethanol) | Fat, vitamin (vitamin A, thiamin, folate, and cobalamin), and mineral (zinc, magnesium) deficiency due to impaired utilization and storage of vitamin A, increased urinary excretion of zinc and magnesium, and a decrease in the absorption of fat, vitamin A, thiamin, cobalamin, and folate absorption. | Provide adequate intake of fruits and vegetables using the Dietary Guidelines for Americans. |
| Anticoagulants (e.g., warfarin [Coumadin]) | Vitamin K and tocopherol intakes decrease the effect of the drug. | Limit foods high in vitamin K, such as broccoli, spinach, kale, turnip greens, cauliflower, and Brussels sprouts, to one serving. Limit vitamin E doses to not more than 400 IU/day. Avoid taking with dong quai, fenugreek, feverfew, excessive garlic, ginger, ginkgo, and ginseng because of their effects. |
| Antihypertensives (e.g., hydralazine) | Pyridoxine antagonist. Increased urinary excretion of manganese and pyridoxine. | Provide adequate pyridoxine and manganese intake and follow Dietary Guidelines for Americans. |
| Antineoplastics (e.g., methotrexate) | Folate antagonist may impair fat, calcium, cobalamin, lactose, folate, and carotene absorption. | Increase green leafy vegetable and folic acid supplements. |
| Cardiac glycosides (e.g., digoxin) | Increased urinary excretion of calcium, magnesium, and zinc. Anorexia. | Avoid excessive intakes of fiber and wheat bran and vitamin D. Avoid the use of hawthorn, milkweed, guar gum, and St. John's wort. |
| Antidepressant (e.g., monoamine oxidase inhibitor such as tranylcypromine, phenelzine, or isocarboxazid) | Hypertension due to interaction with tyramine from cheese and other foods containing tyramine. | Avoid foods high in tyramine (e.g., wine, beer, beef, chicken liver, cured meats such as sausage, salami, game meat, dried fish, avocados, bananas, raisins, miso soup, beans, colas, chocolate, coffee and tea, sauerkraut, etc.). |

## Income Level

Approximately 45 percent of adults 65 and older had incomes below twice the poverty thresholds.[9] The rate of poverty is highest among the oldest of the old, minorities, women, persons living alone, and those with disabilities.[9,54] The poverty rate is higher for the older foreign born than for the older native population.[51] Many older individuals live on a fixed income as they retire from their job, which makes it harder for them to afford medication and a nutritious diet. Due to this situation, they often either reduce the amount of food intake or limit the types of foods they consume.

## ▶ Physiological Changes That Can Affect Nutritional Status

Aging causes multiple physiological changes that affect nutrient needs and nutritional status. Individuals age at different rates, and many of the decreases in physiological functions have an impact on the day-to-day lives of many elders. These changes, both physical and mental,

can occur rapidly in one organ system and slowly in another. For example, by the age of 70, the kidneys lose approximately 28 percent of their weight in comparison with values in young adults, the liver loses 25 percent of its weight and skeletal muscle diminishes by almost half.[48-50,53-56] **BOX 11-2** presents the physiological changes that are often associated with aging.

## Changes in Lean Body Mass

The physiological changes include a decrease in lean body mass (sarcopenia) and total body water. Sarcopenia is due to excessive loss of muscle mass and strength, loss of mobility, neuromuscular impairment, and balance failure. Falls and fractures can lead to immobilization, which induces more loss of muscle mass.[59] Body weight usually decreases after age 60 in men and age 65 in women by an average of 0.5 percent yearly. Many older adults gain body fat and lose about 53 to 60 percent of total body water. Compared to males in their 20s, males in their 70s have approximately 24 pounds less muscle and 22 pounds more body fat.[46,60,61] Intraabdominal fat increases the most and is a risk factor for cardiovascular disease and insulin resistance.[46] The reasons for the age-related gains are not

---

**BOX 11-2** Physiological Changes Due to Aging[25,40,57,58]

**Cardiovascular System**
- Reduced blood vessel elasticity and stroke volume output
- Increased blood pressure
- Decreased cardiac output
- Decreased maximal heart rate

**Endocrine System**
- Reduced levels of estrogen and testosterone
- Decreased secretions of growth hormone
- Reduced glucose tolerance (decreased insulin-like growth factor)
- Decreased ability to convert provitamin D to previtamin D in skin

**Gastrointestinal System**
- Reduced secretion of saliva and mucus
- Dysphagia or difficulty in swallowing
- Reduced secretion of hydrochloric acid and digestive enzymes
- Slower peristalsis
- Reduced vitamin $B_{12}$ absorption

**Musculoskeletal System**
- Reduced lean body mass (bone mass, muscle, and water)
- Decreased bone marrow mass and increased bone marrow fat

- Increased fat mass
- Decreased resting metabolic rate
- Missing or poorly fitting teeth
- Reduced work capacity (strength)

**Nervous System**
- Blunted appetite regulation
- Blunted thirst regulation
- Decreased antibody response
- Decreased brain weight
- Reduced nerve conduction velocity affecting senses of smell, taste, and touch, as well as cognition
- Changed sleep as the wake cycle becomes shorter

**Renal System**
- Reduced number of nephrons
- Less blood flow
- Slowed glomerular filtration rate
- Decreased renal mass

**Respiratory System**
- Reduced breathing capacity
- Reduced work capacity (endurance)
- Decreased elasticity in lung tissue

**Hepatic System**
- Reduced liver volume
- Reduced blood flow

clear, but a longitudinal study shows that lack of exercise could be a factor. Results from the Fels Longitudinal Study showed significant age-related decreases in lean body mass and height and increases in total body fat, weight, and body mass index (BMI). However, a shift in body composition was seen in participants who reported high or moderate physical activity levels. For instance, higher levels of physical activity were associated with higher levels of lean body mass in both men and women.[13,62]

Community nutritionists working with older individuals should consider including physical activities (walking, bicycling, swimming, dancing, etc.) when planning programs for older persons. However, an individual's physician should determine the level of physical activity that is safe. In addition, it is important to correct negative nitrogen balance from increased losses (possibly 2 to 3 grams of nitrogen per day). The usual recommendation is to provide 1.2 g of protein per kilogram body weight and adequate calories to spare protein. In addition, provide adequate fluid intake to help prevent excretion of nutrients.

## Aging Bone

Another feature of biologic aging is a decrease in bone density. After age 40, adults tend to lose stature, with a mean height loss of 4.9 cm (1.9 inches) in women and 2.9 cm (1.1 inches) in men. It is important to note that the rate of bone loss is individualized.[63-65] Excessive loss of bone density increases the risk for osteoporosis, a major cause of morbidity in developed countries. Although hormonal influences account for much of the age-related alteration in bone homeostasis, nutritional factors also play an important role.[66] Several nutrients contribute to bone density, including protein; vitamins C, D, and K; phosphorus; and calcium. Although most North American diets supply an adequate amount of most of these nutrients, calcium intakes are usually below current recommendations. Experts estimate that variations in calcium nutrition in youth may account for a 5 to 10 percent difference in peak adult bone mass, and a 25 to 50 percent difference in hip fracture risk in later life.[67]

Exercises such as walking, running, and dancing and weight-bearing activities are commonly recommended to increase bone density. Evidence suggests that 20 to 30 minutes of moderate to intense physical activity several times per week produces a favorable skeletal benefit.[67]

The New Jersey Department of Health and Senior Services and Rutgers Cooperative Extension collaborated to provide a community program, Project Healthy Bones, at the state level. They provided education on nutrition, osteoporosis prevention and treatment, home safety, and fall prevention to older persons. More than 1,400 older persons participated in the program. Project Healthy Bones focused on the idea that self-esteem, peer support, and incremental successes were important to change behavior and that having fun should be part of the process. Project Healthy Bones used older adults as peer advocate trainers who acted as role models and had a better understanding of the beliefs, limitations, and fears of older participants. Analysis of a 3-day dietary assessment showed that of 57 participants completing 12 to 23 weeks of the program, 39 to 68 percent had increased their calcium intake. The analysis of physical activity levels showed significant progress from exercises in level one (introductory) to level two (advanced) and an increase in amount of weight lifted. These improvements were evident in both participants completing between 12 and 23 weeks of the program and those completing the entire 24-week cycle.[68]

## Changes in Taste, Smell, Appetite, and Digestive Juices

Some physiological changes that occur with age also affect nutritional status. For example, the secretion of certain digestive juices is diminished and gastric acid is reduced, leading to a reduction in the absorption of pH-dependent nutrients such as vitamins C, $B_6$, $B_{12}$, and folic acid.[69] The age-related decreased parietal cell secretion of a glycoprotein called intrinsic factor, which binds vitamin $B_{12}$ and permits its efficient absorption, further impairs its bioavailability. In addition, the decrease in gastric acid can lead to bacterial growth, causing the formation of gas.[69,70]

In some individuals, sensory perceptions of taste, smell, hearing, and vision may change. Food consumption is a complex phenomenon that interrelates to the individual's culture, income, health status, and behavioral characteristics. In older persons, appetite is a critical factor in food intake, which is influenced by medication, the presence of physical (e.g., hypertension, chronic infection) or psychological (e.g., depression) disease, and some physiological sensory functions such as taste and smell. These senses influence appetite and the enjoyment of food and also can influence the amount of food consumed. Because of these reasons, adults need more seasoning of their food.[69]

In older adults, hunger and satiety cues are less than in younger adults. Age has an inverse effect on the variety of foods consumed.[71] The change in palatability of a food once an individual begins to eat it is called **sensory-specific satiety**. This type of satiety is associated with a decreased intake of one food and a switch to another food during an ingestion period. The sensory-specific satiety mechanism promotes more variety and potentially a more well-balanced eating pattern.[72] This mechanism is diminished in older persons compared to younger persons. The reason for the reduced sensory-specific satiety is not clear. The low appetite-regulating mechanism will require older persons to be more aware of their food intake levels and requires them to consume a variety or a combination of foods.

There is a reduction in the ability to taste and smell at about the age of 60, and this reduction becomes more severe in individuals over 70.[73] The reduction of these senses can contribute to impaired nutritional status by decreasing both the appeal and the enjoyment of food. Chemosensory losses that occur with age include the following[74]:

- *Ageusia:* absence of taste
- *Hypogeusia:* diminished sensitivity of taste
- *Dysgeusia:* distortion of normal taste
- *Anosmia:* absence of smell
- *Hyposmia:* diminished sensitivity of smell
- *Dysosmia:* distortion of normal smell

Some research studies show that the reduction in taste acuity is due to a reduction in the number of taste buds on the tongue; other studies suggest that the decrease is the result of changes in sensitivity to specific flavors such as salty and sweet.[75,76] In addition, the ability to distinguish the odors of certain items varies. For instance, the ability to distinguish the odor of breads, vegetables, and coffee reduces significantly with age, but older persons retain the ability to identify green bell peppers and taste sweet foods.[75,76]

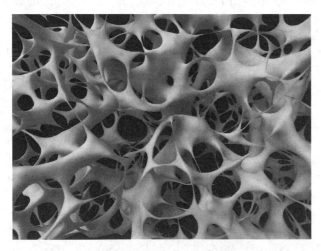

Osteoporosis is porous bone due to reduction in bone mass.
© Sebastian Kaulitzki/Shutterstock

## ▶ Nutrition Screening for Older Persons

To identify malnutrition risk factors among the aging population, the American Academy of Family Physicians, the Academy of Nutrition and Dietetics, and the National Council on Aging collaborated and

developed the Nutrition Screening Initiative (NSI) checklist. This 5-year project focused on nutrition screening and interventions that help prevent and manage nutrition-related problems before a person becomes ill or a condition worsens. **FIGURE 11-4** presents the self-administered Determine Your Nutritional Health checklist. A dietitian, physician, nurse, or other healthcare professional can review the resulting score to determine the person's nutritional risk.

### DETERMINE YOUR NUTRITIONAL HEALTH

Warning signs of poor nutritional health are often overlooked.

Use this checklist to find out if you or someone you know is at nutritional risk.

Read the statements below. Circle the number in the yes column for those that apply to you or someone you know. For each yes answer, score the number in the box. Total your nutritional score.

| | Yes |
|---|---|
| I have an illness or condition that made me change the kind and/or amount of food I eat. | 2 |
| I eat fewer than 2 meals per day. | 3 |
| I eat few fruits or vegetables, or milk products. | 2 |
| I have 3 or more drinks of beer, liquor, or wine almost every day. | 2 |
| I have tooth or mouth problems that make it hard for me to eat. | 2 |
| I don't always have enough money to buy the food I need. | 4 |
| I eat alone most of the time. | 1 |
| I take three or more different prescribed or over-thr-counter drugs a day. | 1 |
| Without wanting to, I have lost or gained 10 pounds in the last 6 months. | 2 |
| I am not always physically able to shop, cook, and/or feed myself. | 2 |
| TOTAL | |

Total your nutrition score. If it's…

0–2   Good! Recheck your nutritional score in 6 months.

3–5   You are at moderate nutritional risk.

See what you can do to improve your eating habits and lifestyle. Your office on aging, senior nutrition program, senior citizens center, or health department can help. Recheck your nutritional score in 3 months.

6+   You are at high nutritional risk.

Bring this checklist the next time you see your doctor, dietitian, or other qualified healthcare or social service professional. Talk with them about any problems you may have. Ask for help to improve your nutritional health.

Remember: Warning signs suggest risk, but do not represent diagnosis of any condition.

**FIGURE 11-4** Determine your nutritional health checklist.

Reproduced from: Nutrition Screening Initiative: Determine your nutritional health checklist. The Nutrition Screening Initiative: Development and implementation of the public awareness checklist and screening tools. The Nutrition Screening Initiative is a joint project of the American Academy of Family Physician and American Dietetic Association, funded in part by a grant from Ross Product Division, Abbott Laboratories, Inc., Columbus, Ohio. 1995. Reprinted with permission.

The checklist uses the word DETERMINE as mnemonic device to communicate basic nutrition information and help users recall the major risk factors and indicators of poor nutritional status. The checklist is not a diagnostic tool, however.

An individual who scored 0 to 2 is considered at good nutritional status, and a recheck in 6 months is recommended. An individual scoring 3 to 5 points, which is considered moderate nutritional risk, is encouraged to recheck his or her nutritional status in 3 months, and a self-help approach to improve nutritional status is encouraged.[77] Individuals with a nutrition score of 6 or more points are regarded as being at high nutritional risk and are encouraged to take the checklist to their physician, dietitian, or other health or social service provider.[78]

A practical approach to nutrition screening recommended by the NSI is presented in **TABLE 11-3**. A Level I Screen is a basic nutrition evaluation tool that can be administered in a community setting. It should be administered annually or if a major change in status occurs. A Level II Screen is administered by a healthcare professional and requires the participation of a physician and dietitian. If problems are identified, the person must be referred to the proper healthcare professional.[77]

Mitchell et al.[77] compared the food group intakes assessed from questions embedded in the NSI Level II Screen with those from a more comprehensive food frequency questionnaire. Results showed that the Level II Screen is a feasible, low-cost tool to screen for determining nutrition risk in older adults. However,

**TABLE 11-3** A Practical Approach to Nutrition Screening

| Level I Screen | | Level II Screen | |
|---|---|---|---|
| Basic nutritional screen completed by social services or health professionals<br>**Measurements:**<br>Height<br>Weight<br>Dietary data (24-hour recall)<br>Living situation<br>Functional status | | Includes laboratory work completed by healthcare professionals in a medical setting<br>**Measurements:**<br>Height<br>Weight<br>Dietary data (24-hour recall)<br>Living situation<br>Biochemical parameters (hemoglobin, albumin, serum cholesterol, glucose)<br>Skinfold measurements<br>Bone density screening | |
| Weight change (underweight) | No nutritional problem but functionally dependent, poor socioeconomic circumstances | Inadequate or inappropriate diet | Obesity<br>Hypercholesterolemia<br>Osteoporosis<br>Protein-energy malnutrition<br>Vitamin deficiency<br>Weight loss (unintentional), etc. |
| Refer to physician | Consider community social services and health programs (Supplemental Nutrition Assistance Program, Meals on Wheels, or Congregate Meals programs); shopping or transportation assistance | Refer to dietitian or community nutrition program | Institute appropriate therapy/management |

**BOX 11-3** Determine: Warning Signs of Poor Nutritional Health

- **Disease:** Any disease, illness, or chronic condition (i.e., confusion, feeling sad or depressed, acute infections) that causes you to change the way you eat, makes it hard for you to eat, or puts your nutritional health at risk.
- **Eating poorly:** Eating too little, too much, or the same food day after day or not eating fruits, vegetables, and milk products daily will cause poor nutritional health.
- **Tooth loss/mouth pain:** It is hard to eat well with missing, loose, or rotten teeth or dentures that do not fit well or cause mouth sores.
- **Economic hardship:** Having less (or choosing to spend less) than $34.30 (female) to $38.60 (male) weekly for groceries makes it hard to get the foods needed to stay healthy (http://www.cnpp.usda.gov). Income below the poverty guideline.
- **Reduced social contact:** Being with people has a positive effect on morale, well-being, and eating.
- **Multiple medicines:** The more medicines you take, the greater the chance for side effects such as changes in taste, increased or decreased appetite and thirst, constipation, weakness, drowsiness, diarrhea, nausea, and others. Vitamins or minerals taken in large doses can act like drugs and can cause harm.
- **Involuntary weight loss or gain:** Losing or gaining a lot of weight when you are not trying to do so is a warning sign to discuss with your healthcare provider.
- **Needs assistance in self-care:** Older people who have trouble walking, shopping, and buying and cooking food are at risk for malnutrition.
- **Elder years above 80:** As age increases, risk for frailty and health problems also rises.

The dollar amounts used in economic hardship were modified by the author using September 2003, U.S. Department of Agriculture low-cost food plan.

Reproduced from: Nutrition Screening Initiative. Determine your nutritional health checklist. The Nutrition Screening Initiative: Development and implementation of the public awareness checklist and screening tools. The Nutrition Screening Initiative is a joint project of the American Academy of Family Physician and American Dietetic Association, funded in part by a grant from Ross Product Division, Abbott Laboratories, Inc., Columbus, Ohio. 1995. Reprinted with permission.

the embedded food group questions in the Level II Screen should be interpreted thoughtfully in the overall screening process. **BOX 11-3** presents the warning signs of poor nutrition health.

Indicators of poor nutritional status in the elderly may be detected by a physical sign, specific symptoms, or measurable parameter that shows that poor nutritional status is present in the person and is causing some symptoms.[77] These can be identified through interview, observation, physical examination, anthropometric measurements, and laboratory tests. Risk factors associated with poor nutritional status include the following[77-82]:

- Inappropriate food and nutrient intake
- Poverty, social isolation
- Dependency and disability
- Acute or chronic diseases or conditions
- Chronic medication use
- Functional disability
- Hunger
- Living alone
- Depression
- Dementia
- Poor dentition and oral health, chewing and swallowing problems
- Minority status
- Advanced age

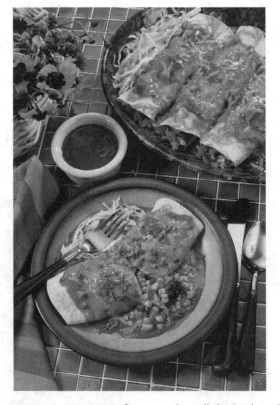

The sensory perceptions of taste and smell diminish with age. Adding adequate spices to foods may motivate an older person to eat.
© Photodisc

## ▶ Anorexia in the Elderly

Although appetite diminishes with advancing age, severe anorexia that leads to significant weight loss (**anorexia of aging**) is not a normal aspect of aging. The standard for serious weight loss used by many nutritionists when monitoring body weight is the loss of 10 pounds or more over a period of 6 months or the loss of 5 percent or more of total body weight over a period of 1 year. Anorexia and weight loss are common in the elderly, especially in individuals with medical or mental illnesses.[83] As mentioned in the previous section, research suggests that many factors contribute to a decline in food consumption with advancing age.[84] With normal aging, men and women may decrease their energy intake as their resting metabolic rate reduces because they are physically less active, their feeding drive (hunger) may decrease, and satiety may occur more easily. This physiological change with aging may be the precursor of pathological anorexia and weight loss that is most commonly due to depression.[85]

*Failure to thrive* is the term used to designate a weight loss condition recognized in older persons. Previously recognized as a syndrome in infants and children who are neglected, failure to thrive in the developing child is characterized by a failure to grow and develop in both physical and social skills. In older persons, the opposite occurs.[86] This condition is characterized as a failure to maintain as the individual regresses in physical well-being and mental function.[36] Weight loss is the first major symptom of failure to thrive in older adults and is followed by increasing physical disability, loss of skills for self-care, social withdrawal, diminished mental function, and, finally, death. In most cases, the individuals are living in the community.

In failure to thrive, there is no biological or physiological explanation for the weight loss and malnutrition. However, in many incidents, the weight loss is due to a lack of financial resources, social isolation, limited ability to obtain adequate groceries or prepare meals, chronic disease and disability, failing eyesight, or other circumstances that limit food intake.[36,87] Prescription drugs also can have a profound impact on appetite through a variety of mechanisms.[88] If detected early, intervention is both possible and effective.

## ▶ Water Requirements

Dehydration is a major problem in older adults, especially in the oldest individuals and those who are institutionalized.[89,90] Morley[83] defined dehydration as losing nearly 2 percent of one's initial body weight; this can occur after not drinking any fluids and consuming only dry foods for 24 hours.[90] This happens because the regulation of body water relies on thirst and an individual's response to that thirst. In general, thirst is reduced in older persons, specifically in those with high serum sodium levels (> 150 milliequivalents per liter) or a high ratio of blood urea nitrogen to creatinine (> 25), which is a good indicator of dehydration.[91,92]

The symptoms of dehydration among older adults include a swollen tongue, constipation, electrolyte imbalance, nausea and vomiting, hypotension, mental confusion, sunken eyeballs, increased body temperature, decreased urine output, pressure ulcers, and urinary tract infections.[93]

A general guideline of total fluid intake for older adults is 3.7 liters per day for men and 2.7 liters per day for women.[94] A research study reported that more than one in three Americans over the age of 60 may not be consuming enough total water from all sources.[95] Good sources of water include tap and bottled water, milk, juice, carbonated beverages, and soups. Valtin[92] suggested that caffeinated drinks (e.g., coffee and soft drinks) and alcoholic beverages also may count toward daily consumption of fluid. However, because of the diuretic effects of these types of beverages, additional tap or bottled water should be consumed to replace the water that is lost.

## ▶ Alzheimer's Disease

**Alzheimer's disease (AD)** is the most common form of dementia in the United States and Europe. It is estimated that in 2007, there were 4.5 million cases of Alzheimer's disease in the United States.[90] Approximately 5 percent of men and women ages 65 to 74 have AD, and nearly half of those age 85 or older may have the disease. It is important that healthcare professionals understand that the incidence of AD increases with age.

AD begins with cognitive loss that becomes worse gradually with the extension of cerebral lesions. Other problems occur such as a loss of independence, orientation impairments, loss of sense of self, loss of meaningful relationship with the world, disordered eating behavior, memory loss, behavior and personality changes, reduced ability to think, and weight loss.[92,96] This weight loss increases the risk for infections, skin ulcers, and falls, and consequently decreases quality of life in individuals with Alzheimer's.[97-99] The disease seems to affect many different cells involving several of the neurotransmitters. Free radical damage is suspected as a mechanism of cell loss in AD, but the cause is unknown.[97]

Individuals with AD often have a chronically poor diet or an increased nutrient need. They often have protein malnutrition and other nutritional deficiencies that improve the status of the individual when corrected. Low blood levels of folate and vitamin $B_{12}$ are often found in individuals with AD.[100] Low folate blood levels may be associated with depressed individuals experiencing a weaker response to antidepressants.[98,101,102] According to research from the Alzheimer's Disease Cooperative Study, large intakes of vitamin E are associated with slowing the progression of AD. The study found that individuals with AD of moderate severity extended the time they were able to care for themselves by consuming 2,000 IU per day of vitamin E compared to those taking a placebo.[101-103]

Vitamin E, thiamine, and vitamin $B_{12}$ have been associated with improved symptoms when blood levels are corrected to normal[101-103]:

- Vitamin E may help by slowing the rate of free radical–induced tissue damage.
- Thiamin may help produce acetylcholine through its participation in the synthesis of acetyl coenzyme A (acetyl CoA), a precursor to acetylcholine, the neurotransmitter most closely associated with AD symptoms.
- Vitamin $B_{12}$ is required for the generation of methyl groups involved in either the synthesis or conservation of choline, the other component of acetylcholine.
- High doses of acetyl-L-carnitine (1,000 mg with breakfast, 1,000 mg with lunch) have also been reported to slow the progression of AD.[73]

AD has three stages, which are presented in **TABLE 11-4**. During stage 1, the individual is encouraged to complete as many tasks as possible, including food preparation and washing dishes. In stage 2, individuals need help keeping track of food intake because they tend to forget. A helper should provide the individual with various stimulating activities such as different types of physical activities. In stage 3, the individual may not recognize foods, may forget to eat, or may forget what to do with the food. In this stage, there is loss of muscle mass and body fat due to the lack of food intake.[104] The individual needs help eating and participating in stimulating activities.

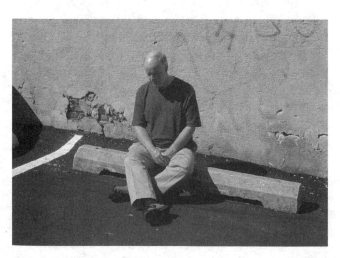

Alzheimer's disease begins with cognitive loss that gradually becomes worse with the extension of cerebral lesions.
© Mel Curtis/Photodisc/Getty Images

**TABLE 11-4** Major Stages of Alzheimer's Disease[90,100,105]

| Stage | Food-Related Symptoms |
|---|---|
| 1 | Purchases and prepares own food, feeds self |
| | Washes dishes |
| 2 | Can feed self, but needs direction and assistance at mealtime |
| | Needs assistance on food intake |
| | Needs to be reminded about eating |
| | Unable to sit still for a long time to eat |
| | May forget how to prepare food |
| 3 | Requires total feeding assistance |
| | Cannot feed self, may refuse to chew and swallow food |
| | Is at risk for malnutrition |
| | May not recognize foods |
| | Forgets what to do with foods |

Nutrition recommendations for individuals with AD are difficult because of limited nutritional data available to healthcare professionals. Additional calories may be needed for increased energy expended by individuals in stages 1 and 2. Foods that are high in antioxidants such as vitamin E, selenium, and vitamin C are recommended; tuna, chicken breasts, cashews, sunflower seed kernels, yellow peppers, papaya, kiwi, oranges, sunflower oil, and enriched grains and cereals are good sources of these nutrients.

AD is difficult for the caregiver and, in many cases, is perceived as a heavy burden to bear. The caregiver, stressed and often depressed, may become socially isolated. This, in turn, can affect the person with AD. It has been reported that the burden AD imposes on the caregiver caused weight loss in the individual with AD.[106] The more stressed, depressed, and tired the caregiver becomes, the more the individual with AD tends to lose weight.

## ▶ Multivitamin and Mineral Supplements

The use of dietary supplements including vitamins, minerals, and herbal and botanical products is growing. Some older persons use supplements to meet their nutrient needs and, in some cases, prolong life. Food contributes more than just its nutrient content; therefore, replacing food with supplements is not an appropriate trade-off.[3] In addition, some nutrients in large amounts can be toxic. Large amounts of one particular nutrient can interact and affect the absorption of other nutrients or interfere with the absorption and metabolism of prescription medications.[80]

The recommendation is to use multivitamin and mineral supplements that do not exceed 100 percent of the Daily Value for any nutrient. This is the safest way to supplement the diet. Supplements containing megadoses or nonnutrient substances may be toxic and should be avoided.[1,28,94] For example, superoxide dismutase, an enzyme that protects against oxidative damage, supposedly slows down aging and can be used to treat AD. However, it is a protein that is broken down to amino acids in the gastrointestinal tract, so oral supplements will not increase blood or tissue levels of this enzyme. Coenzyme Q is a synthetic version of a compound in the electron transport chain and is marketed to older adults as a way to slow aging by improving the immune system.[3] It has been reported that coenzyme Q does not boost immune function and may be dangerous for people with poor circulation.[1]

Healthy dietary patterns including consuming fruits, vegetables, and low-fat dairy products, and following a diet low in total and saturated fat, cholesterol, and sodium are linked to primary prevention and management of nutrition-related health conditions. This presents a challenge for meal planning for older adults diagnosed with diabetes, heart disease, kidney disease, AD and dementia, obesity, and other health issues. Nutritionists providing nutrition intervention to older adults with cardiac disease and/or hypertension may focus on stabilizing blood lipid levels and blood pressure while preserving eating pleasure. The Dietary Guidelines for Americans and/or the Dietary Approaches to Stop Hypertension (DASH) diet, which is high in potassium, magnesium, calcium, protein, and fiber, need to be utilized for the meal planning.[107] In addition, the menus need to include whole-grain breads and cereals, fruits, brown rice, and fresh or frozen vegetables to accomplish these guidelines. More recommendations are available from the Academy of Nutrition and Dietetics Evidence-Based Nutrition Practice Guidelines at http://www.AND evidencelibrary.com.

For the management of clients with chronic kidney disease receiving dialysis, the dietitian may recommend increasing total energy and protein intake to prevent undernutrition, plus individualized attention.[108,109] The recommendation for clients with AD or other types of dementia is to develop an individualized diet that utilizes nutrient-dense foods, plus feeding assistance as needed to achieve the individual's goals.[110] A research study showed that obese older adults losing weight resulted in a loss of both fat mass and lean body mass, which could exacerbate sarcopenia.[109] Therefore, the nutritionist may recommend adequate energy and protein intake plus regular physical activity to preserve lean body mass. In all the conditions discussed, the foods need to be seasoned with salt-free seasonings such as fresh or dried bay leaves, basil, celery seed, thyme, garlic powder, onions, lemon juice, or parsley.[111] Adequate seasoning of the foods will reduce food avoidance and improve the acceptance of the foods.

# ▶ Nutrition Assessment

Nutrition assessment is the interpretation of information from dietary, laboratory, anthropometric, and clinical evaluations. The information can be used to determine the nutrition status of older persons as influenced by the intake and utilization of nutrients.[112] Older populations can be assessed using surveys, surveillance, screening, or interventions. Information obtained through nutrition assessment can be used to determine baseline data. For example, the data from the National Health and Nutrition Examination Survey (NHANES) of noninstitutionalized older adults using the HEI showed that older adults consume poor-quality diets.[113] The HEI consists of 10 components and provides an overall picture of the type and quantity of foods people eat, their compliance with specific dietary recommendations, and the variety in their diets. The mean HEI score for 65 years of age or older was 67.6 out of 100, implying that their diets need improvement. The lowest component scores were for milk and fruit intakes. Approximately 20 percent of people 65 years of age or older had good diets, represented by a score of 81 or above. About 14 percent had poor diets, represented by a score of less than 51. The HEI score was significantly lower for poor older persons than for those with high income.[114]

Another study reported that the presence of children in the household was associated with adults 60 years or older consuming more total fat and saturated fat than adults without children. The foods consumed included whole milk; pizza; salty snack foods; beef (in the form of hamburgers); ice cream, ice milk, and milkshakes; calzones and lasagna; cheese dishes; bacon, sausage, and lunch meat; cakes and brownies; pies, donuts, and pastries; chocolate candy and fudge; margarine; and cookies, all representing convenience foods purchased for near-term consumption.[115] Research results also show that older persons with poor dental health had lower dietary intake levels of vitamin A, carotene, folic acid, and vitamin C, and scored low on a variety of diet, cholesterol, and sodium components of the HEI.[116]

Older adults are a heterogeneous group, with many different health conditions and broad variations in both mental and functional status. Therefore, it is difficult to make general statements that are applicable to all elderly persons. A comprehensive nutrition assessment should include the ABCDs discussed in **TABLE 11-5**.

## ▶ Nutrition Services That Promote Independent Living

Government programs to address nutrition needs and socioeconomic problems for older adults include the USDA's Supplemental Nutrition Assistance Program (SNAP) and Extension program, Adult Day Services food programs, Nutrition Assistance Program for Seniors (NAPS), the Elderly Nutrition Program of the Older Americans Act, and Meals on Wheels and other home-delivered meal programs. The Meals on Wheels program is designed to provide meals to participants who are homebound due to illness or disability and who cannot attend congregate meals. The meals are delivered to participants' homes by volunteers. They meet the nutrition needs of the participant and also provide an opportunity for human contact. In addition, nongovernmental home health programs provide food and nutrition services as part of a broader range of nursing and other support services. For instance, home healthcare nutritionists will shop, prepare food, and clean the kitchen afterward. Home care services allow individuals to receive the necessary support to stay in their homes for as long as possible.

**TABLE 11-5** The ABCDs of Nutritional Assessment for Older Persons[40,117,118]

### A: Anthropometric Measurements

- Height (may be difficult to assess due to poor posture; use knee-to-heel height instead)
- Weight
- Body mass index
- Skinfold measurements (mid-arm muscle circumference, triceps skinfold)

### B: Biochemical Parameters

- Serum albumin, hemoglobin
- Serum nutrient levels (vitamins A, D, C; sodium; potassium; iron; calcium; etc.)
- Serum cholesterol and glucose
- Antigen skin tests
- Urine and fecal analysis
- Fecal analysis for nutrients or metabolites that indicate infection or disease

### C: Clinical Evaluation

- Mental/cognitive status
- Blood pressure
- Medical history and the physical examination
- Gastrointestinal problems (heartburn, constipation, etc.)
- Hair, skin, fingernails shape, eyes, musculature
- Mouth and teeth, gums
- Dentition status
- Oral status (lesions)
- Breast examination status
- Tongue status
- Vision and hearing status
- Protein-energy malnutrition status

| **D: Dietary History and Functional Assessment** |
|---|

**Questions about:**

- Supplements and medication history
- Polypharmacy
- Poor appetite
- Changes in taste, smell, and digestive juices
- Eating alone
- Adequacy of the diet
- Skipping meals
- Special diets
- Lactose intolerance
- Anorexia
- Food security or food insecurity status
- Abnormal eating habits (anorexia)
- Inadequate bowel movement
- Ability to chew and swallow
- Activities of daily living (ADLs) and/or instrumental activities of daily living (IADLs)
- Social assessment (caregivers, annual income and living conditions, lives alone, housebound)
- Sleep deprivation
- Substance and alcohol abuse
- Lack of transportation and/or cooking and food storage equipment

## The Elderly Nutrition Program

Congress first appropriated funds under Title VII of the Older Americans Act of 1965 to begin the Senior Nutrition Program, also called the Elderly Nutrition Program (ENP), created in 1972. Programs such as Meals on Wheels and ENP provide meals to homebound people as well as to those in group settings. Most programs provide meals at least five times per week. The ENP is supported primarily with federal funds, volunteer time, and in-kind donations. Participant contributions make up the remainder.[1]

The Administration on Aging ENP provides grants to support nutrition services to older people throughout the country. The ENP was authorized under Title III, Grants for State and Community Programs on Aging. Title VI grant programs (included in 1978) are similar to Title III funds. It is grants for Native Americans, Alaskan Natives, and Native Hawaiians under the Older Americans Act, that are intended to improve the dietary intake of participants and offer participants opportunities to form new friendships and create informal support networks. These meals and other nutrition services are provided in a variety of settings, such as senior centers, schools, and individual homes.[1]

Meals served under the program must provide at least one third of the daily recommended dietary allowances established by the Food and Nutrition Board of the National Academy of Sciences National Research Council. In practice, the ENP's 3.1 million elderly participants are receiving an estimated 40 to 50 percent of most required nutrients.[1]

The ENP also provides a range of related services, including nutrition screening, assessment, education, and counseling, through some of the network's estimated 4,000 nutrition service providers. These services help older participants identify their general and special nutrition needs as they relate to health concerns such as hypertension and diabetes.

The services help older participants learn to shop for and/or to plan and prepare meals that are economical and help to manage or improve specific health problems as well as enhance their health and well-being. The congregate meal programs also provide older people with positive social contacts with other seniors at the group meal sites.

Volunteers who deliver meals to older persons who are homebound are encouraged to spend some time with the persons. The volunteers also offer an important opportunity to check on the welfare of homebound older persons and are encouraged to report any health or other problems that they may observe during their visits. In addition to providing nutrition and nutrition-related services, the ENP provides an important link to other needed supportive in-home and community-based services such as homemaker home health aide services, transportation, fitness programs, and even home repair and home modification programs.

## Eligibility

The ENP services are targeted to older people with the greatest economic or social need, with special attention given to low-income minorities. In addition to focusing on low-income and other older persons at risk for losing their independence, the following individuals may receive services[1]:

- A spouse of any age
- Disabled persons under age 60 who reside in housing facilities occupied primarily by the elderly where congregate meals are served
- Disabled persons who reside at home and accompany older persons to meals
- Nutrition service volunteers

American Indians, Alaskan Natives, and Native Hawaiians tend to have lower life expectancies and higher rates of illnesses at younger ages, so tribal organizations are given the option of setting the age at which older people can participate in the program.[13]

## Program Results

Research studies of congregate and home-delivered meals participants showed that the programs improved the dietary intake and nutrition status of their clients.[119,120] Participants had greater diversity in their diets and higher intakes of essential nutrients, and they were less likely to report food insecurity than nonparticipants.[121] Additional benefits were derived from the activities associated with the congregate meal services: improved diet counseling, exercise, and more opportunities for improved socialization.

But, regardless of these positive results, there are some gaps in the meal programs, such as a lack of weekend or evening meals for those who cannot afford food or cannot cook; a lack of special diets for people with special dietary needs (e.g., people on a low-sodium, low-fat, high-fiber, or soft diet) and meals that are too high in fat, unappetizing, or lacking in fiber or nutrients (e.g., calcium, selenium, vitamins C and E, or folate).[122] In addition, 41 percent of Title III ENP service providers have waiting lists for home-delivered meals, suggesting a significant unmet need.[1] **TABLE 11-6** shows the Title III-C (formerly known as Title VII) Meal Pattern.

A 3-year follow-up study to evaluate nutrition status and long-term outcome in the elderly living at home showed that about half of the Meals on Wheels participants were malnourished and that the people with a BMI of 28 or more showed the lowest risk for death within 3 years.[124] The special needs of the homebound elderly need to be given greater priority.[125] Their dietary intake might improve if more than one meal per day were provided, if the meal furnished to the client was prepared with greater percentages of the DRI, and if meals were provided 7 days a week rather than 5.

## Other Programs

Low-income individuals who purchase food also may be eligible for hot meals at community "food kitchens" such as Catholic Relief Services and the Salvation Army. These are similar to congregate meals sites, but they serve a broader population. Some food kitchens

| **TABLE 11-6** Title III-C Meal Pattern[123] | |
|---|---|
| **Food Type** | **Recommended Portion Size** |
| Meat or meat alternative | 3 oz cooked portion |
| Vegetables and fruits | Two ½- cup portions* |
| Enriched white or whole-grain bread or alternative | 1 serving (one slice bread or equivalent) |
| Butter or margarine | 1 tsp |
| Milk | 8 oz milk or calcium equivalent |
| Dessert | 1 serving |

*A vitamin C–rich fruit or vegetable is served each day; a vitamin A–rich fruit or vegetable is served at least three times per week.
Reproduced from: U.S. Department of Health and Human Services

and emergency food banks also offer groceries or vouchers to purchase food.[57] SNAP is another option that provides low-income elderly households with the means to purchase food. Unfortunately, because this program carries a "welfare" stigma, some older persons are reluctant to use it.

Although federal nutrition programs for older persons are free, most require determination of eligibility. In some cases, many people who need help buying food cannot meet the eligibility requirements. In 2003, Sharkey[122] found evidence of food insecurity among homebound older women who receive home-delivered meals, regardless of income level.[58] The study also reported that the participants relied on home-delivered meals for long-term food assistance. Visit the Administration on Aging website https://aoa.acl.gov for various nutrition programs that promote health in older persons. Successful Community Strategies at the end of this chapter presents the Senior Farmers' Market Nutrition Program success story.

## ▶ Home Healthcare Services

Home health care is a satisfactory alternative to care and rehabilitation within a hospital or medical setting. Home healthcare services also can help older individuals avoid institutionalization due to illness or recurrence of a previous illness.[50] Approximately 28 percent of individuals older than 65 years who live independently are unable to perform one or more ADLs, and 12.9 percent reported difficulties with IADLs without the assistance of another person or the use of physical assist devices.[50] Homemaker services provide assistance with meal preparation, transportation, bathing, and shopping.

Older persons may need medical nutrition therapy at home involving a variety of health issues, such as heart disease, renal disease, cancer, HIV/AIDS, and/or diabetes, as well as care for one who is on tube feeding such as total parenteral nutrition (TPN). A community nutritionist can make home visits to assess the elders' health status, monitor their nutritional status, and work closely with the home health agencies (speech, physical, or occupational therapists) to improve the lives of these elderly individuals. Usually, community nutritionists who are Registered Dietitians (RDs) may receive reimbursement from some insurance companies if a physician or hospital employs the RD or if services are medically supervised or medically necessary.[51]

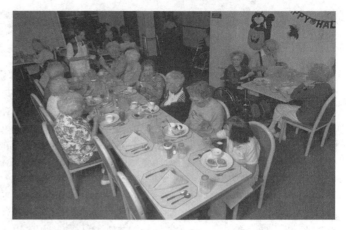

An older person's ability to care for himself or herself is typically evaluated using the instrumental activities of daily living (IADLs), such as preparing meals for oneself.
Courtesy of Ken Hammond/USDA

## Activities of Daily Living

An older person's ability to care for himself or herself is typically evaluated using the **ADLs** and the **IADLs**. The ADLs listed here are used to evaluate a person's ability to perform personal care, either independently, with some help, or with no help at all[13,36]:

- Bathing oneself
- Dressing oneself
- Feeding oneself
- Using the toilet
- Transferring between bed and chair

The IADLs relate to a person's ability to perform housekeeping chores and other activities required to remain independent:

- Prepare meals
- Perform house-cleaning chores
- Handle money and balance a checkbook
- Shop without help
- Use the telephone
- Leave the house without help

The current practice of elder care is community-based. The goal is to provide services that will enable older persons to remain in their own home or in the home of a family member. Older persons who need help with the ADLs or IADLs may receive help from family members; however, increasing numbers of older persons live some distance from their children and others do not have children or other family. To fill this need, services are now being provided by home health agencies, area agencies on aging that receive state and federal funds, and private home care companies.[86]

## Successful Community Strategies

### The Seattle Senior Farmers' Market Nutrition Program[115]

The Senior Farmers' Market Nutrition Program is one of the federal food assistance programs for older persons. In the summer and fall of 2001, the Seattle Senior Farmers' Market Nutrition Program supplied a market basket that contained a variety of seasonal local fresh fruits and vegetables to 480 homebound low-income seniors. The purpose of the intervention program was to increase the fresh fruit and vegetable intake of homebound Meals on Wheels participants and compare their intake with other Meals on Wheels homebound seniors who live outside the project service area.

The program was a collaborative effort with five organizations, including the University of Washington Health Promotion Research Center. Subjects for both the intervention and control groups were recruited via flyers that were delivered by Meals on Wheels drivers. Local farmers were contracted to provide the fruits and vegetables in season. The Meals on Wheels drivers volunteered to deliver the market baskets to the participants' homes every 2 weeks. A newsletter that described the produce, provided recipes for less common seasonal foods, and promoted eating fruits and vegetables accompanied each basket. Each basket contained dark green or orange fruits and vegetables. An average of 1.6 servings of vegetables and 0.67 servings of fruit were provided per day over a period of 5 months. The fruits and vegetables supplied 30 percent of the U.S. Recommended Dietary Allowance for vitamin C, 40 percent for vitamin A, and 8 percent for folate daily for 5 months. Both the basket recipients and control respondents were interviewed by telephone before basket deliveries started and at the end of the intervention. All participants were mailed a serving-size guide with pictures of representative foods. Participants were required to have the guide with them at the time of the telephone survey.

At the end of the intervention period, participants who received the baskets of fruits and vegetables reported consuming an increase of 1.04 servings of fruits and vegetables per day. At baseline, 22 percent of the basket recipients were consuming 5 or more servings of fruits and vegetables per day, but by the end of the season, 39 percent reported consuming 5 or more servings per day. The conclusion was that home delivery of fruits and vegetables is an effective way to increase fruit and vegetable intake in homebound seniors.

## Successful Community Intervention Strategies[126]

### Eat Better & Move More: A Community-Based Program Designed to Improve Diets and Increase Physical Activity Among Older Americans.

This 10-site intervention study was carried out in Florida. The purpose of the intervention was to assess the outcomes of an integrated nutrition and exercise program designed for Older Americans Act Nutrition Program. This program was a part of the Administration on Aging's "You Can! Campaign." Preintervention and postintervention assessments focused on dietary intake and physical activity stages of change, self-reported health status, and program satisfaction.

The program included 620 individuals with an average age of 74.6 years. Eighty-two percent of the participants were women, and 41 percent were members of racial/ethnic minority groups. The lead staff members of this program attended a 1.5-day workshop on protocol implementation, which included eight registered dietitians, one registered nurse, and one Native American program manager at each site.

Mini-talks and activities for group nutrition and physical activity sessions were carried out weekly for 12 weeks. Mini-talks also were used to emphasize the benefits of eating more fruits, vegetables, calcium-rich foods, and dietary fiber, sensible portion sizes, and diet deficiencies or excesses.

Physical activity mini-talks emphasized the benefits of walking. Participants learned how to use a step counter, perform simple stretching exercises, walk more at home and away, dress for all weather, and stay hydrated. Participants checked off food choices and recorded the number of steps taken each day on "Tips & Tasks" sheets.

The questionnaires used for the study included "stage-of-change" questions. To show their current stage, participants selected from five statements reflecting each stage of change. For example:

- *Precontemplation* ("I do not eat 2 to 3 servings of milk, cheese, yogurt, and calcium-rich soy products per day, and I do not intend to begin eating 2 to 3 servings of milk, cheese, yogurt, and calcium-rich soy products per day in the next 6 months.")
- *Contemplation* ("I do not eat; but I intend to begin eating in the next 6 months.")
- *Preparation* ("I do not eat, but I intend to begin eating in the next 30 days.")

## Successful Community Intervention Strategies *(continued)*

- *Action* ("I have been eating, but for less than 6 months.")
- *Maintenance* ("I have been eating for more than 6 months.") The phrase "doing regular physical activity" was substituted in the exercise stage-of-change question.[126]

Results show that 73 percent and 75 percent of the participants made a significant advance of one or more nutrition and physical activity stages of change, respectively.

Twenty-four percent reported improved health status. Daily intake of fruit increased one or more servings among 31% of participants; vegetables, 37%; and fiber, 33%. Daily steps increased 35%; blocks walked increased by 45%; and stairs climbed increased by 24%.

The researchers stated that the program was easy to implement and it improved diets and activity levels of the participants. The researchers also recommended that local providers should offer more such programs with the goal of enabling older Americans take simple steps toward successful aging.

# Learning Portfolio

## Chapter Summary

- The factors that influence aging are interrelated and affect older persons' nutritional status by decreasing their motivation to eat and their ability to acquire and enjoy food.
- Excessive use of over-the-counter and prescription medications can affect nutritional status and contribute to malnutrition.
- According to research from the Alzheimer's disease Cooperative Study, large intakes of vitamin E are associated with slowing the progression of AD.
- The symptoms of dehydration among older adults include swollen tongue, constipation, electrolyte imbalance, nausea and vomiting, mental confusion, sunken eyeballs, increased body temperature, decreased urine output, pressure ulcers, and urinary tract infections.
- The Supplemental Nutrition Assistance Program (SNAP) provides low-income elderly households with the means to purchase food. Unfortunately, because the program carries a "welfare" stigma, some elders are reluctant to use it.
- The Meals on Wheels program is designed to provide meals to participants who are homebound due to illness or disability and cannot attend congregate meals.

## Critical Thinking Activities

- Describe your impression of a typical older person and compare it with the demographic information on older adults given in this chapter.
- Watch television for 1 hour and identify both positive and negative ways in which older persons are portrayed. What types of merchandise are directed toward older persons? How beneficial are these products, including nutrition products, to older persons?
- Interview an older person within your family and ask him or her to list any health problems. Are the health problems nutrition related? Ask him or her to include a typical day's activities in the list. Was physical activity listed and, if so, how often? Ask the older person to keep a 24-hour dietary recall and determine the nutrient intakes, with specific attention to fluid intake. Use the information in this activity to:
  - Develop screening recommendations for your relative.
  - Find resources in your area that would be able to provide meals and other services.
- Volunteer at a congregate meal or home-delivered nutrition program and provide services such as preparing and serving meals.
- Participate in fun activities such as playing bingo with older persons.
- Prepare and present a 10- to 15-minute demonstration/lecture on how using multiple types of over-the-counter and prescribed medicines affects nutrition.
- Divide into groups and create a plan to educate congregate meal participants about the health benefits of being physically active at any size and the possibility of attaining weight reduction.
  - Educate participants on how to use the Nutrition Facts Panel on food products and on how to select appropriate portion sizes for healthful diets, including clarification of the serving size, using the MyPlate Food Guide.

- Provide participants with a list of foods that are high in fiber, saturated fat, and cholesterol.
- Identify the types of assessments that could be used to monitor and determine the impact of a nutrition education program.

- Use the Practical Approach to Nutrition Screening tool (Table 11-3) and Determine: Warning Signs of Poor Nutritional Health (Box 11-3) with at least one congregate meal participant and present the findings.

## 🔍 CASE STUDY 11-1: Nutrition Education for Reducing Chronic Diseases in Older Adults

The Illinois Department of Public Health funded a nutrition education program for persons 60 years or older because they wanted seniors to experience successful aging. The purpose of the education program was to reduce the percentage of obese adults and coronary heart disease deaths. The program's creator, Nikki, was required to recruit and educate at least 300 older adults. She was able to reach the target number of participants by collaborating with the local Illinois Lung and Heart Association. Part of her education program included screening activities. She carried out biochemical and dietary assessments. Results showed that 60 percent of the participants were obese, with a BMI over 30 and a body fat percentage of 46 percent. The average blood pressure was 160/90; 62 percent of the participants had a total blood cholesterol of 340 mg/dl and blood glucose of 110 to 150 mg/dl (tested after fasting). Dietary analysis showed low calcium, fiber, vitamin D, and vitamin A intakes—below the recommended amounts for their age. Total calories from fat was 40 percent, calories from protein 30 percent, and from carbohydrates 30 percent. Some of the participants binge ate, and some had lactose intolerance.

### Questions

1. The majority of Nikki's participants want to experience successful aging. What is the definition of successful aging? What are the four features of successful aging identified by Fisher?
2. Nikki incorporated Healthy People 2010 objectives into her objectives for the program. What are a few examples of the Healthy People 2010 objectives set to promote healthy lifestyles for older adults?
3. One of the goals of the program is to reduce the potential of experiencing chronic diseases evident in this population. What diseases that have an impact on nutritional status are common in the elderly?
4. Nikki read about the theories of aging before providing the education program because she thinks that the participants may ask her about it. What are some of the theories of aging? Briefly describe each.
5. What lifestyle and socioeconomic factors may influence the aging process of Nikki's participants? Briefly describe each.
6. Nikki is aware that some of the participants may be taking several medications, so she included the risk factors for drug–nutrient interactions (DNIs) in her education program. What are the risk factors?
7. The participants were interested in the changes they are experiencing with age. What are some of the physiological changes that occur with aging that Nikki will discuss with the participants?
8. She also explained the changes that occur to the senses due to aging. What are some of the chemosensory losses that may happen with aging?
9. Some of the participants are concerned about Alzheimer's disease. What is Alzheimer's disease? What are the major stages?
10. Nikki carried out an assessment using the Determine Your Nutritional Health checklist. What does it include?
11. Nikki explained the risk factors of poor nutritional status to the participants. What are risk factors associated with poor nutritional status?
12. Several nutrition services are available for the elderly, and Nikki provided her clients with that information. What are the nutrition services that promote independent living among older adults?
13. What are activities of daily living and instrumental activities of daily living? What are some examples of each that Nikki should know?
14. Work in small groups or individually to discuss the case study and practice using the Nutrition Care Process chart provided on the companion website. You can also add other nutrition- and health-related conditions or assessments to the case study to make the case study more challenging and interesting.

## Think About It

**Answer:** The use of over-the-counter and prescription medications can contribute to malnutrition. Drugs can change food intake patterns and interfere with an individual's ability to gather and prepare meals. They also may induce alterations in mental status, blood pressure, urinary continence, coordination, or gait. Drugs may also have a primary effect on diminishing or increasing appetite or may cause an unwanted side effect; for example, drugs that alter taste perception also can cause gastrointestinal discomfort and decrease food intake. The incidence of nausea and vomiting can be common with many medications and, if severe (e.g., with chemotherapy), may result in weight loss and nutrient deficiencies.

## Key Terms

**activities of daily living (ADLs):** Performing personal care, either independently or with help. Determining whether an older person can perform ADLs helps evaluate ability to care for himself or herself.

**Alzheimer's disease (AD; senile dementia of the Alzheimer's type):** A disease that results in the relentless and irreversible loss of mental function.

**anorexia of aging:** The loss of appetite and wasting associated with old age.

**compression of morbidity:** The postponement of the onset of chronic disease such that disability occupies an increasingly smaller proportion of the life span.

**free radicals:** Atoms or molecules that have lost an electron and vigorously pursue its replacement. Free radicals can damage normal cell constituents.

**instrumental activities of daily living (IADLs):** Performing housekeeping chores and other activities required for a person to remain independent.

**life expectancy:** The average length of life span for a population of individuals.

**longevity:** A measure of life's duration in years.

**polypharmacy:** The use or prescription of two or more different drugs to treat one or more health problems.

**sensory-specific satiety:** The change in palatability of a food once an individual begins to eat it.

**successful aging:** Slowing the number and rate of aging changes through positive lifestyle choices or health-related interventions.

## References

1. Administration on Aging, Department of Health and Human Services. The Elderly Nutrition Program. http://www.aoa.gov/. Accessed March 17, 2017.
2. Hoyert DL, Heron MP, Murphy SL, Kung HC. Deaths: final data for 2003. http://www.cdc.gov/. Accessed March 17, 2017.
3. Grosvenor M, Smolin L. *Nutrition: From Science to Life.* Philadelphia, PA: Harcourt College Publishers; 2016.
4. Centers for Disease Control and Prevention. Mortality experience. http://www.cdc.gov/nchs/data/nvsr/nvsr64/nvsr64_02.pdf. Accessed March 17, 2017.
5. Fries JF. *The Compression of Morbidity.* Vol 83. Oxford, UK: Blackwell; 2005:801-823.
6. Hubert H, Eaker E, Garrison R, Castelli W. Life-style correlates of risk factor change in young adults: an eight-year study of coronary heart disease risk factors in the Framingham offspring. *Am J Epidemiol.* 2008;125(5):812-831.
7. Raynaud-Simon A, Lesourd B. Malnutrition in the elderly: clinical consequences. *Presse Med.* 2000;29(39):2183-2190.
8. AARP Organization. Food insecurity. http://www.aarp.org/content/dam/aarp/aarp_foundation/2015-PDFs/AF-Food-Insecurity-2015Update-Final-Report.pdf. Accessed March 17, 2017.
9. The Henry Kaiser Family Foundation. Poverty among seniors. http://files.kff.org/attachment/issue-brief-poverty-among-seniors-an-updated-analysis-of-national-and-state-level-poverty-rates-under-the-official-and-supplemental-poverty-measures. Accessed March 17, 2017.
10. Bowman S. Low economic status is associated with suboptimal intakes of nutritious foods by adults in National Health and Nutrition Examination Survey 1999-2002. *Nutr Res.* 2007;27:515-523.
11. Ervin RB. Healthy Eating Index scores among adults, 60 years of age and older, by sociodemographic and health characteristics: United States, 1999-2002. Centers for Disease Control and Prevention. http://www.cdc.gov/nchs. Accessed March 17, 2017.
12. Bengle R, Sinnett S, Johnson T, Johnson M, et al. Food insecurity is associated with cost-related medication non-adherence in community-dwelling, low-income older adults in Georgia. *J Nutr Gerontol Geriatr.* 2010;29(2):170-191.
13. Fisher B. Successful aging, life satisfaction, and generativity in later life. *Int J Aging Human Dev.* 1995;41(3):239-250.
14. Gary WE, Wethington E, Coleman E. Income health inequalities among older persons. the mediating role of multiple risk exposures. *J Aging Health.* 2008;20(1):107-125.

15. Kerschner H, Pegues J. Productive aging: a quality of life agenda. *J Am Diet Assoc.* 1998;98(12):1445-1448.

16. Ryff C. Beyond Ponce de Leon and life satisfaction: new directions in quest of successful ageing. *Int J Behav Dev.* 1989;12(1):35-55.

17. National Center for Health Statistics. Healthy People 2010: progress review focus area 16 maternal infant and child health. http://www.cdc.gov. Accessed March 17, 2017.

18. Office of Disease Prevention and Health Promotion. Healthy People 2020 objectives. 2016. https://www.healthypeople.gov/2020/data-search/Search-the-Data/page/1/0?nid=&items_per_page=10&pop=&ci=&se=&f%5B%5D=field_topic_area%3A3493. Accessed March 17, 2017.

19. US Dept of Health and Human Services. Healthy People 2020: Maternal, Infant, and Child Health. https://www.healthypeople.gov/2020/topics-objectives/topic/maternal-infant-and-child-health. Accessed March 16, 2017.

20. Gerberding JL. Healthy Aging: *Preventing Disease and Improving Quality of Life Among Older Americans.* 2006. http://www.cdc.gov/. Accessed March 17, 2017.

21. Kennedy ET. Evidence for nutritional benefits in prolonging wellness. *Am J Clinc Nutr.* 2006;83(2):410S-414S.

22. Heilbronn LK, Ravussin E. Calorie restriction and aging: review of the literature and implications for studies in humans. *Am J Clinic Nutr.* 2003;78(3):361-369.

23. Mathers JJ. Nutritional modulation of ageing: genomic and epigenetic approaches. *Mech Ageing Dev.* 2006;127(6):584-589.

24. Abete PP, Della Morte D, Mazzella F, D'Ambrosio D, et al. Lifestyle and prevention of cardiovascular disease in the elderly: an Italian perspective. *Am J Geriatr Cardiol.* 2006;15(1):28-34.

25. Wardlaw G, Kessel M. *Perspectives in Nutrition.* 10th ed. New York, NY: McGraw-Hill; 2016.

26. Brown JE, Sugarman I, Krinke UB, Murtaugh MA, et al. *Nutrition Through Life Cycle.* 5th ed. Belmont CA: Wadsworth Thomson; 2014.

27. Evans PH. Free radicals in brain metabolism and pathology. *Brit Med Bull.* 1993;49:577-587.

28. Yusuf S, Dagenais G, Pogue J. Vitamin E supplementation and cardiovascular events in high-risk patients: the heart Outcomes Prevention Evaluation Study Investigators. *N Engl J Med.* 2000;342(3):154-160.

29. De Grey AD. Free radicals in aging: causal complexity and its biomedical implications. *Free Radic Res.* 2006;40(12):1244-1249.

30. Stadtman EE. Protein oxidation and aging. *Free Radic Res.* 2006;40(12):1250-1258.

31. Harper JM, Leathers CW, Austad SN. Does caloric restriction extend life in wild mice? *Aging Cell.* 2006;5(6):441-449.

32. McCay CM, Crowell MF, Maynard LA. The effect of retarded growth upon the length of life and upon ultimate size. *J Nutr.* 1935;10:63-79.

33. Nnakwe N. The effect of age and dietary restriction on bone strength, calcium and phosphorus contents of male Fischer 344 rats. *J Nutri Health Aging.* 1998;2(3):149-152.

34. Mattison JA, Roth GS, Lane MA, Ingram DK. Dietary restriction in aging nonhuman primates. *Interdisc Top Gerontol* 2007;35:137-158.

35. Kelly DE, Goodpaster BH, Storlien L. Muscle triglyceride and insulin resistance. *Annu Rev Nutr.* 2002;22:325-346.

36. Schlenker E, Gilbert JA. *Williams' Essentials of Nutrition and Diet Therapy.* 11th ed. St. Louis, MO: Mosby; 2015.

37. National Institute on Alcohol Abuse and Alcoholism. Alcohol and nutrition. http://www.alcoholism.about.com. Accessed March 26, 2016.

38. US Dept of Agriculture, US Dept of Health and Human Services. *Nutrition and Your Health: Dietary Guidelines for Americans* (5th ed.). Home and Garden Bull No. 232. Washington, DC: US Dept of Agriculture, US Dept of Health and Human Services; 2005.

39. Dawson DD, Grant BF, Li TK. Quantifying the risks associated with exceeding recommended drinking limits. *Alcohol Clin Exp Res.* 2005;29(5):902-908.

40. Worthington P. *Practical Aspects of Nutritional Support: An Advance Practice Guide.* Philadelphia, PA: Saunders; 2004.

41. Stout CM, Popovich, DJ. Undiagnosed alcoholism and prescription drug misuse among the elderly. *Caring.* 2001;20(1):20-23.

42. Davis SR, Castelo-Branco C, Chedraui P, Lumsden MA, et al. Understanding weight gain at menopause. *Climacteric.* 2012;15(5):419-429.

43. Rigler SK. Alcoholism in the elderly. *Am Fam Physician.* 2000;661:1710.

44. Michel KE, Higgins C. Nutrient-drug interactions in nutritional support. *J Vet Emerg Crit Care.* 2002;12(3):163-167.

45. Nnakwe N. Medication and dietary practices of independent living healthy African-American older persons. *J Nutr Elderly.* 2001;21(1):39-58.

46. Worthington PH. *Practical Aspect of Nutritiona Support: An Advanced Practice Guide.* Philadelphia, PA: Saunders; 2004.

47. Kaufman DW, Kelly JP, Rosenberg L, Anderson TE, et al. Recent patterns of medication use in the ambulatory adult population of the United States: the Slone Survey. *JAMA.* 2002;287(3):337-344.

48. Pronsky ZM, Crowe JP, Young VSL, Elbe D, et al. *Food Medication Interactions.* 15th ed. Birchrunville, PA: Food Medication Interactions; 2015.

49. Davis MA, Murphy SP, Neuhaus JM, Gee L, et al. Living arrangements affect dietary quality for U.S. adults aged 50 years and older: NHANES III 1988–1994. *J Nutr.* 2000;130:2256-2264.

50. Escott-Stump S. *Nutrition and Diagnosis-Related Care.* 8th ed. New York, NY: Wolters Kluwer, Lippincott Williams & Wilkins; 2015.

51. Mahan KL, Escott-Stump S. *Krause's Food, Nutrition, and Diet Therapy.* 11th ed. St. Louis, MO: Mosby; 2012.

52. Stanfield PS, Hui YH. *Nutrition and Diet Therapy Self-Instructional Modules.* 12th ed. Sudbury, MA: Jones & Bartlett; 2012.

53. Lee J, Frongillo EA. Nutritional and health consequences associated with food insecurity among US elderly persons. *J Nutr.* 2001;131(5):1503-1509.

54. US Dept of Health and Human Services, Association on Aging. Profile of older Americans. https://aoa.acl.gov/aging_statistics/profile/index.aspx. Accessed March 16, 2017.

55. Beers MH, Porter RS, Jones TV, Kaplan JL, et al, eds. *The Merck Manual of Geriatrics.* 19th ed. Whitehouse Station, NY: Merck Research Laboratories; 2011.

56. ASPEN Board of Directors, Clinical Guidelines Task Force. Guidelines for the use of parenteral and enteral nutrition in adult and pediatric patients. *J Parenter Enteral Nutr.* 2000;26:(1 suppl):1SA-138SA.

57. Saltzman JR, Russell RM. The aging gut: nutritional issues. *Gastroenterol Clin North Am.* 1998;27(2):309-324.

58. Seals DR, Monahan KD, Bell C, Tanaka H, et al. The aging cardiovascular system: changes in autonomic function at rest and in response to exercise. *Int J Sport Nutr Exerc Metab.* 2001;11(suppl):S189-S195.

59. McGee M, Binkley J, Jensen GL. *The Science and Practice of Nutrition Support.* Dubuque, IA: Kendall/Hunt; 2001.

60. Harris TB, Visser M, Everhart J, Cauley J, et al. Waist circumference and sagittal diameter reflect total body fat better than visceral fat in older men and women: The Health, Aging and Body Composition Study. *Ann NY Acad Sci.* 2000;904:462-473.

61. Guo SS, Roche AF, Chumlea WC. Tracking of body mass index in children in relation to overweight in adulthood. *Am J Clin Nutr.* 1999;70(suppl):145S-148S.

62. Van den Beld AW, de Jong FH, Grobbee DE, Pols HA, et al. Measures of bioavailable serum testosterone and estradiol and their relationships with muscle strength, bone density, and body composition in elderly men. *J Clin Endocrinol Metab.* 2000;85(9):3276-3282.

63. Khosla S, Melton LJ, Atkinson EJ, O'Fallon WM. Relationship of serum sex steroid levels to longitudinal chnages in bone density in young versus elderly men. *J Clin Endocrinol Metab.* 2001;86(8):3555-3561.

64. Sahota O, Hosking DJ. The contribution of nutritional factors to osteopenia in the elderly. *Curr Opin Clin Nutr Metab Care.* 2001;4(1):15-19.

65. Vicente-Rodriguez G, Ara I, Pérez-Gómez J, Dorado C, et al. Muscular development and physical activity as major determinants of femoral bone mass acquisition during growth. *Brit J Sport Med.* 2005;39:611-616.

66. Klotzbach-Shimomura K. Project Healthy Bones: an osteoporosis prevention program for older adults. *J Exten.* 2001;39(3):293-303.

67. Brownie S. Why are elderly individuals at risk of nutritional deficiency? *Int J Nurs Pract.* 2006;12(2):110-118.

68. National Heart, Lung, and Blood Institute. Disease and conditions index: pernicious ancmia. http://www.nhlbi.nih.gov. Accessed March 17, 2017.

69. Yukawa H, Takao S. Aging-related changes of food intake in elderly subjects living in an urban community and relation with vital prognosis: results of an 8-year longitudinal study (TMIG-LISA). *Geriatr Gerontol Int.* 2003;3(S1):S55-S62.

70. Mayo Clinic. Malnutrition and seniors: when a relative doesn't eat enough. *Senior Health.* http://www.mayoclinic.com/. Accessed March 17, 2017.

71. Pribitkin ER, Cowart BJ. Prevalence and causes of severe taste loss in a chemosensory clinic population. *Ann Otol Rhinol Laryngol.* 2003;112(11):971-978.

72. University of Connecticut, Taste and Smell Center. General information. http://www.uchc.edu. Accessed March 17, 2017.

73. Schiffman SS. Intensification of sensory properties of foods for the elderly. *J Nutr.* 2000;130(4S suppl):927S-930S.

74. Drewnowski A. Sensory control of energy density at different life stages. *Proc Nutr Soc.* 2000;59:239-244.

75. Takahashi RR. Nutritional risk in community-dwelling elderly long-term care insurance recipients. *Nippon Ronen Igakkai Zasshi.* 2006;43(3):375-382.

76. Guigoz YY. The Mini Nutritional Assessment (MNA(R)): review of the literature—what does it tell us? *J Nutr Health Aging.* 2006;10(6):466-487.

77. Mitchell DC, Smiciklas-Wright H, Friedmann JM, Gordon J. Dietary intake assessed by the nutrition screening initiative level II screen is a sensitive but not a specific indicator of nutrition risk in older adults. *J Am Diet Assoc.* 2002;102(6):842-844.

78. Peng CC, Glassman PA. Incidence and severity of potential drug–dietary supplement interactions in primary care patients. *Arch Intern Med.* 2004;164(6):630-636.

79. Shahar DD, Shai I, Vardi H, Fraser D. Dietary intake and eating patterns of elderly people in Israel: who is at nutritional risk? *Eur J Clin Nutr.* 2003;57(1):18-25.

80. Sharkey JJ. Variation in nutritional risk among Mexican American and non-Mexican American homebound elders who receive home-delivered meals. *J Nutr Elder.* 2004;23(4):1-19.

81. Huffman GB, Grove B. Evaluating and treating unintentional weight loss in the elderly. *Am Fam Physician.* 2002;65(4):640-650.

82. Morley JE, Baumgartner RN, Roubenoff R, Mayer J, et al. Sarcopenia. *J Lab Clin Med.* 2001;137(4):231-243.

83. Morley J. Anorexia, body composition, and ageing. *Curr Opin Clin Nutr Metab Care.* 2001;4(1):9-13.

84. White R, Ashworth A. How drug therapy can affect, threaten and compromise nutritional status. *J Human Nutr Diet.* 2000;13(2):119-129.

85. American Dietetic Association. Position of the American Dietetic Association: nutrition, aging and the continuum of care. *J Am Diet Assoc.* 2000;100:580-595.

86. Armstron-Esther CA, Browne KD, Armstrong E, Sander L. The institutionalized elderly: dry to the bone! *Int J Nurs Stud.* 1996;33(6):619-628.

87. Lindeman RD, Romero LJ, Liang HC, Baumgartner RN, et al. Do elderly persons need to be encouraged to drink more fluids? *J Gerontol Bio Sci Med Sci.* 2000;55(7):M361-M365.

88. Bhalla A, Sankaralingam S, Dundas R, Swaminathan R, et al. Influence of raised plasma osmolality on clinical outcome after acute stroke. *Stroke.* 2000;31(9):2043-2048.

89. Wingate DD, Phillips SF, Lewis SJ, Malagelada JR, et al. Guidelines for adults on self-medication for the treatment of acute diarrhoea. *Aliment Pharmacol Ther.* 2001;15(6):773-782.

90. National Institute of Aging, US National Institutes of Health. Alzheimer's disease fact sheet. http://www.nia.nih.gov. Accessed March 26, 2016.

91. Juan WY, Basiotis PP. More than one in three older Americans may not drink enough water: insight 27 September 2002. *Fam Econ Nutr Rev.* 2004;16:49-51.

92. Valtin H. "Drink at least eight glasses of water a day." Really? Is there scientific evidence for '8x8'? *Am J Physiol Regul Integr Compar Physiol.* 2002;283(5):R993-R1004.

93. Andorn A, Pappolla MA. Catecholamines inhibit lipid peroxidation in young, aged, and Alzheimer's disease brain. *Free Radic Viol Med.* 2001;31(3):315-320.

94. Giannakopoulos PP, Gold G, Kövari E, von Gunten A, et al. Assessing the cognitive impact of Alzheimer disease pathology and vascular burden in the aging brain: the Geneva experience. *Acta Neuropathol.* 2007;113(1):1-12.

95. Farias ST, Mungas D, Reed BR, Harvey D, et al. MCI is associated with deficits in everyday functioning. *Alzheimer Dis Assoc Disord.* 2006;20(4):217-223.

96. Otsuka M, Yamaguchi K, Ueki A. Similarities and differences between Alzheimer's disease and vascular dementia from the viewpoint of nutrition. *Ann N Y Acad Sci.* 2002;977:155-161.

97. Morris MM, Evans DA, Schneider JA, Tangney CC, et al. Dietary folate and vitamins B-12 and B-6 not associated with incident Alzheimer's disease. *J Alzheimers Dis.* 2006;9(4):435-443.

98. Abou-Saleh MM, Coppen A. Folic acid and the treatment of depression. *J Psychosomat Res.* 2006;61(3):285-287.

99. Morris MM, Evans DA, Bienias JL, Tangney CC, et al. Dietary intake of antioxidant nutrients and the risk of incident Alzheimer disease in a biracial community study. *JAMA.* 2002;287(24):3230-3237.

100. Young KK, Greenwood CE, van Reekum R, Binns MA. A randomized, crossover trial of high-carbohydrate foods in nursing home residents with Alzheimer's disease: associations among intervention response. *J Gerontol A Biol Sci Med Sci.* 2005;60(8):1039-1045.

101. Mittelman MM, Haley WE, Clay OJ, Roth DL. Improving caregiver well-being delays nursing home placement of patients with Alzheimer disease. *Neurology.* 2006;67(9):1592-1599.

102. Mayo Clinic. Nutrition and healthy eating. http://www.mayoclinic.org/healthy-lifestyle/nutrition-and-healthy-eating/basics/nutrition-basics/hlv-20049477. Accessed March 16, 2017.

103. Niedert KC, Dorner, B. *Nutrition Care of the Older Adult.* 2nd ed. Chicago, IL: American Dietetic Association; 2004.

104. Miller SL, Wolfe RR. The danger of weight loss in the elderly. *J Nutr Health Aging.* 2008;12(7):487-491.

105. Alzheimer's Association. Stages of Alzheimer's. http://www.alz.org/alzheimers_disease_stages _of_alzheimers.asp. Accessed March 26, 2016.

106. Young KWH, Green CE. Shift in diurnal feeding patterns in nursing home residents with Alzheimer's disease. *J Gerontol.* 2001;56:700-706.

107. American Dietetic Association. Position of American Dietetic Association: practice paper of the American Dietetic Association—individualized nutrition approaches for older adults in health care communities. *J Am Diet Assoc.* 2010;110(10):1554-1563.

108. Gibson RS. *Principles of Nutritional Assessment.* 2nd ed. Dunedin, New Zealand: Oxford University Press; 2005.

109. Dixon LB, Winkleby MA, Radimer KL. Dietary intakes and serum nutrients differ between adults from food-insufficient and food-sufficient families: Third National Health and Nutrition Examination Survey, 1988-1994. *J Nutr.* 2001;131(4):1232-1246.

110. Lin BH. Nutrition and health characteristics of low-income populations: Healthy Eating Index. Agriculture Information Bull. 796–796-1. 2005. US Dept of Agriculture Economic Research Services. http://www.ers.usda.gov. Accessed March 17, 2017.

111. Laroche HL, Hofer TP, Davis MM. Adult fat intake associated with the presence of children in households: findings from NHANES III. *J Am Board Fam Med.* 2007;20(1):9-15.

112. Sahyoun NR, Lin CL, Krall E. Nutritional status of the older adult is associated with dentition status. *J Am Diet Assoc.* 2003;103(1):61-66.

113. Blecher L. Using forecasting techniques to predict meal demand in Title IIIc Congregate Lunch Programs. *J Am Diet Assoc.* 2004;104(8):1281-1283.

114. Millen BE, Ohls JC, Ponza M, McCool AC. The elderly nutrition program: an effective national framework for preventive nutrition interventions. *Am Diet Assoc.* 2002;102(2):234-240.

115. Gollub EA, Weddle DO. Improvements in nutritional intake and quality of life among frail homebound older adults receiving home-delivered breakfast and lunch. *J Am Diet Assoc.* 2004;104(8):1227-1235.

116. Bartali B, Frongillo E, Bandinelli S, Lauretani F, et al. Low nutrient intake is an essential component of frailty in older persons. *J Gerontol A Biol Sci Med Sci.* 2006;61(6):589-593.

117. Insel PT, Ross D, McMahon K, Bernstein M. *Nutrition: 2002 Update.* 5th ed. Sudbury, MA: Jones & Bartlett Publisher; 2014.

118. Lutz C, Przytulski K. *Nutrition and Diet Therapy.* 5th ed. Philadelphia, PA: F.A. Davis Company; 2010.

119. Fey-Yensan N, English C, Ash S, Wallace C, et al. Food safety risk identified in a population of elderly home-delivered meal participants. *J Am Diet Assoc.* 2001;101:1055-1057.

120. Saletti A, Johansson L, Yifter-Lindgren E, Wissing U, et al. Nutritional status and a 3-year follow-up in elderly receiving support at home. *Gerontology.* 2005;51:192-198.

121. Eppich S, Fernandez C, Study finds Chapel Hill, NC soup kitchen serves nutritious meals. *J Am Diet Assoc.* 2004;104(8):1284-1286.

122. Sharkey J. Risk and presence of food insufficiency are associated with low nutrient intakes and multimorbidity among homebound older women who receive home-delivered meals. *J Nutr.* 2003;133(11):3485-3491.

123. US Dept of Agriculture Food and Nutrition Service. Nutrition Services Incentive Program. 2007. http://www.fns.usda.gov/fdd/programs /nsip/. Accessed March 17, 2017.

124. Fox MK, Hamilton W, Lin BH. Effects of food assistance and nutrition programs on nutrition and health. Vol 4. Executive summary of the literature review. FANRR-19. Economic Research Service, US Dept of Agriculture; 2016.

125. Johnson DB, Beaudoin S, Smith LT, Beresford SA, et al. Increasing fruit and vegetable intake in homebound elders: the Seattle Senior Farmers' Market Nutrition Pilot Program. *Prev Chronic Dis.* 2004;1(1):AO3.

126. Wellman NS, Kamp B, Kirk-Sanchez J, Johnson M. Eat Better & Move More: a community-based program designed to improve diets and increase physical activity among older Americans. *Am J Public Health.* 2007;97(4):710–717.

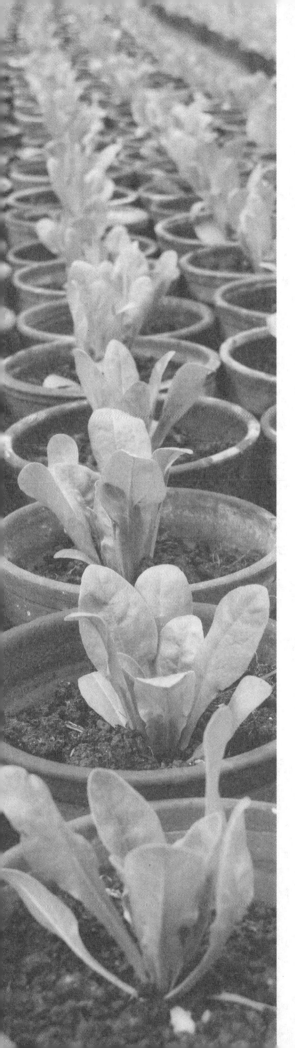

# PART III
# Delivering Successful Nutrition Services

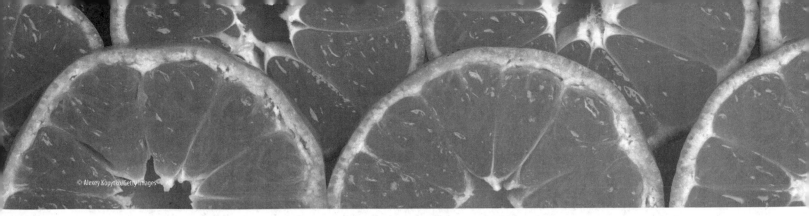

© Alexey Kopytko/Getty Images

# CHAPTER 12

# Principles of Planning Effective Community Nutrition Programs

## CHAPTER OUTLINE

- Introduction
- Identifying Issues
- Analyzing Subjective and Objective Data
- Developing a Program Plan
- Program Implementation
- Program Evaluation
- Data Sources and Collection Methods
- Program Assessment
- Reporting Program Success

*plan*
↓
*implement*
↓
*evaluate*

## LEARNING OBJECTIVES

- Explain the programming processes of planning, implementation, evaluation, and assessment.
- Explain the different types of evaluation.
- Discuss the different data collection methods.

## ▶ Introduction

The term *program* has a variety of meanings. For our purposes, a **program** is a collection of activities intended to produce a particular outcome.[1] In community nutrition programs, activities focus directly on nutrition issues or on health problems. The overall purpose is to improve the health of the community or public. **Program planning** is an act of formulating a program for a definite course of action, a process of exploring a situation, deciding on the circumstance, and designing actions to create the desired outcome.[2] Planning can be more exciting than carrying out the activities related to the program itself. The nutritionist must recognize the importance of continuously critiquing and reevaluating the services that are being provided. This chapter focuses on the practicalities of program planning, **program implementation**, and **program evaluation**, with high-quality health and well-being as the ultimate goal.

# ▶ Identifying Issues

In program planning, it is essential to identify issues of interest or concern. Surveys are useful for identifying issues of importance and achieving consensus when it is not practical for people to meet face to face.[3] Community nutritionists also can use data collected from community nutrition assessments, demographic data, maternal and infant mortality rates, and medical records to create a problem list.[4] The problem list compares and ranks perceived needs or those identified by the assessment data. It may reflect a community-wide concern, including ethnic or age groups that are at high nutritional risk. The needs of the groups can be compared and contrasted with the capacity of existing agencies to meet the desired outcome. The problem list can be used to request more funds, plan programs, and evaluate existing programs, as well as to determine delivery plans so the community can directly benefit from the program.[5] In addition, community assessment can identify the percentage of low-income individuals, the cost of housing in the community, cultural differences, language barriers, housing needs, the location and kinds of local markets, and the quality and prices of the foods they offer. To assess the extent of hunger in the community, data are needed on local food costs, household resources to obtain and prepare food, and barriers that constrain individuals or families from obtaining adequate food, such as language barriers and cultural differences.[6]

## Factors That Prompt Program Planning

The nutrition-related health issues that have been identified through a community needs assessment may trigger the decision to develop a nutrition program. For example, the community needs assessment may show that many newly immigrated Hispanic people are not aware of the Special Supplemental Nutrition Program for Women, Infants, and Children (WIC) or that the majority of the children living in a poor neighborhood are not enrolled in the National School Lunch Program.

Additional factors that may prompt program planning include research findings. For example, research shows that the number of women reaching menopause and postmenopausal age has increased, as has the incidence of nutrition-related conditions such as heart disease, osteoporosis, and cancer in women. Hence, the Illinois Department of Public Health Office of Women's Health funded education programs to address these health issues. Other factors that may trigger program planning include government policy, such as increasing nutritious foods in schools; the availability of funds to improve an existing program or to create new programs; and federal or state mandates.

At the national level, health problems are changing. Epidemiological data show high mortality and morbidity rates due to nutrition-related issues (i.e., malnutrition, obesity, heart disease, cancer, and diabetes).[7-9] Hence, the Hearts N' Parks Magnet Centers in 11 states became part of the well-known community-based program that works to reduce some of the nutrition-related health conditions. Hearts N' Parks is an innovative program that aims to reduce the trend of obesity and the risk for coronary heart disease in the United States by encouraging Americans of all ages to aim for a healthy weight, follow a heart-healthy eating plan, and engage in regular physical activity. Hearts N' Parks is supported by the National Heart, Lung, and Blood Institute (NHLBI) of the National Institutes of Health and the National Recreation and Park Association (NRPA). Some of the program activities include nutrition and fitness, stress reduction, and family life programs. Typically, the programs for children or adolescents are provided during summer camps or after-school activities for 7 to 11 weeks. The program also serves seniors and women and ends after an average of 12 weeks.

An evaluation of the Hearts N' Parks program showed that children learned to identify nutritious foods and reported being more willing to choose nutritious foods over less nutritious foods. On average, 26 percent of the children increased their heart-healthy eating knowledge and 15 percent increased their heart-healthy eating intention. Children also increased their interest in various forms of physical activity.[10]

Another national program is the U.S. National Cancer Institute's (NCI's) Fruits and Veggies—More Matters Campaign (formerly known as 5 A Day for Better Health). In 2003, the NCI initiated this campaign to motivate African American men to eat nine servings of fruits and vegetables a day. This campaign was trigged by the high incidence of cancer in the African American population. The campaign used a series of national radio spots that reached more than 17 million listeners a week for 4 months. Currently, the campaign offers an eight-page brochure designed specifically for African American men, and a 9-a-Day website (http://www.fruitsandveggiesmatter.gov/downloads /AA_Mens_Brochure.pdf) that explains the impact of diet on African American men's health. This successful community strategy features the Colorado State University Nutrition Education Program. **FIGURE 12-1** presents additional factors that may prompt program planning.

# ▶ Analyzing Subjective and Objective Data

Subjective and objective data are very important in program planning. **Subjective data analysis** involves

**The Community and Public Needs Assessment Revealed:**

- Infant malnutrition and mortality
- An increase in the low-income minority population
- An increased incidence of obesity in school-age children
- An increased rate of measles in the Hispanic and Asian communities
- An increased rate of osteoporosis in older women living in a retirement community
- Research findings about the high incidence of diseases such as heart disease and cancer
- Concerns of well-known community leaders or stakeholders
- Government policy changes related to health
- The availability of resources from the government and/or private organizations for new programs or to expand existing programs

The public or community acknowledges that the health issues need attention or upgrading.

New programs are developed or revised, or existing programs are expanded.

**FIGURE 12-1** Factors that may prompt program planning.

Data from: Boyle M. *Community Nutrition in Action: An Entrepreneurial Approach.* 4 ed. Belmont, CA: Thomson Wadsworth; 2005.

the collection and analysis of data on the various clients' perceived needs. This includes clarification of community values and analysis of the community (external) and agency (internal) environments in which the nutrition program plan will operate.[5,11,12] Community nutritionists can obtain subjective data by studying the mass media, such as reading local newspapers, including those that serve local neighborhoods or ethnic groups; listening to area radio stations, including those that target ethnic groups or special interests; and watching local television coverage.[12,13] The media typically reflect local values, political views, interests, educational levels, and lifestyles. It is possible to identify and determine current critical issues in the community via media coverage of meetings of local, state, national, or international governmental bodies and their opposing views.[5] In addition, perceived problems and needs for nutrition services can be obtained by interviewing professional colleagues (public health physicians, nurses, community health educators, and clinical dietitians) in health agencies to ascertain their perspectives on the community. Also, the use of in-depth narrative interviews is effective in collecting data. An in-depth interview is a nondirective research technique in which the participant is invited to "tell me the story about your health condition, starting with when you first noticed anything was wrong," and the only prompts used are "tell me more about that" or "what happened next?"[13,14] Informant interviews, which consist of direct conversations with selected members of a community about community members or groups and events, are an effective method of data collection. Holding informant interviews and involving stakeholders are good ways to generate information about community beliefs, norms, and values.

**Objective data analysis** involves collecting and analyzing data from available demographic and health statistics to prepare the community diagnosis and problem list. For example, vital statistics on births and deaths that are reported to the state health agency can be used in community assessment. All births and deaths are recorded through a local registrar or clerk, usually in the city or county health department. Death certificates provide information on primary and secondary causes of death (mortality). Objective data are collected to determine what is known about the community's population in total compared with what is known about individuals.[5,12] **TABLE 12-1** presents examples of subjective and objective data.

**TABLE 12-1** Examples of Subjective and Objective Data[5]

| Subjective Data | Sources |
|---|---|
| Beliefs<br>Values<br>Lifestyles<br>Political views | Media (local newspapers, radio stations, television)<br>Stakeholders<br>Informants<br>Physicians<br>Nurses |

| Objective Data | Sources |
|---|---|
| Demographic statistics (age, gender, race, ethnicity, income, and educational level)<br>Vital and health statistics (births, deaths, infant mortality rate, and marital status)<br>Physical environment (mild climate, inner-city neighborhood, size of neighborhood, public spaces, roads, and older homes) | Birth and death certificates<br>U.S. Census Bureau<br>Medical records<br>Centers for Disease Control and Prevention<br>National surveys (e.g., National Health and Nutrition Examination Survey [NHANES]) |

A community nutritionist can assess clients' nutritional status and collect observable data using generally accepted parameters, which are described in Chapter 2. For example, researchers at Ohio University used the subjective method of data collection to assess food insecurity. Food insecurity in rural Southeast Ohio was reported to be about two to three times higher than for the rest of the nation. Funding from the University of Ohio and the support of community agencies helped students enrolled in a community nutrition course to conduct a needs assessment and identify factors influencing food insecurity in rural Appalachian Ohio. The students collected data through a review of literature on food insecurity and hunger and interviews with area agencies. They focused the interviews on the agencies' missions/goals and funding sources, and gathered information from annual reports.

Their assessment confirmed the need for additional emergency food resources, and they developed a program, "Halt Hunger on the Hocking," to address this need. A food drive was planned as a service-learning project, which improved the community's food security status.[15,16]

# Successful Community Strategies

## The Colorado State University Nutrition Education Program[17-23]

Hispanics are projected to be the largest minority group within the United States by the year 2010. Colorado has a large Hispanic population representing about 14 percent of the state's total population. Additionally, there are approximately 21,000 migrant farm laborers who work in agricultural capacities throughout the state. Studies suggest that low-income Hispanics often demonstrate low intakes of vitamins A and C, calcium, iron, and protein and high rates of diabetes, obesity, and infections.

It is very difficult to provide effective nutrition education programs because these individuals are among the poorest in the state, especially when considering the migrant farm worker families. The obstacles to effective nutrition programs involve mainly limited financial resources on the part of both the agencies providing the education and the individuals being served. Other obstacles include lack of transportation, childcare, and time needed for educational endeavors as well as low education levels, low literacy rates, limited opportunities to learn English if English is the second language, culture, health beliefs, and, in some cases, if the nature of the population is especially transient. These factors have severely restricted participation in and success of the nutrition education endeavors. Translation issues, reading level considerations, and complexities of program content have become critical considerations for educators. Community agencies have found these obstacles to be major challenges in providing effective nutrition education programs.

A nutrition education program entitled *La Cocina Saludable* was designed according to the Stages of Change Model and implemented in 10 southern Colorado counties. The objectives of the program were to improve the nutrition-related knowledge, skills, and behaviors that lead to healthy lifestyles in a low-income Hispanic population. The contents of the program included nutrition information designed to help mothers of preschool children provide for their children's nutritional needs. Materials developed for this program included the following:

- A free-standing, color photograph, bilingual flip chart
- Corresponding bilingual *La Cocina Saludable Resource Guides*
- A three-dimensional, free-standing, bilingual Food Guide Pyramid
- Coordinating plastic kitchen utensils used as incentives
- Brochures representing the bilingual Food Guide Pyramid
- Food Guide Pyramid magnets

The *Resource Guide* was written in both English and Spanish and included scripted teaching pages corresponding to text background pages. This guide was designed to provide the abuela (Hispanic grandmother) educators, who were minimally trained in nutrition and teaching, with a resource for the nutrition information as well as a script to follow while they taught the classes, thus improving the consistency and accuracy of information presented to participants. The program attempted to overcome barriers by incorporating a flexible program format carried out by abuela educators using the processes described in the Stages of Change Model. The program was evaluated using knowledge, skills, and behavior pretest, posttest, and 6-month follow-up surveys on both the abuela educators and the actual class participants. The materials focused on five units:

- "Make It Healthy" discussed basic nutrition knowledge, including use of the Food Guide Pyramid.
- "Make It Fun" provided tips on making food fun to encourage preschool children to eat healthful foods.
- "Make a Change" explained techniques for lowering fat, lowering salt, lowering sugar, and increasing fiber in diets.
- "Make It Safe" discussed food safety techniques, including cleanliness, the safe cooking of foods, and properly storing foods.
- "Make a Plan" provided tips on choosing healthy foods and on making food resources last longer.

*(continues)*

## Successful Community Strategies (continued)

Each of the five units included an experiential and behavioral learning activity designed to reinforce the messages presented in the unit and to use the specific kitchen utensil designated for that unit. The kitchen utensil was then given to the participants as a reward for participating and to encourage them to return for the next class meeting.

Results show that the training program was an effective means of disseminating nutrition information and skills to abuela educators, particularly in the areas of healthful eating and the Food Guide Pyramid, in which the educators were the most deficient in knowledge and skills. In addition, the results suggested that the five class units led to significant gains in knowledge, skills, and retention of this knowledge. At 6 months, the program participants improved their survey scores after attending the program compared to the control group, who did not attend the program. Additionally, the results suggest that this type of program can be effective in changing selected nutrition-related knowledge, skills, and behaviors leading to healthy lifestyles for low-income Hispanic mothers of preschool children.

## Writing a Mission Statement

The data collected through subjective and/or objective methods can be used to help write a mission statement. The mission statement is a statement of clear direction for the health program.[24] This statement must be clear, brief, concise, realistic, and inspirational. It is important to choose and rank the most critical issues in order of priority in the mission statement as well as in the subsequent steps of writing the objectives and the **action plan** or activities.[5] When wording the mission statement for nutrition service needs, consider the organization's philosophy, products, services, markets, values, and concern for the public. It is important to review the mission statement of the organization before writing a mission statement for a specific program. Reviewing the organization's mission statement and matching it with the program's goals will accomplish the following[25,26]:

- Make sure the program is implementing the organization's directive
- Justify the resources, time, and expense the program utilized
- Generate support from supervisors

If the program's goals do not match the organization's mission statement, it will be difficult for the nutritionist to justify use of the organization's resources. He or she will not receive support from supervisors or obtain internal funds and approval for the new program. **BOXES 12-1** and **12-2** present samples of mission statements.

---

**BOX 12-1** Cornell Cooperative Extension Mission Statement

The Cornell Cooperative Extension mission statement is to enable people to improve their lives and communities through partnerships that put experience and research knowledge to work.

---

**BOX 12-2** The Cooperative State Research, Education, and Extension Service

The Cooperative State Research, Education, and Extension Service (CSREES) mission statement is to advance knowledge for agriculture, the environment, human health and well-being, and communities by supporting research, education, and extension programs in the Land Grant University System and other partner organizations. CSREES does not perform actual research, education, and extension but rather helps fund it at the state and local level and provides program leadership in these areas.

## Clarifying Goals

Regardless of the type of data collection method used (subjective or objective), it is important to clarify the program goals because communities often express their goals broadly, which may affect data collection and analysis as well as the program outcome. Goals are general statements about what the program should accomplish (e.g., to improve the health of children, older persons, and pregnant women).[27] For example, the community may want children to grow up healthier. In this case, further exploration is required to identify factors that influence the growth of children in the community (e.g., poor food or a lack of safe places to play and learn).[28]

In the United States, nutritionists can use the national goals and objectives outlined in Healthy People 2010 to plan their programs. The goals are very helpful because they target specific priority needs of the U.S. population identified by a cross-section of practitioners and interested citizens.[28,29] For example, Objective 19-4 is to promote health and reduce chronic diseases associated with diet and weight. To use the Healthy People 2010 and 2020 objectives, a community might evaluate how well they meet national or state objectives, decide on the significance of the objectives, and then use gaps as starting points for action.

Goals are different from objectives. Goals are broad statements of desired outcome or changes, whereas objectives are specific, measurable actions of the desired outcome to be completed within a specified time frame.[2] For instance, the McLean County Public Health Department identified a high incidence of iron-deficiency anemia in their county and aimed to decrease the prevalence of iron-deficiency anemia in low-income minority children.

*Goal:* To reduce iron-deficiency anemia in McLean County

*Objective:* By the end of the nutrition and health promotion program:

Eighty percent of low-income minority children ages 2 to 5 years will be enrolled in the WIC program.

The number of anemic children in McLean County will be reduced by 95 percent.

Another approach for writing well-designed objectives described is to incorporate the A to E method of writing objectives, as follows.[30,31]

- **A = Audience:** Who is the target audience? For example, pregnant women, infants, children, elderly, and others.
- **B = Behavior:** What behavior do you want your target audience to adopt? For example, eat more fruits and vegetables, participate in physical activities for 30 minutes, 5 days a week.
- **C = Condition:** How? Under what situations or framework will the learning occur? After what intervention or new program will the audience or participants be expected to improve their performance? For example, after Fruit and Veggies—More Matters' Health Program utilizing the media and other methods of encouraging the consumption of fruits and vegetables.
- **D = Degree:** What is the acceptable minimum level of performance? How much will be accomplished. For example, does the nutritionist want the participant to consume the exact recommended servings of fruits and vegetables (100 percent) or 85 percent or the recommended amount?
- **E = Evaluation:** How to assess the outcome of the education program. Which tool or methods will be used to measure behavior change? For example, a 24-hour food recall, food frequency survey, or food record may be used to assess how many fruits and vegetables the participants consumed in a day.

In addition, when writing objectives some of the words to avoid are as follows:

- Understand
- Be familiar with
- Appreciate
- Be aware of
- Have a knowledge of
- Realize
- Believe
- Be interested in

**Appropriate words to use when writing an objectives are as follows:**

- List
- Define
- Calculate
- Identify
- Plan
- Describe
- Select
- Differentiate
- Make

## ▶ Developing a Program Plan

It is important to develop a program only after reviewing existing programs and talking with other health professionals such as nurses and other dietitians who have worked with comparable programs or with the target population. Examples of ways to make connections with other professionals are by attending professional conferences, contacting experts in the area, searching the literature, networking via word of mouth, searching the Internet, and becoming a member of an Academy of Nutrition and Dietetics practice group. The following are the six important factors to consider when writing or designing a program plan[5,32,33]:

- The established and emerging scientific evidence from research findings in nutrition and food science that apply to the public's health and/or issues relevant to the community that have not been addressed adequately.
- The organization's mission and philosophy.
- Federal and state legislation either requiring or permitting nutrition services in the community's health and human services system.
- Federal, national, state, local, public, or private sector organizations that provide funds for nutrition services.
- Opportunities to contract with other community health and human services agencies to provide nutrition services.
- Model nutrition objectives or standards published by expert groups that are pertinent to the community.

In addition, community nutritionists can utilize various models or theories to implement a program. The nutritionist can determine which models or theories, if any, provide a good explanation or understanding of the problems that have been selected. For example, the Stages of Change Model can be used to work with people who may not be aware they are affected by a nutrition-related health condition (such as high blood pressure); another model (Social Learning Theory) can help people acquire skills and motivate them to take preventive action. Depending on the type of health condition, some theories or models may be more useful than others. For many health conditions, especially complex ones, a single theory may not fully address the problems, and it may be necessary to consider and combine multiple theories or parts of a theory.[34]

To continue the previous example, to achieve the goals and objectives related to iron-deficiency anemia in low-income minority children, the community nutritionist could develop a program plan that would accomplish the following[2]:

- Evaluate the developmental levels of 95 percent of low-income minority children by contacting the health department and the neighborhood free clinics that will evaluate the children's developmental levels. WIC program eligibility will be determined for 90 percent of the children observed by the health department and neighborhood free clinics. This will involve WIC program personnel, the health department, and the neighborhood free clinics as the principal change agents.
- Implement an outreach program to identify at-risk infants not identified by the healthcare providers. This activity will involve using key informants, community and public health nurses, community leaders, and clinical dietitians in the community.
- Have as a goal that 85 percent of all the children who are eligible for WIC food supplements will enroll in the program.
- Teach mothers so that 70 percent of the mothers of the children enrolled in WIC will show four different methods of incorporating WIC supplements into their children's diet. The nutritionist will develop the nutrition education components and the marketing plan for the program. The local health department will provide the facilities, teaching rooms, materials, training, equipment, and funds for the program.

## Designing Actions

The action plan is a concise statement of the methods, activities, or intervention strategies for a primary, secondary, and/or tertiary prevention program.[27] Interventions must be sufficiently intensive or forceful to achieve the objectives by the target date. Two examples of interventions are nutrition education and social marketing (e.g., public awareness campaigns), which are associated with social planning; these strategies are used in nationwide school and media initiatives in the United States to promote the consumption of fruits and vegetables (e.g., the Fruits and Veggies—More Matters program). Social action uses lobbying strategies such as writing letters or making telephone calls to legislators to change a school lunch policy.[28] Community development organizations can use strategies such as community forums and key informants where critical discussion is supported. The following should be considered when designing a program's action plan[27,28,35]:

- Creating a more desirable environment and using communication as a technique
- The resources that are needed and the sources of funding
- The staff needed for the program and their responsibilities
- The theoretical framework appropriate for the program

Another action that must be taken when carrying out a program is keeping accurate records that are designed specifically to support the programming processes and program activities. The nutritionist needs to be responsible for certain tasks[36]:

- Keeping a journal that can assist in tracking the actions and critically reflecting on the outcome.
- Establishing criteria for reviewing the methodologies using statistics. A systematic review is a useful method for summarizing the effectiveness of public health and other population-based interventions.
- Planning nutritional and dietary classes.
- Providing nutritional/dietary guidelines.
- Writing nutrition prescriptions.
- Documenting all activities to save time and prevent conflict.
- Coordinating, controlling, managing, and directing the program.
- Using documentation as a source of data for program evaluation.

## Management System

There are two aspects to any management system. The first is the personnel who will manage and organize the program and make sure its goals and objectives will be adequately addressed. The skills and qualification of the staff will influence the quality of the nutrition program. The second aspect is the data system. The nutritionist needs to determine the method the program will use to measure and record data about the participants, their use of the program, and the program outcomes.[11] The use of quantitative methods, qualitative methods, or a combination of data collection methods provides the overall organizational structure needed for an efficient data system.[11,27]

## Resources, Budgets, and Feasibility

A feasibility study occurs during the program initiation phase and must be accomplished before significant expenses are carried out. Determining the costs of a program is an essential part of program planning. It is important to calculate the actual cost of a program by determining both the direct and indirect costs. It is also important to plan for situations that may increase the cost of the program, such as an increase in the number of participants or the length of the education program; a need for additional equipment, staff, or space; and so on. Cost analysis, like other components of programming, becomes easier with practice. The community nutritionist who adds the skill of cost analysis to his or her repertoire will be well prepared to carry out a very effective program.[11,27]

Community and public health nutritionists working in nonprofit organizations and government agencies often encounter challenges in obtaining funds for all the components of a program. It is important that nutritionists link the budget to the program activities. This will reduce unnecessary activities, increase the efficiency of carrying out the program, and reduce costs. Funds may be available to pay personnel salaries, reimburse their travel, buy equipment, and plan a marketing campaign in the present year's budget, but there may not be enough funds to pay for supplies, conduct screening tests, and develop the educational materials.[37] At this stage in the program planning process, the community nutritionist needs to review the budget and other program elements (e.g., travel, marketing campaign) and decide whether outside funding such as cash grants or in-kind funds are available for the program.[11] Once the areas of need are identified, the nutritionist can then prepare and submit grant proposals for funding.

Funding sources include grants and contracts from local, state, or federal agencies; foundations; and private contributions. Grants are a source of initial and ongoing funding. The funding organization generally releases guidelines as to what the organization will fund. The guidelines are frequently released as a request for proposals. These proposals specify how the nutrition center or program would meet the goals of the granting organization in a given time line. They describe the services and planned client outcomes. See Chapter 14 for more information on grant writing.

Contracts are another source of funding and can be with the local government, state agencies, or private organizations. Contracts are drawn up for a particular service with project outcomes and a given time line. They provide opportunities for nutrition centers and programs to advance services, practices, and education. For example, the local WIC program may ask for a contract from the local government to perform nutrition screening for admission into the WIC program.

Resources should be sought both within and outside the community. Organizations within the community may serve as resources and can promote community self-reliance. These need to be considered before looking for resources outside the community.[11] For example, students enrolled in a food and nutrition program may collaborate with experienced retired nutritionists and take turns teaching adolescent parents, instead of bringing in outside assistance. Possible sources of support both within and outside the community include businesses, social and professional clubs, volunteers, community institutions, and agencies such as churches, schools, and colleges.

The Public Health Service of the U.S. Department of Health and Human Services, as well as the U.S. Department of Agriculture, have been the principal government sources of funding for food and nutrition programs. To take advantage of the funding provided by these agencies, community nutritionists must link their programs to the types of projects or research these agencies fund. Examples of private philanthropic foundations who may provide funding include the W.K. Kellogg Foundation and the Rockefeller Foundation.

## Managing Tasks and Time

Program planning needs to be linked with time estimates and task specifications. In the case of a comprehensive nutrition and health program, the time frame necessary for development may be a year or more.[27] For new individual programs, it may require up to 6 months of planning to implement a health promotion effort. To promote success in planning a project, some type of time framework must be established.[27] For example, if students are involved, let the students know when they need to complete their work; if elders need immunizations prior to flu season, note when the immunizations should be finished; or if the project is funded by an agency, state clearly when a final report is expected.[28,38] From these fixed time requirements, the nutritionist and community can work backward to the present; however, if there are no time requirements, working forward from the present is possible.

Time and task management tools can be used during all phases of programming and are helpful when a number of people are working on different aspects of the program. All tools can be modified, such as modifying the language to match the needs of the targeted audience.[28] These tools should list goals, objectives, action strategies, and time lines that indicate tasks or activities that must be done, by whom, and when. Creating two time lines—an optimistic time line as well as an alternative one (for if things take longer)—may be a wise choice.

## ▶ Program Implementation

Program implementation is the process of putting a program into action or executing a plan.[28,39] An intervention program's implementation must be based on program goals, objectives, and outcomes. The nutritionist must consider the following[3]:

- The quality of the program implementation
- How to handle unexpected situations
- How to keep the program on track
- The back-up plans for unexpected situations

In the implementation phase of the program planning process, the clients, providers, and administrators must select the best plan to solve the original problem. This stage of the process involves work and activities aimed at achieving the stakeholders' expectations.[40] The person or group who established the goals and objectives may make the implementation efforts, or they may be delegated to others. Providing reasons why a particular solution or model was chosen will help the nutritionist get the administration's approval for the plan. It is important to involve clients and administrators throughout the planning process; this helps promote acceptance of the plan.

It is very important to state clearly how the program will be implemented. The implementation of a program may be time limited, such as a 10-month program for women's health issues or a 1-year letter-writing campaign to reduce fat intake in school-age children. Tasks, time, and resources must be carefully monitored during implementation to best utilize the program's funds.

Implementation is shaped by the nutritionist's chosen roles, the type of health or nutrition problem selected as the focus for intervention, the community's readiness to take part in problem solving, and the characteristics of the social change process.

Community nutritionists should not be surprised at unexpected situations. There may be glitches in carrying out the program, such as failure to ensure that the promotional materials (handouts, fliers, and illustrations) are culturally appropriate or there were too few public transportation routes to the program site. The need to make changes during the implementation period does not mean that the program was not well planned—changes are inevitable. The nutritionist must anticipate the unexpected, such as reallocation of funds during the program, clients not responding to the invitation to participate in the intervention program, clients not cooperating fully (e.g., not completing a questionnaire for evaluation of the program), or presentation slides not working.[11] Community nutritionists need to continuously consider how things can be improved.

The people who are the hardest to reach are sometimes neglected in the planning phase. These people, who often do not come to events such as community forums, may be the most marginalized or at risk and may be the people the program is most intended to benefit. Bracht and Kingsbury[41] argue that it is the practitioner who finds it "hard to hear" rather than the client who is "hard to reach." It is important to make meaningful connections with these people. If the planning phase is not appropriately planned and friendly, people will not be receptive to intervention strategies.

A method of increasing participation (and voice) among seniors was incorporated into one community development project. Hitchcock et al.[28] formed a steering committee with a balance of seniors and practitioners. Community forums were held in settings frequented by seniors. Those who came to community forums were invited to join a networking process whereby they designed questions, practiced interviewing, and then went into the community to interview other seniors. Through this procedure, interviewees suggested additional names of people who had not participated (e.g., homebound seniors). The interviewers were paid as research assistants from a government grant. Opportunities for empowerment and increased community competence among seniors were obvious in this method, and, amazingly, meaningful information was gained about the seniors' views and goals.

## ▶ Program Evaluation

Evaluation is defined as the methods used to determine whether a service is needed and likely to be used, whether it is conducted as planned, whether the service actually helps the purpose, and whether objectives are carried out or planned activities are completed.[42] The first item listed also is referred to as formative evaluation. This type of evaluation begins with an assessment of the need for a program. The evaluation conducted to assess program outcomes or as a follow-up to the results of the program activities is called summative evaluation. An allocation of 10 percent of the program budget is recommended for evaluation.[6]

# Evaluation Types

As mentioned earlier, evaluation may be formative, occurring throughout all programming processes, or summative, occurring at an end point. Formative evaluation is ongoing and provides information to those planning and implementing the program during the program implementation. The purpose of this type of evaluation is to strengthen or improve the program being evaluated, to determine the quality of its implementation, and to permit improvements to the program while activities are in progress.[28,43] Health promotion programs also conduct a formative assessment to do the following[43,44]:

- Understand the perspective in which the intervention will take place and the development of consensus on goals.
- Assess participants' reactions to the program and improve the health promotion programs.
- Identify specific behaviors of concern and the cause of these behaviors.
- Identify community attitudes that might inhibit or promote program goals.
- Identify resources available to the program. Formative assessment is the key to improving the relevance, sustainability, and effectiveness of community-based public health programs.[45]

Summative evaluation, on the other hand, provides retrospective information about the performance of the program and is conducted at the completion of the program.[7,43] It assesses changes in behaviors, attitudes, knowledge, or health status indicators such as morbidity, mortality, risk behaviors, and others.

# Why Program Evaluation and with Whom

Program evaluation is an ongoing process from the beginning of the planning phase until the program ends. The goal of the evaluation must be clear to everyone involved in the program. Program evaluation provides critical information (e.g., the number of participants enrolled, outcomes, and impact) for funding agencies, top-level decision makers, program accreditation reviewers, and the community at large.[2] Evaluation of an intervention is carried out from the following perspectives[11,46]:

- To see whether the objectives have been achieved
- To determine whether the procedures were carried out according to expectations
- To identify the strengths and weaknesses of the program materials
- To determine the impact of the program
- To test new methods and approaches
- To justify expanding the program, reducing the program, or even closing it

In addition, it shows whether the program is fulfilling its purpose. The major goal of program evaluation is determining the following[2,27,47]:

- *Relevance:* The need for the program
- *Progress:* Tracking of program activities to meet program objectives; assessing whether the program is functioning as planned
- *Efficiency:* The relationship between program outcomes and the resources spent
- *Effectiveness:* The ability to meet program objectives and the results of program efforts
- *Impact*: Long-term changes in the client population
- *Standards:* Determining whether the program staff have the needed credentials; making sure the staff is trained to provide the program

All persons involved in implementing a program need to be a part of the plan for program evaluation. The individuals concerned with evaluation may be divided into four categories[28,43]:

- *The population/community itself*: The community must be invited to participate in the evaluation process, because the actions to be evaluated concern them directly.
- *The change agents (e.g., the community nutritionists, the physician)*: These people will play an important role in the evaluation process. Moreover, this evaluation will help them improve their performance.
- *The evaluation specialists internal or external to the planning team*: They will provide technical expertise for the evaluation.
- *The sponsors and government representatives*: This will allow them to see the impact of the activities they have promoted and to consider further expansion of the program.

In addition, the results of program evaluation can be used to influence public policy, distribute resources, and persuade politicians and community leaders who have the power to change policies or address a health issue. For example, the high rate of cancer deaths in two rural towns in northeast Colorado prompted community leaders to take action and request an intervention by their local university nutrition department. A research study identified that the rate of cancer incidence was higher (14 percent above the state norm) in these two counties. Citizens, aware that nutrition and eating practices could lower cancer risk, contacted their Colorado State University Cooperative Extension agent for program possibilities. A team was formed to work in these remote small towns to improve nutrition, diet, and health using the 5-a-Day message. The intervention also included fruit and vegetable demonstrations, newspaper articles, pamphlets, discussions, taste testing, and fruit and vegetable puppet shows explaining 5-a-Day and the importance of fruits and vegetables to grades K through 6. The nutritionist evaluated the program using 24-hour food recall and before and after questionnaires to assess fruit and vegetable consumption.

Results showed that the children had an increased awareness of fruits and vegetables in their diet. The residents of the counties stated that they liked the newspaper articles, pamphlet, and demonstrations and would like the 5-a-Day nutrition and cancer prevention program to continue.[48]

According to the World Health Organization's European Working Group, evaluation of health promotion programs should be participatory. In participatory evaluation, community leaders or participants in the program decide what to evaluate, select the methods and data sources, carry out the evaluation, analyze the data, and present the findings. Participatory evaluation approaches increase the likelihood that results will be directly useful in creating community change.[6] In general, program evaluation consists of the following three integral parts[28,49]:

1. *Responsiveness:* How well the program performed with the problem concerning the program
2. *Effectiveness:* How well the desired outcomes were achieved
3. *Efficiency:* How much was achieved with the minimum use of resources

## The Program Process Evaluation

Program evaluation is often conceptualized in terms of process, structure, impact, and outcomes. Process describes all the activities conducted to produce change.[2] Process evaluation answers the question: Was the program implemented as planned? It centers on program activities instead of outcome. This includes items such as the budget, the program organization, distributing educational materials to all the participants in a timely manner, accurately anticipating the number of people attending a lunch or after-hours workshop, and whether the facilities were accessible.[27,28] Programs are not often implemented exactly as planned. For example, a program activity may be altered based on midterm feedback from the participants, such as changing the time the program is offered because working parents could not participate or excuse themselves from work to attend the program. The nutritionist could use either open-ended or closed-ended questionnaire or both to evaluate program perception or outcome. Examples of an open-ended question include but not limited to: Explain some reasons for attending the breastfeeding program. What did you like or dislike about the program? A close-ended question asks participants to rate the program. For example, rate your satisfaction with the breastfeeding program (satisfied, very satisfied, unsatisfied, and very unsatisfied).[16]

Structural evaluation consists of assessing the resources used in providing the nutrition program. Process and structural evaluations provide support for outcome evaluation because the interpretation of program outcomes depends on an understanding of the program as it happens.[2] Structural evaluation also refers to evaluating the settings in which the program is carried out and includes materials, qualifications of the staff, organizational structure, and factors related to program delivery, such as the training of personnel and equipment (e.g., blood pressure apparatus, skinfold caliper, and bone densitometry).[2,11] This evaluation approach is based on the assumption that, given a proper setting with adequate equipment, good nutrition programming will be achieved.

Outcome evaluation (also known as summative evaluation) is the result of the program. The value of outcome evaluation is that it provides the best information possible about program performance. It evaluates whether the program achieved the stated goals and objectives. Outcome evaluation is the most difficult type of evaluation because it involves an assessment of health status indicators and quality of life that were identified in the planning stage.

In one example of outcome evaluation, Rivera et al.[50] studied the nutritional outcome of a large-scale, incentive-based development program on 373 intervention groups in Mexico. Children and pregnant and lactating women in participating households received fortified nutrition supplements, and the families received nutrition education, healthcare, and cash transfers. The outcome measures showed better growth rates in children and lower rates of anemia in low-income, rural infants and children in Mexico.[50] Another example of outcome indicators includes epidemiological statistics such as mortality, morbidity, and disability rates. For instance, a cohort study showed that children who were exposed to methylmercury from traditional seafood diets that include pilot whale meat were significantly associated with deficits in motor, attention, and verbal tests.[51] Additional examples of indicators include safety, behavior, health-related policies, individual and population health status, and use of resources.[52] The satisfaction of stakeholders may or may not be a good indicator of program success (e.g., parents of teens may not be satisfied about after-school physical activities, but the program may help prevent obesity and heart disease).

The terms *outcome* and *impact evaluation* are sometimes used interchangeably, but sometimes are used differently to reflect time differences.[28] Impact evaluation measures the immediate effects of the program on participants' knowledge, attitudes, and behaviors. It assesses changes in the well-being of individuals, households, or communities that can be attributed to the nutrition program. For example, immediate and short-term outcomes are assessed shortly after completion of a program to determine whether the results were as expected (impact). The important impact evaluation question is: What would have happened to the participants receiving the intervention if they had not received the program? For example, upon completion of a Fruits and Veggies—More Matters program, the number of participants who consumed fruits and vegetables increased (impact). In the longer term, outcomes are assessed after a certain amount of time has elapsed (e.g., 1 year later) to determine whether changes occurred as anticipated. For example, the number of participants who consumed fruits and vegetables increased and the incidence of high blood pressure and high blood cholesterol decreased (impact) 1 year after the health promotion program. Long-term outcome evaluation is difficult because it requires resources for longitudinal tracking. Also, participants' cooperation and compliance can be difficult to obtain.

## ▶ Data Sources and Collection Methods

After the type of evaluation and overall evaluation questions have been decided, the next step is the selection of data sources and data collection methods. Several data sources on health and nutrition are available for public use, particularly from government surveys. These data sources can be used to design community and public health programs. The data may represent information collected at the national, state, or local level on health issues such as diabetes, tobacco use, obesity, nutrient consumption, hypertension, or heart disease. One example of existing data that nutritionists may use is the National Health and Nutrition Examination Survey (NHANES), which examines the dietary practices of the U.S. population and the relationship between diet and health. Another example source of data is the Behavioral Risk Factor Surveillance System (BRFSS), which is the world's largest telephone survey; it tracks health risks of adults (persons over 18) in the United States. (Tables 2-3 and 2-4 in Chapter 2 present examples of secondary and demographic datasets that could be sources for a community needs assessment.)

Some granting agencies may specify their preferred method or source of data collection, or the nutritionist may need to collect data from a specific target population in the community that may not be available from government sources. Data sources usually include people and documents. Collection methods include the following[5]:

- Interviews (face-to-face or telephone)
- Focus groups
- Observations
- Surveys (questionnaire mailings)
- Medical record reviews

Telephone and mail surveys are less expensive than face-to-face interviews and are easier to use for a population-based survey. Not all clients, especially low-income persons, have telephones, however, and this method may produce skewed results.[53] Information about the percentage of the population with telephones is available from the local telephone company for land lines and possibly cell phone companies. Chart or record reviews are an effective method of collecting data when clinic or program participants are the population of interest or are an appropriate convenience sample.

Standardized surveys may be used, or they may be created specifically for the program.[54,55] An example of a questionnaire created for a program is shown in **FIGURE 12-2**. In the field of nutrition, two commonly used survey methods are the 24-hour recall and the food frequency list. Obtaining accurate 24-hour recall information requires a highly skilled interviewer who uses visual prompts, such as measuring cups or spoons, food models, and different-sized cups and bowls. It is important that the nutritionist reconcile the advantages and disadvantages of the dietary assessment instruments, which are presented in Chapter 2 in Table 2-10.

## Cost—Benefit Analysis

**Cost—benefit analysis (CBA)** of a nutrition program is the evaluation of the costs of a program in relation to health outcomes. CBA converts program inputs and outputs into monetary terms and then determines whether there is a net benefit to the program by subtracting costs from benefits.[55] It also evaluates program efficiency.[42] Costs are the value of the resources that must be used to develop, implement, and operate the program being analyzed. Community nutritionists must estimate the tangible and intangible and the direct and indirect costs of the program. The activities in a program that are valued in dollars are referred to as tangible; those that cannot be valued easily in dollars are referred to as intangible. Direct costs are the resources budgeted for or assigned to the program. Direct costs can be directly associated with the project with a high degree of accuracy. Examples of direct costs include personnel salaries, travel reimbursement, equipment,

Date Today: _____  Name: _____  ID Number: _____

Date of Birth: _____  Female _____  Male _____

**INSTRUCTIONS:** Here are some questions about your health and feelings. Please read each question carefully and check (✓) your best answer. You should answer the questions in your own way. There are no right or wrong answers. (Please ignore the small scoring numbers next to each blank.)

| | Yes, describes me exactly | Somewhat describes me | No, doesn't describe me at all |
|---|---|---|---|
| 1. I like who I am | 12 | 11 | 10 |
| 2. I am not an easy person to get along with | 20 | 21 | 22 |
| 3. I am basically a healthy person | 32 | 31 | 30 |
| 4. I give up too easily | 40 | 41 | 42 |
| 5. I have difficulty concentrating | 50 | 51 | 52 |
| 6. I am happy with my family relationships | 62 | 61 | 60 |
| 7. I am comfortable being around people | 72 | 71 | 70 |

**TODAY** would you have any physical trouble or difficulty:

| | None | Some | A lot |
|---|---|---|---|
| 8. Walking up a flight of stairs | 82 | 81 | 80 |
| 9. Running the length of a football field | 92 | 91 | 90 |

During the **PAST WEEK:** How much trouble have you had with:

| | None | Some | A lot |
|---|---|---|---|
| 10. Sleeping | 102 | 101 | 100 |
| 11. Hurting or aching in any part of your body | 112 | 111 | 110 |
| 12. Getting tired easily | 122 | 121 | 120 |
| 13. Feeling depressed or sad | 132 | 131 | 130 |
| 14. Nervousness | 142 | 141 | 140 |

During the **PAST WEEK:** How often did you:

| | None | Some | A lot |
|---|---|---|---|
| 15. Socialize with other people (talk or visit with friends or relatives) | 150 | 151 | 152 |
| 16. Take part in social, religious, or recreation activities (meetings, church, movies, sports, parties) | 160 | 161 | 162 |

During the **PAST WEEK:** How often did you:

| | None | 1–4 Days | 4–7 Days |
|---|---|---|---|
| 17. Stay in your home, a nursing home, or hospital because of sickness, injury, or other health problem | 172 | 171 | 170 |

**FIGURE 12-2** Duke Health Profile.

**PHYSICAL HEALTH SCORE**

| Item | Raw Score* | |
|---|---|---|
| 1 | = _____ | |
| 4 | = _____ | |
| 5 | = _____ | |
| 13 | = _____ | |
| 14 | = _____ | |
| Sum | = _____ | × 10 = |

**MENTAL HEALTH SCORE**

| Item | Raw Score* | |
|---|---|---|
| 1 | = _____ | |
| 4 | = _____ | |
| 5 | = _____ | |
| 13 | = _____ | |
| 14 | = _____ | |
| Sum | = _____ | × 10 = |

**SOCIAL HEALTH SCORE**

| Item | Raw Score* | |
|---|---|---|
| 2 | = _____ | |
| 6 | = _____ | |
| 7 | = _____ | |
| 15 | = _____ | |
| 16 | = _____ | |
| Sum | = _____ | × 10 = |

**GENERAL HEALTH SCORE**

| | | |
|---|---|---|
| Physical Health score | = _____ | |
| Mental Health score | = _____ | |
| Social Health score | = _____ | |
| Sum | = _____ | ÷ 3 = |

**PERCEIVED HEALTH SCORE**

| Item | Raw Score* | |
|---|---|---|
| 3 | = _____ | × 50 = |

**SELF-ESTEEM SCORE**

| Item | Raw Score* | |
|---|---|---|
| 1 | = _____ | |
| 2 | = _____ | |
| 4 | = _____ | |
| 6 | = _____ | |
| 7 | = _____ | |
| Sum | = _____ | × 10 = |

To calculate the scores in this column the raw scores must be revised as follows: If 0, change to 2; if 2, change to 0; if 1, no change.

**ANXIETY SCORE**

| Item | Raw Score* | Revised |
|---|---|---|
| 2 | = _____ | _____ |
| 5 | = _____ | _____ |
| 7 | = _____ | _____ |
| 10 | = _____ | _____ |
| 12 | = _____ | _____ |
| 14 | = _____ | _____ |
| Sum | = _____ | × 8.333 = |

**DEPRESSION SCORE**

| Item | Raw Score* | Revised |
|---|---|---|
| 4 | = _____ | _____ |
| 5 | = _____ | _____ |
| 10 | = _____ | _____ |
| 12 | = _____ | _____ |
| 13 | = _____ | _____ |
| Sum | = _____ | × 10 = |

**ANXIETY-DEPRESSION (DUKE-AD) SCORE**

| Item | Raw Score* | Revised |
|---|---|---|
| 4 | = _____ | _____ |
| 5 | = _____ | _____ |
| 7 | = _____ | _____ |
| 10 | = _____ | _____ |
| 12 | = _____ | _____ |
| 13 | = _____ | _____ |
| 14 | = _____ | _____ |
| Sum | = _____ | × 7.143 = |

**PAIN SCORE**

| Item | Raw Score* | Revised |
|---|---|---|
| 11 | = _____ | _____ × 50 = |

**DISABILITY SCORE**

| Item | Raw Score* | Revised |
|---|---|---|
| 17 | = _____ | _____ × 50 = |

**\*Raw Score** = last digit of the numeral adjacent to the blank checked by the respondent for each item. For example, if the second blank is checked for item 10 (blank numeral = 101), then the raw score is "1," because 1 is the last digit of 101.

**Final Score** is calculated from the raw scores as shown and entered into the box for each scale. For physical health, mental health, social health, general health, self-esteem, and perceived health, 100 indicates the best health status, and 0 indicates the worst health status. For anxiety, depression, anxiety-depression, pain, and disability, 100 indicates the worst health status and 0 indicates the best health status.

**Missing Values:** If one or more responses is missing within one of the eleven scales, a score cannot be calculated for that particular scale.

**FIGURE 12-2** (continued)

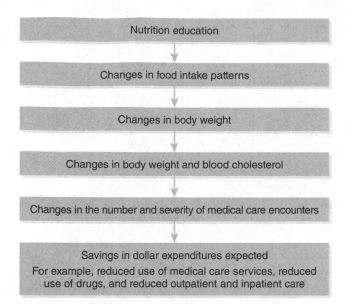

**FIGURE 12-3** Potential economic benefits associated with nutrition education on obesity and blood cholesterol.

supplies, and continuing education for nutrition personnel, printing, and marketing the program. Indirect costs are resources that allow the program to operate, but are not directly attributable to a specific program. Examples include time lost from work by recipients participating in a program, childcare costs, utilities, building and grounds, and janitorial services.

Benefits are the positive outcomes or consequences of a program. It is easier to determine costs than benefits, which are more complex. For example, if a program benefit is a change in an individual's food purchasing patterns, then that benefit can be valued as the money saved from the new mix of foods purchased. However, intangible costs and benefits, especially benefits, can be measured more directly without using a dollar value.[56] Some examples could include knowledge gained, attitudes changed, skills acquired, practices adopted, and individual and societal end results. **FIGURE 12-3** presents potential economic benefits associated with nutrition education on obesity and blood cholesterol.

### ☑ Think About It

After conducting a needs assessment, a community nutritionist decided to design and provide nutrition education programs to pregnant women in his community. What must he consider when determining the cost of a program?

## ▶ Program Assessment

Assessment of health promotion and disease prevention programs—which includes data gathering, analysis, and reporting—is used to determine program outcomes and measure overall program effectiveness. Most external agencies also require that program directors assess program effectiveness to justify the program's cost.

A wide variety of assessment instruments are used to appraise health promotion programs. Some instruments focus on assessing general health status, whereas others focus on more specific health behaviors such as diet. A health risk appraisal can be used to assess current health behaviors, judge the impact of behaviors on health status, and also predict future outcome. An example of a health status assessment is the Duke Health Profile (shown earlier in Figure 12-3).[57] It is designed to assess functional health status over a 1-week time period.[58] It has 11 scales: physical health, mental health, social health, general health, perceived health, self-esteem, anxiety, depression, anxiety-depression, pain, and disability.[27]

Nutrition assessment instruments are used in health promotion programs to assess dietary habits and nutrition-related health conditions such as heart disease, obesity, osteoporosis, and diabetes. It is essential to choose a valid and reliable instrument to collect the needed information. In addition to validity and reliability, assessment instruments need to be usable by the intended audiences. A 24-hour recall, food frequency checklist, and 3-day food record are the most widely used nutrition assessment tools and are effective in most cases. These instruments are discussed in Chapter 2.

Nutrition assessment is also used to monitor the progress of national programs. For example, studies show that some modifiable maternal behaviors and experiences before, during, and after pregnancy are associated with undesirable health outcomes for the mother and her infant (e.g., physical abuse, insufficient folic acid consumption, smoking during pregnancy, and improper infant sleep position).[59,60] The Pregnancy Risk Assessment Monitoring System (PRAMS) is an ongoing, state- and population-based surveillance system designed to monitor selected maternal behaviors and experiences that occur before, during, and after pregnancy among women who deliver live-born infants.[61] Between 2000 and 2003, PRAMS mailed a sample of three self-administered surveys to mothers and interviewed nonresponders by telephone. The survey data were linked to selected birth certificate data to create annual PRAMS analysis datasets that can be used to produce statewide estimates of perinatal health behaviors and experiences among women delivering live infants. The data from 19 states measured progress toward achieving HP 2010 objectives for the following eight perinatal indicators[62]:

- *Pregnancy intention:* Results show that in 2003, the prevalence of intended pregnancy among women having a live birth ranged from 48.1 percent in Louisiana to 66.5 percent in Maine.
- *Multivitamin use:* In 2003, the prevalence of multivitamin use at least four times per week during the month before pregnancy ranged from 23.0 percent in Arkansas to 45.2 percent in Maine. During 2000 to 2003, multivitamin use increased significantly in three states (Illinois, North Carolina, and Utah).
- *Physical abuse:* In 2003, the prevalence of physical abuse by a husband or partner during the 12 months before pregnancy ranged from 2.2 percent in Maine to 7.6 percent in New Mexico; during 2000 to 2003, significant decreases were recorded in three states (Alaska, Hawaii, and Nebraska).
- *Cigarette smoking during pregnancy:* In 2003, the prevalence of abstinence from cigarette smoking during the last 3 months of pregnancy ranged from 72.5 percent in West Virginia to 96.1 percent in Utah.
- *Cigarette smoking cessation:* In 2003, the prevalence of smoking cessation during pregnancy ranged from 30.2 percent in West Virginia to 65.8 percent in Utah.
- *Drinking alcohol during pregnancy*: In 2003, the prevalence of abstinence from alcohol during the last 3 months of pregnancy ranged from 91.3 percent in Colorado to 98.0 percent in Utah.
- *Breastfeeding initiation:* In 2003, the prevalence of mothers who breastfed their babies in the early postpartum period ranged from 51.2 percent in Louisiana to 90.3 percent in Alaska. During 2000 to 2003, significant increases were recorded in six states (Arkansas, Illinois, Louisiana, Nebraska, North Carolina, and South Carolina).
- *Infant sleep position:* In 2003, the prevalence of healthy full-term infants who were placed to sleep on their backs ranged from 50.0 percent in Arkansas to 78.7 percent in Washington. During 2000 to 2003, significant increases were recorded in eight states (Alaska, Colorado, Illinois, Louisiana, Maine, Nebraska, North Carolina, and West Virginia).

Some health promotion program assessments such as PRAMS are continuous. **FIGURE 12-4** presents five phases of a continuous inquiry and learning process. Each phase comprises two or three concrete steps. Some

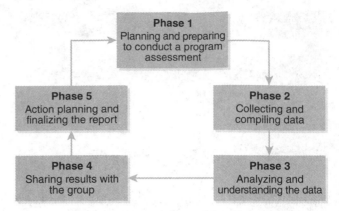

**FIGURE 12-4** The five phases of the continuous assessment.

Reproduced from: O'Connor C, Zeldin S. Program assessment and improvement through youth-adult partnership: The YALPE Resource Kit. *J Extension*. 2005; 43(5), Article 5T0T4.

steps are to be carried out in assessment team meetings and some in meetings with all program participants. The entire process takes about 24 hours to complete over a period of 1 to 4 months, depending on the needs and structure of the program. However, the process is flexible; it allows programs and organizations to carry out the implementation process as needed. The guides for action planning based on assessment results, included in Phase 5 of the process, make the link between the assessment process and program improvement to promote a continuous inquiry cycle.

## ▶ Reporting Program Success

Results and recommendations from the various program evaluations need to be summarized, analyzed, and interpreted at regular intervals in statistical, graphic, and narrative reports written according to agency requirements and outlines. The program director is often responsible for writing the report. There should be a list of who will receive the report and a strategy for distribution.[42] One aspect of reporting should be weekly, monthly, or quarterly informal feedback to the staff. Quarterly or semiannual written and verbal reports should be reviewed with the staff and administrators, and annual written reports should be sent to the agency board, funding agencies, and the public.

Most agencies publish annual reports that summarize their work during the year and that are disseminated to the community.[63] Nutrition services should be highlighted in these reports and successful programs showcased to the community through media coverage. **TABLE 12-2** presents an example of a formal report format. See **BOX 12-3** for a sample of a program report.

**TABLE 12-2** Formal Report Format[11,63-65]

| Report Elements | Content |
|---|---|
| Prefatory section | *Title Page/Front Cover*<br>■ The title of the report (for some reports, this must be centered, all in capital letters, and about 1½ inches from the top of the page).<br>■ The name and title of the person for whom the report is intended.<br>■ The name, position, and business address of the writer.<br>■ The date the report is issued.<br>■ The fiscal year of the report.<br>■ Begin pagination with the title page.<br>■ Prefatory parts are paginated with small Roman numerals (i, ii, iii, iv).<br><br>*Table of Contents*<br>■ The table of contents provides a map of the structure of the complete report, from the cover page to the appendix.<br><br>*Table of Figures*<br>■ Use to list three or more visual aids such as tables and/or figures and their page numbers.<br><br>*Abstract/Executive Summary*<br>■ The summary of the entire report.<br>■ Write the abstract after the report has been written. |
| Body section | *Background Information*<br>■ State the objective of the program.<br>■ Provide background information on the issue or program.<br>■ Discuss the type of theoretical framework that was used.<br>■ Describe the equipment (skinfold caliper, blood pressure apparatus, etc.)<br>■ Provide results/outcomes of the program.<br>■ Describe how the program was carried out.<br>■ Use the visual aids to summarize the findings/outcomes.<br>■ Refer to visual aids within the text before presenting them.<br>■ Discuss the results.<br>■ Show how certain outcomes were achieved.<br>■ Include the strengths and weaknesses of the program. |
| Terminal section | *Conclusion*<br>■ Summarize the major findings/outcome of the program.<br><br>*Recommendations*<br>■ Recommend specific courses of action (to take or avoid).<br>■ List the recommendations in order of priority.<br><br>*Work Cited*<br>■ List all your sources of information.<br><br>*Optional Appendix*<br>■ Contains any other data that would clarify the report.<br>■ This is supplementary material that would interrupt the flow of the body of the report (such as charts, figures, maps, and pictures). |

Modified from: Kamalani P, Hurley, Leeward CC. A guide to the document: The formal report. University of Hawaii. http://emedia.leeward.hawaii.edu/hurley/eng209w/booklet/pages/unit2/frguide.pdf. Accessed July 27, 2016.

**BOX 12-3** A Sample of a Program Report

**Prefatory Section**

*Understanding Menopause*

By

*Dr. Nweze Nnakwe*

Program Director

To

Illinois Department of Public Health

Office of Women's Health

June 30, 2006

**Table of Contents**

Background Information

Conclusion

Recommendations

Work Cited

Appendix

**Table of Figures**

Abstract/Executive Summary

**Body Section**

*Background Information*

The objective of this program was to increase the knowledge of physiological and emotional changes that often may be experienced during perimenopause and menopause in women 40–60 years old. This program utilized the Health Belief Model. Participants were recruited through a variety of strategies such as distributing flyers throughout McLean County in various businesses and organizations, fitness centers, churches, and newsletters. The program was advertised in newspapers, local TV stations, and radio stations. The local CNN Headline News interviewed the director, which aired for 2 weeks. Gift giveaways such as Boca coupons were one of the strategies utilized to recruit participants. The nutritionist developed a website and educational materials, including a brochure, PowerPoint slides, handouts including nutritional recipes, and posters on how to increase women's knowledge of the physiological and emotional changes that often may be experienced during perimenopause and menopause. The nutritionist conducted 15 workshops and/or seminars to educate women about menopause and health-related issues such as heart disease and osteoporosis, obesity, and stress management. The director initiated a Health Night Fair at an African American church. The program reached the targeted population of 280 for the first year. A 3-month follow-up survey showed that there were some behavior changes such as improved nutrition knowledge, improved level of physical activity, increased number of women beginning hormone replacement therapy, and increased use of soy products. The difficulty associated with the program is low attendance at the sessions.

**Terminal Section**

*Conclusion*

The targeted population of 280 was reached for the first year. The first quarter of the first year was used to develop the program. Implementation of the program started fully in the second quarter. Eighty-five percent of the participants reported behavior change.

*Recommendation*

In addition to the first year's strategies, utilizing personal contact with businesses, women's organizations, and churches for the recruitment of participants will be helpful. Continued collaboration with wellness programs and other organizations such as the Heart and Lung Association will be important.

Works Cited and Appendix were not used.

# Learning Portfolio

## Chapter Summary

- Community and public health nutritionists use programs to improve the health of communities.
- Factors that may trigger program planning include research findings, a change in existing policy, and availability of resources.
- Formative evaluation provides information to those planning and implementing the program and permits improvements to the program while activities are in progress.
- Summative evaluation provides retrospective information about the performance of the program when the program has been completed.

- Funding sources for nutrition programs include grants and contracts from local, state, and federal agencies or foundations and private contributions.
- Data collection methods include interviews, focus groups, observations, and surveys.

## Critical Thinking Activities

- Divide into groups and perform assessments (on a child and/or an adult) that include body fat measurements using a skinfold caliper, body mass index, and 24-hour-dietary recall.

- Survey participants (college students, older adults, or high school students) to determine their knowledge of MyPlate food guide.
- Use the educational methods and materials presented in the success story of the Colorado State University education program to determine other strategies that could be used to provide a more effective nutrition education program in the Hispanic community.

---

## 🔍 CASE STUDY 12-1: Nutrition Education in Multicultural Communities

During an initial survey of a community, Ikechi, a public health nutritionist, discovered that migrant and other minority students in the local schools were consuming foods for lunch that are high in fat and calories, and low in essential nutrient such as iron; calcium; protein; vitamins C, A, and D; and folate. He also observed that about 20 percent of the students were obese, 30 percent were overweight, and some had chapped, red, swollen lips and tooth decay. In addition, most of the students did not have enough money to purchase nutritious foods. The following barriers to weight management were identified:

- Lack of awareness about the need for and benefits of weight management
- Belief that weight restriction in children can be harmful
- Belief that engaging in a weight management program is expensive and time consuming
- Ikechi was asked to develop a nutrition education program.

### Questions

1. Before Ikechi could carry out the activities, he decided to learn more about nutrition programming and program planning. What is the definition of a program in relation to community nutrition, and what is the overall purpose? What is program planning?
2. Ikechi knew that he must collect and analyze different types of data. What are subjective and objective data analyses?
3. Ikechi needed to know the mission of the community regarding nutrition and health. What is a mission statement and action plan? Why is it important to review the mission statement and match it with the program goals?
4. Ikechi must design and plan the program before carrying out nutrition education. What are the factors to consider when writing or designing a program plan?
5. What is program implementation? What are some of the factors that Ikechi must consider when implementing a program?
6. Ikechi conducted different types of evaluations. What are the reasons for conducting a program evaluation? What are the evaluation aspects?
7. Determining the cost of a program is very important in providing a nutrition education program. What is a cost—benefit analysis? How is it used in relation to a nutrition program?
8. Reporting program success requires continuous assessment. What are the five phases of a continuous assessment?
9. Work in small groups or individually to discuss the case study and practice using the Nutrition Care Process chart provided on the companion website. You can also add other nutrition and health-related conditions or assessments to the case study to make the case study more challenging and interesting.

---

## Think About It

**Answer:** Determining the cost of a program is an essential part of program planning. It is important to calculate the actual cost of a program by determining both the direct costs (personnel salaries, travel reimbursement, equipment, supplies, continuing education for nutrition personnel, printing/postage, and marketing the program) and indirect costs (time lost from work by recipients participating in a program, childcare costs, utilities, building and grounds, and janitorial services). It is also important to plan for situations that may increase the cost of the program, such as an increase in the number of participants or the length of the education program; a need for additional equipment, staff, or space; and so on.

## Key Terms

**action plan:** A concise statement of the methods, activities, or intervention strategies to be undertaken.

**cost—benefit analysis:** The analytic process whereby the costs and benefits of a program are identified and measured in monetary (dollar) terms.

**objective data analysis:** The collection and analysis of available demographic and health statistics to prepare a community diagnosis and problem list.

**program:** A collection of activities intended to produce particular results.

**program evaluation:** An ongoing process from the beginning of the planning phase until a program ends.

**program implementation:** The process of putting a program into action.

**program planning:** The process of exploring a situation, deciding on a more desirable situation, and designing actions to create the desired situation.

**subjective data analysis:** The collection and analysis of data on various clients that are observable and measurable, such as listening to radio stations, watching local television coverage, and interviewing key informants/community leaders.

# References

1. Dignan MB, Carr PA. *Program Planning for Health Education and Promotion.* 2nd ed. Philadelphia, PA: Lea & Febiger; 1992.

2. Stanhope M, Lancaster J. *Community and Public Health Nursing: Population-Centered Health Care in the Community.* 9th ed. New York, NY: Elsevier; 2015.

3. Wilson MM, Thomas D, Rubenstein LZ, Chibnall JT, Anderson S, Baxi A. Appetite assessment: simple appetite questionnaire predicts weight loss in community-dwelling adults and nursing home residents. *Am J Clin Nutr.* 2005;82(5):1074-1081.

4. Shannon J, Shikany JM, Barrett-Connor E, Marshall LM, et al. Demographic factors associated with the diet quality of older US men: baseline data from the Osteoporotic Fractures in Men (MrOS) study. *Public Health Nutr.* 2007;10(8):810-819.

5. Kaufman M. *Nutrition in Promoting the Public's Health: Strategies, Principles, and Practice.* Sudbury, MA: Jones and Bartlett; 2009.

6. Caravella J. A needs assessment method for Extension educators. *J Extension.* 2006;44(1):1-7.

7. Bramley DD, Hebert PP, Jackson RR, Chassin MM. Indigenous disparities in disease-specific mortality: a cross-country comparison—New Zealand, Australia, Canada, and the United States. *N Z Med J.* 2004;117(1207):U1215.

8. Bryce J, Boschi-Pinto C, Shibuya K, Black RE. WHO estimates of the causes of death in children. *Lancet.* 2005;365(9465):1147-1152.

9. Caulfield LE, Richard SA, Black RE. Undernutrition as an underlying cause of malaria morbidity and mortality in children less than five years old. *Am J Trop Med Hyg.* 2004;71(2 suppl):55-63.

10. National Institute of Health. Hearts N' Parks Program continues to help participants of all ages adopt Hearty-Healthy behaviors. http://www.nhlbi.nih.gov/. Accessed March 16, 2017.

11. Boyle MA, Holben D. *Community Nutrition in Action: An Entrepreneurial Approach.* 4th ed. Belmont, CA: Thomson Wadsworth; 2013.

12. Adler NE, Castellazzo GG, Ickovics JR. Relationship of subjective and objective social status with psychological and physiological functioning: preliminary data in healthy white women. *Health Psychology.* 2000;19(6):586-592.

13. Jensen CJ, Finifter DH, Wilson CE, Koenig BL. Community assessment of senior health using a telephone survey and supplementary methods. *J Appl Gerontol.* 2007;26(1):17-33.

14. Greenhalgh T, Chowdhury M, Wood GW. Story-based scales: development and validation of questionnaires to measure subjective health status and cultural adherence in British Bangladeshis with diabetes. *Psychol Health Med.* 2006;11(4):432-448.

15. Dahlberg JC, Holben DH. Halt hunger on the Hocking: a service-learning project developed in response to a needs assessment of a rural Appalachian Ohio Community. *J Am Diet Assoc.* 2004;104(8 suppl):S58.

16. Clark CC. *Health Promotion in Communities: Holistic and Wellness Approaches.* New York, NY: Springer Publishing; 2002.

17. Taylor TT, Serrano E, Anderson J, Kendall P. Knowledge, skills, and behavior improvements on peer educators and low-income Hispanic participants after a stage of change-based bilingual nutrition education program. *J Community Health.* 2000;25(3):241-262.

18. US Census Bureau. *The Official Statistics.* Washington, DC: US Government Printing Office; 1996. https://www.census.gov/. Accessed March 17, 2017.

19. Colorado Migrant Health Department. *Colorado Migrant Health Program 1996 Report Denver.* Denver, CO: Colorado Migrant Health Department; 1996.

20. Diehl AK, Stern MP. Special health problems of Mexican Americans: obesity, gallbladder disease, diabetes mellitus, and cardiovascular disease. *Adv Intern Med.* 1989;34:79-96.

21. Lopez L, Masse B. Income, body fatness, and fat patterns in Hispanic women from the Hispanic Health and Nutrition Examination Survey. *Health Care Women Int.* 1998;14:117-128.

22. US Census Bureau. *Statistical Abstract of the United States.* 110th ed. Washington, DC: US Government Printng Office; 1990.

23. US Census Bureau. *Current Population Survey.* Washington, DC: US Government Printing Office; 1996. https://www.census.gov/. Accessed March 17, 2017.

24. Valente T. *Evaluating Health Promotion Programs.* New York, NY: Oxford University Press; 2002.

25. McNamara C. Basics of developing mission, vision and values statements. In: *Field Guide to Nonprofit Strategic Planning and Facilitation.* Minneapolis, MN: Authenticity Consulting; 2007.

26. Cooperative State Research E, Extension Service. Expanded food and nutrition education program success stories: collaboration. http://www.csrees.usda.gov/nea/food/efnep/success-collaboration.html. Accessed March 16, 2017.

27. Anspaugh DJ, Dignan MB, Anspaugh SL. *Developing Health Promotion Programs.* 2nd ed. Long Grove, IL: Waveland Press; 2006.

28. Hitchcock J, Schubert PE, Thomas SA. *Community Health Nursing.* 2nd ed. Clifton Park, NY: Thomson Delmar Learning; 2003.

29. US Dept of Agriculture, US Dept of Health Human Services. *Nutrition and Your Health: Dietary Guidelines for Americans.* 8th ed. Home and Garden Bull. US Dept of Agriculture, US Dept of Health Human Services; 2015.

30. PennState. Archive of Learning Design Instructional Guides. *Writing Objectives.* http://archive.tlt.psu.edu/learningdesign/objectives/writing.html. Accessed March 17, 2017.

31. Heinrich R, Molenda M, Russell JD, Smaldino SE. *Instructional Media and Technologies for Learning.* Englewood Cliffs, NJ: Merrill; 1996.

32. Nelson D. The Health Information National Trends Survey (HINTS): development, design, and dissemination. *J Health Comm.* 2004;9(5):443-460.

33. Glasgow RE, Lichtenstein E, Marcus AC. Why don't we see more translation of health promotion research to practice? Rethinking the efficacy-to-effectiveness transition. *Am J Public Health.* 2003;93(8):1261-1267.

34. Kreuter MW, Lezin NA, Green LW. *Community Health Ideas That Work.* 2nd ed. Boston, MA: Jones & Bartlett; 2003.

35. Gregory J. Using message strategy to capture audience attention: readers' reactions to health education publications *J Nonprofit Public Sector Market.* 2006;15(12):1-23.

36. Briss PA, Brownson RC, Fielding JE, Zaza S. Developing and using the guide to community preventive services: lessons learned about evidence-based public health. *Annu Rev Public Health.* 2004;25:281-302

37. Serritzlew S. Linking budgets to activity: a test of the effect of output-purchase budgeting. *Public Budg Financ.* 2006;26(2):101-120.

38. Russell LB, Dong-Churl S, Safford MM. Time requirements for diabetes self-management: too much for many? *J Fam Pract.* 2005;54(1):52-56.

39. Bisset S, Potvin L. Expanding our conceptualization of program implementation: lesson from the genealogy of a school-based nutrition program. http://her.oxfordjournals.org. Accessed March 16, 2017.

40. Chen H. *Practical Program Implementation: Assessing and Improving Planning, Implementation, and Effectiveness.* London, UK: Sage; 2004.

41. Bracht N, Kingsbury L. Community organization principles in health promotion: a five stage model. In: Bracht N, ed. *Health Promotion at the Community Level.* Newbury Park, CA: Sage; 1990.

42. Valente TW, Fosados R. Diffusion of innovations and network segmentation: the part played by people in promoting health. *Sex Transm Dis.* 2006;33(7 suppl):S23-S31.

43. Edelstein S. *Nutrition in Public Health: A Handbook for Developing Programs and Services.* 3rd ed. Sudbury, MA: Jones & Bartlett; 2011.

44. Gittelsohn J, Evans M, Story M. Multisite formative assessment for the Pathways study to prevent obesity in American Indian schoolchildren. *Am J Clin Nutr.* 1999;69(4 suppl):767S–772S.

45. Merzel C, D'Afflitti J. Reconsidering community-based health promotion: promise, performance, and potential. *Am J Public Health.* 2003;93(4):557-574.

46. Health Canada. First Nations and Inuit Home and Community Care (FNI HCC) Program: evaluation guide. *The Purpose of Evaluation.* http://www.hc-sc.gc.ca/. Accessed April 14, 2016.

47. Williams J. *Introduction to Health Services.* 7th ed. New York, NY: Wiley; 2007.

48. Ryan L, Anderson J. The effect of nutrition education on improving fruit and vegetable consumption of youth. *J Extension.* 1995;33(5):1-5.

49. Kaufman M. *Nutrition in Public Health A Handbook for Developing Programs and Services.* Rockville, MD: Aspen; 2007.

50. Rivera JA, Sotres-Alvarez D, Habicht JP, Shamah T, et al. Impact of the Mexican Program for Education, Health, and Nutrition on rates of growth and anemia in infants and young children *JAMA.* 2004;291(21):2563-2570.

51. Frodi D, Esben BJ, Pal W, White RF, et al. Impact of prenatal methylmercury exposure on neurobehavioral function at age 14 years. *Neurotoxicol Teratol.* 2006;28(3):363–375.

52. Nemcek MA, Sabatier R. State of evaluation: community health workers. *Public Health Nurs.* 2003;20(4):260-270.

53. Floyd JF, Gallagher P, Stringfellow V, Zaslavsky AM, et al. Using telephone interviews to reduce

nonresponse bias to mail surveys of health plan members. *Medical Care.* 2002;40(3):190-200.

54. Ariza AJ, Chen EH, Binns HJ, Christoffel KK. Risk factors for overweight in five-to six-year-old Hispanic-American Children: a pilot study. *J Urban Health.* 2004;81(1):150-161.

55. Lambur M, Rajgopal R, Lewis E, Cox RH. Applying cost benefit analysis to nutrition education programs: focus on the Virginia Expanded Food and Nutrition Education Program. Pub. No. 490-403. http://www.ext.vt.edu/pubs/nutrition/490-403/490-403.html#L7. Accessed March 16, 2017.

56. Rein DB, Constantine RT, Orenstein D, Chen H, et al. A cost evaluation of the Georgia Stroke and Heart Attack Prevention Program. *Prev Chronic Dis.* 2006;3(1):A12.

57. Parkerson GR, Broadhead WE, Tse CK. The Duke Health Profile: a 17-item measure of health and dysfunction. *Medical Care.* 1990;28(11):1056-1072.

58. Baró E, Ferrer M, Vázquez O, Miralles R, et al. Using the Nottingham Health Profile (NHP) among older adult inpatients with varying cognitive function. *Quality Life Res.* 2006;15(4):575-585.

59. Bell JF, Zimmerman FJ, Mayer JD, Almgren GR, et al. Associations between residential segregation and smoking during pregnancy among urban African-American women. *J Urban Health.* 2007;84(3):372-388.

60. Mosley BB. Folic acid and the decline in neural tube defects in Arkansas. *J Arkansas Med Soc.* 2007;103(10):247-250.

61. Collier SA, Hogue CJ. Modifiable risk factors for low birth weight and their effect on cerebral palsy and mental retardation. *Matern Child Health J.* 2007;11(1):65-71.

62. Suellentrop K, Morrow B, Williams L, D'Angelo D, Centers for Disease Control and Prevention (CDC). Monitoring progress toward achieving maternal and infant Healthy People 2010 objectives: 19 states, Pregnancy Risk Assessment Monitoring System (PRAMS), 2000–2003. *MMWR Surveill Summ.* 2006;6(55):1-11.

63. Kamalani Hurley P, Leeward CC. A guide to the document: the formal report. 2005. http://emedia.leeward.hawaii.edu/hurley/eng209w/booklet/pages/unit2/frguide.pdf. Accessed March 16, 2017.

64. Kirmse DW. Formal technical report organization. 2001. http://pie.che.ufl.edu/guides/reports/formal_report.html. Accessed April 24, 2011.

65. Fischer A, Northey M. Formal reports and proposals. In: *Impact: A Guide to Business Communiction.* 1993. http://www.pearsoned.ca/highered/divisions/virtual_tours/northey/sample_chapter_9.pdf. Accessed March 16, 2017.

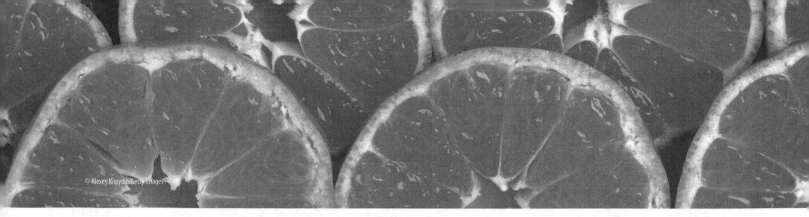

# CHAPTER 13

# Theories and Models for Health Promotion and Changing Nutrition Behavior

## LEARNING OBJECTIVES

- Identify different theories and models that community nutritionists can use to provide effective nutrition programs.
- Discuss each theory and its application to community and public health nutrition.
- Explain how behavioral models can provide positive nutrition messages.

## ▶ Introduction

Several behavior change theories indicate how to tailor messages so they are more relevant to individuals or communities. For example, using the Transtheoretical or Stages of Change Model to tailor a health message would involve considering areas of concern in the client's diet (e.g., inadequate milk consumption) and physical activity (e.g., sedentary lifestyle), as well as the client's level of readiness or motivation to change their behavior.[1]

Conversely, tailoring based on the Health Belief Model (HBM) would center on the client's perception of the risks and benefits associated with changing behavior. For example, Fitzpatrick et al.[2] carried out a statewide community-based intervention program based on the HBM. The aim of the program was to improve physical activity and physical function in older adults attending senior centers throughout Georgia. Examples of how the main concepts of this framework were incorporated into the program include[2]:

- *Perceived susceptibility and severity*: Emphasizing the health conditions that occur frequently in older adults that are associated with low physical activity
- *Perceived benefits*: Defining how to take action by increasing physical activity
- *Perceived barriers*: Providing information and correcting misinformation about physical activity
- *Cues to action*: Providing "how-to" information illustrating 16 chair exercises
- *Self-efficacy*: Demonstrating and reinforcing the various ways to include physical activity in daily life

In this Georgia Senior Center program, participants completed a pretest and posttest that assessed physical activity and physical function, which were categorized as poor, moderate, or good. The 4-month physical activity intervention included 16 sessions that focused on educator-led chair exercises, promotion of walking, using a pedometer, and recording daily steps. Results showed that participants improved their physical function on all four items.

This chapter discusses evidence-based types of models shown to be effective in program planning and strategies as they relate to behavior change, nutrition, and health.

## ▶ Program Planning Using Theories and Models

In the past, program planning, implementation, and evaluation activities were frequently based on the premise that communities were the recipients of programs rather than partners in programming. There is now value in considering other ways of programming that can create opportunities for processes that empower the community (i.e., create opportunities for community control).[3] *Program paradigms* are defined as representations of approaches to programming that offer explanations of the processes involved. To provide guidance throughout programming processes, communities and nutritionists together may either create their own model or use an already-tested programming or planning model. Sometimes a model is recommended by a funding agency. Because all models are based on values and assumptions, the nutritionist needs to ensure that the chosen model is either consistent with the nutrition ideas or can be adequately adapted.[4]

When concepts and constructs are related to each other and purposely combined to form a unit, the resulting entity may be labeled a *framework*, a model, or a theory.[5] In this perspective, a framework refers to a scheme that specifies the steps in a process.[5,6]

For example, community nutritionists could use a framework that includes listening, critical reflection, participatory dialogue, theme recognition, action, and reflection on action. Regardless of the programming framework the community nutritionist prefers, knowledge of a variety of frameworks is helpful because he or she will be working with people from diverse backgrounds. Generally, a framework is a planning tool. It can incorporate theories, models, or parts thereof, and it allows for the organization of a large and unspecified number of potentially predictive or explanatory variables.

Program *models* are ways of viewing real events, and they can be physical, symbolic, or mental. A program model describes what the nutritionist should do to provide both effective instruction and the support services needed to persist in the learning process long enough to create a behavior change.[7] A physical model is a specific, observable replica of a real structure (e.g., chemical equations, anatomic models, and food models). Symbolic models have a higher level of abstraction than do physical models. For example, signs have symbolic meanings to those who read them. A "No Smoking" sign signifies that the readers should refrain from smoking. Mental models have an even greater level of abstraction than both physical and symbolic models because they convey a mental image, not a real picture. For example, the term *nutrition* has different meanings for different people.[6] To provide guidance throughout programming processes, communities and nutritionists together may either create their own model or theory or use an already-tested programming or planning model. Sometimes a model is recommended by a funding agency. Because all models are based on values and assumptions, the nutritionist needs to ensure that the chosen model or theory is either consistent with the nutrition ideas or can be adequately adapted.[4] Community nutritionists can use different models or theories to provide effective nutrition education.

A *theory* is a construct that accounts for or organizes events. A nutrition theory explains or describes a specific event of nutrition. Theories provide nutritionists with different lenses through which to see situations; each lens provides a different view and understanding. In general, the most effective programs are those that are theory based.[4]

The quality of the working relationships among participants is very important to the success of any program. Many frameworks have been designed to guide this relationship in health promotion programs. This section will discuss the P-Process, PRECEDE-PROCEED, and several other frameworks that community nutritionists can utilize to design health promotion programs.

## Health Belief Model

The Health Belief Model (HBM) emphasizes perceived threat as a motivating force and perceived benefits (fewer barriers) as a preferred path to action.[8] It asserts that readiness to take action to avoid an illness or condition is possible because people will do the following[8-10]:

- Perceive themselves as threatened by the condition, which in turn is determined by a perception of personal vulnerability ("How likely am I to get heart disease and how soon?") and perceived severity of the condition ("How bad would it be to have heart disease?")
- Perceive that the recommended course of action to reduce the threat is feasible and efficacious ("Will I feel better if I change the fats or the diet that I eat?") and that the barriers or costs to it are low ("How hard will it be to make these changes in my diet or fat intake?")
- Believe that they have the ability to successfully perform the recommended behavior ("How confident am I that I can succeed in changing my diet and fat intake?")

## Application

Wallace[11] studied personal characteristics associated with the practice of osteoporosis-protective behaviors among nontraditional college women using HBM. The participants responded to a questionnaire about their osteoporosis knowledge, weight-bearing exercise, and dietary calcium intake. Results show that 50.7 percent of the participants did not follow the exercise guidelines and 67.8 percent did not follow the guidelines for calcium. The author stated that HBM was helpful in predicting exercise and calcium behavior.[11] Similarly, Strychar[12] examined the relationship among knowledge, health beliefs, and dietary behaviors of participants using the HBM. A total of 3,432 individuals' ages 18 to 74 participated in a screening program conducted in 54 supermarkets in Montreal and Quebec. This program identified participants' risk for cardiovascular disease by measuring total serum cholesterol, blood pressure, height, weight, level of physical activity, and tobacco use. A 10-minute debriefing counseling session interpreted risk factors and recommended follow-up. Seventy percent ($n = 2,420$) also completed a nutrition questionnaire on knowledge, health beliefs, and frequency of consumption of high-fat foods. Respondents increased their knowledge and reduced the frequency of consumption of high-fat foods following the screening program, particularly individuals with higher blood cholesterol levels and high blood pressure. Depending on the relative strength of benefits and barriers, program strategies could target either the benefits of change or overcoming the barriers.

## Knowledge-Attitude-Behavior Model

The Knowledge-Attitude-Behavior Model (KABM) stresses that a gain in new knowledge leads to changes in attitude, which, in turn, result in improved dietary behavior or practices.[13] For changes in attitude and behavior to occur, the knowledge provided must be motivational. Research suggests that some types of knowledge are more motivating than others. Rogers[14] refers to "awareness" knowledge as the kind that captures people's attention, increases awareness, and enhances motivation, whereas "how-to" knowledge is the kind people need when they are already motivated. Social psychological research makes a similar distinction, with "anticipated consequences" or expectancies as the kind of knowledge that is likely to enhance motivation to take action (motivational knowledge), whereas "behavioral capabilities" (or knowledge and skills) are needed by people in order to act on their motivations (instrumental knowledge). In addition, it is important to consider the acquisition of attitudes. For example, an attitude can be acquired passively by observation (e.g., watching a TV program on how to prepare a low-fat food) or acquired actively by the integration of beliefs about the consequences of an action (e.g., reducing sodium intake to lower blood pressure).[15,16]

General nutrition education interventions have used a stated or implied KABM, which emphasizes dissemination of "how-to" (e.g., how to reduce fat intake) or "skills" information (e.g., shopping with a grocery list). Topics that have been covered include food groups, balanced diets, label reading, high-fat or high-fiber foods, food shopping and preparation skills, managing food budgets, and food sources of nutrients. This kind of instrumental knowledge is essential for those already motivated to eat nutritiously, but for others it is just "information."[10,17] On the other hand, knowledge can be motivating when it is about the potential positive or negative consequences of behavior, particularly if these are of personal relevance or when they tap into other motivators and reinforcers of change.[18] Both motivational and instrumental, or how-to, knowledge are needed for effective nutrition education designed to promote behavioral change.

## Application

KABM is an educational strategy that uses an intervention approach. For example, a list of foods that are good sources of calcium or public announcements of good sources of calcium may be a motivational factor to dietary improvement for individuals who are concerned about the incidence of osteoporosis. However, memorizing a list of foods that are high in calcium does not result in a change in behavior.[19]

## Social Learning Theory

The Social Learning Theory (SLT) (also called Social Cognitive Theory (SCT) or Social Influence Theory) emphasizes the interactive nature of the effects of cognitive and other personal factors and environmental events on behavior.[6] The three major constructs/concepts in SLT are behavioral capacity (having the skills necessary for the performance of the desired behavior, such as quitting excessive alcohol drinking), efficacy expectations (beliefs regarding one's ability to successfully carry out a course of action or perform a behavior), and outcome expectations (beliefs that the performance of a behavior will have the desired effects or consequences).[6,20,21]

The main idea in SLT is "reciprocal determinism." This means that behavior is determined by the interaction among three elements: the person, the person's behavior, and the environment.[6,22] The person's actions contribute to creating the environment, and the actions and environment contribute to the person's cognitions or "expectancies." There are three types of expectancies: beliefs about how events are connected, beliefs about the consequences of one's actions (outcome expectations), and beliefs about one's competence to perform the behavior needed to influence the outcomes (efficacy expectations). Incentives also contribute to behavior; incentive or reinforcement is the value of a particular outcome to a person.[6,23]

## Application

When problem behaviors are closely tied to social or economic motivations, more comprehensive theories and models, such as the SLT, may be effective tools for planning nutrition interventions.[24] For instance, if a community nutritionist needs to promote milk-based foods as sources of dietary calcium, SLT would support an educational intervention addressing behavioral capability (knowledge and skills needed to select and prepare milk-based foods), reciprocal determinism (availability of milk-based foods in vending machines and restaurants), expectations (beliefs about osteoporosis as a consequence of avoiding milk-based foods), self-efficacy (confidence in one's ability to use more milk-based foods), observational learning or modeling (seeing peers and other role models drinking milk), and reinforcement (positive or negative feelings that occur when milk drinking is practiced).[25]

In the United States, few children fulfill the current national dietary recommendations to eat five servings of fruits and vegetables per day to promote optimal health and prevent chronic diseases.[26,27] A study examined the effectiveness of a 10-week classroom-based nutrition intervention program that combined child-focused interactive lessons and skill-building activities, repeated food tasting opportunities, and interactive parent-focused lessons on child-feeding strategies to increase children's fruit intake. The change in the children's knowledge, preference, and intake of fruit and parents' use of controlling child-feeding strategies were measured in a pretest or posttest manner. Lessons consisted of 1 hour of instruction provided to children and parents devoted to enhancing knowledge about a fruit, skills necessary to incorporate the fruit into the diet, and techniques to enhance goal-directed behaviors. The sessions included interactive discussions, case studies, brainstorming activities, and games. Topics covered in the classes included exposure (increasing the availability of healthful foods), monitoring (understanding that the children can self-regulate the amount of food they need each day), restriction (learning how to present a variety of foods to children without restricting access to certain foods), rewarding or punishing (understanding that using food as a reward or punishment can be counterproductive), and encouragement (learning how to present food to a child in a less aggressive manner without using verbal prompting).[11] Seventeen parent–child pairs who participated in the first class session, which consisted of an orientation and preevaluation session, but were unable to attend any follow-up classes, served as the control.

Parents were taken into a separate room, where they were given instruction on child-feeding strategies to enhance fruit acceptance. In the final half-hour of the session, parents rejoined their children in the food laboratory. During this period, parents and children were given the opportunity to sample 10 different fruits (apple, orange, banana, grape, pear, star fruit, mango, papaya, kiwifruit, and cantaloupe). The same 10 fruits were used in each class to give children several opportunities to taste them. Also during this segment of the class, parents were encouraged to practice feeding strategies they had learned earlier. There was a significant increase in knowledge scores and fruit intake by children in the experimental versus the control group. Fruit preference scores were similar between groups. Additionally, there was a significant decrease in the use of controlling child-feeding strategies by parents in the intervention versus the control group. This study showed that a nutrition intervention program consisting of extensive food exposure and parent-focused lessons on child-feeding strategies is feasible and can be effective.[28]

An additional example of a nutrition program utilizing the SLT was carried out by Miller et al.[29] to evaluate an intervention to improve food label knowledge and skills in diabetes management among older adults with diabetes mellitus. The program used a randomized pretest and posttest control group design. The participants were ages 65 years and older with type 2 diabetes for 1 year or longer. Forty-eight participants were assigned to the experimental group, and 50 participants served as the control group. The program was conducted in an outpatient setting.

A dietitian conducted the intervention of 10 weekly group sessions. Information processing, learning theory, and SCT principles were used in the program development and evaluation.

The main outcome measures assessed were as follows:

- Participant knowledge
- Outcome expectations (expected results of behavior)
- Self-efficacy
- Decision-making skills

The researchers identified two factors in their findings for outcome expectations (positive and negative) and for self-efficacy (promoters of and barriers to diabetes management). The experimental group had higher improvement in knowledge scores than the control group. They had higher:

- Positive outcome expectations
- Promoters of diabetes management and decision-making skills
- Reduction in barriers to diabetes management

The posttest showed no significant difference in negative outcome expectations between groups.

Applications: Older adults with diabetes can benefit from nutrition education designed to improve the knowledge and skills essential for diabetes management.

**FIGURE 13-1** presents an example of how behavioral models can be used to provide positive nutrition messages for increasing consumption of fruit juice. Each level of the figure adds important concepts addressed by the models discussed in this section.

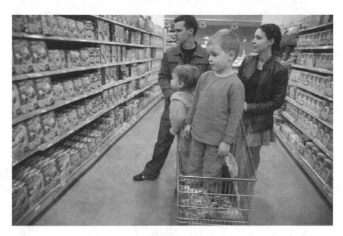

Proper display of nutritious foods can motivate consumers to select nutrient-dense foods.
© Losevsky Pavel/ShutterStock, Inc.

## Theory of Reasoned Action

The Theory of Reasoned Action (TRA) is a highly specific theory outlining cognitive and attitudinal determinants of behavior.[6,30] Attitudes and subjective norms determine an individual's intentions, which are foretelling of behavior. Behavior is likely to follow the stated intentions when there is a shorter time span between intentions and behavior. The TRA is related to the Theory of Planned Behavior (TPB). According to the model, behavior is determined directly by a person's intention to perform the behavior. Intentions are the instructions people give to themselves

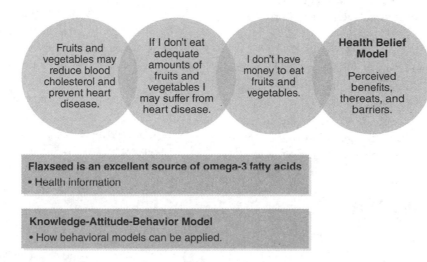

**FIGURE 13-1** How behavioral models can provide positive nutrition messages.

Modified from Freeland-Graves J, Nitzke S. Position of the American Dietetic Association: Total diet approach to communicating food and nutrition information. J. Am. Diet. Assoc. 2002; 102(1):100-108.

to behave in certain ways.[31] People use this principle for their future behavior. In forming intentions, people tend to consider the outcome of their behavior and the opinion of significant others before committing themselves to a particular action.[32] In other words, attitudes and subjective norms influence an individual's belief that a certain behavior will have a given outcome, and this determines his or her attitudes by evaluating the actual outcome of his or her ability to control the behavior.[33]

## Application

Interventions that aim to change dietary behavior provide the possibility for significant public health impact. Theory-based approaches to public health interventions are useful for designing, implementing, and evaluating research. At West Virginia University, Booth-Butterfield and Reger[34] used TRA to conduct an intervention study targeting high-fat (whole and 2 percent) milk users.

The intervention was composed of systematic combinations of either 1) paid advertising (professionally produced TV, radio, and newspaper advertisements) played with heavy frequency and strategic placement, 2) public relations (events produced to garner extensive free or "earned" media coverage in local news), or 3) community education (in-store activities such as blind taste testing and school promotions such as poster design contests). Supermarket milk sales data were collected, and randomly selected intervention and comparison community residents were surveyed via telephone to assess milk use. TRA constructs were used in the surveys that were conducted immediately before and after a 6-week mass media campaign. Campaign messages were aimed at changing behavioral rather than normative beliefs.

Results showed significant and predicted changes in intervention participants on intention, attitude, and behavioral beliefs, but not subjective norm outcomes. The message-based intervention that focused upon a specific behavior produced statistically and practically significant public health effects. People reported more switching, and supermarkets showed increased low-fat milk sales. The study also showed that the combination of paid advertising with public relations produced the strongest effects. One of the strongest features of the theory is that it functions as a practical guide for producing behavior change.

## Diffusion of Innovation Theory

Diffusion of Innovation Theory examines the process in which an innovative idea or practice achieves acceptance.[6,35] Behavior change in specific cultural groups or populations may be seen as the adoption of an innovative

behavior (e.g., starting physical activity, eating unfamiliar food). Diffusion of Innovation Theory has the following key components[6,36,37]:

- *Compatibility*: If innovations are consistent with the economic, sociocultural, and philosophical value system of the adopter, adoption is more likely to happen.
- *Flexibility*: Innovations that can be unraveled and used as separate components will be applicable in a wider variety of user settings.
- *Reversibility*: It is desirable that innovation has the capability of termination in case the adopting individual (or organization) wants to revert to his or her (or its) previous practices. Innovations that are not capable of termination are less likely to be adopted.
- *Relative advantage*: Adoption is more likely if innovation seems more beneficial when compared to previous methods.
- *Complexity*: Complex innovations are more difficult to communicate and understand and are, therefore, less likely to be adopted.
- *Cost efficiency*: Innovation is desirable if its perceived benefits, both tangible and intangible, outweigh its perceived costs.
- *Risk*: The degree of uncertainty introduced by an innovation helps determine its potential for adoption. Innovations that involve higher risk are less likely to be adopted.

## Application

The mass media are an immediate and effective way of introducing new information or trying to influence attitudes, especially during the early stages of reaching audiences susceptible to accepting new ideas.[38] However, at the point of adoption, interpersonal channels are more influential.[39] A communications strategy could consist of using the mass media to introduce the message, provide knowledge, influence attitudes, and reinforce behavior and using interpersonal intervention to teach and encourage the adoption of the behavior.[40] When using the Diffusion of Innovation Theory to promote systemic change within WIC, for example, it is important to talk about the relative benefits of the innovation (e.g., a decrease in iron-deficiency anemia in children) rather than mandating use of a new system or process.

### ✍ Think About It

What is a framework, and how can community nutritionists use it in program planning?

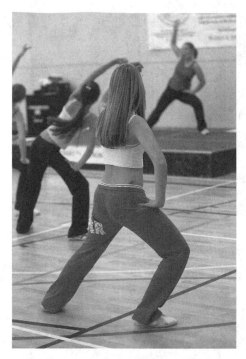

Adopting and maintaining regular aerobic activity is an important part of any health regimen.
© John Lumb/ShutterStock, Inc.

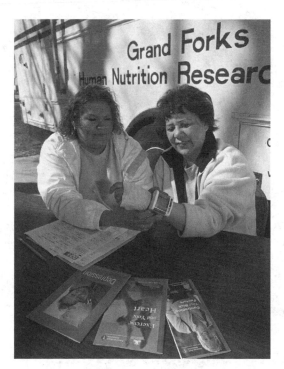

Presenting a positive organizational climate is a significant factor in the success of a program.
Courtesy of Peggy Greb/USDA

## Transtheoretical or Stages of Change Model

Another useful model for planning behavioral intervention programs is the Transtheoretical or Stages of Change Model. According to this conceptual model, the health behavior change process is gradual, continuous, and dynamic.[41,42] People do not immediately change from old to new behaviors; instead, they progress through a sequence of five discrete states, as follows[6,43]:

1. *Precontemplative:* Individuals in this stage have no intention of changing their behavior. They are not aware of the risk and deny that adverse outcomes could happen to them or they are aware of the risk but have made a decision not to change their behavior.
2. *Contemplative:* Individuals in this stage have the intention to change, but have no specific plans to change soon.
3. *Preparation:* Individuals in this stage have plans to change their behavior and may have taken the first step of changing their behavior.
4. *Action:* Individuals in this stage have started to change their behavior, but the behavior change is fairly recent and may be inconsistent.
5. *Maintenance:* These individuals have maintained consistent behavior change for a long time. The newly acquired behavior has become a part of their lives.

This model suggests that individuals engaging in a new behavior go through the stages of precontemplation, contemplation, preparation, action, and maintenance, but not always in a linear manner; it also may be cyclical because many individuals must make several attempts at behavior change before their goals are realized. The amount of progress people make as a result of intervention tends to be a function of the stage they are in at the start of treatment.[6] **TABLE 13-1** presents the changes and techniques community nutritionists and participants can use to address each stage. The Successful Community Strategies feature in this chapter presents the approach used by the University of North Carolina Chapel Hill.

## Application

The Transtheoretical or Stages of Change Model has direct application to nutrition intervention. Program strategies are more effective when designed to match the individual's stage in the change process. For example, individuals in the precontemplation stage would lack awareness or intent to adopt a behavior, such as reducing dietary fat and losing weight. Educational programs for these individuals would put more emphasis on the benefits of making a change. The more practice-oriented "how-to" tips would be diverted to programs and materials targeting individuals in advanced stages, such as action or maintenance.[44] **BOX 13-1** outlines interviewing processes that can be used to identify and assist individuals at different stages of change.

**TABLE 13-1** Stages of Change Model

| Stage of Change | Characteristics | Techniques |
|---|---|---|
| Precontemplation | Not currently considering change: "Ignorance is bliss." | Validate lack of readiness. Clarify that the decision is theirs. Encourage reevaluation of current behavior. Encourage self-exploration, not action. Explain and personalize the risk. |
| Contemplation | Ambivalent about change: "Sitting on the fence." Not considering change within the next month. | Validate lack of readiness. Clarify that the decision is theirs. Encourage evaluation of pros and cons of behavior change. Identify and promote new, positive outcome expectations. |
| Preparation | Some experience with change and are trying to change: "Testing the waters." Planning to act within 1 month. | Identify and assist in problem solving regarding obstacles. Help identify social support. Verify that he or she has underlying skills for behavior change. Encourage small initial steps. |
| Action | Practicing new behavior for 3 to 6 months. | Focus on restructuring cues and social support. Bolster self-efficacy for dealing with obstacles. Combat feelings of loss and reiterate long-term benefits. |
| Maintenance | Resumption of old behaviors: "Fall from grace." | Evaluate trigger for relapse. Reassess motivation and barriers. Plan stronger coping strategies. |

Reproduced from: Prochaska JO, DiClemente CC. Stages and processes of self-change of smoking: Toward an integrated model of change. J. Consult. Clin. Psychol. 1983; 51:390. Reprinted with permission.

## Social Marketing Theory

Social marketing is the use of marketing concepts and tools to increase the acceptability of social ideas or practices. Social Marketing Theory (SMT) employs a consumer orientation, audience analysis and segmentation, and aspects of exchange theory in seeking to increase the acceptability of a behavior in a target group.[6,45] An example of a program using SMT is Project LEAN (Low-Fat Eating for America Now), a national campaign whose goal was to reduce dietary fat consumption to 30 percent of total calories through public service advertising, publicity, and point-of-purchase programs in restaurants, supermarkets, and school and worksite cafeterias. Project LEAN successfully demonstrated the use of the media, market segmentation, effective spokespersons, and successful partnerships.[46]

## Application

Another example of the use of SMT in public health campaigns is Fruits & Veggies—More Matters, which was one of the first major health campaigns to follow the principles of SMT. Using data from a variety of research interviews and surveys, designers of this campaign studied the preferences and habits of various audience segments and developed messages that would be perceived as relevant, comprehensible, and actionable by people in those subgroups. By distributing messages based on the needs of consumers in a variety of settings, such as supermarkets, restaurants, and the Internet, the campaign made progress toward the goal of increasing Americans' consumption of fruits and vegetables.[47]

## Healthy Communities: The Process

Another program framework model is Healthy Communities: The Process. This is a grass-roots community development process. This model is useful when diverse members of a community come together to work on health issues.[48] The phases of the model are entry, needs assessment, planning, doing, and renewal.[49] The entry phase focuses on existing situation, and need assessment focuses on health needs, for example, *determine Hispanic community norms for infant bottle-feeding*. The planning

**BOX 13-1** Motivational Interviewing Algorithm

1. Assess and personalize individual's risk status:
   - "Based on your body mass index (BMI), physical examination, family history, and symptoms, I am concerned about the following: _____, _____, and _____."
   - "I want to talk to you about how your weight may be affecting your health."
2. Stages of change evaluation:
   - "How do *you* feel about your weight?"
   - "What concerns do *you* have about health risks?"
   - "Are *you* considering/planning weight loss now?"
   - "Do the pros of changing outweigh the cons?"
3. Educate, risks, and advice: Weight goal:
   - Educate: Medical Consequences Tip Sheet (longevity and quality of life).
   - Advice: Establish a reasonable goal for weight loss using a clear statement. "A 5 percent to 10 percent weight loss over 6 months for a total loss of _____ to _____ pounds."
4. Assess patient's understanding and concerns:
   - "How do you feel about what I've said?"
   - "On a scale of 1 to 10, with 10 being 100 percent ready to take action, how ready are you to lose weight?"
5. Facilitate motivation depending on the individual's level of contemplation:
   *Facilitate Motivation for Precontemplators*
   - Validate the individual's experience.
   - Acknowledge the individual's control of the decision.
   - In a simple, direct statement, give your opinion on the medical benefits of weight loss for the individual.
   - Explore potential concerns.
   - Acknowledge possible feelings of being pressured.
   - Validate that the individual is not ready.
   - Restate your position that the decision to lose weight is up to the individual.
   - Encourage reframing of current state of change as the potential beginning of a change rather than a decision to never change.

   An answer between 1 and 4 means the individual has very little intention to lose weight.

   An answer between 5 and 7 means the individual is ambivalent about taking action to lose weight. The goal is to move the individual from "No" to "I'll think about it."

   *Facilitate Motivation for Those in Preparation*
   - Praise the decision to change behavior.
   - Prioritize behavior change opportunities.
   - Identify and assist in problem solving regarding obstacles.
   - Encourage small initial steps.
   - Assist individuals in identifying social supports.

   **Goal:** Provide direction and support.

6. Schedule follow-up:
   - Tell the individual when you would like to see him or her again.
   - Give the individual a referral to a health specialist (e.g., dietitian, exercise specialist, therapist), if appropriate.

Modified from: Ockene JK. Providing Training for Patient-Centered Alcohol Counseling in a Primary Care Setting. Arc Intern Med. 1997;157:2334-2341; Simkin-Silverman L, Wing R. Management of Obesity in Primary Care. Ob Res. 1997;5:603-612; and Taylor S. St. Anthony Family Medicine Residency, Denver, CO.

phase focuses on responding to health needs For example: *Explore WIC program eligibility. Investigate the likelihood of qualifying for Supplemental Nutrition Assistance Program. Determine the availability of culturally acceptable foods.* The doing phase focuses on action. For example: *Locate all county infants, children, and their mothers seen by the Public Health Department for WIC and other programs. Locate or form an outreach program for the community.* The renewal phase focuses on evaluation.

For example: *75 percent of the infants and 80 percent of the children were eligible for WIC food supplements and will be enrolled in the program. Mothers and children who were not qualified due to immigrant status were directed to other food assistance programs, such as food pantries and/ or Catholic Social Services.*[50]

Near the completion of each phase, a pause is recommended so the community group can reflect on several questions: Were the goals accomplished? What is the status of the project? What worked? What did not and why?[48,49,51]

This model has been used in grass-roots community development and Healthy Cities and Healthy Communities projects. Now that community development is becoming more familiar in healthcare, the model is gaining further acceptance with grantors and with evaluators who use participatory research methods. This model could be used for planning community-based nutrition programs, but the nutritionist may want to change the terminology in the model from "needs" to "issues or interests" to better match a strength-oriented focus.

## P-Process

In 1983, the first Population Communication Services project team, which included staff from Johns Hopkins University, developed the framework known as the P-Process.[52] The P-Process provides a communication campaign framework for strategy development, project implementation, technical assistance, institution building, and training.[53] Public health nutritionists can use the P-Process when planning programs for populations such as those with HIV/AIDS, older persons, pregnant women, or the homeless.

The P-Process has been used around the globe for over 25 years and consists of six steps followed in sequence to develop and implement effective communication strategies, programs, and activities[52]:

1. *Analysis:* Listen to potential audiences; assess existing programs, policies, resources, strengths, and weaknesses; and analyze communication resources.
2. *Strategic design:* Decide on objectives, identify audience segments, position the concept for the audience, clarify the behavior change model, select channels of communication, plan for interpersonal discussion, draw up an action plan, and design evaluation.
3. *Development, pretesting and revision, and production:* Develop message concepts, pretest with audience members and gatekeepers, revise and produce messages and materials, and retest new and existing materials.
4. *Management, implementation, and monitoring:* Mobilize key organizations, create a positive organizational climate, implement the action plan, and monitor the process of dissemination, transmission, and reception of program outputs.
5. *Impact evaluation:* Measure the impact on audiences and determine how to improve future projects.
6. *Plan for continuity:* Adjust to changing conditions and plan for continuity and self-sufficiency.

The P-Process is a well-tested framework that specifies the major steps needed to implement a health communication campaign. It provided the framework for Strategic Communication Planning and Evaluation (SCOPE), which is a CD-ROM–based training tool.

## Application

The P-Process is used mainly in developing countries and is not widely used in the United States. However, funding agencies such as the U.S. Agency for International Development (USAID) may require nutritionists to use the P-Process to carry out their programs. For example, the Mother Care Project intervention program in India was funded by USAID. The intervention program used information, education, and communication to increase pregnant women's knowledge about anemia. The purpose of the program was to improve the hematological status between each of the three trimesters of pregnant women in a rural community. Iron supplementation was carried out using ferrous sulfate tablets containing 60 mg of elemental iron. Deworming was provided through administration of 100 mg mebendazole tablets taken twice daily for 3 days. A total of 117 family care volunteers were responsible for an average of 200 households each; they were trained to use flash cards to impart knowledge about anemia.

Results showed a significant decrease in the prevalence of anemia by 31, 21.2, and 12 percent, respectively in the first, second, and third trimesters in the intervention groups.[54]

## Precede-Proceed

The PRECEDE-PROCEED model is another framework that community and public health nutritionists can adopt when planning effective nutrition programs. This model provides a comprehensive guide to planning and implementing health promotion activities in nine phases; the first five involve diagnosis or needs assessment, and the last four involve implementation and evaluation.[53] This framework could be used for planning, implementing, and evaluating many large and small health programs. The long-term use of the model has permitted testing and refinement. It has been modified to ensure more community viewpoints and full participation.[52]

PRECEDE-PROCEED is an acronym for the components of the model. PRECEDE stands for Predisposing, Reinforcing, and Enabling Constructs in Educational/Environmental Diagnosis and Evaluation. As its name implies, it represents the process that precedes, or leads up to, an intervention. PROCEED stands for Policy, Regulatory, and Organizational Constructs in Educational and Environmental Development. **BOX 13-2** presents the PRECEDE-PROCEED Model.[4]

The Planned Approach to Community Health (PATCH) programs were based on PRECEDE, and the results led to the development of PROCEED. In the model, social, epidemiological, behavioral, environmental, educational, ecological, policy, and administrative dimensions are assessed and multilevel strategies are designed to improve health status and quality of life.

**BOX 13-2** Precede-Proceed Model

**Phase 1.** *Social assessment:* A targeted segment of the population in a self-study was asked to identify their needs and desires related to their quality of life.

*Program/Application:* College students were interviewed and then surveyed about their health interests. Concerns were expressed about unplanned pregnancy and sexually transmitted diseases (STDs).

**Phase 2.** *Epidemiological assessment:* Epidemiological data were used to identify and rank the health goals or problems that might contribute to quality-of-life issues.

*Program/Application:* Sexually active students reported a lack of condom use. STD and pregnancy rates in national data were similar to those reported by students in the self-study (relates to Healthy People 2010 Objectives 7-3 [health risk behavior information for college and university students] and 23-11 [responsible adolescent sexual behavior]).

**Phase 3.** *Behavioral and environmental assessment:* Participants were asked to identify and rank health-related behavioral risk factors and environmental risk conditions related to the goals/problems.

*Program/Application:* Risk factors and conditions included embarrassment, cost, accessibility, partner trust, and partner refusal.

**Phase 4.** *Educational and ecological assessment:* In relation to the goals/problems, identify factors that have the potential to influence behavior or environment and categorize factors as predisposing (knowledge, attitudes, values, beliefs, perceptions of individuals that can be altered through direct communication), enabling (skills, resources, or barriers controlled largely by societal forces and systems that make possible a change in behavior or environment), or reinforcing (feedback and rewards given to support changes made).

*Program/Application:* Predisposing factors were relationship skills, sexual health knowledge, and skills in condom use. An enabling factor was readily available condoms at low cost. Feedback and rewards were social support and college credit for involvement in peer education programs.

**Phase 5.** *Administrative and policy assessment:* Determine capabilities and resources available to develop and implement the program.

*Program/Application:* Campus health departments were willing to collaborate and provide funds, teaching time, educational materials, and condoms for 2 years. The college administration agreed to support the program (e.g., physical plant staff assistance).

**Phase 6.** *Implementation:* Based on resources, select methods and strategies of interventions and implement.

*Program/Application:* Students, nurses, family and consumer scientists, and faculty developed and implemented peer educational strategies for relationship skill building and sexual health knowledge, including condom use. Faculty arranged credit for students involved. Condom machines ($0.25 per condom) were installed in all washrooms.

**Phases 7, 8, and 9.** *Process, impact, and outcome evaluation:* Respectively evaluate the implementation of the program, the immediate results, and the long-term results in terms of changes in quality of life for the target population.

*Program/Application:* Many issues emerged during implementation (e.g., the maintenance of condom machines, unplanned pregnancies, iron-deficiency anemia, and low-birth-weight babies). Throughout implementation, opportunities to evaluate program activities were provided and activities were adjusted accordingly. At the end of 2 years, students were again interviewed and surveyed. The results were used to determine whether the program should be continued, changed, or stopped.

The depth developed in each phase of the model depends upon resources as well as goals. An advantage is that the model is well recognized by government agencies and grantors.

Modified from: Hitchcock J, Schubert PE, Thomas SA. Community Health Nursing. 2nd ed. Clifton Park, NY: Thomson Delmar Learning; 2003.

# Successful Community Strategies

## University of North Carolina Chapel Hill Nutrition Education CD-ROM Program for Women Receiving Food Assistance[55]

Community and public health nutritionists use different modalities to deliver nutrition education to their clients. The use of Internet technology has provided these professionals a new modality. Campbell et al.[55] utilized a computer-based interactive program to test the efficacy of interactive nutrition education for Special Supplemental Nutrition Program for Women, Infants, and Children (WIC) participants and to address their unique needs, interests, and concerns. The survey

*(continues)*

## *Successful Community Strategies* (continued)

sample comprised 307 respondents to the follow-up survey. Participants were mostly female (96 percent), 20 percent were pregnant, and 50 percent were minorities (African American and other).

Measures were obtained at baseline, immediately postprogram, and at a 1- to 2-month follow-up. Dietary intake of fat, fruits, and vegetables was assessed using a brief validated 26-item food frequency questionnaire (FFQ) administered at baseline and at the 1- to 2-month follow-up. Participants were asked how often they ate a medium-sized serving of each food. A photograph of each food was also shown on the computer. Participants entered all of their own baseline and postprogram data using a touchscreen monitor. Participants were provided with headphones and audio narration to make the program more accessible for those with low literacy skills. The intervention group completed the baseline survey, received the intervention, and answered immediate postprogram questions, but the control group completed the surveys and did not receive the intervention until after follow-up. The participants completed the survey within 15 minutes and the intervention in about 20 to 25 minutes on the computer. After completing the intervention, participants received small gifts, including a refrigerator magnet, one or two wallet-sized brochures with healthful eating tips and recipes, and a $2 gift coupon to a local supermarket chain.

The program's conceptual framework was based on health behavior theories, mainly Social Cognitive Theory and the Transtheoretical Model. The conceptual model was similar to that designed for a previous project, StampSmart.[56] The FoodSmart intervention included four main components: a full-motion video soap opera, interactive infomercials, tailored dietary and psychosocial feedback determined by baseline assessment questions, and take-home print materials (recipe book and a nutrition education newsletter). Following is a description of each component.

*Video soap opera:* A video soap opera, titled *Baby Oh Baby,* was created by project staff based on popular television soap opera plots. The soap opera was designed to engage the attention of the participants, used vicarious persuasion to model positive behavior changes, and emphasized the importance of good prenatal, infant, and child nutrition. The staff centered the plot on a woman who pretended to be pregnant to swindle money from her former boyfriend. Subsequently, she learned that she really was pregnant with her fiancé's child. She initially learned about prenatal nutrition to help her make her faked pregnancy seem genuine. Later, she improved her diet for the sake of her baby and husband-to-be. The soap opera was divided into five segments, interrupted by infomercials and tailored feedback "breaks."

*Infomercials:* Interactive infomercials were designed to assess nutrition knowledge and skills and provide feedback tailored to participant gender and baseline knowledge. Infant feeding, choosing low-fat foods, healthful menu choices, meal planning, and the Food Guide Pyramid were included as part of the topics. Popular television commercial themes and humor were used to increase interest in the infomercials. For example, the infant feeding feedback featured babies talking to each other about what they needed to be fed, tailored to participant knowledge of infant feeding and the age of the participant's infant.

*Tailored dietary feedback:* Based on the results of the FFQ, participants received immediate feedback about their diet and specific strategies to improve their eating habits. Dietary feedback about fat and fruit and vegetable consumption was tailored to participants' gender, pregnancy or breastfeeding status, interest in weight control, and stage of readiness to decrease fat. Strategies for lowering fat were focused on the participant's dairy, meats, or snacks consumption. For pregnant or breastfeeding women, feedback focused on increasing fruits, vegetables, and calcium-rich foods instead of focusing on lowering dietary fat or losing weight.

### Results

There was no difference between the intervention and control groups in terms of *knowledge level* for either low-fat choices or infant feeding recommendations at baseline. The majority of participants knew the correct answer at baseline, except for the fast food item. However, at follow-up, the intervention groups' mean score for low-fat knowledge and infant feeding knowledge increased significantly more than the control group.

The participants' *self-efficacy* (confidence) for healthful eating was similar between groups at baseline, but the intervention group's self-efficacy immediately after the intervention increased significantly for all items except for baking or broiling meat rather than frying.

*Stages of change* (differences in the stages of change model): Participants in precontemplation consumed the highest mean fat, at 90 g/day; contemplators and preparers consumed slightly less fat (contemplators 78 g/day, preparers 80 g/day). Those in the action and maintenance states consumed the least fat (action 42 g/day, maintenance 41 g/day). There was no intervention effect through stages of change between baseline and follow-up.

## Successful Community Strategies *(continued)*

*Dietary behavior:* The intervention group consumed slightly more servings of fruits and vegetables and slightly more fat compared with the control group, but the results were not statistically significant.

*Process measures:* Immediately postintervention, participants in the intervention group were asked questions about the helpfulness of, their interest in, and the length of the FoodSmart program. A total of 63.7 percent of participants thought the program was very helpful or helpful, and 88.6 percent said that they would be very or somewhat interested in using a similar program in the future. In terms of length, however, 51.3 percent indicated that the 30- to 40-minute program was too long.

# Learning Portfolio

## Chapter Summary

- Community nutritionists can plan an effective nutrition education program using one model or a combination of models.
- Communities and the nutritionists together may either create their own model or use an existing programming or planning model.
- When concepts and constructs are related to each other and combined to form a unit, the resulting entity may be labeled a framework, a model, or a theory.
- The PRECEDE-PROCEED model provides a comprehensive guide to planning and implementing health promotion activities in nine phases; the first five involve diagnosis or needs assessment, and the last four involve implementation and evaluation.
- Social marketing is the use of marketing concepts and tools to increase the acceptability of social ideas or practices.
- The three major constructs/concepts in Social Learning Theory are behavioral capacity (having the skills necessary for the performance of the desired behavior, such as quitting excessive alcohol drinking), efficacy expectations (beliefs regarding one's ability to successfully carry out a course of action or perform a behavior), and outcome expectations (beliefs that the performance of a behavior will have the desired effects or consequences).
- A nutrition theory explains or describes a specific event of nutrition.

## Critical Thinking Activities

- Review the general theories of learning summarized in the chapter. Decide which one would most effectively fit the learning needs of a community in which adolescent cigarette smoking is on the rise. Explain the theory you chose.
- Obtain, read, and present at least two research articles that utilized any of the models or theories discussed in this chapter for in-class discussion.

## 🔍 CASE STUDY 13-1: Abnormal Eating Disorders in Female Athletes

A group of high-achieving, 19- to 20-year-old female athletes (dancers, long-distance runners, figure skaters, and gymnasts) were referred to the university dietitian for dietary counseling. These students were members of the university athletic team for the past 2 years. Some of the athletes complained of episodes of fainting, weakness, and fatigue while they were competing or during the events. Prior to fainting they felt dizzy and had episodes of muscle cramping and headaches over the past 4 weeks. Some of them also reported experiencing abdominal pain and a burning sensation in their chest 4 months ago, but the use of antacids and a change in eating habits, such as consuming smaller, more frequent meals, reduced the symptoms. All of the students have lost an average of 17 pounds (7.7 kg) during the past year because their coaches strongly recommended weight loss. Their current friends are only school athletes. The students expressed concern over recent changes in their body, such as breast development and widening hips. They want to maintain a trim, muscular physique and fear excessive weight gain will affect their speed and athletic performance. They reported a normal menstrual cycle every 30 days until 5 to 10 months ago, when

*(continues)*

## CASE STUDY 13-1: Abnormal Eating Disorders in Female Athletes

(continued)

menses abruptly ceased. The dietitian decided to use HBM and screened the students for eating disorders. The students were then provided a sheet of paper to draw themselves. Almost all of the students:

- Depicted themselves as having a large neck, a disconnected neck, or no neck
- Emphasized their mouth
- Depicted wide thighs
- Created pictures without feet or with disconnected feet

The students completed a nutrition questionnaire on knowledge, health beliefs, and frequency of consumption of food according to MyPlate guideline and completed a dietary history questionnaire. The students' diet history showed that they were consuming a high-protein (90 to 120 g/day), low-fat, and low-carbohydrate diet for the past month. They typically consume low-fat or high-sugar drinks. They reported no vomiting or abuse of laxatives, enemas, or diuretics. They skip meals often and compensate by snacking. They expressed concern about being overweight and not muscular enough. Based on a 24-hour dietary recall, the students were consuming about 800 to 900 kcal per day and did not abide by MyPlate guideline.

Anthropometric measurement showed an average height of 66 inches, weight of 90 pounds, and a BMI of 15.6 kg/m$^2$. Laboratory data showed low serum potassium (2.5 mEq/L), calcium (8.0 mg/dl), phosphate (4.2 mg/dl), albumin (3.4 g/L), and hemoglobin (11.0 g/dl).

The dietitian provided nutrition counseling to the students and recommended a 2-week follow-up. She also referred them for medical management, cognitive-behavioral intervention, and nutrition counseling.

### Questions

1. What are the clues in the students' history and report that showed that they may have an eating disorder?
2. Based on the students' laboratory values, what are the possible causes of their fainting spells and muscle cramps?
3. Is their current caloric intake adequate for their age and physical activity levels?
4. What nutrient deficiencies could the students develop by skipping meals and consuming too few calories daily?
5. Review the Stages of Change Model and discuss the stage that some of these students may be experiencing.
6. The dietitian decided to provide nutrition education targeting student athletes using Social Marketing Theory (SMT). Discuss the advantages of using SMT.
7. This chapter discussed different types of models and theories. Which of these models could the dietitian use to provide nutrition counseling to the students beside the Health Belief Model?
8. Why is normal menstrual cycle important? Discuss the relationship between menstrual cycle and osteoporosis.

## Think About It

**Answer:** A framework is a scheme that specifies the steps in a process. For example, community nutritionists could use a framework that includes listening, critical reflection, participatory dialogue, theme recognition, action, and reflection on action to plan a nutrition program.

## Key Terms

**frameworks:** Schemes that specify the steps in a process.

**models:** Physical, symbolic, or mental ways of viewing a real object.

**program paradigms:** Representations of approaches to programming that offer explanations of the processes involved.

**self-efficacy:** The belief in one's capabilities of making a behavior change.

**theory:** A construct that accounts for or organizes events.

## References

1. Realine BF. *Nutrition Education and Change: Education in a Competitive and Globalizing World Series.* New York, NY: Nova Science; 2009.
2. Fitzpatrick SE, Reddy S, Lommel TS, et al. Physical activity and physical function improved following a community-based intervention in older adults in Georgia senior centers *J Nutr Gerontol Geriatr.* 2008;27(1-2):135-154
3. Bateson MC. *Composing a Life.* 3rd ed: New York, NY: Penguin Books; 2011.

4. Hitchcock J, Schubert PE, Thomas SA. *Community Health Nursing.* 2nd ed. Clifton Park, NJ: Thomson Delmar Learning; 2003.

5. Kline MV, Huff RM. *Promoting Health in Multicultural Populations: A Handbook for Practtioners.* 3rd ed. New Delhi, India: Sage; 2015.

6. Stanhope M, Lancaster J. *Community and Public Health Nursing: Population-Centered Health Care in the Community.* 9th ed. New York, NY: Elsever; 2015.

7. Comings JP, Soricone L, Santos M. *An Evidence-based Adult Education Program Model Appropriate for Research.* Boston, MA: National Center for the Study of Adult Learning and Literacy (NSCALL); 2006.

8. Sapp SG, Weng CY. Examination of the health-belief model to predict the dietary quality and body mass of adults. *Int J Consum Stud.* 2007;31(3): 189-194.

9. Owen A, Splett PL, Owen GM. *Nutrition in the Community: The Art and Science of Delivering Services.* 4th ed. New York: McGraw-Hill; 1999.

10. Contento I, Balch G, Bronner YL, et al. The effectiveness of nutrition education and implications for nutrition education policy, programs, and research: a review of research. *J Nutr Educ.* 1995;27(6):284-418.

11. Wallace LS. Osteoporosis prevention in college women: application of the Expanded Health Belief Model. *Am J Health Behav.* 2002;26(3): 163-172.

12. Strychar IM. Changes in knowledge and food behaviour following a screening program held in a supermarket. *Can J Public Health.* 1993;84(6):382-388.

13. Freeland-Graves J, Nitzke S. Position of the American Dietetic Association: total diet approach to communicating food and nutrition information. *J Am Diet Assoc.* 2002;102(1):100-108.

14. Rogers EM. *Diffusion of innovations.* 5th ed. New York, NY: The Free Press; 2003.

15. Bagozzi RP, Moore DJ, Leone L. Self-control and the self-regulation of dieting decisions: the role of prefactual attitudes. *Basic Appl Soc Psychol.* 2004;26(273):199-213.

16. Maiman LA, Becker MH. The Health Belief Model: origins and correlates in psychological theory. In: Becker MH, ed. *The Health Belief Model and Personal Health Behavior.* Thorofare, NJ: Charles Slack; 1974.

17. Dickin KL, Dollahite JS, Jean-Pierre H. Nutrition behavior change among EFNEP participants is higher at sites that are well managed and whose front-line nutrition educators value the program. *J Nutr.* 2005;135:2199-2205.

18. Pittet D, Simon A, Hugonnet S, Pessoa-Silva C, Sauvan V, Perneger TV. Hand hygiene among physicians: performance, beliefs, and perceptions. *Ann Intern Med.* 2004;141:1-8.

19. Monneuse MO, Bellisle F, Koppert G. Eating habits, food and health related attitudes and beliefs reported by French students. *Eur J Clin Nutr.* 1997;51(1):46-53.

20. Durkin KF, Wolfe KF, Clark GA. College students and binge drinking: an evaluation of social learning theory *Sociol Spectr.* 2005;25(3):255-272

21. Spahn JJ, Reeves RS, Keim KS, et al. State of the evidence regarding behavior change theories and strategies in nutrition counseling to facilitate health and food behavior change. *J Am Diet Assoc.* 2010;110(6):879-891.

22. Bodenmann G, Schaer M. Social learning theories. *Sprache Stimme Gehör.* 2006;30:17-20.

23. Tian PS, Morawska OA. A cognitive model of binge drinking: the influence of alcohol expectancies and drinking refusal self-efficacy. *Addict Behav.* 2004;29(1):159-179.

24. Fulkerson JA, French SA, Story M, Nelson H, Hannan PJ. Promotions to increase lower-fat food choices among students in secondary schools: description and outcomes of TACOS (Trying Alternative Cafeteria Options in Schools). *Public Health Nutr.* 2004;7(5):665-674.

25. Rogers LQ, Matevey C, Hopkins-Price P, Shah P, Dunnington G, Courneya KS. Exploring social cognitive theory constructs for promoting exercise among breast cancer patients. *Cancer Nurs.* 2004;27(6):462-473.

26. Hansona N, Neumark-Sztainera D, Eisenberga ME, Storya M, Walla M. Associations between parental report of the home food environment and adolescent intakes of fruits, vegetables and dairy foods. *PublicHealth Nutr.* 2005;8:77-85

27. Boynton-Jarrett RR. Impact of television viewing patterns on fruit and vegetable consumption among adolescents. *Pediatrics.* 2003;112(6 pt 1): 1321-1326.

28. Gribble LS, Falciglia G, Davis AM, Couch SC. A curriculum based on social learning theory emphasizing fruit exposure and positive parent child-feeding strategies: a pilot study. *J Am Diet Assoc.* 2003;103(1):100-103.

29. Miller CK, Edward L, Kissling G, Sanville L. Evaluation of a theory-based nutrition intervention for older adults with diabetes mellitus. *J Am Diet Assoc.* 2002;102:1069-1107.

30. Ajzen I, Fishbein M. *Understanding and Predicting Social Change.* Englewood Cliffs, NJ: Prentice Hall; 1980.

31. Ross L, Kohler CL, Grimley DM. The theory of reasoned action and intention to seek cancer information. *Am J Health Behav.* 2007;31(2):123-134.

32. Carroll LJ, Whyte A. Predicting chronic back pain sufferers' intention to exercise. *Br J Ther Rehab.* 2003;10(2):53-58.

33. Folta SC, Bell R, Economos C, Landers S, Goldberg JP. Psychosocial factors associated with young elementary school children's intentions to consume legumes: a test of the theory of reasoned action. *Am J Health Promot.* 2006;21(1):13-15.

34. Booth-Butterfield S, Reger B. The message changes belief and the rest is theory: the 1% or less milk campaign and reasoned action. *Prev Med.* 2004;39(3):581-588.

35. Britto M, Pandzik GM, Meeks CS, Kotagal UR. Combining evidence and diffusion of innovation theory to enhance influenza immunization. *Jt Comm J Qual Patient Saf.* 2006;32(8):426-432.

36. Elder JP, Lytle L, Sallis JF. A description of the social-ecological framework used in the trial of activity for adolescent girls (TAAG). *Health Educ Res.* 2007;22(2):155-165.

37. Sanson-Fisher RW. Diffusion of innovation theory for clinical change. *Med J Austral.* 2004;180(6):S55-S566.

38. Valente TW, Fosados R. Diffusion of innovations and network segmentation: the part played by people in promoting health. *Sex Transm Dis.* 2006;33(7 suppl):S23-S31.

39. Burgoon JK, Bonito JA, Ramirez A, Dunbar NE, Kam K, Fischer J. Testing the interactivity principle: effects of mediation, propinquity, and verbal and nonverbal modalities in interpersonal interaction. *J Comm Health.* 2002;52(3):657-677.

40. Bandura A. Social Cognitive Theory of Mass Communication. *Media Psych.* 2001;3(3):265-299.

41. Prochaska JO, DiClemente CC. Stages and processes of self-change of smoking: toward an integrated model of change. *J Consult Clin Psychol.* 1983;51(3):390-395.

42. Herzog TA. Are the stages of change for smokers qualitatively distinct? An analysis using an adolescent sample. *Psychol Addict Behav.* 2007;21(1):120-125.

43. Canales MK, Rakowski W. Development of a culturally specific instrument for mammography screening: an example with American Indian women in Vermont. *J Nurs Meas.* 2006;14(2):99-115.

44. Greene GG, Rossi SR, Rossi JS, Velicer WF, Fava JL, Prochaska JO. Dietary applications of the Stages of Change Model. *J Am Diet Assoc.* 1999;99(6):673-678.

45. Dearing JW, Maibach EW, Buller DR. A convergent diffusion and social marketing approach for disseminating proven approaches to physical activity promotion. *Am J Prev Med.* 2006;31(4):S11-S23.

46. Samuels S. Project LEAN: A national campaign to reduce dietary ft consumption. *Am J Health Prom.* 1993;4:435-440.

47. Lefebvre RCD, Johnston L, Loughrey C, et al. Use of database marketing and consumer-based health communication in a message design: an example from the Office of Cancer Communication's "5 A Day for Better Health" program. In: Maibach EW, Parrott RL, eds. *Designing Health Messages: Approaches from Communication Theory and Public Health Practice.* Thousand Oaks, CA: Sage; 1995:217-246.

48. Grier S, Bryant C. Social marketing in public health. *Ann Rev Pub Health.* 2005;26:319-339

49. Anspaugh DJ, Dignan MB, Anspaugh SL. *Developing Health Promotion Programs.* 2nd ed. Long Grove, IL: Waveland Press; 2006.

50. British Columbia Ministry of Health. *Healthy Communities: The Process.* Victoria, BC, Canada: British Columbia Ministry of Health; 1989.

51. Curran S, Gittelsohn J, Anliker J. Process evaluation of a store-based environmental obesity intervention on two American Indian Reservations. *Health Educ Res.* 2005;20(6):719-729.

52. Valente T. *Evaluating Health Promotion Programs.* New York, NY: Oxford University Press; 2002.

53. Green L, Kreuter MW. *Health Promotion Planning: An Education and Environmental Approach.* Mountain View, CA: Mayfield; 1991.

54. Abel R, Rajaratnam J, Kalaimani A, Kirubakaran S. Can iron status be improved in each of the three trimesters? A community-based study. *Eur J Clin Nutr.* 2000;54:490-493.

55. Campbell MK, Carbone E, Honess-Morreale L, Heisler-Mackinnon J, Demissie S, Farrell D. Randomized trial of a tailored nutrition education CD-ROM program for women receiving food assistance. *J Nutr Educ Behav.* 2004;36(2):58-66.

56. Campbell MK, Honess-Morreale L, Farrell D, Carbone E, Brasure M. Effects of a tailored multimedia nutrition education program for low income women receiving food assistance. *Health Educ Res.* 1999;14(2):246-256.

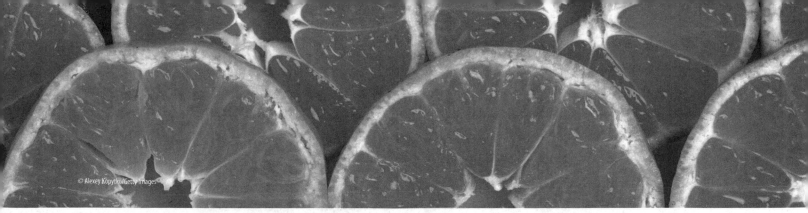

# CHAPTER 14

# Acquiring Grantsmanship Skills

## LEARNING OBJECTIVES

- Define *grant proposal.*
- Specify major items in a grant application.
- Identify potential collaborators for a grant proposal.
- Discuss the parts of a grant proposal.
- Discuss the sources for funding community and public health nutrition.

## ▶ Introduction

Many community and public health **programs** have experienced reductions in their **budget**. Because of these reductions, they are compelled to become more creative with existing resources and/or obtaining grant funds to develop, expand, or continue their programs. Although many agencies are accomplishing more with less money, several are seeking grant funds to accomplish the organization's goals. For these reasons, grant applications have become very competitive, and the number of individuals and organizations seeking funds has increased significantly.[1,2] A **grant** is a fund awarded to individuals or an organization for **research**, educational, or demonstration programs. The grant monies are used to support new innovative programs or expand existing programs to meet community healthcare needs.[3]

Both the grantor and the nutritionist seeking a grant need each other. Community nutritionists can identify community needs and develop creative methods to address them, and foundations, corporations, and other donors have the financial resources necessary to make a program work. The two groups often form productive collaborations, but the grant seeker must take the initiative.

It is important for community nutritionists to acquire grant-writing skills in order to be successful in obtaining money for their research or community-related programs. The elements to consider when writing a grant proposal include ethical issues, sources of funds (foundations; federal, state, and local agencies), the length of the proposal, time to write the proposal, and the staff required to carry out the project. Preparing a research study or organizing a community education program and writing a grant proposal are complex endeavors, not only because of the many elements that go into research and program design, but also because each element plays an essential role in the success of the program or research.[4]

One of the elements nutritionists encounter in grant writing and in other aspects of dietetics is ethical issues. The Academy of Nutrition and Dietetics has provided a set of guidelines for registered dietitians, licensed nutritionists, and registered dietetic technicians entitled the *Code of Ethics for the Profession of Dietetics*. These ethical guidelines are a set of principles that dietitians and nutritionists must apply in every situation coupled with their personal judgments, experience, knowledge, and skills. See Chapter 15 for details on the American Dietetic Association's (ADA's) Code of Ethics. This chapter discusses grant writing and the different components of a grant proposal.

## ▶ Laying the Foundation for a Grant

A **grant proposal** is a written request for money (and occasionally for other resources). Writing a grant proposal compels the nutritionist to create, define, and refine the research idea or community education program.[5] An excellent grant proposal requires very good organization and a strong foundation. To get adequate resources for a program, community nutritionists need to submit a proposal to an agency or foundation that grants funds for health promotion programs. Sometimes nutritionists may need to submit proposals to their own employing agency for funding such as **travel grants** to conferences, **training grants** to learn how to prepare a grant proposal, **demonstration grants** to demonstrate a new approach to delivering community health programs, or **equipment grants** to acquire small tools for a program.[6,7] In addition, the nutritionist may submit proposals for **service grants** to support activities and services to the community over and above those outreach programs that are already funded.[8] This also could be accomplished through a **block grant**, which is a sum of money the federal government gives to a state or local government while suggesting a general purpose for the money's use. However, the federal government permits the state or local government to spend the money without meeting specific conditions.

Writing a grant proposal is a systematic, step-by-step process that requires the following:

- Identifying stakeholders
- Generating ideas
- Establishing the need for the grant
- Locating collaborators
- Identifying barriers to overcome (understanding the language of the proposal)
- Locating grant money
- Describing goals
- Finding out how to apply
- Writing a request (i.e., a proposal)

## ▶ Identifying Funding Sources

The nutritionist or grant-seeking organization should look for funding from an agency that funds a specific type of need in the community. For example, a community service group, such as Kiwanis or the March of Dimes Birth Defects Foundation, may focus on helping pregnant women and children and may be willing to fund a program to improve youth health or prevent folic acid deficiency in a community. Similarly, the American Heart Association (AHA) may fund a smoking prevention program and the National Dairy Council may fund an osteoporosis prevention program. It is also important to recognize small corporations and businesses in the community as potential sources when seeking grant support. Examples of local funding sources are businesses such as Wal-Mart, K-mart, State Farm Insurance and other insurance agencies, banks, and others in the community. Sources at the state level include the public health department and the state branches of the AHA, National Dairy Council, and others. At the national level, the National Institutes of Health (NIH), U.S. Department of Agriculture, National Science Foundation (NSF), and other federal agencies should be consulted. See http://nutrition.jbpub.com/communitynutrition for an inventory of U.S., Canadian, and other national funding sources as well as for a sample request for a proposal from the *Federal Register*.[9]

After locating a potential funding source, it is a good idea to contact the funding agency to discuss whether the nutrition program idea matches the agency's interests and to clarify the agency's requirements (such as questions to be answered, deadlines for submission, and submission format). Guidelines differ among agencies, mainly in the amount of details required; however, the grant writer must answer the following questions in order to be successful[6]:

- What are the objectives/aims, how much will it cost, and what is the time line?
- How is the proposed project related to the grantor's interests?
- What is the maximum amount of money the applicant can request?
- What has already been accomplished in the research project or program?
- What would be the benefits if this project/program were carried out?
- What are the methods and procedures for the project/program?
- How would the project/program be evaluated?
- Why is the applicant the most qualified person to carry out this research project or nutrition program?
- Is collaborative work required?

The search for funding is a step-by-step process. First, the nutritionist/grant seeker must have a clear idea of the project or program needing funding. Second, he or she must search for and locate potential grantors. Third, he or she must contact and apply for financial support. Although the grant seeker may modify the program plan later on, it is a good idea to design the project before starting a funding search. The following will help build the proposal[10,11]:

- Start as early as possible.
- Put together a strong, representative grant writing team.
- Identify someone in the community who has grant writing experience.
- Consider all of the people whose skills or knowledge will be needed.
- Involve the major partners early.
- Locate available health data through the Centers for Disease Control and Prevention (CDC) for research information and data (e.g., obesity, heart disease, osteoporosis, mortality and morbidity rates) in your state or community.
- Search for research articles related to the topic.
- Show that the applicant is aware of and plans to work toward local, state, and national standards (if applicable).

Most philanthropic organizations and many corporations are prepared ahead of time for requests for money. They have readymade grant applications and guidelines describing the kinds of programs they are interested in funding. It is important to not waste these organizations' time if your needs do not match their guidelines. Grantors seldom make exceptions to their grant policies.[10]

After locating the funding source, the next step is to make an initial contact. Potential grantors respond to initial contacts in different ways. Some grantors will fund a project, with a small grant, directly from a letter of intent. Others will ask for expanded aspects of the letter of intent. The majority of foundations and corporations who regularly fund programs will send out a request for proposal (RFP) grant application form.[12] These forms are usually very clear about what and how much information the foundation needs from applicants. It is important not to exceed the maximum amount of information; give them exactly what they ask for—no more, no less.

Regardless of the form it takes, a typical grant proposal will include the following elements: an introductory overview of the proposal or background information, a statement of need, a project description, and a budget. In addition, grantors may ask for a mission statement (i.e., the rationale and goals of the program), a list of important personnel, and a description of any project partnerships.[10,13]

## ▶ Identifying Possible Collaborators

**Collaboration** is a mutual sharing and working together to achieve common goals in such a way that all persons or groups are recognized and growth is enhanced.[14] Many funding agencies look for programs that use a collaborative approach. The proposal has greater potential of being funded if the grant writer seeks partners such as community agencies, local businesses, and individuals who could provide financial backing or an **in-kind** or **matching grant** to support the grant proposal during the planning stage.[15] For example, a service-learning project that can raise matching funds or in-kind donations from a local community member confirms to a grantor that there is community "buy-in." Partnering with another school or community organization on a program can provide additional funding leverage for both partners.

Preparing a grant proposal is very time consuming and labor intensive. Therefore, a professional grant writer may be needed to coordinate the activities and gather materials needed to complete the grant application. Forming a grant writing committee may be beneficial when submitting a grant application for a large sum of money, especially for federal or block grants (such as maternal and child health grants, preventive health and health services grants, and community development grants).[14] The committee may consist of the agency epidemiologist, a nurse, a nutritionist, an accountant, community leaders, a statistician, and a physician. In addition, the grant seeker can partner with other health-care professionals, such as those at a college of nursing, school of public health, or college of dentistry. These professionals also engage in community-based health research and community intervention efforts to reduce morbidity and mortality from diseases and conditions ranging from infant mortality to chronic and genetic diseases.[15-19]

Skills in networking, coordination, and cooperative learning are also necessary in forming a successful partnership.[2,20] You can gain networking experience by attending grant writing workshops and professional development events as well as associating with colleagues in and outside your local community.

## ▶ Writing the Grant

Writing a grant is a systematic process. The components of a proposal vary from one grant sponsor to another; therefore, it is very important to read and follow the grantor's instructions very carefully. The components include the items listed in the following sections. However, the sequence of the items may vary according to the needs of the granting agency. It is also very important to make the proposal clear and concise. Funding agencies' guidelines usually put a limit on the number of pages for the entire proposal; it is essential to adhere to the page limit and all the requirements stipulated in the RFPs.

### Letter of Intent

The application procedure for writing a research or grant proposal may start with a letter of intent to the funding organization, prior to an invitation to submit a full proposal. The first letter of intent may be sent to indicate to a funding agency the plan to submit a grant proposal. The letter of intent follows many of the same procedures as a proposal, but it is limited to a few pages. Some letters of intent include a limited literature review, but some agencies prefer to receive a more extensive proposal at the beginning. In either case, each step of the proposal must be supported by data. The letter of intent may include the following nine items[21,22]:

- Names of the principal and co-investigators, organization/institution/community center, address, telephone and fax numbers, and e-mail address
- Title of the proposed project (brief information about the project)
- Purpose/aim of the project
- Brief description of the project design
- Results of preliminary data
- Time requirements for the project
- Estimated annual and total project budget
- Résumé (of the investigators)
- Impact or significance of the project to the community

The letter of intent is a good opportunity to describe the positive outcome of a funded grant and the impact this program or research will have on the community if it is funded.

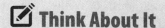
**Think About It**

Ann, a community nutritionist, wrote a grant proposal for providing nutrition intervention to Native American men, women, and children. The purpose of the grant proposal was to reduce fat intake and increase physical activity in this community. At the end of writing the grant proposal, she asked, "How can I assemble this proposal to maximize the potential of receiving the funds for this project?"

### Request for Proposal

After the letter of intent is accepted and the organization asks for submission of a proposal, the detail work of writing the proposal starts. The proposal may begin with the concise summary of one to three pages that was included in the letter of intent.

The grant writer should read the request very carefully and follow the guidelines because the proposal may be disqualified if it is submitted in an improper format.[23] The two major challenges that a grant seeker must address are clarity and consistency within the grant. Assembling a **research grant** or project application is similar to using building blocks. The foundation and structure for the proposal are the specific aims. From the specific aims, the project design and methods are chosen to answer the identified research or program questions and hypotheses. A **hypothesis** is a supposition or question that is raised to explain an event or guide investigation.[24,25] The community project design and aims are then used to formulate appropriate statistical analyses and evaluation.

Organizing the proposal by the specific aims is one way to promote clarity among hypotheses, variables, instruments, and data analyses. For example, you could use special font styles such as bold or italics to highlight these variables consistently throughout the sections of the grant; however, make sure that these formatting options are allowed by the funding agency.[20]

The individual parts of a research/project grant are discussed in the following sections. Major components of a proposal grant application include[21]:

- Abstract
- Research/project plan
- References

- Budget
- Curriculum vitae or résumé
- Other support (collaboration with business or community organizations)
- Resources (matching funds)
- Institutional review board approvals (as needed)
- Appendix
- Dissemination of findings
- Capability

## Title

The proposal title should be short, explicit, and informative. It should project the idea of the proposal and inform the grant reviewers as to what they are about to read. Some grantors may limit the number of characters and spaces allowed in the title. It is beneficial to use a catchy project title; it may not be the decisive factor in the grant application, but it may help reviewers remember the proposal better than others reviewed. Some examples of catchy titles might be:

- Nutrition for Fitness
- 21st-Century Nutrition
- Fit for Life
- Fitness Education: In Shape
- Healthy Hearts
- Building Better Bones

## Abstract

An abstract is a short summary of the proposed research project/program. It persuades the reviewer to read the proposal and allows busy reviewers to learn the main ideas without reading the entire proposal. It is advisable to write the abstract last and use it to summarize the specific aims or objectives, background, significance, research/project design, and method sections. One of the challenging aspects of writing an abstract is adhering to the word limit required by the grantor.[25] An editor can help in reducing unnecessary words and phrases.

It is important to bear in mind that the abstract sets the stage for the remainder of the proposal. Be sure to include any changes that were made in the body of the proposal if the abstract was written early in the grant writing process. (This is one reason to write the abstract last.) Attention to detail, especially in the abstract, to catch readers' attention is very important.[20]

## Literature Review and Background Information

This section discusses not only what is currently known related to the proposed area of the study, but also, and more importantly, the significance of the research project or program. This section justifies the project,

builds the case for the project, and highlights the need for the project.[5] It is vital to convince the reviewers that this project or program is the next logical step based on the state of the science or the community needs. It is also important to show how this program addresses a widespread or significant health concern. Linking the proposed program to national health objectives such as Healthy People 2010 and 2020 or federal or professional organizational research priorities will strengthen the likelihood of funding for the proposal.[20,26]

In addition, the literature review should focus on the specific aims of the proposal. Critically evaluate existing knowledge and identify gaps in the scientific evidence. Link the conceptual framework to the project. A **conceptual framework** is a way of showing relationships that are known and ones that have not been investigated but may be the focus of the project.[27] The literature reviews found in many journal articles are good examples you can follow when writing your proposal. Strategies that may enhance the literature review include the following[28]:

Provide current relevant facts and statistics about the intervention program for the community or population.

- Describe your experience in the area/topic.
- Explain the significance of this project to the community or population.
- Provide a clear statement about the connection among the program and research objectives, methodologies, and outcome.
- Preempt and answer all the reviewer's questions.
- Describe the advantages of this project to the community.
- Tailor the proposal to the grant agency's priorities.
- Explain how this project fits and supports existing programs, if any.
- Provide subsections as needed.
- List pilot or preliminary findings, if available.

This section should not include the following:

- Acronyms common to your area of expertise (many reviewers may not be familiar with them)
- Research that does not support the grant proposal
- Jargon or slang
- The same literature review for different grant proposals

## Specific Aims

This part of the proposal describes the purpose(s) of the project, what the project intends to accomplish, and the potential value of the research project or program. Although the organization of this section may vary, most nutritionists start with the purpose(s) of the program. The statement of purpose includes the main project variables, their possible interrelationships, and the nature of the population of interest. For example, "The purpose of this research project is to assess the relationship among four sets of variables: 1) the prevalence of obesity in schoolchildren, 2) the eating patterns of schoolchildren, 3) the physiological effects of obesity, and 4) the effects of culture on breastfeeding."[12,20] Another example is: "The aim of this program is to increase the number of fruits and vegetables that men age 55 years or older consume."

The following example is taken from a grant proposal titled "Perinatal Alcohol Users: Identification and Intervention." The specific aims of this study were as follows[12,20,29]:

- Identify alcohol users and abusers at risk for delivering an infant with fetal alcohol syndrome/fetal alcohol effects
- Educate pregnant women's health professionals regarding the identification of any adverse effects of alcohol on the women and their offspring
- Evaluate the effectiveness of interventions by comparing this group of mothers and infants to those randomly selected as a control group and to those followed in the Perinatal, Newborn Division, and Child and Family Health Services Pediatric Tracking databases

Another example of a grant proposal is the program supported by the Illinois Public Health Department Office of Women's Health titled "Understanding and Managing Menopause." The goals were the following:

- Increase the participants' knowledge of the options available to manage menopause.
- Increase the participants' knowledge of physiological and emotional changes that often may be experienced during perimenopause and menopause.
- Reinforce health practices that will maintain lifelong good health and vitality.
- Increase the participants' knowledge of the options available to ensure well-being and good health and increased assertion to advocate for each woman's individual needs.

After the statement of purpose, the **grantee** can include a description of the problem that the project intends to solve or help solve, for example, "Interventions are needed to increase the identification of women at risk for delivering infants with spina bifida and fetal alcohol syndrome. Once identified by healthcare practitioners, the participants will be referred to a dietitian who can then enroll and maintain the women in prenatal care."[12]

## Research or Program Method

This section must answer the research or program questions. It should contain critical information needed to evaluate the quality of the proposal, independent of any other document. It must be concise and thorough, and specify what the researcher or program coordinator intends to achieve. Although the format for the plan may differ depending on the funding source, most project plans include certain sections: specific aims, background and significance, preliminary results, methods and procedure, and references.[5] The nutritionist must provide a full description of how the objectives will be achieved; how success or outcome will be assessed (e.g., an evaluation plan and the number of participants that will be recruited for the program); a description of the participants (or sample or subjects), including who will be involved; the order and time frame of the program activities (time and activity charts, see **TABLE 14-1**); and the duties and qualifications of the project staff.[30] Citing preliminary results relevant to the project will be a feature unique to the proposal.

Six basic elements comprise the research project design: setting and sample; description of intervention, if applicable; instruments; data collection procedures; data analyses; and time line. These elements are briefly discussed in the following sections.[12]

**Setting and Sample.** The nutritionist must describe the location chosen for the program and the rationale for the selection over other possible locations. Describe the typical client population (older persons, minority groups, infants, etc.). Additionally, if a distant site was selected over a local site, it is important to provide a rationale for that decision. Address how distance will affect data collection, participation, and quality of data collection or the intervention.[12]

Describe the criteria for inclusion and exclusion of participants in the project. It is unethical to exclude any segment of the population that is willing to participate. In addition, the nutritionist has an obligation to convince the reviewer of the adequacy of the site to produce a sufficient number of subjects based on inclusion and exclusion criteria. To address the issue, include in narrative text or table format the number of participants available per month or year for the project at the data collection site who meet the inclusion criteria.[12] In addition to the number of subjects, federal grants such as **formula grants** often require the principal investigator to address the recruitment of special populations, including gender and racial/ethnic groups as well as women and children.[31]

**Intervention.** The proposal must describe in detail the intervention procedure and administration. Include how the treatment condition differs from the control or comparison group.[12] One example of an intervention is the Brief Intervention Model (BIM), which includes

| Task | January | February | March | April | May | June | July |
|---|---|---|---|---|---|---|---|
| Develop ideas, needs assessment, proposal goals, objectives, and title. Determine the target audience. Establish need. | X | X | | | | | |
| Plan marketing strategies, review related literature, seek collaborators, and determine methods and procedures. | X | X | | | | | |
| Analyze preliminary data; submit letter of intent; and determine instruments, equipment, and materials. | | | X | X | | | |
| Write proposal and seek second opinion to review the proposal. | | | | | X | X | |
| Recruit participants and submit proposal. | | | | | | X | |
| Write results. | | | | | | X | |
| Implement and evaluate. | | | | | | X | X |

**TABLE 14-1** Grant Activity Chart and Time Line for Nutrition Education Programs

a 10-minute interview with a person in the study. Using the Perinatal Alcohol Users example, following an intervention, the nutritionist and the pregnant women would set a mutual goal for reducing the amount of alcohol the women consume.[12]

**Instruments.** This part of the proposal describes each of the study or project variables and their measurements. It is essential to describe the population, method of administration, reliability, and validity for each instrument (e.g., bone densitometry, blood pressure apparatus, skinfold caliper) that will be used for the program. If alternative instruments are available, the grantee/nutritionist needs to discuss the rationale for the selection of a particular instrument. Describe any necessary training of project personnel in the use of each instrument. It is helpful to report pilot data or whether any pilot study is planned for the new instruments.[12] Finally, in an appendix include lists of all instruments needed.

**Data Collection Procedures.** The writer can start describing how potential participants will be identified and recruited into the program in this section of the proposal. This is followed by a clear description of how and when the intervention will be carried out. Also, include an explanation of the control group. It is important to explain the data collection method, and the aspects of how, when, where, and who uses the instruments. Include a description of how the study personnel will

be trained in the data collection process.[12] The nutritionist must address any potential problems that may be encountered during the project protocol and should include a plan for how problems will be managed. If the study is complex, the nutritionist should develop a step-by-step procedural checklist that will be used by data collectors to ensure no procedural item is omitted during the course of the research project.[32]

**Data Analysis.** This part of the proposal must describe the plans for data management, refinement, and reduction. It is important to describe how the data will be collated, coded, keyed, and verified. This section describes how the data collected will be analyzed to determine the success or outcome of the project. The investigator must provide the name of the statistical test that will be used.[12,32] The principal investigator/nutritionist may want to consider including a statistician on the planning team.

It is important to separate the database of respondents from the results to maintain confidentiality. Also, provide a plan on how to disseminate the findings of the project.[33]

**Time Line.** This part of the proposal describes the anticipated time frame for project activities, such as the hiring and training of project personnel, identification and recruitment of participants, data collection, data preparation, analysis, marketing the program, and writing the report. It is better to propose an adequate period for some aspects of the grant, such as recruitment of participants and hiring personnel. Sometimes, it is better to provide the information in the form of a chart or graph of time relationships and sometimes in a narrative form. See example in Table 14-1.[34]

## References

This part of the proposal is the last part of the project plan and consists of references to journal articles, books, and other materials that were quoted in the grant proposal. It is important to provide bibliographic information in a consistent referencing format such as the American Psychological Association (APA) style or any other format the grantor suggested.[35]

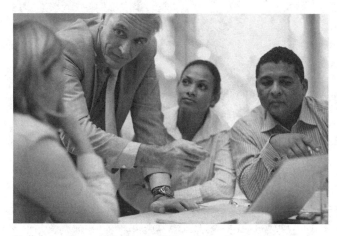

Collaborating with other healthcare professionals may increase the potential for being funded.

© Yuri Arcurs/ShutterStock, Inc.

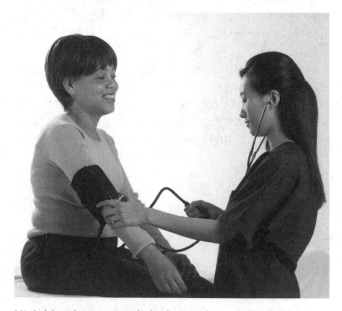

High blood pressure is linked to cardiovascular disease.

© iofoto/ShutterStock, Inc.

## Budget

This section of the proposal is very important. The proposed budget and any matching funds must be related to the proposed program activities. It is important for the grant writer to review the grantor's budget criteria meticulously. Grantors typically specify allowable expenses and those that are not fundable.[36] For example, some grants will not allow funding for indirect costs or the salary of the principal investigator, but will allow salaries for consultants and research assistants. Some federal grants do not allow for meals and travel costs related to the presentation of the results, whereas others may. It is essential to link budget items to grant activities (research personnel, consultants, equipment, supplies, travel, computer costs, and other related expenses). The goal is to request exactly what is needed to conduct the project. The funding agencies often require budget justification. Budget justification is a description of the budget items requested and a rationale for why this expense is needed.[12]

**TABLE 14-2** presents a sample budget. This sample budget serves only as a general model and would vary according to the type of research project or program. Also, as already mentioned, some funding agencies do not pay indirect costs. Below are additional strategies that may enhance the budget section[28]:

- Do not ask for more or less money than the project requires.
- Provide a narrative on how the money will be spent.
- Do not exceed the amount specified by the granting agency.
- Explain how matching funds will be used.
- Obtain the administrators' support by involving them in the budget preparation.
- Obtain the correct price for each item on the budget.

## Curriculum Vitae or Résumé

This part of the proposal will highlight the relevant professional accomplishments of the project directors such as their educations, professional experiences, research, publications, honors, and previous grant awards. It is essential to highlight the achievements related to the proposed project first, because most grantors typically request an abbreviated résumé. Check the guidelines; most agencies restrict the résumé to two or three pages.[37] The curriculum vitae should include a listing of all publications from the past 3 to 5 years and any additional references specifically related to the topic area of the proposed research/program. Membership in professional organizations or involvement in community service is usually omitted unless it helps demonstrate the experience or leadership ability to carry out the proposed project.[12]

**TABLE 14-2** Sample Budget for One Year

| Items | Funding Agency/Month | University or Agency/Month | Total/Year |
|---|---|---|---|
| **Personnel Salary/Wages** | | | |
| Principal investigator/senior personnel (director) | $6,000.00 | $2,000.00 | $96,000.00 |
| One graduate assistant/staff (assists in data collection and processing) | $500.00 | -0- | $6,000.00 |
| **Subtotal** | **$6,500.00** | **$2,000.00** | **$102,000.00** |
| **Fringe Benefits** | | | |
| Life insurance, retirement at 0.33 percent multiplied by salaries | $214.00 | $66.00 | $2,568.00 |
| Medical insurance, $120 multiplied by the number of months | $120.00 | -0- | $1,440.00 |
| **Travel** (for data collection and for the dissemination of information) | | | |
| Mileage (800 @ $0.35) | $280.00 | -0- | $280.00 |
| Lodging (5 nights @ $60/night) | $300.00 | -0- | $300.00 |
| Per diem (10 days @ $42/day) | $420.00 | -0- | $420.00 |
| **Equipment** | $15,000.00 | -0- | $15,000.00 |
| HP computer printer (for preparing flyers, letters) | | | |
| Bone density measurement (scanner) | | | |
| **Supplies** | $300.00 | -0- | $300.00 |
| Office supplies (pens, paper, etc.) | | | |
| Computer printer supplies (ink cartridges) | | | |
| **Contractual Services** | | | |
| Telephone | $100.00 | -0- | $100.00 |
| Postage | $500.00 | -0- | $500.00 |
| Printing | $500.00 | -0- | $500.00 |
| **Total Direct Costs for the University/Agency** | -0- | $2,066.00 | $2,066.00 |
| **Total Direct Costs for the Funding Agency** | $24,234.00 | -0- | $125,474.00 |
| **Indirect Costs** (for program administration) 8 percent of total direct costs from the funding agency | $1,938.00 | $165.00 | $2,103.00 |
| **Subtotal** | **$26,172.00** | **$2,231.00** | **$127,577.00** |

## Dissemination of Findings

Dissemination of findings constitutes the final outcome of a funded research project. This section describes how the community, stakeholders, and other interested individuals will learn about the project and its findings. Disseminating the findings increases the body of knowledge unique to the discipline of nutrition. It is important to describe a possible, effective, and appropriate dissemination plan and indicate who will be responsible for this activity.[12,35] There are many opportunities for disseminating the findings, including publication in a related journal, professional meetings, and online presentation. The information that can be presented includes the theory you developed, pilot data, and any instruments that were developed.[38]

The dissemination of findings offers benefits to both the sponsor and the grantee. For example, the community will become aware of the grantor's priorities and commitment. They also become cognizant of the mission and activities of the organization receiving the funds.[12]

## Capability

This part of the proposal shows the capacity and dependability of the grantee and his or her organization. The project director (principal investigator) must have the expertise needed to direct all the activities of the grant. The director also must specify the qualifications and abilities of the project staff. He or she must show that the organization has the capability to support the proposed project and that the project can be carried out on time and within the proposed budget. In addition, it is important to include any collaborators' resources and capabilities. The nutritionist must persuade the reviewers that he or she has access to the segment of the population that will be recruited for the project (e.g., older persons, children, pregnant women, postmenopausal women). This can be achieved by providing the number of the targeted audience living in the community (using census data). It is also necessary to include and show that participants are available for the study or project. (Provide a list with the volunteers' signatures, if possible.[39]) Also, describe how you will sustain the program after the funding has ended.[40]

The grantee must include the organization's goal, mission statement, activities, previous achievements, and any unique characteristics that position them for the funding. The nutritionist also should include the facilities, matching funds, equipment, materials, and any other resources that will contribute significantly to the success of the proposed project.

**BOX 14-1** presents the steps to grant funding success. The Successful Community Strategies feature in this

> **BOX 14-1** Steps to Grant Funding Success
>
> - Start early.
> - Ask someone else to read the grant before sending it.
> - Work off a preliminary budget; it helps to reduce expansiveness.
> - Look for community partnerships.
> - Involve a professional grant writer.
> - Establish the need for the grant.
> - Use national research and statistics to support the application (e.g., CDC data).
> - Incorporate state and national standards.
> - Understand the language for the proposal.
> - Do not exceed the page limits, and use 12-point font.
> - If the proposal was not funded initially, use the reviewer's comments to revise the proposal.

chapter describes a successful proposal that received a small grant program award.

## Assembling the Final Product

Once all parts of a grant proposal are written and spell-checked, the whole thing can be assembled: the cover sheet (containing the name of the principal investigator or project manager, including his or her address, telephone number, and e-mail address), the proposal itself, the budget, and the supplementary materials. Add a cover letter, and be sure to note whether the grantor wants multiple copies or if a cover sheet needs to be signed by staff or board members.[18,40] It is important to observe the grantor's deadline because late applications are automatically disqualified.

## Reviewing the Grant Proposal

The grantors typically send a letter to the grantee acknowledging receipt of the proposal and informing him or her of when they plan to announce which proposals will be funded. The grantee can call, e-mail, or send a letter to the grantor if the letter of acknowledgment was not received within 2 to 3 weeks of submission.

Reviewing a grant proposal is a time-consuming activity. The reviews are typically performed by expert committees known as study sections.[41] It may take longer than expected to announce the recipients of the grant because of time constraints, a delay in budget approval by the state or federal government, or availability of the reviewers. Therefore, grant writing requires a great deal of persistence, creativity, and patience.

# ▶ Funded Proposals

The grant seeker/nutritionist may receive a check with a cover letter if the proposal is funded, or he or she may receive a full-blown **contract** that could stipulate any number of things, such as that the grantee must submit a quarterly and/or final report when the project is completed, that there was a reduction in the amount requested, or that the president of the organization must sign the contract. In all cases, the grantee should write immediately to acknowledge the award. It is important to read the contract first before signing it and note when and what kinds of reports are due.[35]

After receiving the award, check to see whether the grantor has specific reporting forms and guidelines. If the grantor does not ask for a report, send one anyway. Show the grantor how well the money was utilized. If the project generated a newspaper article or other publication, send a copy to the grantor. If it includes a public event, invite the grantor to attend. If you received heartfelt letters of thanks from participants, send samples of the letters to the grantor.[28,42]

It is important to submit the report on time or send a letter or call to inform the grantor that the report will be late if there are extenuating circumstances that prevent the grantee from submitting the report on time.

## If a Proposal Is Rejected

The letter of rejection will probably be a form letter. It is appropriate to contact the grantor and ask for anything that will help when submitting in the future. Perhaps they liked the proposal but did not have enough money or it was not a priority topic at that time.[43] It is important to be cordial when requesting more information. After an objective review of the grantor's guidelines, if the grant seeker believes there is still the potential to receive the award, he or she can apply again in about a year.[35] Many applicants are only successful on their second or third attempt. The Successful Community Strategy presents UCLA's successful grant strategy.

# Successful Community Strategies

## The UCLA Small Grant: Are Economic Incentives Useful for Improving Dietary Quality Among WIC Participants and Their Families?[44,45]

The Economic Research Service (ERS) of the U.S. Department of Agriculture created a small grant program in 1998 (titled the Food Assistance and Nutrition Research Program) to stimulate new and innovative food assistance and nutrition issues and to broaden the participation of social science scholars in these issues. These projects focused on the economics of obesity, food insecurity and childhood obesity, food assistance program participation and household well-being, and community influence on food assistance and dietary choices. Several of the projects focused on specific populations, such as people living in the rural South and those living on American Indian reservations.

The grant award selection process included peer review panels composed of experts from the academic, government, and private sectors. In addition to reviewers' comments, the selection process considered coverage of priority research/program areas, overlap between proposals and ongoing projects, program needs, and potential benefits from research/program collaborations on particular projects.

To administer the small grant program, the ERS formed partnerships with five academic institutions and research institutes. Partner institutions had the advantage of being closer to the particular regional and state environments that influenced program delivery and outcomes. Each partner institution provided a different emphasis on food and nutrition assistance research.

Dena Herman and colleagues at the University of California Los Angeles received one of the grant awards to investigate whether providing supplemental financial support explicitly for the purchase of fresh fruits and vegetables would result in high uptake of the supplement and whether the individuals would continue to consume more fruits and vegetables after the financial support was removed.

To carry out this project, the researchers/nutritionists provided vouchers for fresh fruit and vegetable purchases to low-income women participating in the Public Health Foundation Enterprises (PHFE) WIC program in Los Angeles. A total of 602 women who enrolled for postpartum services at three selected WIC program sites (about 200 per site) in Los Angeles were recruited. Sites were assigned to either intervention with vouchers redeemable at a local supermarket, intervention with vouchers redeemable at a nearby year-round farmers' market, or a control site with minimal nonfood incentive for participation interviews. Vouchers were issued bimonthly at the level of $10 per week. Interventions were carried out for 6 months, and participants' diets were followed for an additional 6 months following the intervention. Quantitative 24-hour dietary recalls were conducted at four interviews for all participants; in addition, at the

*(continues)*

## Successful Community Strategies (continued)

intervention sites, two extra interviews spaced 2 months apart were conducted to obtain information on the fruits and vegetables purchased with the vouchers. Specifically, participants were asked to respond to the question, "What did you buy with your fruit and vegetable coupons last week?" Voucher redemption rates were obtained from scanned data from the supermarket's corporate headquarters. In the farmers' market, vouchers presented for purchase were collected by the farmers' market manager and submitted to the city government's accounting department for tallying; vouchers were then mailed to the study's research staff, who recounted the redeemed vouchers and logged the tallies into an electronic database.

In total, $44,000 worth of vouchers were issued for the supermarket and $44,960 for the farmers' market. Redemption rates were 90.7 percent for the farmers' market and 87.5 percent for the supermarket. Overall, participants reported purchasing 27 and 26 different fruits and 34 and 33 different vegetables in the farmers' market and supermarket outlets, respectively. Five fruits and five vegetables accounted for about 70 percent of the items reported for each group, with only minor differences in items. The 10 most frequently reported items were oranges, apples, bananas, peaches, grapes, tomatoes, carrots, lettuce, broccoli, and potatoes. A larger number of item purchases were reported for the farmers' market condition, though the total number of types of fruits and vegetables did not differ significantly between the two conditions.

Participants in the intervention conditions increased their consumption of fruits and vegetables with use of the supplement and sustained that increase 6 months after the intervention was completed. At baseline, participants at the farmers' market site reported eating 2.2 servings/1,000 kcal on average, at the supermarket site 2.9 servings/1,000 kcal, and at the control site 2.6 servings/1,000 kcal. Six months after the intervention, this same comparison was made and the increase in fruit and vegetable intake reported by the intervention sites was sustained. Both the farmers' market and supermarket sites reported eating 4.0 servings of fruits and vegetables/1,000 kcal on average, whereas the control site reported eating 3.1 servings/1,000 kcal on average. The difference in consumption between each of the intervention sites and the control site was statistically significant even after adjusting for multiple comparisons. These results were identical when evaluating consumption of fruits and vegetables, excluding beans and potatoes, and of fruits and vegetables, excluding juices. Increases in vegetable consumption were mainly responsible for the overall increases in fruit and vegetable intake. The researchers concluded that the sustained intake of fruits and vegetables may be reflective of the positive cultural habits that the participants have retained as well as the timing of the study at a critical point in the life course. They also attributed the high intake of fruits and vegetables to the large proportion of Latinos included in the study.

# Learning Portfolio

## Chapter Summary

- Writing a grant proposal is a systematic process.
- Grant-seeking organizations or individuals should look for funding from an agency that funds a specific type of need in the community.
- Partnering with another school or community organization on a program can provide additional funding leverage for both partners.
- Many funding agencies look for programs that use a collaborative approach.
- Grant seekers must have a clear idea of the project or program that needs funding.
- Once a funding source that looks promising is located, the next step is to make an initial contact. Potential grantors respond to initial contacts in different ways. Some grantors will fund a project directly from a letter of intent, whereas others will ask for expanded aspects of the letter of intent.

- The grant writer should read the request for proposals very carefully and follow the guidelines because the proposal may be disqualified due to improper format.
- The research plan is the most critical component of the proposal. It should contain vital information needed to evaluate the quality of the proposal, independent of any other document.
- The grantors usually send a letter to the grant seeker acknowledging the receipt of the proposal and informing him or her of when they plan to announce which proposals will be funded.
- Many applicants are successful only on their second or third attempt.

## Critical Thinking Activities

- Speak with a community member, a community or public health nutritionist, a researcher, and an administrator who have been involved in research. Ask them about their roles and functions in the research.

- Divide into groups and identify funding sources for research in community and public health nutrition for minority groups in the community.
- Identify and write a small grant proposal that may be submitted to a granting agency for funding about a weight loss program for a group of minority children.
- Identify a nutrition problem that has relevance to the community and public health nutrition in your area that could be used to develop a grant proposal.

## 🔍 CASE STUDY 14-1: Nutrition Research in American Indian Community

Debra Parrish at Keweenaw Bay Ojibwa Community College received funding from the Economic Research Service of the U.S. Department of Agriculture to conduct nutrition screening and other health assessments with the Keweenaw Bay Indian Community, a federally recognized Indian tribe located on the L'Anse Indian Reservation in Baraga County, Michigan. The project developed nutrition surveys for families of children ages 1 to 4 years. Distribution of the surveys proved difficult because tribal operations do not have mailing lists for these children. So collecting the data was very time consuming. The goals of the project included the following:

- Documenting the prevalence of nutrition-related diseases (anemia, dental caries, protein-energy malnutrition, stunted growth, high fat intake, and obesity) among tribal youth.
- Reducing the incidence of chronic diseases—for example, diabetes.
- Creating programs that integrate Ojibwa culture to enhance learning that, in turn, would bring about healthy lifestyle changes.

### Questions
1. Writing and receiving a grant is very important in the field of nutrition. What is a grant? Briefly explain at least three different types of grants.
2. Writing a grant proposal is a systematic, step-by-step process. What are the steps Debra needs to take in writing a grant proposal?
3. Debra identified collaborators for matching and in-kind grants. What is an in-kind grant? What is a matching grant?
4. Her granting agency required Debra to conduct research with the funds she received. What is a research grant? What are the major components of a grant proposal application?
5. Work in small groups or individually to discuss the case study and practice using the Nutrition Care Process chart provided on the companion website. You can also add other nutrition and health-related conditions or assessments to the case study to make the case study more challenging and interesting.

## Think About It

**Answer:** Once all parts of a grant proposal are written and spellchecked, the entire thing can be assembled. The following need to be included: the cover sheet (containing Ann's name as project manager, including her address, telephone number, and e-mail address), the proposal itself, the budget, and the supplementary materials. She needs to add a cover letter and be sure to note whether the grantor wants multiple copies or if a cover sheet needs to be signed by staff or board members. It is important to observe the grantor's deadline because late applications are automatically disqualified.

## Key Terms

**block grant:** A sum of money the federal government gives to a state or local government. The fed-eral government suggests a general purpose for the use of the money (e.g., community services or social services) as authorized by legislation, but permits the state or local area to spend the money without meeting specific conditions.

**budget:** A financial plan that shows expenses and income related to a specific service.

**collaboration:** Mutual sharing and working together to achieve common goals in such a way that all persons or groups are recognized and growth is enhanced.

**conceptual framework:** A visual way of demonstrating relationships that are known and ones that have not been investigated but that may be the focus of the project.

**contract:** A written agreement between a grantee and a third party to acquire routine goods and services. The contract could stipulate any number of things, such as that the grantee must submit a quarterly and/or final report when the project is completed, that there was a reduction in the amount requested, or that the president of the organization must sign the contract.

**demonstration grant:** A grant given to show a new approach to delivering a community health program or to demonstrate a technique.

**equipment grant:** A grant for small instruments for a start-up fund.

**formula grant:** Noncompetitive awards based on a predetermined formula provided to grantees. The amount is established by a formula based on certain criteria (e.g., population, per capita income, poverty, service needs, or number of substandard housing units in a community) that are written into the legislation and program regulations. These are directly awarded and administered in a department's program offices. These programs are sometimes referred to as state-administered programs.

**grant:** Money given to an individual or an organization for a need and that does not require repayment. Grants can be given out by foundations, governments, and the like. Grants to individuals can be either scholarships or donations.

**grant proposal:** A written request for money (and occasionally for other resources).

**grantee:** The organization or individual awarded a grant or cooperative agreement by the grantor and who is legally responsible and accountable for the use of the funds provided and for the performance of the grant-supported project or activities.

**hypothesis:** A supposition or question that is raised to explain an event or guide investigation.

**in-kind:** Contribution of equipment, supplies, or other tangible resources, as distinguished from a monetary grant. Some organizations may also donate the use of office space or staff time as an in-kind contribution.

**matching grant:** The amount of project costs that the organization, other sponsors, or the institution will contribute toward the project. Support may consist of money, equipment needed for the project, personnel (in-kind), or supplies.

**program:** A healthcare service designed to meet identified healthcare needs of individuals.

**research:** A systematic investigation, including development, testing, and evaluation, designed to develop or contribute to generalizable knowledge.

**research grant:** Grant money to support an ongoing research study, develop new hypotheses, or improve existing ideas. Normally there are no, or only very few, conditions associated with the award. The researcher is free to decide on the course of his or her research and to use the funds accordingly, subject only to the general conditions of the sponsor and the policies of the university or organization.

**service grant:** Grant money that supports activities and services to the community over and above those outreach programs already funded. This also could be accomplished through a block grant.

**training grant:** Grant money to learn how to prepare a grant proposal and/or learn new techniques.

**travel grant:** Grant money funding travel and related expenses outside of the state, community, or local area for the purposes of research, both basic and applied; to attend conferences; or to attend a workshop on how to write a grant proposal.

## References

1. Marshall MI, Johnson A, Fulton J. Writing a successful grant proposal. *Purdue Extension.* EC-737. 1990. https://www.extension.purdue.edu/extmedia/ec/ec-737.pdf. Accessed March 16, 2017.
2. Stanhope M, Lancaster J. *Community and Public Health Nursing: Population-Centered Health Care in the Community.* 9th ed. New York, NY: Elsevier; 2015.
3. DeHaven T. Community development. CATO Institute. http://www.downsizinggovernment.org/hud/community-development#Overview. Accessed March 17, 2017.
4. Bordage G, Dawson B. Experimental study design and grant writing in eight steps and 28 questions. *Med Educ.* 2003;37(4):376-385.
5. Inouye SK. An evidence-based guide to writing grant proposals for clinical research. *Ann Intern Med.* 2005;142(4):274-282.
6. Karsh E, Fox AS. *The Only Grant-Writing Book You'll Ever Need.* 5th ed. New York, NY: Carroll & Graf Publishers; 2014.
7. Bartlett S, Burstein N, Andrews M. Food Stamp Program Access Study eligible nonparticipants. 2004. http://www.ers.usda.gov/. Accessed April 20, 2016.
8. Grants.Gov. Grant categories. http://www.grants.gov/aboutgrants/grant_categories.jsp. Accessed May 17, 2017.
9. Hitchcock J, Schubert PE, Thomas SA. *Community Health Nursing.* 2nd ed.Clifton Park, NY: Thomson Delmar Learning; 2003.
10. Colwell JC, Bliss DZ, Engberg S, Moore KN. Preparing a grant proposal: part 5—organization and revision. *J Wound Ostomy Continence Nurs.* 2005;32(5):291-293.
11. Watts ML. Ryan White CARE Act reauthorization: opportunities for patients and dietetics professionals. *J Am Diet Assoc.* 2004;104(11):1661-1662.

12. Kenner C, Walden M. *Grant Writing Tips for Nurses and Other Health Professionals.* Washington, DC: American Nurses Association; 2001.

13. Ryan B, Eng M. Make your grant proposal successful. *Pharm J.* 2004;272:475-477.

14. Edelstein S. *Nutrition in Public Health: A Handbook for Developing Programs and Services.* 3rd ed. Sudbury, MA: Jones & Bartlett; 2011.

15. Examining Community-Institutional Partnerships for Prevention Research Group. Building and sustaining community-institutional partnerships for prevention research: findings from a national collaborative. *J Urban Health.* 2006;83(6):989-1003.

16. Fisher EB Jr. The results of the COMMIT trial. *Am J Public Health.* 1995;85(2):159-160.

17. Farquhar JW, Fortmann SP, Flora JA, et al. Effects of community wide education on cardiovascular disease risk factors: the Stanford Five-City Project. *JAMA.* 1990;264(3):359-365.

18. Elder JP, Schmid TL, Dower P, Hedlund S. Community heart health programs: components, rational, and strategies for effective interventions. *J Public Health Policy.* 1993;14(4):463-479.

19. Sullivan M, Kelly JG. *Collaborative Research: University and Community Partnership.* Washington, DC: American Public Health Association; 2001.

20. Rummel N, Spada H. Learning to collaborate: an instructional approach to promoting collaborative problem solving in computer-mediated settings. *J Learn Sci.* 2005;14(2):201-241.

21. Lofir D, Date AR. Reading and writing education research grants program. http://www.ed.gov /programs/readingresearch/2006-305g.pdf. Accessed March 16, 2017.

22. Philbrick DA. Writing a successful grant application. https://www.joe.org/joe/1990summer/tt3 .php. Accessed March 16, 2017.

23. Lusk SL, Sally L. Developing an outstanding grant application. *West J Nurs Res.* 2004;26(3):367-373.

24. Bliss DZ, Savik K, Whitney JD. Writing a grant proposal: research methods. *J Wound Ostomy Continence Nurs.* 2005;32(4 pt 2):226-229.

25. Cummings PP, Rivara FP, Frederick P, Koepsell TD, et al. Writing informative abstracts for journal articles. *Arch Pediatr Adolesc Med.* 2004; 158(11):1086-1088.

26. Gray M, Bliss DZ. Preparing a grant proposal: reviewing the literature. *J Wound Ostomy Continence Nurs.* 2005;32(2 pt 2):83-86.

27. Murray CJ, Ezzati M, Lopez AD, Rodgers A, et al. Comparative quantification of health risks: conceptual framework and methodological issues. *Popul Health Metr.* 2003;1(1):1478-7954.

28. SchoolGrant. Grant writing tips. http://www .schoolgrants.org. Accessed March 17, 2017.

29. Kenner C. *Perinatal Alcohol Users: Identification.* Grant funded by the Centers for Disease Control and Prevention. Atlanta, GA; 1991.

30. Grove LK. Writing winning proposals for research funds. *Tech Comm.* 2004;51(1):1-8.

31. Xuehao C. Ridership accuracy and transit formula grants. *Transportation Res Rec.* 2006;1986:3-10.

32. Heibert SM. The strong-inference protocol: not just for grant proposals. *Adv Physiol Educ.* 2007;31(1):93-96.

33. Carlson S, Anderson B. What are data? The many kinds of data and their implications for data re-use. *J Comput Mediated Commun.* 2007;12(2):635-651.

34. Burke MA. *Simplified Grant Writing.* Thousand Oaks, CA: Corwin Press; 2002.

35. International Council of Nurses. Guidelines for writing grant proposals. 2006. http://www.icn .ch/. Accessed March 17 2017.

36. Van Zant S. Successful grant-writing strategies. *Leadership.* 2003;32(4):6.

37. Barrett KE. Preparing your curriculum vitae. *J Pediatr Gastroenterol Nutr.* 2002;34(4):362-365.

38. Fain JA. *Reading Understanding, and Applying Nursing Research.* 6th ed. Philadelphia, PA: F.A. Davis; 2014.

39. Boyle MA, Holben D. *Community Nutrition in Action: An Entrepreneurial Approach.* 4th ed. Belmont, CA: Thomson Wadsworth; 2013.

40. Fredalene B. Securing funds through grant writing. *Exchange Early Child Leaders.* 2006;168: 66-69

41. Schwartz DA, Mastin JP, Martin MM. Improving grant application peer review for the NIEHS. *Environ Health Perspect.* 2006;114(5):A270.

42. School Grant. http://www.pearsonschool.com /index.cfm?locator=PSZuEb. Accessed March 16, 2017.

43. Locke L, Spirduso W, Silverman S. *Proposals That Work: A Guide for Planning Dissertations and Grant Proposals.* 6th ed. Thousand Oaks, CA: Sage; 2013.

44. Parrish D. Assessing nutritional habits of Ojibwa children. In: Stommes E, ed. *Food Assistance and Nutrition Research Small Grants Program: Executive Summaries of 2004 Research Grants.* Vol 2011. Washington, DC: US Dept of Agriculture, Economic Research Service; 2004.

45. Herman D, Harrison GG, Jenks E, Afifi AA. Are economic incentives useful for improving dietary quality among WIC participants and their families. http://nutrition.ucdavis.edu/. Accessed March 17, 2017.

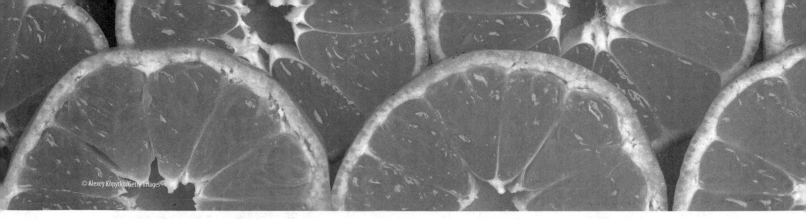
© Alexey Kopytko/Getty Images

# CHAPTER 15

# Ethics and Nutrition Practice

## CHAPTER OUTLINE

- Introduction
- What Is Ethics?
- Nutrition and Ethics
- Conflicts of Interest in Research
- Basic Principles of the Protection of Human Subjects
- Basic Ethical Principles
- Business Conflicts
- Ethics in Health Promotion
- Ethical Decision Making
- *Code of Ethics for the Profession of Dietetics*

## LEARNING OBJECTIVES

- Define ethics.
- Discuss the possible conflicts of interest between research and business.
- Discuss ethical dilemmas in health promotion.
- Discuss the basic ethical principles.
- Discuss factors to consider in moral decision making.

## ▶ Introduction

It is important that community nutritionists understand ethical issues that may affect their practice of nutrition. To address this need, the Academy of Nutrition and Dietetics' (AND's) *Code of Ethics for the Profession of Dietetics* covers most aspects of the dietetic practice. The purpose of the Code of Ethics is to assist dietitians in decision making in areas of moral conflict. There are potential conflicts of interest in providing accurate nutrition information to the public, conducting research,

securing grant funds, and other aspects of professional life. This chapter discusses different ethical issues as they apply to nutrition and the *Code of Ethics for the Profession of Dietetics*.

## ▶ What Is Ethics?

Hitchcock et al.[1] defined **ethics** as the study of the nature and justification of **principles** that guide human behaviors and are applied when moral problems arise.

Ethical actions involve decisions about which actions, relationships, and policies should be considered right or wrong.[2] The word *ethics* is derived from the Greek *ethos*, "the distinctive character of acting" or the manner of action that contributes to a person's growth.[3] In the literature, both ethics and morality are, at times, used interchangeably, but distinction can be made between the two. Morality is derived from the Latin *mosmoris*, which means "the customary way of acting," in the sense that the nutritionist has the self-discipline to produce proper attributes. Morality can be viewed as the ability to distinguish moral problems from other problems. To be able to differentiate among feelings, facts, and values and reflect on them is a cognitive ability preconditioned by a moral motivation to do good, as it relates to nutrition and health practitioners. Ethics, on the other hand, refers to the methodical analysis of what is right or wrong, good or bad.[3,4]

## ▶ Nutrition and Ethics

The interests of grant funding agencies, such as food industries and private agencies, can create opportunities for conflicts of interest when conducting grant-related research and reporting findings. A community nutritionist involved in research is prone to conflicts of interest.[5] For example, he or she has an obligation to the funding agency, but also obligations to the profession of dietetics and to the public and the community to provide accurate and complete information that is not misleading.

Ethical codes apply when implementing a community nutrition program just as they do in all other aspects of dietetic practice.[6] The protection of human health involves ensuring adequate nutrition, prevention of malnutrition, and defense against unsafe foods. Healthy people are more able to participate in human affairs and are more able to live productive and meaningful lives if credible scientific knowledge is utilized to adequately improve their lives. Government, private agencies, and healthcare professionals are obligated to ensure that human health is improved by providing reliable scientific information.

The ethical questions community and public health nutritionist's encounter are similar to those encountered in other disciplines. **Moral obligation** is the duty to act in a particular way in response to moral norms. For instance, the community nutritionist must be honest when communicating diet and health information to clients and must ascertain whether scientific findings are sufficient and credible before being translated into dietary advice.[7] The role of community nutritionist requires practices that accept moral responsibility for the growth and development of individuals, families, and communities.

The following is an example of an ethical dilemma encountered by a nutritionist. A community nutritionist was hired to categorize those in the community according to health needs and decide who should receive first priority for nutrition education and medical nutrition therapy. The categories were as follows[7,8]:

- Those who cannot survive due to lack of food and who are severely malnourished (African American and Hispanic infants, and older persons)
- Those who can be assisted to prevent long-term disability (European American populations at high risk for obesity and individuals experiencing mild hypertension)
- Those who do not have an acute disabling illness or are not at risk for long-term disability (school-age children who are not obese, women with uncomplicated pregnancies, and elderly individuals with adequate healthcare coverage but who need nutrition education)

This example is connected to two ethical principles in the AND's Code of Ethics, presented later in this chapter: No. 1, which addresses honesty, integrity, and fairness, and no. 11, which addresses efforts to avoid bias in any kind of professional evaluation of others. The community nutritionist first selected those who were severely malnourished and then those who were at risk for obesity. Finally, he or she provided nutrition education to the school-age children, women with uncomplicated pregnancies, and elderly individuals.[9]

## ▶ Conflicts of Interest in Research

Due to a reduction in government funding, increased university overhead expenses, and other reasons, many nutrition scientists obtain research support or funding from nongovernment sources. These sources can include corporations (e.g., food, drug, biotechnology, and nutrient supplement companies), commodity groups (e.g., walnut or peanut growers, beef or soybean farmers, sugar cane or beet growers, corn growers, etc.), health organizations (e.g., American Heart Association, American Cancer Institute, March of Dimes), and other nonprofit groups (e.g., foundations and research or policy institutes).[10] Dietitians must be cautious about potential conflicts of interest because their research is commonly funded by some of these organizations, along with their employer, and the funding agency's interests may conflict with their own.[11] For example, a nutrition scientist may decide to conduct research on osteoporosis (with funding from the dairy council) because the funds are available instead of researching a topic that is more widely needed by society, such as effective nutrition education methods, but for which funding is limited (funding from local county).

Another aspect of conflict of interest involves the dissemination of the research findings to the public, media, scientific meetings, and interviews with journalists. The interests of the agencies paying for the research may conflict with the actual outcomes of the research and how the results are presented.[12] For instance, the nutrition scientist may be pressured to delay or suppress the outcomes of the research or be pressured to reinterpret the results in a way that is more favorable to the funding source.[10] The Code of Ethics of the American Society for Nutritional Sciences (ASNS) states that when members are speaking to the public on a topic with which they may be perceived as having a potential conflict of interest, members should reveal those interests to their audience or the person with whom they are speaking. The ASNS Code of Ethics also states that it is unethical to conduct research if the results determine whether the findings will be published or not.[13]

There may be consequences when nutrition scientists exaggerate the importance of research findings or suppress the outcome of research in favor of the funding agency. The consequences include, but are not to limited to, the following[10,14-16]:

- What is said or not said may add to public confusion on nutrition topics.
- People may be misled about how to select a healthful diet.
- Genuine findings and inferences may be discarded.
- The public's confidence in nutrition science may be undermined.
- Worthwhile treatments/therapy may not be pursued because the original research was discredited.
- Science-based public policy decisions may be affected.

Another possible area of conflict is if nutrition scientists serve on research proposal review boards in their area of expertise and at the same time conduct research on topics related to the proposals being reviewed. A conflict of interest exists if a reviewer's judgment regarding the quality of someone's research proposal is unfairly influenced by his or her own research hypothesis or by the interests of his or her own funding source. Researchers, such as those on review committees, should avoid even the appearance of unfairness in conflicts in the review and evaluation of research and research proposals of other dietitians.[12,17] This is important because such review processes are usually "blind," consequently making potential unfairness hidden. The recommendation is to exempt oneself from the decision making when there is potential for

a conflict of interest. Visit http://www.eatrightpro.org/resources/career/code-of-ethics/what-is-the-code-of-ethics, for examples of scenarios about the principles of the code of ethic.

McKnutt[10] suggested the following safeguards to reduce the possibility of conflicts of interest related to sources of research funding[10,12,18,19]:

- What is expected of nutrition scientists when they receive government or nongovernment funds should be spelled out in a written agreement that is reviewed by a committee of the nutrition scientists' employers/organizations. This process decreases the likelihood of investigators doing research that may conflict with the interests of society or the interests of the university.
- Some funding-acceptance policies do not consider it to be a conflict of interest for nutrition scientists to receive funds to do studies if both the researchers and the agency agree before the research starts that results will not be published because the research may be related to a patent application. However, the ASNS Code of Ethics forbids members from accepting money to do research if the grantor has the right to forbid publication of findings if the results are not favorable to the grantor's business or social-marketing objectives. Many other codes, rules, and policies have similar positions. In most contracts between research scientists and grantors, the scientists retain full responsibility for all data and analysis.[13]
- When results are published in a scientific journal, editors and reviewers have an opportunity to assess whether the scientist's relationship with the funding source has influenced the design of a study or interpretation of results. In addition, most nutrition journals publish as part of a research report the source of the investigator's funding, thereby alerting journalists who report scientific findings and other readers to consider whether a study may be influenced by whomever funded it.

## ▶ Basic Principles of the Protection of Human Subjects

Scientific research has produced substantial social benefits. It has also created some troubling ethical questions. Public attention was particularly drawn to the reported abuses of human subjects in biomedical experiments during the Second World War. During the Nuremberg War Crime Trials, the Nuremberg Code was drafted as a set of standards for judging physicians and scientists who had conducted biomedical experiments on concentration camp prisoners. This code became the prototype of many later codes intended to guarantee that research involving human subjects would be carried out in an ethical manner.[20]

Research is defined as a systematic investigation, including research, development, testing, and evaluation, designed to develop or contribute to generalizable knowledge.[21] It also includes activities that meet this definition, whether conducted under a program considered "research" or for other purposes.[22] A **human subject** is defined as a living individual about whom an investigator is conducting research to obtain data through intervention or interaction with the individual or to obtain identifiable private information.[22]

The Nuremberg Code consists of rules, some general and others more specific, that guide investigators or the reviewers of research in their work. These rules are usually inadequate to cover complex situations; at times they conflict and are often difficult to interpret or apply. Therefore, on July 12, 1974, the National Research Act (Public Law 93-348) was signed into law, creating the National Commission for the Protection of Human Subjects of Biomedical and Behavioral Research. The commission was asked to identify the basic ethical principles that should form the foundation of the conduct of biomedical and behavioral research involving human subjects and to develop guidelines to ensure that such research is conducted in accordance with those principles.

The Belmont Report is the outgrowth of an intensive 4-day period of discussions that were held in February 1976 at the Smithsonian Institution's Belmont Conference Center, supplemented by the monthly deliberations of the commission that were held over a period of nearly 4 years. The Belmont Report summarized the basic ethical principles identified by the commission in the course of its deliberations. It is a statement of basic ethical principles and guidelines that should assist in resolving the ethical problems that surround conducting research with human subjects. The report is published in the *Federal Register* and reprints are available upon request. The two-volume appendix (DHEW Publication No. [OS] 78-0013 and No. [OS] 78-0014), containing the lengthy reports of experts and specialists who assisted the commission in fulfilling this part of its charge, is available for purchase from the Superintendent of Documents, U.S. Government Printing Office, Washington, DC 20402.[20] Also, the preliminary papers can be found on the Internet at https://www.hhs.gov/ohrp/regulations-and-policy/belmont-report/index.html.

## ▶ Basic Ethical Principles

The phrase **basic ethical principles** refers to those general judgments that serve as a basic justification for the particular ethical prescriptions and evaluations of human actions. Three basic principles, among those generally accepted in the U.S. cultural tradition, are relevant to the ethics of research involving human subjects and are presented in **BOX 15-1**: the principles of respect for persons, beneficence, and justice.[20]

---

**BOX 15-1** The Three Basic Ethical Principles

*Respect for persons:* Respect for persons incorporates at least two ethical convictions: first, that individuals should be treated as autonomous representatives (individuals with deliberation capacity about personal goals and acting under the direction of such deliberation) and second, that persons with diminished autonomy (children, prisoners, the frail elderly, etc.) are entitled to protection. The principle of respect for persons thus divides into two separate moral requirements: the requirement to acknowledge autonomy and the requirement to protect those with diminished autonomy. In research involving human subjects, participation must be voluntary, and adequate information such as the aim, procedures, risks, and benefits must be disclosed to the participants before they consent for the research. The participants must have the opportunity to ask questions and be informed that they can withdraw from the study at any time.

*Beneficence:* People are treated in an ethical manner, not only by respecting their decisions and protecting them from harm, but also by making efforts to secure their well-being. Such treatment falls under the principle of beneficence. The term *beneficence* usually includes acts of kindness or charity that go beyond strict obligation. Two general rules have been formulated as complementary expressions of beneficent actions in this sense: 1) do no harm and 2) maximize possible benefits and minimize possible harms.

*Justice:* Justice is the sense of "fairness in distribution" or "what is deserved." An injustice occurs when some benefit to which a person is entitled is denied without good reason or when some burden is imposed unduly. There are several accepted formulations of just ways to distribute burdens and benefits. Each formulation mentions some relevant property on the basis of which burdens and benefits should be distributed. These formulations are 1) to each person an equal share, 2) to each person according to individual need, 3) to each person according to individual effort, 4) to each person according to societal contribution, and 5) to each person according to merit.

Community nutritionists almost always involve human subjects in their work. Sometimes their activities involve limited practice, and other times they involve a combination of practice and research. Principally, the term *practice* refers to interventions designed exclusively to enhance the well-being of an individual patient or client and that have a reasonable expectation of success.[21] In contrast, the term *research* refers to an activity designed to test a hypothesis, set procedures designed to reach that objective, and permit conclusions to be drawn (e.g., expressed in theories, principles, and statements of relationships).[23] It includes interviewing; surveying, testing, or observing individuals for the purpose of collecting data and changing the individuals' physical, psychological, and environmental status.

The protection of human subjects is important whether it is for behavioral or biomedical research. The Belmont Report should be used as a guide whenever human beings are involved in any research. Many organizations, universities, and hospitals have an institutional review board (IRB) that is responsible for educating and monitoring research activities for protecting human subjects. Both the participant and the investigator must sign a consent form (see **FIGURE 15-1**) with accurate and adequate information about the research. Research involving incomplete disclosure

is not justified.[20] For instance, an observational study known as the Tuskegee study was a long-term observation of the "natural" course of syphilis in African American men who were recruited into the study without **informed consent**. The men were observed for several decades but did not receive penicillin, although its effectiveness in the treatment of syphilis was established several years after the initiation of the study.[2] Information about the use of human subjects in research can be found on the National Institutes of Health's website (http://www.nih.gov).

## ▶ Business Conflicts

Many companies in the food industry hire Registered Dietitians (RDs) or support their research activities. Dietitians who are employed by the food industry (such as cereal, dairy, or fast food companies) often encounter moral dilemmas. First, they have obligations to their employer because it is their source of livelihood, and, second, they have obligations to the public to do no harm. Society has recognized the field of dietetics as a profession because of its perceived service in public welfare.[12] Dietitians can serve the interests of the public and the employer by looking for acceptable alternatives. For example, a dietitian was hired to educate women

**(Insert the organization's logo here)**

**Building Better Bones**

**Description and Explanation of Procedure:** A bone density test is indicated because you have some risk for developing osteoporosis, and you may not already have a diagnosis of osteoporosis. This procedure will be performed using a Hologic Sahara Clinical Bone Sonometer. It is a painless, noninvasive test of the bone mineral density of the heel that takes only a few minutes to perform. The test will be performed by a licensed, trained operator.

**Risk:** There is little or no discomfort associated with this method of measuring bone density. With this ultrasound machine, there is no radiation involved.

**Benefits:** I understand that this procedure will provide me with basic information about my bone mineral density.

**Confidentiality:** I have been assured that information regarding my identity and bone mineral density measurement will be given only to me, my physician, or (organization's name). I understand that any data or answers to questions will remain confidential with regard to my identity.

I have been given an opportunity to ask questions, and all such questions have been answered satisfactorily.

I further understand that I am free to withdraw my consent and terminate my participation at any time.

**Signed Consent:** I have read the above information and agreed to undergo the procedure to measure my bone mineral density.

_____ _____
Date            Participant's Name (Print)

_____ _____
Date            Participant's Signature

_____ _____
Date            Witness's Signature

**FIGURE 15-1** Sample consent form.

55 years or older about how to prevent osteoporosis. Part of her responsibility was to acquire bone densitometry to measure bone density. A nutrient supplement company provided the Sahara Clinical Bone Sonometer, but asked her to sell their vitamin and mineral supplements to the women and said that the dietitian would receive a commission when she sold these products. This ethical dilemma is addressed by the AND's Code of Ethics Principle No. 14, which addresses endorsement of products, and Principle No. 12, which addresses conflicts of interest. In this scenario, the dietitian should not allow financial gain to cloud her professional obligations as stated in the code, should not endorse products, and should not participate in situations leading to conflicts of interest.[19,24]

The suggestion is to avoid compromising relations as far as is practical, and when that cannot be done, to disclose the circumstances to all parties that could be affected.[12] When dietitians and other healthcare professionals respect clients as moral agents, they are acting in agreement with the requirements of the moral principle of autonomy. The **principle of autonomy** is the freedom for an individual to choose which actions to take.[25]

## ▶ Ethics in Health Promotion

The purpose of health promotion is to enable people to increase control over factors that affect their personal health and prevent the incidence of chronic health conditions. One of the distinctive elements of any profession is the acknowledgment by professionals and the public of the need to keep up-to-date with the latest advances in the field.[26,27] Community dietitians must continue to learn new techniques and the latest evidence-based information and to provide high-quality services in current and future work settings in order to remain competent with changing public health issues.[28] They also have the responsibility to determine the limits of their competence. A community nutritionist implementing a new program must become competent in that area of practice. For example, he or she may need to learn the latest electronic communication techniques (such as those found on the Internet) as well as legal and ethical issues that may arise when conveying information using the Internet or e-mail for nutrition education programs.[9,29]

Benner[26] defined *competence* as the ability to demonstrate appropriate professional behaviors with desirable outcomes.[26] Dietitians who are competent use up-to-date knowledge and skills, make accurate assessments based on appropriate data, critically evaluate their own practice, communicate effectively with clients and other professionals, and improve performance based on advice from others.[30,31] Therefore, they are uniquely placed to make moral judgments when translating scientific knowledge or information into dietary messages to the public and clients. As promoters of nutrition, it is important to avoid a paternalistic approach, which is a liberty-limiting principle often used to overrule for their own good people's actions or expressed desires.[25] Paternalism is justified if the issues that would be prevented are greater than the violation of the moral rule and if the dietitian is willing to allow the violation of the moral rule in all similar circumstances and be able to publicly advocate this kind of violation. For example, a community nutritionist may override a pregnant woman's wish to use illegal drugs and alcohol by referring her to an alcohol and drugs treatment center so that fetal damage can be prevented. Paternalism seems to be limited to acts that prevent people from committing some serious bodily harm to themselves or others. Additionally, it is morally justified to restrict a person's liberty when not doing so could cause life-threatening physical or mental harm; for example, asking parents to immunize their children against childhood diseases or asking pregnant women to avoid using cocaine.[25]

Similarly, moral sensitivity is a genuine concern for the well-being and dignity of clients that may become a moral burden because they have the right to determine their own plan of life. Moral sensitivity involves a conflict-laden situation and a self-awareness of one's own responsibility in the situation.[32] An example of a moral burden is a community nutritionist not being able to feed animal products to an anemic Hindu pregnant woman because of her religious beliefs, which restrict all animal products. Another example is an attempt to feed a client who is suffering from anorexia nervosa who refuses to eat any food.

One ethical conflict is how to achieve the goal of protecting and promoting public health while ensuring individuals' freedom of choice. The principle of **beneficence** states, "we ought to do good and prevent or avoid doing harm."[33] However, there may be limits on the amount of benefits clients should expect from nutrition education. Surely, nutrition education should not be expected to benefit individuals who continue to put themselves at risk by consuming foods high in fat, calories, and saturated fat and practicing a sedentary lifestyle. The ethical dilemma is how to balance harms and benefits while ensuring freedom of choice. Services that provide the greatest balance of good over bad, or benefit over harm, are in accordance with the **rule of utility**.[25,34]

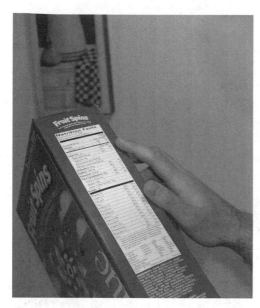

Including genetically modified ingredients is required in such countries as Japan and many European countries.

© Jones & Bartlett Learning. Photographed by Christine McKeen.

## ▶ Ethical Decision Making

In community nutrition, the main component in **ethical decision making** is focusing on the best interests of the clients while allowing every stakeholder to share in the decision. Ethics is not only about doing what the rules require or making sure that every good goal or value has been carried out. Ethics is about balancing rules, goals, and values to achieve moral justification of decisions. This is the duty of all who participate in making choices.[35]

The skills in making ethical decisions tend to increase over time and with experience for community nutritionists and those in clinical practice. This moral development typically changes as the individual matures.[36] A higher level of ethical consideration is achievable where ethical codes are used only as tools in soul-searching and in culturally sensitive decision-making processes.[37]

Ethical decision making involves several variables. It can be enhanced by an orderly process that considers clients' values, professional obligations, and ethical principles. The following are ways to make ethical decisions[3,25,38,39]:

- *Identify the problem.* The community nutritionist should clarify the issue (e.g., values, conflicts, and matters of principles) and gather all the relevant data (facts, norms, principles, rules, and interpretations of the rules).
- *Collect additional information.* The community nutritionist should decide who will be the main decision makers and what the clients or their families want.

- *Identify all the options available to the decision makers.* The community nutritionist should consider all possible courses of action and their outcomes and evaluate the probability that future decisions may have to be made. He or she should realize that all personal judgments contain subjectivity and no one can claim to be totally objective.
- *Understand.* The community nutritionist should understand that all personal judgments have shared dimensions. Human existence is coexistence; therefore, consultation of the many opinions in the community is critical, and reflection on the possible consequences of a decision on the community is very important.
- *Think the situation through.* The community nutritionist should consider the basic values and the professional obligations involved, investigate the ethical principles and relevant rules, and realize that every human judgment is fallible.
- *Make the decision.* The community nutritionist should choose the course of action that reflects his or her best judgment.
- *Assess the decision and its outcomes.* The community nutritionist should compare the actual outcomes of the situation with the expected outcomes. He or she should determine whether the process of decision making used can be improved for future situations having similar characteristics.

In addition, the AND's position paper on ethical issues provides assumptions that may form the basis for ethical deliberation. Community nutritionists may consider using these assumptions when making good moral judgments[36,39-41]:

- *Autonomy:* Respect for the autonomy of the individual is a very strong value in U.S. culture. Adults with decisional capacity should be free to make their own choices about their concerns. There is a limit to freedom, but that limit has to be defined with each situation and should strongly favor the individuals.
- *Nonmaleficence:* "Do no harm." This basic demand has succeeded as a guide to action in clinical medicine. It is the warning to ensure that whatever is done to help the individual does not also hurt the individual (i.e., the balance of "help" and "hurt" must favor helping the individual).
- *Beneficence:* Doing good for clients is the goal of community nutrition. Whatever action is taken should be the right action.
- **Justice**: "Fairness" is the main formula used to describe justice in clinical decision making and can be applied in community nutrition. Moral action is the fair action that treats each person equally in similar circumstances.[35]

## Think About It

A community nutritionist was designing a nutrition program for a multiethnic group with different income levels. She wondered how important it was to treat each person equally, and then she remembered hearing about ethical decision making. She wondered what ethics really is and whether there was an ethical principle that related to fairness.

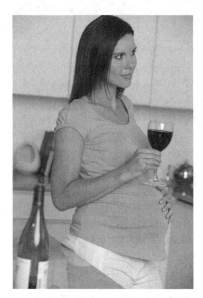

Consuming harmful substances during pregnancy poses grave danger for the developing fetus.

© Monkey Business Images/ShutterStock, Inc.

## ▶ Code of Ethics for the Profession of Dietetics

The January 1999 *Journal of the Academy of Nutrition and Dietetics* stated that the AND and its Commission on Dietetic Registration (CDR) had adopted a voluntary, enforceable **code of ethics**. In 2009, the AND Board of Directors, House of Delegates, and CDR approved the current Code of Ethics. This code, entitled the *Code of Ethics for the Profession of Dietetics*, challenged all members, RDs, and registered dietetic technicians to uphold ethical principles. The enforcement process for the Code of Ethics establishes a fair system to deal with complaints about members and credentialed practitioners, peers, or the public.[20]

The House of Delegates adopted the first code of ethics in October 1982 and enforcement began in 1985. The code applied only to members of the AND. A second code was adopted by the House of Delegates in October 1987 and applied to all members and CDR-credentialed practitioners. A third revision of the code was adopted

by the House of Delegates on October 18, 1998, and began being enforced on June 1, 1999, for all members and CDR-credentialed practitioners.[42]

The Ethics Committee is responsible for reviewing, promoting, and enforcing the code. The committee also educates members, credentialed practitioners, students, and the public about the ethical principles contained in the code. Support of the Code of Ethics by members and credentialed practitioners is vital to guiding the profession's actions and to strengthening its credibility. Visit the AND's Code of Ethics Preamble and Principles at: http://www.eatrightpro.org/resources/career/code-of-ethics.

## Public Health Nutrition Code of Ethics

In relation to public health nutrition, the publication entitled *Principles of the Ethical Practice of Public Health* established the Public Health Leadership Society, which is founded on ethics.[43] The society created 12 principles that mirrored morality and human rights as a part of its framework. Dietitians employed in a public health setting should utilize both the *Code of Ethics for the Profession of Dietetics* and the *Principles of the Ethical Practice of Public Health* in their practice.

## Violating the Academy of Nutrition and Dietetics Code of Ethics

If a member or credentialed practitioner has violated the *Code of Ethics for the Profession of Dietetics*, an appropriate form must be submitted to the Ethics Committee. The complaint must be made within 1 year of the date that the complainant (the person making the complaint) first became aware of the alleged violation.[24] The complainant does not have to be a member of the AND or a practitioner credentialed by the CDR. The complaint must provide details on the violation; the basis for the complainant's knowledge of the violation; names, addresses, and telephone numbers of all persons involved or who might have knowledge of the activities; and whether the complaint has been submitted to a court, an administrative body, or a state licensure board. The complaint must also cite the section(s) of the *Code of Ethics for the Profession of Dietetics* allegedly violated. The complaint must be signed and sworn to by the complainant(s).[24,42]

After a hearing on an appeal and citing the provision(s) of the *Code of Ethics for the Profession of Dietetics* that may have been violated, the committee may decide that the dietitian be censured, placed on probation, suspended, or expelled from the AND or that the credential of the dietitian be suspended or revoked by the CDR. The decision of the Ethics Committee is sent to the dietitian and the complainant as soon as possible.[24]

## Licensure

Many state licensure boards accept the RD credential from the CDR. Credentialing is the formal recognition of professional or technical competence.[44,45] Fellow of the Academy of Nutrition and Dietetics (FAND), Certified Nutrition Support Dietitian (CNSD), and Board Certified Specialist in Renal Nutrition (CSR) are other certifications that may be required by the state or an employer. Some states have a practice act, which requires that a license be held by the practitioner in order to perform the professional duties allowed in that state by law. Other states have a title act, which specifies that practitioners cannot describe themselves as "dietitians" unless they are licensed in that state. The CDR website (http://www.cdrnet.org) lists of all the states with state licensure requirements.[46] State licensing boards have the legal authority to enforce the scope of practice in their state and outline those duties that the practitioner can conduct. Generally, the state board will require that practitioners are certified by a national organization (CDR) in order to meet the requirements for licensure. States often have their own requirements for renewal, and licensees may have to meet the state requirements for continuing education to remain licensed.[47] In states that require certification, it is a violation of state law to practice dietetics without a license.

## Successful Community Strategies

### Get Fit with the Grizzlies: A Community-School-Home Initiative to Fight Childhood Obesity[48]

The Memphis Grizzlies, the city's National Basketball Association franchise, launched "Get Fit with the Grizzlies," a 6-week curricular addition focusing on nutrition and physical activity in Memphis city schools (MCS). The research population consisted of every fourth- and fifth-grade student in MCS during the 2006 to 2007 school year ($n = 17,066$). These grades were chosen due to MCS data that revealed these grade levels possessed extremely high body mass index (BMI) statistics compared with other grade levels, and because this age range has been shown to be more reliable to give commentary as well as establish an evaluation on this pilot program.

A new six-lesson supplemental mini-unit focusing on nutrition and exercise was written for the fourth and fifth grades by veteran MCS elementary physical education teachers. Parents/caregivers were included in the lessons via homework (i.e., exercising with their child, discussing healthy foods, eating dinner together), and their signature was necessary on their child's Get Fit activity/food log. The Memphis Grizzlies' community investment department worked closely with MCS administration and teachers to finalize the program, and the Grizzlies' marketing staff successfully secured sponsors to help fund the initiative.

The Get Fit with the Grizzlies program was evaluated using a pretest and posttest. The 18-item Get Fit with the Grizzlies Student Questionnaire was created using objectives drawn directly from the Get Fit curriculum's six lessons and questions from the CDC's Youth Risk Behavior Survey (YRBS).[49]

The first 8 questions dealt with knowledge-based information delivered in the lessons, and the last 10 questions asked for the student's current health-related behavior information, specifically eating and physical activity habits within the previous 24 hours. In order to achieve face and content validity, the questionnaire was examined by a panel of experts consisting of a Registered Dietitian, an exercise physiology professor, three veteran elementary physical education teachers, a university elementary education specialist, and a university-level statistician. Modifications were made based on the panel's feedback.

Results showed significant health knowledge acquisition (7 of 8 questions), with odds ratios confirming moderate to strong associations. Of 10 health behavior change questions, 7 improved significantly after intervention. The only knowledge test item that did not show increased performance was based on the recommended amount of time that children should engage in daily physical activity.

# Learning Portfolio

## Chapter Summary

- A human subject is a living individual about whom an investigator (professional, student, etc.) is conducting research to obtain data through intervention or interaction with the individual or to obtain identifiable private information.

- The phrase *basic ethical principles* refers to those general judgments that serve as a basic justification for the particular ethical prescriptions and evaluations of human actions.

- Respect for persons incorporates at least two ethical convictions: first, that individuals should be treated as autonomous individuals (individuals with deliberation capacity about personal goals and acting under the direction of such deliberation) and, second, that persons with diminished autonomy (children, etc.) are entitled to protection.
- Ethical codes apply in implementing a community nutrition program just as they do in all other aspects of dietetic practice.
- Ethical actions refer to decisions about which actions, relationships, and policies should be considered right or wrong.
- A conflict of interest exists if a reviewer's judgment regarding the quality of someone's research proposal is unfairly influenced by their own research hypothesis or by interests of their own funding source.
- In community nutrition, the main component in ethical decision making is focusing on the best interests of the clients while allowing every stakeholder to share in the decision.

- The Academy of Nutrition and Dietetics and its Commission on Dietetic Registration have adopted a voluntary, enforceable code of ethics. This code, entitled the *Code of Ethics for the Profession of Dietetics*, challenges all members, Registered Dietitians, and registered dietetic technicians to uphold ethical principles.

## Critical Thinking Activities

- Divide into groups and suggest three ways that community nutritionists can utilize the *Code of Ethics for the Profession of Dietetics* when delivering nutrition care services to certain segments of the U.S. population (e.g., older persons, children, minority groups).
- Identify two research studies in the literature relevant to community and public health nutrition, and describe the strengths and limitations of the research and the potential ethical issues that may occur during the research study.
- Interview a childcare center staff member and obtain information about how they keep children's records confidential and possible ethical issues that may happen in handling the children's records.

## ⌕ CASE STUDY 15-1: Type 2 Diabetes Mellitus and Ethical Issues

A group of Hispanic women 40 to 55 years old were referred to a community nutritionist, Anthony, for counseling because the majority of them had a history of fatigue and lethargy, mostly noticeable after meals and in the evening, and they have a very sedentary lifestyle. Recently some of these women began to take black cohosh for hot flashes. A dietary record from the participants revealed that they seldom ate breakfast, and bought tortilla chips and a sandwich at work for lunch. Dinner consisted of store-bought refried beans with Mexican sausage three times a week, which was often accompanied by a dessert. They drank about two glasses of sweetened soft drink daily and two glasses of wine twice per month. The BMI of 60 percent of the women on average was about 32, with blood pressure of 140/90. Laboratory analysis showed that plasma glucose was 135 mg/dl, LDL cholesterol was 125 mg/dl, HDL cholesterol was 45 mg/dl, and triglycerides were 255 mg/dl for 62 percent of the participants. The nutritionist's recommendations included that the women replace all their ethnic foods with the foods typically consumed in the United States. He asked them to return in 4 weeks for a follow-up on the nutrition intervention. The women refused to attend the follow-up session. One day, a journalist called Anthony to interview him about his nutrition education program in the community. During the interview, Anthony revealed the medical history of these women to the journalist without their consent. In addition, most of the women qualify for Supplemental Nutrition Assistance Program (SNAP), but Anthony refused to inform them about this assistance because of their ethnicity.

### Questions

1. What medical conditions and risks do these women's symptoms and laboratory values represent?
2. What evidence-based nutrition recommendations would you offer these women for their current diagnosis?
3. Based on their history and laboratory data, what medical conditions and risks do the symptoms and laboratory values represent?
4. What is the role of exercise in clients with prediabetes and type 2 diabetes?
5. Which of the principles of the AND Code of Ethics did the nutritionist violate?
6. Identify the basic ethical principles observed in this scenario that were discussed in BOX 15-1.

## Think About It

**Answer:** Ethics is the study of the nature and justification of principles that guide human behaviors and are applied when moral problems arise. The ethical principle that relates to fairness is justice. Justice is the sense of fairness in distribution or what is deserved.

## Key Terms

**basic ethical principles:** General judgments that serve as a basic justification for the particular ethical prescriptions and evaluations of human actions.

**beneficence:** Ethical principle stating that one should do good and prevent or avoid doing harm.

**code of ethics:** A set of statements encompassing rules that apply to people in professional roles.

**ethical decision making:** Making decisions in an orderly process that considers ethical principles, individual values, and professional obligations.

**ethics:** The science or study of moral values; also a code of principles and ideals that guides action.

**human subject:** A living individual about whom an investigator (e.g., professional or student) is conducting research to obtain data through intervention or interaction with the individual or to obtain identifiable private information.

**informed consent:** When an individual agrees to a treatment plan after receiving sufficient information concerning the proposal, its incumbent risks, and the acceptable alternatives.

**justice:** Ethical principle that claims people should be treated equally. It is the standard of fairness served when an individual is given what is due, owed, or deserved.

**moral obligation:** Duty to act in a particular way in response to moral norms.

**principle of autonomy:** The freedom of an individual to act as he or she chooses.

**principles:** The foundations for rules.

**rule of utility:** Derived from the principle of beneficence; this includes a moral duty to weigh and balance benefits against harms in order to increase benefits and reduce the occurrence of harms.

## References

1. Hitchcock J, Schubert PE, Thomas SA. *Community Health Nursing.* 2nd ed. Clifton Park, NY: Thomson Delmar Learning; 2003.
2. Monsen ER, Vanderpool HY, Halsted CH, McNutt KW, et al. Ethics: responsible scientific conduct. *Am J Clin Nutr.* 1991;54(1):1-6.
3. Edelman M. *Health Promotion Throughtout the Lifespan.* 8th ed. St. Louis, MO: Mosby; 2014.
4. Lutzen K. *Moral Sensitivity: A Study of Subjective Aspects of the Process of Moral Decision Making in Psychiatric Nursing* [dissertation]. Stockholm, Sweden: Karolinska Institute; 1993.
5. Holler H. Resources for ethical dilemmas in dietetics. *J Am Diet Assoc.* 2002;102(12):1817-1818.
6. Winterfeldt EA, Ebro LL. *Dietetics: Practice and Future Trends.* Sudbury, MA: Jones and Bartlett; 2005.
7. American Dietetic Association. ADA report: practice paper of the American Dietetic Association—dietary supplements. *J Am Diet Assoc.* 2005;105(3):460-470.
8. Fornari A. Promoting professionalism through ethical behaviors in the academic setting. *J Am Diet Assoc.* 2004;104(3):347-349
9. Rodriguez JC. Legal, ethical, and professional issues to consider withtin communicating via the internet: a suggested response model and policy. *J Am Diet Assoc.* 1999;99:1428-1432.
10. McNutt K. Conflict of interest. *J Am Diet Assoc.* 1999;99:29-30.
11. McCaffree J. Characteristics of ethical issues versus poor business practices *J Am Diet Assoc.* 2003;103(10):1380-1381.
12. Waymack MH. Ethical conflicts of interest. *J Am Diet Assoc.* 2003;103(5):555-560.
13. American Society for Nutrition Sciences. *Code of Professional Responsibility for Members of the American Society for Nutritional Sciences.* Bethesda, MD: American Society for Nutrition Sciences; 1998.
14. Rosenstock L, Lee L. Attacks on science: the risks to evidence-based policy. *Am J Public Health.* 2002;92(1):14-18.
15. Kassirer J. Financial conflict of interest: an unresolved ethical frontier. American Society of Law, Medicine and Ethics and Boston University School of Law. *Am J Law Med.* 2000;27:149-162.
16. Cohen JJ. Trust us to make a difference: ensuring public confidence in the integrity of clinical research. *Acad Med.* 2001;76(2):209-214.
17. Rock C. An important issue in nutrition research and communications. *J Am Diet Assoc.* 1999;99:31-32.
18. Andrews M, Marian M. Ethical framework for the registered dietitian in decisions regarding withholding/withdrawing medically assisted nutrition and hydration. *J Am Diet Assoc.* 2006;106(2):206-208.
19. Academy of Nutrition and Dietetics. Code of ethics for the profession of dietetics. *J Am Diet Assoc.* 1999;99(1):109-113.

20. National Institutes of Health. Regulations and ethical guidelines. http://ohsr.od.nih.gov. Accessed March 17, 2017.

21. Monsen ER. *Research: Successful Approaches.* 2nd ed. Chicago, IL: American Dietetic Association; 2003.

22. US Dept of Education. Information about the protection of human subjects in research supported by the Department of Education: overview. 2006. http://www.ed.gov/. Accessed March 17, 2017.

23. Côté-Arsenault D, Morrison-Beedy D. Maintaining your focus in focus groups: avoiding common mistakes. *Res Nurs Health.* 2005;28(2):172-179.

24. Academy of Nutrition, Dietetic Commission on Dietetic. Registration code of ethics for the profession of dietetics and process for consideration of ethics issues. *J Am Diet Assoc.* 2009;109(8): 1461-1467.

25. Stanhope M, Lancaster J. *Community and Public Health Nursing: Population-Centered Health Care in the Community.* 9th ed. New York, NY: Elsevier; 2015.

26. Benner P. Issues in competency-based testing. *Nurs Outlook.* 1982;30(5):303-309.

27. Manore MM, Myers EF. Research and the dietetics profession: making a bigger impact. *J Am Diet Assoc.* 2003;103(1):108-112.

28. Houle CO. *Continuing Learning in the Professions.* San Francisco, CA: Jossey-Bass; 1981.

29. Gate G. Ethics opinion: dietetics professionals are ethically obligated to maintain personal competence in practice. *J Am Diet Assoc.* 2003; 103(5):633-635.

30. Epstein RM, Hundert EM. Defining and assessing professional competence. *JAMA.* 2002;287(2): 226-235.

31. Hampl J, Hill R. Dietetic approaches to US hunger and food insecurity. *J Am Diet Assoc.* 2002; 102(7):919-923.

32. Lützén K, Dahlqvist V, Eriksson S, Norberg A. Developing the concept of moral sensitivity in health care practice. *Nursing Ethics.* 2006;13(2): 187-196.

33. Frankena WK. *Ethics.* Cliffs, NJ: Prentice Hall; 1973.

34. Beauchamp TL, Childress JF. *Principles of Biomedical Ethics.* 5th ed. New York, NY: Oxford Press; 2001.

35. O'Sullivan J, Potter RL, Heller L. Position of the American Dietetic Association: ethical and legal issues in nutrition, hydration, and feeding. *J Am Diet Assoc.* 2002;102(5):716-726.

36. Neukrug E, Lovell C, Parker R. Employing ethical codes and decision-making models: a developmental process. *Counsel Values.* 1996;40:103.

37. Curry KR, Jaffe A. *Nutrition Counseling and Communication Skills.* Philadelphia, PA: W.B. Saunders; 1998.

38. Watley LD, May DR. Enhancing moral intensity: the roles of personal and consequential information in ethical decision-making. *J Bus Ethics.* 2004;50(2):105-126.

39. Clayman ML, Roter DD, Wissow LS, Lawrence S, et al. Autonomy-related behaviors of patient companions and their effect on decision-making activity in geriatric primary care visits. *Social Sci Med.* 2005;60(7):1583-1591.

40. Elger BS. [Ethics in clinical routine care: example of prognosis information]. *Med Klin.* 2002;97(9):533-540.

41. Kennedy WW. Beneficence and autonomy in nursing: a moral dilemma. *Br J Perioper Nurs.* 2004;14(11):500-506.

42. Kieselhorst KJ, Skates J, Pritchett E. American Dietetic Association: standards of practice in nutrition care and updated standards of professional performance. *J Am Diet Assoc.* 2005;105(4): 641-656.

43. Public Health Leadership Society. *Principles of the Ethical Practice of Public Health.* Vol 2.2. Chicago, IL: American Public Health Association; 2002.

44. American Dietetic Association, Commission on Accreditation for Dietetics Education. *Accreditation Manual for Dietetics Education Programs.* 4th ed. Chicago, IL: American Dietetic Association; 2000.

45. Commission on Dietetic Registration. CDR certifications and state licensure. http://www.cdrnet .org. Accessed March 17, 2017.

46. Myers EF, Barnhill G, Bryk J. Clinical privileges: missing piece of the puzzle for clinical standards that elevate responsibilities and salaries for registered dietitians? *J Am Diet Assoc.* 2002;102(1): 123-132.

47. Parrish D. Assessing nutritional habits of Ojibwa children. In: Stommes E, ed. *Food Assistance and Nutrition Research Small Grants Program: Executive Summaries of 2004 Research Grants.* Vol 2011. Washington, DC: US Dept of Agriculture, Economic Research Service; 2004.

48. Irwin CC, Irwin RL, Miller ME, Somes GW, et al. Get fit with the Grizzlies: a community-school-home initiative to fight childhood obesity. *J Sch Health.* 2010;80(7):333-339.

49. Centers for Disease Control and Prevention. Youth risk behavior surveillance: United States, 2005. *Morb Mortal Wkly Rep.* 2006;55(SS-05):1-108.

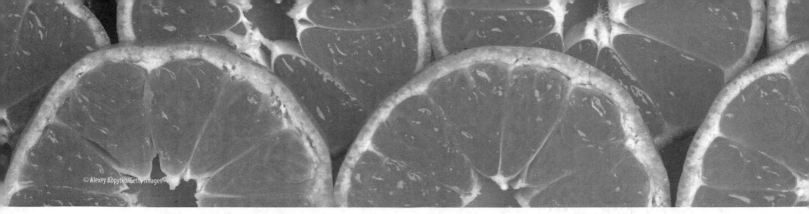
© Alexey Kopytko/Getty Images

# CHAPTER 16
# Principles of Nutrition Education

## LEARNING OBJECTIVES

- Define nutrition education.
- Discuss different educational strategies that may be effective in providing nutrition education throughout the life span.
- List the different components of a nutrition education lesson plan.
- Identify strategies to consider when providing nutrition education to participants with different cultural backgrounds.
- Identify ways to encourage participation in a health promotion program.

## ▶ Introduction

**Nutrition education** is an essential major component of health promotion and disease prevention strategies, and most major policy documents require integration of nutrition education into healthcare, worksites, colleges, and elementary and secondary schools. In the food marketplace, nutrition education, or the dissemination of food and nutrition information, has also increased in importance.[1,2] Successful nutrition messages are essentially consumer-oriented. The basic principle of the consumer-oriented communication technique is to

457

understand what consumers know, believe, value, and do relating to food, diet, and nutrition.[3] This chapter discusses the principles of nutrition education and how community nutritionists can design and implement the nutrition education aspect of an intervention.

# ▶ Educational Principles

Different types of educational principles can be utilized to guide the selection of nutrition and health information for individuals, families, and the public. The most useful categories of educational principles include those associated with the theory of learning, the nature of learning, and the events of instruction.[4]

## The Theory of Learning

The theory of learning explains the processing, storage, and retrieval of knowledge in the mind in which informational processing is based.[5] **Learning** is defined as the process leading to relatively permanent behavioral change or potential behavioral change.[6] For example, as clients learn about nutrition, they can alter their eating habits and subsequently change their nutrition or dietary behavior. It is also important to know that behavior is influenced by the clients' environment, how they learn new behaviors, and what motivates them to change or remain the same.

## The Nature of Learning

One way to consider the nature of learning is by examining the cognitive, affective, and psychomotor domains of learning. Each domain has explicit behavioral components that form a hierarchy of steps or levels that build on the previous one.[4,7] Understanding these three learning domains is essential in providing effective nutrition education.

**Cognitive domain**: This involves knowledge and the development of intellectual skills, including the recall or recognition of specific facts, procedural patterns, and concepts that serve in the development of intellectual abilities and skills.[8,9] It also consists of comprehension, understanding, and application and is divided into a hierarchical classification of behaviors. The clients learn each level of cognition in order of difficulty.[7] For nutrition education to be effective, community nutritionists must first assess the cognitive abilities of their clients so expectations and plans are directed toward the correct level. Teaching above or below the participants' or individuals' level of understanding may lead to frustration and discouragement.[4]

**Affective domain**: This includes the way individuals deal with things emotionally, including feelings, values, appreciation, enthusiasm, motivation, and attitude. It also consists of changes in attitude and the development of values.[4,10] In affective learning, nutritionists consider and try to influence what individuals, families, and communities think, value, and feel about nutrition and health. It is important that dietitians listen carefully to detect clues to feelings that may influence learning because their values and attitudes may be different from those of their clients. As with cognitive learning, affective learning consists of a series of steps.[7] A comparison of the affective and cognitive domains is presented in **TABLE 16-1**. The domains help the nutritionist determine what he or she should evaluate/identify and how to react/adapt based on client status. It is hard to change well-established characteristics such as values, attitudes, beliefs, and interests. People need support and encouragement from health professionals and those around them to reinforce new behaviors to make changes.

**Psychomotor domain**: This includes the performance of skills that require some level of neuromuscular coordination and use of motor skills. Clients can be taught a variety of psychomotor skills, including preparing foods, measuring blood pressure and blood glucose levels, bathing infants, breastfeeding, and so on.[4] The levels of psychomotor learning, from the simplest to the most intricate level of observable movements, are outlined in **BOX 16-1**. Three conditions must be achieved before psychomotor learning occurs[4,7,10]:

---

**BOX 16-1** Levels of Psychomotor Learning

- *Imitation:* The clients were able to peel a carrot after observing a demonstration by a community nutritionist.
- *Manipulation:* Diabetic clients followed instructions and practiced how to measure blood glucose levels.
- *Precision:* Diabetic clients measured blood glucose levels using a hand-size meter.
- *Articulation:* The clients planned and prepared a well-balanced diabetic meal.
- *Naturalization:* Diabetic clients is capable of measuring their blood glucose levels plan their meals and eat three nutritious meals and snacks each day.

**TABLE 16-1** Steps in the Cognitive Domain Compared with the Affective Domain

| Step | Cognitive Domain | Affective Domain |
| --- | --- | --- |
| Knowledge | A Women, Infants and Children Program (WIC) client remembered how to wash hands before preparing foods; for example, knows the food safety rules. | Clients appreciated knowing the food safety rules |
| Comprehension | Older adults participating in a community health workshop understood the importance of consuming foods that are high in calcium; for example, stated that milk is a good source of calcium. | The participants were motivated to learn about sources of calcium. |
| Application | The clients purchased low-fat milk after learning about the link between saturated fat intake and heart disease. | Clients informed their family members the value of low fat diet. |
| Analysis | The clients remembered the different type of fat; for example, compares the fat content of different types of milk. | Clients related the consumption of low fat diet to reducing heart disease. |
| Synthesis | The clients plans a low-fat and high-calcium diet. | Clients collected and organized low fat and high calcium recipes. |
| Evaluation | The clients evaluates/analyzes the fat and calcium content of a meal | The clients changed their behaviors and are consistent in consuming low fat and high calcium diets. |

Modified from: Stanhope M, Lancaster J. *Community and Public Health Nursing.* 5th ed. New York, NY: Mosby; 2000; and Dembo MH. *Applying Educational Psychology.* 5th ed. Published by Allyn and Bacon, Boston, MA. Copyright © 1994 by Pearson Education.

- The participants must have the needed ability. For example, the nutritionist may find out that a client participating in the Special Supplemental Nutrition Program for Women, Infants, and Children (WIC) may be capable of following instructions containing one or two steps on how to feed her newborn infant. Therefore, the nutritionist needs to adapt the education plan to fit the client's abilities.
- The client must have a sensory image of how to carry out the skill. For instance, when educating a group of obese young adults about the skills for managing their weight, the nutritionist may ask them to picture themselves losing weight.
- The client must have opportunities to practice these new skills. It is important to provide practice sessions during the program because many clients may not have the facilities, motivation, or time to practice what they have learned. For example, a new mother needs to practice breastfeeding until she has learned how to feed her baby.

For a community nutritionist to facilitate skill learning, he or she needs to demonstrate the skills to clients, either in person, electronically, or by using visual aids such as posters, pictures, or food models.[4,11] After the demonstration, the nutritionist needs to allow the clients to practice and correct any errors in carrying out the skill.

The following six principles can help the nutritionist carry out effective nutrition education programs[4,12]:

- *Message:* Send a clear message to the learner. Assess the learner's readiness at various stages of the learning process and be cognizant of factors that may affect the learning process (e.g., emotional, physical, or environmental stressors).
- *Format:* Select the most appropriate learning format (e.g., lecture, small group, storytelling methods).
- *Environment:* Create the best possible learning environment (room, furniture, visual aids, flyers, and other materials).
- *Experience:* Organize positive and meaningful learning experiences (create a pleasant atmosphere, present materials in a well-organized and logical manner).
- *Participation:* Engage the learner in participatory learning (use role-play, storytelling, hands-on training, case studies, and critical thinking activities).
- *Evaluation:* Evaluate and give objective feedback to the learner (use quizzes, demonstrations of skills gained). The nutritionist can use the feedback from the learners to improve the education program.

## Events of Instruction

To provide effective nutrition education, nutritionists need to utilize the nine basic steps of instruction. These nine steps of instruction that follow can help clients gain more information from the nutritionist[4,13]:

*Gain attention:* How can the nutritionist gain the attention of the client? One method is to convince the clients that the information is important and beneficial to them.

*Inform the learners/clients of the objectives of instruction:* What are the goals and objectives of the education program? It is important to outline the major goals and objectives of the instruction. Stating the objectives of the program will develop the clients' expectations of what they need to learn.

*Stimulate recall of prior learning:* What is the clients' previous knowledge of the topic? The nutritionist needs to help the client remember previous knowledge related to the topic of interest. This will help the client link the new knowledge with prior knowledge. For example, find out how much the clients know about the topic by asking them questions related to the topic.

*Present the material:* How should the nutritionist present the information? It is important to present the essential elements of the topic first in a clear, organized way that considers the clients' strengths, needs, and limitations.

*Provide learning guidance:* How can the nutritionist help clients learn? Provide clear direction to clients so they can convert general information that has been presented into meaningful information they can remember. The nutritionist can use demonstration and visual aids to help clients learn.

*Elicit performance:* How can the nutritionist elicit performance from clients? Encourage clients to demonstrate what they have learned.

*Provide feedback:* Is feedback necessary? Providing feedback to clients will help them improve their knowledge and skills. The feedback will help them modify their thinking patterns and behaviors.

*Assess performance:* Why assess the clients' performance? Evaluate clients to determine if they acquired new knowledge and skills. For example, the nutritionist can administer a pretest and posttest to assess how much information the clients were able to learn.

*Enhance retention and transfer of knowledge:* How can the nutritionist increase retention and transfer of the new knowledge? Once the new skill has been acquired, the nutritionist can help the clients apply the information to new situations (using case studies and critical thinking activities).

Nutritionists may help clients maximize their learning experiences by using these nine steps. Omitting any of the steps may impede the learning process.

## ▶ Applying Educational Principles to Program Design and Interventions

Nutrition education has many definitions. For the purpose of this discussion, nutrition education is a learning experience designed to increase the acceptance of eating and other nutrition-related behaviors contributing to health and well-being.[14] This definition and others suggest that behavioral change is the ultimate criterion for effective nutrition education. The term **behavior** does not mean measuring nutrient intake by dietary recalls, records, or food frequency questionnaires. It means the effects of nutrition education (such as the intake of specific foods) or actual behaviors (such as eating five fruits and vegetables per day, having fruits available and visible at home, reducing salting of foods, taking the skin off of chicken, having one's bone density or serum cholesterol checked, quitting smoking, exercising five times a week, limiting alcohol intake, or reading a food label).[14-16]

Research studies show that nutrition education works.[15,17,18] It is a significant factor in improving dietary practices when behavioral change is set as the goal and the educational strategies used are designed with that intention.[18] It is also important to note that interventions often do not achieve across-the-board success. Generally, nutrition education works on one criterion but not necessarily on another, with one gender but not with the other, or with one ethnic group but not another. Everyone has a different mixture of backgrounds, cultures, health risks, health beliefs, motivators, learning styles, environment, goals, and expectations.[19] Research studies show that the more effective education programs are behaviorally focused and are based on appropriate theories and prior research.[15,20] Behaviorally focused nutrition education encourages the adoption of food and nutrition-related behaviors that are conducive to health and well-being. The behaviors addressed are identified based on the needs, perceptions, motivations, and desires of the target audience as well as from research-based nutrition and health goals.[21]

Studies also show that effective nutrition programs use a combination of modern models of individual, social, and environmental change.[14,22,23] Additionally, effective programs integrate good instructional design and learning principles and use the mass media (television, radio, newspapers, the Internet, etc.) to facilitate a high degree of individualization.[19] Educational research intervention studies show that the degree of the intervention's effect on knowledge and behavior could be predicted based on a quality rating of the intervention's application of the six principles of education[18]:

- *Consonance:* The degree of fit between a program and its objectives. For example, an intervention to improve proper breast pump usage; teaching the benefits of using breast pumps without showing how to use them would be insufficient.
- *Relevance:* The degree to which an intervention is geared toward individuals, including the appropriate reading level and visual acuity. For example, design programs tailored to the individual's knowledge, beliefs, circumstances, cultural background, and prior experiences as determined by pretests.
- *Individualization:* Allows individuals to have personal questions answered or instructions paced according to their individual learning progress. The education should be tailored to individual needs.
- *Feedback:* Determine how much progress the clients have made, if any.
- *Reinforcement:* Reward the desired behavior. The use of praise and congratulations are very effective in rewarding changed behavior.
- *Facilitation:* Take actions to measure accomplishments or eliminate obstacles. For example, a blood glucose monitoring hand-size meter that facilitates clients' ability to adhere to a prescribed diet.[19,18,24]

Communication models and expectancy-value theories, such as the Health Belief Model (HBM) or Theory of Reasoned Action (discussed in Chapter 13), have been used to increase awareness and motivation, whether in direct interpersonal interventions or indirect interventions through media.[14] Lately, the most commonly used planning and implementation tool is social marketing.[4] In social marketing, commercial marketing techniques and principles are used to plan, implement, and evaluate programs designed to change health or social behaviors. The process, also termed consumer-based health communications, transforms scientific recommendations into message strategies that are relevant to the consumer.[25]

## Identify Educational Needs

Community nutritionists learn about the needs of their clients by performing a systematic and thorough client needs assessment. Needs assessments should be part of the education plan because they help the nutritionist develop a level of awareness and anticipate how the target audience will receive the program activities. In addition, the nutritionist needs to create environmental realms that can create a positive and supportive atmosphere and maximize the learning process. **BOX 16-2** provides the environmental realms that can be considered. The steps for needs assessments are listed in **BOX 16-3** and Chapter 2. Once the needs have

---

**BOX 16-2** Environmental Realms

**Physical Realm**

This realm includes setting up the program and positioning the presenter and the clients in a physical relationship to one another. It also includes lighting and temperature of the room, volume of amplification equipment, furniture, and bathroom facilities. The more subtle effects of environment are those that create a stimulating setting, allow for few external distractions, and assist the learner in concentration and attention.

**Interpersonal Realm**

This realm consists of human relationships and should be therapeutic, supportive, and conducive to producing quality educational interactions. The interpersonal dynamic should be one in which learners experience a clear sense that the educator cares about their progress and needs. Learners also can contribute to the interpersonal environment by showing interest in the subject and remaining responsible for both peer and group interactions.

**Organizational Realm**

This realm entails the administrative aspects of the educational program. Beginning with scheduling, announcements, and other preparations, this is the realm that makes the components of the program merge into an effective learning session. Arrangements for parking, delivery of audio-visual materials, ensuring readability of printed or projected materials, and responsiveness to ongoing learner needs and requests are a few examples of the organizational aspects of environment.

Reproduced from Stanhope M, Lancaster J. Community and Public Health Nursing. 5th ed. New York: Mosby, 2000. Reprinted with permission from Elsevier.

---

been identified, they should then be prioritized to address the most critical educational needs first.[26]

For a nutrition education program to be effective, the nutritionist must establish a comprehensive time table.[12] This can be accomplished by creating a task development time line like the one presented in **TABLE 16-2**. The task development time line identifies the tasks needed to complete the project and the month or period in which those tasks will be accomplished.[12] This time line may be modified according to the activities of other programs.

## ▶ Education Across the Life Span

Nutrition education that has personal meaning for a particular population group is essential. Educational strategies with individuals and groups are more likely to be effective if they address people's specific nutrition

<table>
<tr><td colspan="2">**BOX 16-3** Steps of a Needs Assessment</td></tr>
</table>

1. Identify what the clients want to know.
2. Establish how the clients want to learn, what they think, and what they feel.
3. Identify what will improve the clients' ability and motivation to learn.
4. Collect data from the family, community, and other sources to assess learning needs, willingness to learn, and situational and psychosocial factors that would influence learning. Do precession surveys.
5. Provide a data-based context for the program.
6. Analyze assessment data to identify cognitive, affective, and psychomotor learning needs. Encourage clients' participation in the process. Provide on-the-spot assessments.
7. Help the clients prioritize learning needs.

Reused courtesy of Oncology Nursing Society from "Patient Education: Needs Assessment and Resource Identification" by D.L. Volker, 1991, Oncology Nursing Forum, 18(1), p. 119. Copyright © 1991 by ONS. All rights reserved.

concerns. It is also important to examine the different intervention strategies that may be effective in providing nutrition education throughout the life span.

## Adult Learners

**Adult learning** is defined as adults gaining knowledge and expertise.[4] Many older adults are interested in measures they perceive will help them remain healthy or that will manage chronic conditions they may be experiencing. This interest motivates them to implement more health-promoting behaviors.[27] Many older people are enthusiastic readers and are familiar with the current nutrition issues in the media. Health-conscious older persons accept nutrition education offered through the radio, television, local newspapers, magazines, journals, the Internet, or the American Dietetic Association and Cooperative Extension Services hotlines that they can call for answers to nutrition questions. In addition, adult education programs such as peer or shared learning groups and Cooperative Extension Programs provide nutrition education to older adults.[28]

**TABLE 16-2** A Task Development Timeline for a Comprehensive Health Promotion Program

| Month | Task | Month | Task |
|---|---|---|---|
| **January** | ▪ Determine financial commitment<br>▪ Interview/survey client groups<br>▪ Conduct needs assessment<br>▪ Determine target audience<br>▪ Determine program identifier<br>▪ Form employee committee | **September** | ▪ Develop program marketing<br> Comprehensive program<br> Individual components<br>▪ Implement program<br> Program I<br> Program II<br> Program III |
| **February** | ▪ Form employee committee<br>▪ Develop mission statement<br>▪ Develop goals and objectives<br>▪ Determine programs<br>▪ Determine format | **October** | ▪ Develop program marketing<br> Comprehensive program<br> Individual components<br>▪ Implement program<br> Program I<br> Program II<br> Program III |
| **March** | ▪ Determine staff needs<br>▪ Determine equipment needs<br>▪ Train staff<br>▪ Determine partnerships<br>▪ Plan program evaluation | **November** | ▪ Develop program marketing<br> Comprehensive program<br> Individual components<br>▪ Implement program<br> Program I<br> Program II<br> Program III<br>▪ Evaluate program<br> Program I<br> Program II<br> Program III |

| April | ■ Train staff<br>■ Determine nutrition messages<br>■ Determine partnerships | December | ■ Develop program marketing<br>Comprehensive program<br>Individual components<br>■ Plan program evaluation<br>■ Evaluate program<br>Program I<br>Program II<br>Program III |
|---|---|---|---|
| May | ■ Determine nutrition messages<br>■ Develop lesson plan<br>Program I<br>Program II<br>Program III | | |
| June | ■ Develop lesson plan<br>Program I<br>Program II<br>Program III | | |
| July | ■ Develop lesson plan<br>Program I<br>Program II<br>Program III | | |
| August | ■ Develop program marketing<br>Comprehensive program<br>Individual components | | |

Data from: Anspaugh DJ, Dignan MB, Anspaugh SL. *Developing Health Promotion Programs.* Boston, MA: McGraw-Hill; 2000.

Educational interventions exist in which a major goal is improving the knowledge of older adults. The nutrition intervention strategies that have been effective in increasing nutrition knowledge for improved nutritional adequacy in this population include[14,29-31]:

■ Personalized approaches such as self-assessment of nutritional status or behaviors and comparison of these with recommendations. Cholesterol and bone density screenings and dietary intake assessments are effective starting points for nutrition education.
■ Behavioral approaches include individual self-assessments followed by behavioral self-management techniques, such as goal setting, problem solving, and social support.
■ Attention to motivators and reinforcements include an interest in maintaining health, providing opportunities for social interaction and social support, enhancing self-efficacy, and recognizing the need for good taste and ease of food preparation.

The following are some tips to consider when providing nutrition education to older adults[32,33]:

■ Use previous experiences as learning resources. Collaborate with the adult learner by sharing life experiences and knowledge. Use direct experience such as family health history and past experiences. It also is important to note that adults tend to learn in stages. See **FIGURE 16-1** for the adult learning stages.
■ Modify the presentation of learning resources to the learner's level of experience. Consider the impact of chronic conditions/disease and emotional and cultural factors on the client's ability to communicate or learn the materials.

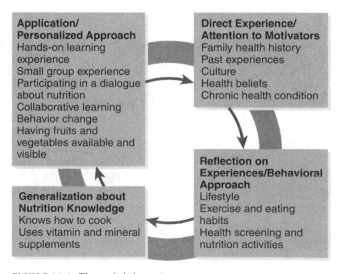

**FIGURE 16-1** The adult learning stages.

- Provide feedback about the client's achievement of objectives at periodic intervals. This will help maintain the client's attention span.
- Guide the adult learner to reflect on the learning experiences that lead to lifestyle change, such as an increase in physical activities and improved eating habits.
- Connect the adult learner's previous health experiences (such as hypertension, diabetes, or heart disease) to the nutrition education.
- Arrange for a comfortable physical environment conducive to interaction with and among adult learners. Provide hands-on learning experiences using small groups and collaborative learning.

## Child Learners

Nutrition education for young children is an area of high priority because of the severe consequences hunger and malnutrition can have on this group. Anemia, obesity, dental caries, and growth retardation are nutritional concerns for preschool-age children.[14,34,35] Children are not born with the natural ability to choose nutritious foods, but they are born with a preference for sweet tastes.[36] They also show negative reactions to bitter and sour tastes and a neutral response to salty tastes. It has also been found that preference for a food is a major determinant of food intake in young children.[37] Involving children in meal planning and preparation will increase their food acceptance and intake. Successful nutrition education programs for children have used the following intervention strategies[14,38-41]:

- Involving parents and families as the main recipients of the program or in combination with a program offered to preschool and school-age children. Children have shorter attention spans than adults. They tend to learn more through adult active participation.

- Using a behaviorally focused approach that targets children's behaviors using a social modeling of peer and adult role models eating nutritious meals and snacks. Adults should offer food to children in a positive social environment and not as rewards.
- Using developmentally appropriate learning experiences and materials for children ages 4 to 7 so they understand concepts such as having energy and a strong heart, eating low-fat foods, and keeping germs out of the body.
- Presenting food-based activities such as tasting parties, food preparation, vegetable and fruit gardens, engaging the five senses with food, eating nutritious meals and snacks, and interactive activities (games, songs, role-playing, stories, puppets, and puzzles).
- Incorporating a self-evaluation or self-assessment and feedback component is effective in interventions for older children with personalized computer-assisted feedback.
- Using abstract thinking as a learning tool for adolescents. Like adults, adolescents are able to reason deductively. Using peer groups is a significant method of enhancing adolescents' learning.

The following are additional tips to consider when providing nutrition education to children[40,41]:

- Create a positive attitude toward food.
- Build children's self-esteem by serving cultural and ethnic foods.
- Introduce a variety of unfamiliar nutritious foods.
- Have children participate in mealtime activities, such as setting the table, preparing food, serving food, and cleaning up.

**TABLE 16-3** presents motivating factors for nutrition learning and how adults and children learn.

| **TABLE 16-3** Motivating Factors and How Adults and Children Learn | | | |
|---|---|---|---|
| **How Adults Learn** | **Adult Motivators** | **How Children Learn** | **Child Motivators** |
| Reading | Health condition | Role models | Parents |
| Media (television, radio, magazines, and the Internet) | Health consciousness | Role play/observation | Teachers |
| | Family history | Stories and songs/music | Peers |
| Social interaction | Health beliefs | Demonstration | Media (television and magazines) |
| Stories | Friends | Hands-on experience | |
| Hands-on experience | Relatives/family | Media (videotape, television, and the Internet) | Food tasting |
| Demonstration and dialogue | | | Curiosity |
| Observation and reflection | | | |
| Small group discussions | | Peers | |
| Focus groups and role-play | | Games and fieldtrips | |

## Pregnant and Lactating Women

The goal of nutrition education for pregnant women is relatively clear: appropriate maternal weight gain, nutritional adequacy of the maternal diet, and positive infant outcomes, such as satisfactory birth weight. The goals are similar for lactating women (see Chapter 8 for more information on pregnant and lactating women.) The methods and timing of interventions are very important. The following are some effective intervention strategies[14,42,43]:

- Nutrition counseling and classes that focus on pregnant women's specific behaviors using individualized assessment. The follow-up sessions should reinforce and maintain behavior.
- Prenatal exposure to information about the benefits of breastfeeding with respect to health benefits using group classes and peer breastfeeding classes. Peer education involves inspiring a group of pregnant and lactating women to express health and nutritional messages to each other. The group becomes active participants in the educational process instead of passive recipients.
- Incentives for participation are very successful for the Special Supplemental Nutrition Program for Women, Infants, and Children (WIC) population. For example, grocery store discount coupons can motivate participation.

Additional tips for providing an effective nutrition intervention include the following[4,14,40]:

- Using pamphlets to address the benefits of breastfeeding for mothers and infants
- Asking open-ended questions
- Facilitating cooperative learning skills and group processes
- Being friendly
- Sending clear messages to clients
- Engaging the learner in participatory learning
- Organizing positive and meaningful learning experiences

## ▶ Education and Culture

How a person interprets messages is based on his or her cultural framework; interpretation of visual elements varies considerably by ethnic group. What may be attractive, appealing, or acceptable to one ethnic group or subgroup may not be so to others.[14] When designing nutrition education materials, it is important to use cultural images that people of the target ethnic group view as positive. It is also important to use those images or symbols within a framework that the target audience feels is appropriate. For example, one educational program created an initial version of a booklet for American Indians on reducing dietary fat that portrayed an eagle on the cover. Although the contents of the booklet were understood and accepted by the target audience, the use of the eagle, a sacred and positive image for this group, was considered inappropriate for the cover of a nutrition education booklet. The cover was redesigned and retested.[14]

Equally important is geography, because it influences dietary choices. With regard to dietary practices, the accessibility, affordability, and acceptability of available foods play a more important role than ethnicity in the use of those foods.[44] For example, a sample poster developed for a Nigerian group with pictures of romaine lettuce, bananas, Brussels sprouts, beets, bean sprouts, seaweed, and peas was used in an area where some of these foods, such as Brussels sprouts, bean sprouts, and seaweed, were not readily available; the group therefore showed poor recognition and acceptance of these items. But these foods were acceptable to another group that had access to them. See Chapter 5 for more information on the influence of culture on the acceptability of foods. The following are additional strategies for nutrition education interventions that may be used for a multicultural group[14,45,46]:

- Review revised materials for illustration and content issues.
- Modify materials based on input from working groups.
- Be knowledgeable about appropriate reading levels (literacy).
- Have an understanding of the cultural appropriateness of vocabulary.
- Limit the number of messages in each educational piece.
- Put people into partnerships—pair up, discuss, and share ideas to engage the participants.
- Use the HBM when organizing messages.
- Make note of visual appropriateness (with particular attention to cultural preferences and taboos).
- Incorporate an interactive style.
- Use quality visuals.
- Use bilingual interpreters.

## ▶ Developing a Nutrition Education Plan

To plan means to develop a method for achieving a particular outcome. People learn or receive new information in different ways; therefore, having a basic understanding of differences in learning styles and planning programs that address these differences can contribute to successful outcomes or behavior change.[47] Dialogue is one of the educational methods or styles that Vella[48] has used in the community under diverse circumstances. This approach is based on the principle that adults have had sufficient life experiences to maintain a dialogue with any teacher about various subjects and can relate the topics to life experiences. The core concept of the dialogue approach is helping teachers become co-learners and learners become co-teachers and providing opportunities for participants to apply what they have learned. This approach encourages learners to use interaction to achieve the program objectives.

Joye Norris,[49] the author of *From Telling to Teaching*, introduced the concept of learning through dialogue to paraprofessional educators and learners in the Expanded Food and Nutrition Education Program (EFNEP) in Massachusetts. EFNEP audiences are typically diverse, including pregnant women, families with children, youth, the homeless, people in shelters and institutions, and people from different cultures.

For the Massachusetts EFNEP program, Norris[49] worked with paraprofessionals and learners to determine the lesson topics after several meetings and discussions. Their first step after determining the topics was to incorporate a unique element of the curriculum into the topics' names to reinforce each lesson; for example, "Moving to the Mambo" for the movement lesson (physical activity or exercise), "Foods a Go-Go" for eating on the run, "Whole Grain Twist," "5-A-Day Salsa," "Low-Fat Limbo," "Kitchen Calypso," and "Food Safety 4-Step." The titles gave the lessons energy and a sense of the cultural diversity that characterized the audience. In addition, music that was consistent with the title of each lesson was used to reinforce the elements in the curriculum. The next step was to develop the nutrition education materials; for instance, seven festive color logos, one for each lesson; posters; sorting cards; food safety bingo; food labels; stickers; three-dimensional models; and other educational materials that reinforced the learning objectives were developed. The lessons began with participants sharing their activities in pairs. The participants were given charts (a small one for personal use and a large one for the group) on which they could monitor their progress.

The following are the five learning principles that Norris[49] used to conduct successful nutrition education programs:

- *Respect*: Respect the learners as decision makers of their own learning. It is also important to respect their characteristics (who they are, where they have been, and what they know).
- *Inclusion*: The learner must be actively involved in the organization and implementation of the activities. Learners are highly motivated and involved when they are working in small groups or teams. Therefore, it is important to make them feel a part of the group and equal to others in the group.

- *Engagement*: Learners must do more than just listen. They must be involved in what they are learning.
- *Relevancy*: Determine why the information is important to the learner and how it has personal meaning for them.
- *Safety*: Create an environment that makes the learner feel free to participate in the activities without fear.

Another way a nutritionist can provide an effective nutrition education program to the community is to use an appropriate theoretical model. For example, when providing educational programs to communities, the nutritionist may decide to use the PRECEDE-PROCEED model to organize the teaching program. However, when delivering education to individuals or families, the nutritionist may choose to use the HBM to identify the specific beliefs, behaviors, or cultural factors that need to be modified to change behaviors.[4] See Chapter 13 for detailed information on these models and how they can be used to provide a nutrition education program.

The focus of community nutrition education should be on health promotion for population aggregates. Such education may happen at the local, state, national, or international level. People of all ages and socioeconomic and sociocultural backgrounds should be included. Education can occur in schools, clinics, prisons, worksites, shelters, and community forums. Education programs may be directed toward a specific population, such as diabetic pregnant women, or toward a specific community, such as a town in Mexico with a high incidence of anemia where people want to learn about reducing iron-deficiency anemia. Either way, the education plan must address the needs of the specific population. **TABLE 16-4** presents the skills and strategies community nutritionists can utilize to develop successful nutrition education for communities and individuals.

Examples of behaviors to be addressed by an education program include those related to food, such as adding less salt to food, eating lower fat foods, or adding two vegetables and two glasses of milk a day; those related to other nutritional concerns, such as breastfeeding; or those related to the environment that have an impact on dietary practices, such as using impure water or buying minimally processed foods.[14,50] Studies show that variations or combinations of several theories, such as the Social Learning Theory and social marketing, have been effective in producing behavioral change.[51,52] **BOX 16-4** presents effective research-based educational strategies.[52,52-55] However, a program can still be successful if cognitive and affective domains are addressed. A short-term nutrition program cannot expect behavior change outcomes but may create awareness of the nutrition issue.

**TABLE 16-4** Skills Recommended for Successful Nutrition Education in Communities and Individuals

| | |
|---|---|
| **Community Nutritionist/ Manager Skills** | Community and public health nutritionists need to possess certain skills to be successful in educating communities and individuals about nutrition issues. The skills include, but are not limited to, the ability to create and conduct needs assessment; develop the mission statement, objective, and goal; and have the skills to hire, train, evaluate, and supervise staff. They need to have the ability to purchase equipment; understand the departmental culture, legal and ethical regulations for health, nutrition, and fitness/wellness programs; and communicate effectively with higher authorities. |
| **Marketing/ Promotional Skills** | Community and public health nutritionists need the ability to design and plan nutrition programs. Be able to develop marketing strategies, choose the promotional materials (CDs, DVDs, handouts, instructional materials, etc.), and be able to carry out the educational programs. |
| **Educator/ Motivator Skills** | Community and public health nutritionists need the ability to develop educational materials, create assessment tools and lesson plans, and form wellness committees. They need the skills to inspire clients, encourage behavioral change, provide support to the clients, and know how adults learn. |
| **Evaluator Skills** | Community and public health nutritionists need the skills to design programs and conduct staff evaluation tools. They need the ability to collect, analyze, and interpret data to higher authorities. They also need to be able to serve as a role model to the staff and clients. |
| **Counselor Skills** | Community and public health nutritionists need the ability to consult and counsel clients, interpret assessment results, and effect behavioral change. |

Data from: Anspaugh DJ, Dignan MB, Anspaugh SL. Developing Health Promotion Programs (page 10). McGraw Hill Higher Education, 2000.

**BOX 16-4** Effective Theoretical Research-Based Educational Strategy

**Program Title:** Dietary Fat and Heart Disease Intervention Strategy[29]
**Objective:** To recognize the fat content of commonly consumed food items
**Theory Used:** Health Belief Model

### Activities

- Display food models (interactive) such as food packages, fat-filled test tubes, syringes filled with shortening, whole and nonfat milk, French fries, baked potatoes, croissants, and potato chips.
- Include in the food models foods that are popular with the target audience.
- Create a table tent for each food item in the display by printing the food's name, serving size, and fat content in teaspoons (5 grams fat = 1 tsp) on a 3- × 5-inch index card folded in half width-wise.
- To make fat-filled plastic test tubes, fill 12 or more test tubes with different amounts of fat in each (i.e., from ¼ to 3 tsp in ¼-tsp increments).
- Fill plastic test tubes by placing the tubes upright in a test tube rack and pouring melted shortening into the tubes through a funnel.
- Set up the display by grouping similar food types together (e.g., place fast foods in one area, dairy products in another area, etc.). Beside each item, place its table tent and a test tube filled with the amount of fat found in one serving. Combine test tubes until the correct amount of fat is displayed.
- Give each visitor a paper plate and a fat-filled syringe. Ask the participant to plan a meal or snack using the foods displayed. Then have the participant squeeze the amount of fat in the meal or snack from the syringe onto the plate. (The syringes can be refilled with shortening and used again. Keep paper towels and spatulas (for mixing, spreading, or lifting) available.

**Program Title:** Using Food Calendars to Self-Monitor: Got 5? Nutrition for Kids Program (5 A Day Intervention)[27]
**Objective:** To help establish enhanced lifestyle practices
**Theory Use:** Transtheoretical Model/Stages of Change Model

*(continues)*

**BOX 16-4** Effective Theoretical Research-Based Educational Strategy *(continued)*

## Activities

- Provide each child with a guide containing colored pictures and the names of the top 20 fruits and a similar guide for the top 20 vegetables.
- Provide a total of four 2-week calendars. Use colored fruit and/or vegetable calendars.
- Ask students to write down the names of all the fruits and/or vegetables they consumed for four consecutive 2-week color fruit and/or vegetable calendars.
- Review serving sizes during the first lesson.
- Ask students to complete a tally sheet (provided) for each calendar to assist them in self-evaluation.
- Ask parents to sign each calendar once completed.
- Provide incentives for completing each calendar, such as a jump rope for the first calendar, a Beanie baby for the second, a hula-hoop for the third, and a $5 book fair gift certificate for the fourth.

**Program Title:** Feed Your Mind: An Interactive Nutrition Evaluation for Teenagers (*Jeopardy*-Like Interactive Activity)[28]
**Objectives:** To detect knowledge and behavior changes that occurred after the nutrition intervention
**Theory:** Social Learning Theory and Knowledge-Attitude Behavior Model

## Activities

- Provide six examples of nutrition topics, such as calcium; food label reading; fat, weight, and exercise; fast foods; and My Plate.
- Use colorful, eye-catching graphics displayed on exhibit boards at the front of a classroom.
- Set game card values at 20, 40, 60, 80, and 100.
- Group game cards into categories to reflect the objectives (Funny Bones, Label Lingo, Skinny on Fat, Movin' and Munchin', Think Fast, and Grab Bag).
- List one nutrition question for 27 of the 30 game cards. List "Go To" on the remaining game cards, which will direct them to the nutrition questionnaire with "yes/no," multiple choice questions.
- Divide participants into teams of four to six players and distribute questionnaires.
- Read aloud 15 questions in section 1 while participants individually mark their responses on the questionnaire (provided).
- Teams will take turns answering game questions after section 1.
- When a "Go To" card is selected, the educator will read the question aloud and direct participants to answer questions individually.
- The game ends when all game card questions are answered.
- The team with the most points wins a nonperishable food item such as juice box.

Data from: Byrd-Bredbenner CF, M. Dietary fat and heart disease intervention strategies. J. of Nutrition Education. 2000; 32 (1):60A; Kuczmarski MF, Aljadix L. Using food Calendars to Self-Monitor: Got 5? Nutrition for kids program. J of Nutrition Education. 2003; 35:269-270; Struempler BJ, Cobrin S. Feed your mind: An interactive nutrition evaluation for teenagers. J of Nutrition Education. 2002; 34(1):59.

## ▶ Developing a Lesson Plan

An effective nutrition education program requires thorough planning. The nutrition education **lesson plan** needs to describe the desires of the target population. It is the blueprint for organizing a class.[56] A well-designed lesson plan ensures a clear focus and articulates specific learning outcomes. The nutrition messages of a particular educational program may be designed to change the learners' behavior. For example, the nutritionist plans to use the MyPlate chart to demonstrate how to achieve the Fruits and Veggies—More Matters message to "Eat Five to Stay Alive." The chart will portray different types of fruits and vegetables. Fruits and Veggies—More Matters is a national media program designed to encourage the U.S. population to eat five or more servings of fruits and vegetables daily. The program is a joint venture of the National Cancer Institute (NCI) and the Produce for Better Health Foundation.[57]

Lesson plans encourage advanced planning and organization. They help the educator prepare and have instructional materials ready. They also help the nutrition educator think carefully about matching methods and outcomes and think about how to present new information in interesting ways while meeting the needs of different learning styles. See Table 16-5 (later) for methods that can be used to plan a successful nutrition education program.

The written format of the planned activities should be as individualized as the target audience, but all activity plans should include these basic features[58]:

- Subject/lesson title or concept to be presented
- Specific objectives
- Format
- Materials list

- Procedure/step-by-step learning activities
- Target audience
- Duration
- Evaluation and suggestions for improvement

## Components of a Lesson Plan

Each individual lesson should be planned in advance, contain enough information so another person can use it, and follow a consistent format. Activities can then be modified to address the needs of a particular segment of the population. Lesson plans usually include the following[58]:

- *Title of the lesson:* The title captures the audience's attention. It is very important because it can make the difference between attendance and nonattendance of the health promotion program. The title is the main concept/component of the marketing plan and should be 10 words or less; for example, "Building Better Bones."
- *Target audience:* It is important to identify the clientele at the beginning of the lesson plan. The target audience determines the communication formats that will be used and the type of promotional strategy. For example, if the target audience is of low literacy, the nutritionist will use an alternative method (e.g., videotapes, demonstration) to ensure the message is understood.
- *Duration:* Determine the time that will be most acceptable to the target audience to get the greatest number of participants. Determine how long the program will take, including break time. Some nutrition education programs may take from one to three class periods.
- *Program goal:* The lesson plan should contain a general statement(s) about the desired outcome of the health promotion program; for example, plan a nutritious diet that can reduce the risk for cancer. Each goal should be linked to the objective of the program.
- *Objective:* This establishes the content to be addressed in the lesson and identifies the behavior to be practiced that will yield a successful outcome. It indicates observable clients' behavior and serves as the basis for evaluation of the lesson; for example, the clients will be able to increase the number of fruits and vegetables eaten from two a day to five a day.
- *Procedure:* It is important to determine how the program activities will be carried out in the lesson plan. Include how the activities will be introduced and any background information. List each step sequentially. Include a clear outline of the sequence of activities to be used in a class session. Also include the conclusion/closure of the program.
- *Learning experiences or activities:* It is essential to determine the instructional strategies in the lesson plan. Strategies are methods that can help participants personalize information. They encourage interaction among participants and help them assess their personal feelings about the health promotion information. Examples of strategies include discussion groups, overhead transparencies, participant worksheets and the instructor's answer key, puzzles, games, Power-Point slides, video clips and discussion, and small group exercises. These activities can give the clients the content and concepts of the program. Outline the different activities/events and tasks that must be accomplished during the learning experience.
- *Method of evaluation:* This helps the instructor see whether the participants have achieved the objective. List the strategies for evaluating the effectiveness of the educational program, the amount or level of knowledge acquired, the attitude affected, or the behavioral changes made due to the educational program. Determine how the program outcomes will be evaluated, such as using a questionnaire that asks the participants to write down what they liked or disliked about the program and whether it helped them. Another strategy could be to administer a pretest and posttest.
- *Materials needed:* It is important to list all the materials needed for the educational program in the lesson plan. The materials are the tools needed for accomplishing the program's goals and objectives, such as videotapes, foods (e.g., different sizes, colors, and shapes of fruits and vegetables), disposable plates and napkins, an overhead projector, computer, handouts, food models, and so on.

The following section presents a sample lesson plan on bone health.

## Lesson Plan Sample

**Title:** Bone Health

**Target Audience:** Women 55 years and older in the community

**Program Goals:** The participants will learn the content of MyPlate to reduce the risk for osteoporosis.

**Objectives:** The participants will be able to:
- Identify the main food groups and list foods that are high in calcium and fat
- Distinguish between a fruit and a vegetable
- Learn how to select a low-fat, high-calcium diet

**Materials and Equipment:**
- Food models
- Paper plates
- Packages from a variety of healthy and "junk" foods

- MyPlate diagram
- Projector
- Restaurant menu
- Table

**Duration:** One hour (with one 15-minute break)

**Procedure:**
- Display MyPlate chart on the overhead projector.
- Exhibit food groups according to similarity using food models; for example, place the dairy products on one area of the table.
- Introduce the activities enthusiastically and encourage participation at the beginning of the session.
- Summarize the session by either summarizing the discussion points or encouraging the participants to try the new strategies from the educational program.

**Learning Activities:**
- Give each participant a paper plate.
- Allow participants to select a total of five fruits and vegetables for their plate.
- Conduct a discussion about the differences of the foods they have selected.

- Ask the participants to brainstorm all of the foods they can think of that are made with milk.
- Ask the participants to analyze the menu from a popular restaurant and see if the menu contains food from each group.

**Evaluation Method:**
- Ask the participants to list three high-calcium foods.
- Ask the participants to list two low-fat foods.
- Ask the participants to list the MyPlate food groups.

## Specify the Nutrition Messages

In a lesson plan, it is important to identify nutrition issues and what motivates the audience. The message should go beyond demographics such as race/ethnicity, age, gender, education level, and income level.[58] It is important that the nutrition educator specifies the actions or behavioral change(s) he or she wants the target audience to adopt. It also is important to use straightforward language relevant and compelling to the audience; for example, take a brisk 10-minute walk on your lunch break to encourage physical activity. See **TABLE 16-5** for communication guidelines for educational

**TABLE 16-5** Communication Guidelines for Educational Interactions

| Communication Method | Action |
|---|---|
| Be prepared and start with confidence | Be straightforward |
| Use clear, and precise pronunciation | This helps the audience pay attention |
| Requires active pleasant, and intensity of voice. | For example, the nutritionist could say, we will discuss the Dietary Guidelines instead of "Dietary Guidelines will be discussed. |
| Be optimistic | For example, the nutritionist could say, the majority of individuals are able to lose weight with a well-balanced diet and exercise, instead of a few people have not been able to lose weight with a well-balanced diet and exercise. |
| Don't use medical terminology or jargon, or data. | Use examples, case studies |
| Mention credible sources. | For example, Academy of Nutrition and Dietetics journal. Instead of unprofessional web site. |
| Be aware of your audience's knowledge level of nutrition. | Ask the audience probing questions about the topic, encourage interaction |
| Emphasize important point | Determine relevant topic to the audience |
| End with a smile | Control your emotion, allow time for questions. |

Modified from Stanhope M, Lancaster J. Community and Public Health Nursing. 5 ed. New York: Mosby; 2000.

interaction. More information on nutrition messages is provided later in this chapter.

## Choose a Program Identifier

Choosing a **program identifier** that expresses the main idea of the program is important. A program identifier is a logo, slogan, motto, or tagline that communicates the main concept of the education program.[58] Typically, these make claims about providing an important benefit or solution or about being most suitable for the target audience. The idea behind the concept is to create a memorable phrase that sums up the educational program or reinforces the target audience's memory of the issue. These can be used in promotional materials such as brochures, flyers, and posters. It is important to share the initial logo and promotional materials' concepts with members of the target audience or colleagues for their input.

## Develop a Marketing Plan

An effective marketing program is crucial for the nutrition education program to be successful. The main purpose of the marketing plan is to attract the attention of the target audience. Consequently, it is important that the community nutritionist knows the target audience, keeps the message simple and to the point, and avoids clutter. Cluttered media, mainly too many words and pictures, can overpower the program's messages.[12]

## Form Partnerships

When developing the marketing plan, it is beneficial to form partnerships with entities such as local businesses, healthcare organizations, and government agencies. For example, local businesses may donate giveaway materials for prizes (e.g., T-shirts, cookbooks, gym bags, gift certificates, restaurant certificates, movie certificates) that can be used as incentives to stimulate interest in the program.[12] The community nutritionist also can form partnerships with other health promotion organizations, such as the American Heart Association or American Cancer Institute, during their health promotion kick-off events. This is a good way to initiate the program and reduce the program's cost. Events can include ribbon cuttings, local celebrity events, drawings, food tasting, or other activities.

## Establish Educational Goals and Objectives

Once the clients' needs are determined, the goals and objectives to guide the educational program should be established and stated. **Objectives** are written statements of intended outcomes. They are specific, short-term measures that should be accomplished in steps toward achieving the long-term goal. Objectives are stated in terms of expected outcomes—an end result that must be achieved or an expected change in behavior. The expected outcomes need to be defined in measurable terms[4]; for example, participants are expected to identify high-fat foods from a list provided.

## Determine Which Methods to Use

The educational methods chosen for the program need to accomplish the program's goals and objectives. Choose methods that match the clients' strengths and needs. Use the strategies previously listed for adults and children that match the target audience. The lesson plan may require cooking demonstrations, small group sessions, mass media techniques (radio, posters, etc.), case studies, and lectures. You will need to select the appropriate teaching tools, such as audio-visual aids, DVDs, handouts, health assessment equipment, and PowerPoint presentations.[4]

## Implement the Program

After the educational methods have been established, they need to be implemented. Implementation entails the following[4,59]:

- Control the starting and stopping of each method and strategy at the most appropriate time and manner (e.g., arrive early, start with greeting the clients first to capture their attention, use warm-ups or icebreakers to get people involved).
- Coordinate and control the environmental factors, the flow of the presentation, and other contributory facets of the program to set the stage for a positive learning environment (e.g., noise, arrange for a babysitter, set a break time).
- Keep the materials logically related to the overall program goals.
- Listen before starting to teach. Encourage participation and acknowledge different viewpoints.
- Edit information. Provide important information first.

## Evaluate the Educational Process

Evaluating a nutrition education program is as important in the educational process as it is in the nutrition practice, and it must be included in the lesson plan. Educational evaluation includes[4]:

- Educator evaluation
- Process evaluation
- Product evaluation

Educator evaluation allows for modifications in the teaching process and enables the nutritionists to adequately address the learners' needs.[4,60] The evaluation may occur throughout (formative evaluation) or at the end of the program (summative evaluation). Ongoing evaluation allows the teacher to correct misinformation, misinterpretation, or confusion. The educator may receive feedback verbally or nonverbally. Process evaluation examines the components of the education program[59] to determine whether goals and objectives were being addressed throughout the program. The process can be measured qualitatively and quantitatively.[61] For example, a qualitative assessment answers the question, "How well does the learner appear to understand the content?" A quantitative assessment answers the question, "How much of the content does the learner retain?"[61] The product evaluation evaluates the outcome of the educational process.[62]

Different approaches can be used to evaluate nutrition and behavioral changes. These include questionnaires, surveys, skills demonstrations, testing, subjective client feedback, and direct observation of improvements in client mastery of materials.

## Gather, Organize, and Structure Knowledge

The nutrition educator serves as the facilitator of the education process. Therefore, selecting plans appropriate for the target audience that support the stated objectives is very important (see Table 16-5). Despite the educator's level of knowledge or the quality of the interpersonal relationship that the educator has developed with the learner, good organization of the material is important for learning to happen. Materials need to be presented in a logical and integrated manner, from simple introductory concepts to more complex ideas. As part of the lesson plan, the educator needs to locate, evaluate, and validate the sources of the health and nutrition information being communicated to the clients. It is also essential to make the concepts/ideas clear to the participants. The speed of the presentation should match the ability of the learner and leave enough pauses for the learner to absorb the information.[4] The following questions can help the nutrition educator structure the educational concept[58]:

■ *What are the contents/concepts to be addressed in the lesson?* Define the objective of the activities; for example, 5-year-old children can name at least two foods that are good for teeth. Make sure the material is culturally sensitive.

■ *Where is the location of the activity?* Make sure it is accessible to the target audience.

■ *When will the program start and how often will it take place?* Establish the length of the activity.

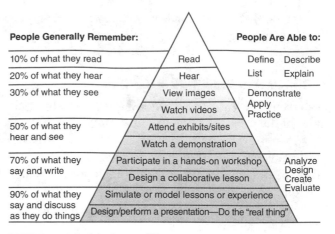

| People Generally Remember: | | People Are Able to: |
|---|---|---|
| 10% of what they read | Read | Define  Describe |
| 20% of what they hear | Hear | List  Explain |
| 30% of what they see | View images | Demonstrate |
| | Watch videos | Apply  Practice |
| 50% of what they hear and see | Attend exhibits/sites | |
| | Watch a demonstration | |
| 70% of what they say and write | Participate in a hands-on workshop | Analyze  Design |
| | Design a collaborative lesson | Create  Evaluate |
| 90% of what they say and discuss as they do things | Simulate or model lessons or experience | |
| | Design/perform a presentation—Do the "real thing" | |

**FIGURE 16-2** Dale's Cone of Experience.

Adapted from: Edgar Dale's Cone of Experience, Audio-Visual Methods in Teaching, 3rd ed. (New York Holt, Rinehart, and Winston, 1969). Reprinted with permission from Raymond S. Pastore Bloomsburg University, Bloomsburg, PA 17815-1301.

■ *Which segment of the population/target audience is participating in the activities?* What is the audience's profile (age, gender, race/ethnicity, socioeconomic status, education, and religion)?

■ *How will the activities be carried out effectively?* For adult learners, case studies, small group work, computer interactive activities, panel presentations, and demonstrations are very effective; for children, games, demonstration, role playing, and fieldtrips are effective methods; and for large-group presentations, lectures, demonstrations, groups, and panel presentations are effective.[63] It is also essential to use visual aids such as flipcharts, transparencies, handouts, or slides.

**FIGURE 16-2.** Dale's Cone of Experience presents some active learning experiences that can be utilized to carry out educational activities.

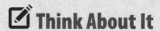

**Think About It**

What factors can promote the progress and success of a nutrition program?

## ▸ Enhancing and Achieving Program Participation

It is reported that effective programs to promote improved dietary practices among low-income families depend on the motivation and performance of the educator. Motivating clients to participate is essential to the progress and success of nutrition and health promotion programs.[64] Hence, the activities of the program require a variety of appealing strategies and an awareness of the practical and psychosocial concerns of potential participants. **Participation**, as it pertains to this discussion, is when clients join others in health promotion activities. One of the strategies for encouraging participation is including health risk assessments, such as screening for blood pressure and other preventive health screenings, as a tool to attract potential participants into health promotion activities. Also, matching clients with partners may increase participation.

For example, Liberman et al[65] investigated potential factors affecting decisions to engage in a cardiac rehabilitation program (CRP). A total of 129 attendees and 61 nonattendees completed the study. Results showed that physician recommendation was the most important factor influencing both women's and men's decisions to participate in CRP, followed by encouragement from family members. For women who attended the CRP, encouragement from their adult children was significantly more influential than it was for men. Attention to health promotion was also a significantly more powerful motivator for women.

In addition, more clients will participate in health-promoting activities or programs if they are accessible, affordable, and convenient. Other practical strategies that community nutritionists may use to encourage clients to join health promotion programs include the following[26,58]:

- Adapting the program literature or educational materials to the demographic characteristics of the target audience
- Considering the educational level of the participants
- Finding convenient class times and locations (e.g., grocery stores, worksites)
- Distributing promotional materials (e.g., newsletters, flyers, radio, e-mail, TV)
- Providing incentives (e.g., T-shirts, magnets, gym bags, headbands, cookbooks, restaurant certificates)

In addition, program planning that addresses identified barriers, including insufficient incentives, inconvenient locations, and time limitations, may facilitate higher participation in worksite wellness opportunities.[66]

## Successful Community Strategies

### Social Marketing Nutrition Education Campaign[67]

The 5 A Day for Better Health program utilizes the media and other channels to encourage individuals to consume five servings of fruits and vegetables every day. A significant amount of information has been disseminated using this program. It is reported that within 1 month, 1,800 media messages were disseminated, all governors signed proclamations of support in 1 year, 225 newspapers carried the stories, and 1 million brochures about the program were distributed. Reports show that the campaign and its principal message had substantial penetration during the 2 years of the campaign; the percentage of Americans who knew that five or more was the number of servings of fruits and vegetables to eat every day for good health increased from a baseline of 8 percent to 29 percent, and the percentage who believed that eating fruits and vegetables would potentially help prevent cancer increased from 45 to 64 percent. However, 13 percent reported that it would be very hard to eat five or more servings of fruits and vegetables each day.

Data from Lefebvre RCD, Johnston L, Loughrey C et al. Use of database marketing and consumer-based health communication in a message design an example from the Office of Cancer Communication's "5 A Day for Better Health Program." In: Maibach EP, RL. eds., Designing health messages. Approaches from communication theory and public health practice. Thousand Oaks, CA: Sage Publications; 1995:217-246.

## ▶ General Ideas for Designing Messages

Health and nutrition messages must be consumer oriented. The community will choose to work with the nutritionist based on the benefits to be gained. Few people will attend a workshop or planning session just out of curiosity.

Many organizations, such as the Academy of Nutrition and Dietetic Association, the U.S. Department of Agriculture, the U.S. Department of Health and Human Services, and others, have combined efforts to develop positive nutrition messages. In 1998 and 1999, the International Food Information Council (IFIC) conducted focus group research with consumers to determine the barriers that consumers experience in adopting healthy diets. IFIC developed tips for communicating nutrition messages that resonate with consumers.[68] These tips are available at http://www.foodinsight.forg/articles/2015-dietary-guidelines-for-americans-resources. Community nutritionists can incorporate these messages into different nutrition and education promotion programs. One of this chapter's Successful Community Strategies showcases a successful social marketing message.

One role of the community nutritionist is to clarify mixed messages that consumers receive from various sources (family, friends, professional colleagues, the media, the Internet, etc.) and tailor the health messages according to the client's specific needs and health situations. One of the positive aspects of being a nutrition and health educator is that the majority of the U.S. population is interested in nutrition and health messages. For example, research shows that four in five persons surveyed agreed that there is a relationship between diet and health,[55,68-70] 57 percent became more aware of the benefits of a healthy diet in the previous year,[70] and more than half of consumers reported searching for diet and nutrition information in the last month.[71] In addition, 41 percent felt that they were doing all they could to eat healthfully.[72]

The task of educating consumers without overwhelming them is challenging. It means presenting the information in ways consumers want to hear it. For example, positive messages can help prevent the confusion that occurs due to conflicting information. It is reported that the news media disseminate more positive messages than negative ones about food.[68] This positive approach enables consumers to achieve the principles of a healthy diet and physical activity as part of their overall lifestyle. For example, take a 10-minute brisk walk on your lunch break. It will help you feel better, and you will become more energetic.

It is the responsibility of the educator to provide information that is understandable. Medical jargon and technical terms may hinder the clarity of the intended message.[73] For example, when helping clients understand diet control for hypercholesterolemia, the dietitian might use the phrase "high blood cholesterol" rather than the term "hypercholesterolemia."

# Successful Community Strategies

## The Partners for Life Nutrition Education Program for Pregnant Women[74]

The Freedom from Hunger Foundation joined the Mississippi Cooperative Extension Service and the State Department of Health to establish the Partners for Life Program (PFLP). The purpose of this joint venture was to address the maternal nutrition problems in the Delta region. Leflore County, a county representative of the Delta region, was selected as the pilot site for a formative evaluation of a nutrition education program for high-risk pregnant women prior to implementation of the PFLP in the other five Delta counties. The investigators' and program planner's goal was to collect data that would answer the following questions:

- Could the Expanded Food and Nutrition Education Program (EFNEP) curriculum be adapted to meet the nutritional needs of pregnant women?
- Could peer educators be trained to deliver an effective intervention?
- Could pregnant women be successfully recruited to participate in the program?
- Would the adapted curriculum produce sufficient data in a pilot study to determine its potential for changing dietary knowledge and behavior in pregnancy?
- What are the reactions of pregnant women regarding participation in the program and usability of the nutrition program?

To accomplish this goal, an advisory committee consisting of physicians, nurses, nutritionists, health educators, and other health professionals with a maternal and child health viewpoint was formed. The advisory committee provided guidance to the PFLP staff about the development and adaptation of the EFNEP nutrition education program. The investigators adapted EFNEP's methodology for pregnant clients in the local WIC program receiving maternity care at the county health department. The nutrition education lessons were delivered in a sequence of eight consecutive weekly sessions of 60 minutes each. The main teaching format was discussion and observational learning in the clients' homes.

This approach created an interactive education/teaching style. The content areas of the lessons were:

- Maternal and infant nutrition
- Health problems and solutions
- Eating healthy and healthy baby
- How to make decisions
- Saving for mother and baby
- Food, friends, and fun
- Caring for the baby
- Preparation for delivery

Results of the formative evaluation showed both positive and negative outcomes. Positive outcomes were 1) the recruitment and training of the peer educators to provide the intervention had a positive outcome; 2) the recruitment of the targeted population for the pilot study was successful; 3) the project questionnaires and measuring forms were successfully completed; and 4) the improvement in nutrition knowledge and dietary behavior was statistically significant. Two negative outcomes in this formative study were 1) the program experienced problems retaining participants it recruited, and 2) deviation of the time frame for intervention delivery. Participants identified program length as the main reason for their dissatisfaction. The authors recommended that nutrition educators and planners can use the results from this formative evaluation to make changes in problem areas (participant retention and length of the program) prior to implementation of a full-scale impact evaluation.

# Learning Portfolio

## Chapter Summary

- Nutrition education is any set of learning experiences designed to facilitate the voluntary adoption of eating and other nutrition-related behaviors conducive to health and well-being.
- It is important to note that interventions often do not achieve across-the-board success. Generally, nutrition education works on one criterion, but not necessarily on another, or with one gender, but not with the other.
- One way to consider the nature of learning is by examining the cognitive, affective, and psychomotor domains of learning. Each domain has explicit behavioral components that form a hierarchy of steps or levels that build on the previous one.
- The nutrition intervention strategies that have been effective in increasing nutrition knowledge for improved nutritional adequacy in older populations include personalized approaches, behavioral approaches, attention to motivators, and reinforcements.
- The goal of nutrition education for pregnant women is relatively clear: appropriate maternal weight gain, nutritional adequacy of the maternal diet, and positive infant outcomes, such as satisfactory birth weight. The goals are similar for lactating women.
- A lesson plan needs to describe the desires of the target population. It is the blueprint for organizing a class. A well-designed lesson plan ensures a clear focus and specific learning outcomes.

- The program identifier conveys the key theme of the program.
- In developing the marketing plan, it is beneficial to form partnerships with local businesses, healthcare organizations, government agencies, and the like.
- Objectives are written statements of intended outcomes in measurable terms.
- The nutrition educator serves as the facilitator of the education process.

## Critical Thinking Activities

- Develop a lesson plan, including writing at least two measurable objectives, for a nutrition education program on fitness and exercise for high school students. Include all the components of a lesson plan presented in this chapter.
- Provide two examples of incentives that can motivate high school students to participate in a health promotion program.
- Identify at least four skills essential to a successful nutrition education program and why they are essential.
- Plan a nutrition education program using the theoretical framework presented in Box 16-4. Also, identify two levels of psychomotor skills the clients may possess.
- Identify four strategies to motivate participation.
- Identify two organizations or businesses that can be partners for a nutrition education program. Include their roles in the program.

## 🔍 CASE STUDY 16-1: The Impact of Using Different Nutrition Education Methods

Elon, a community nutritionist, used different methods of delivering nutrition education to three different geographic areas in Chicago. Reports show a high prevalence of high-fat, high-calorie dietary practices. Some of the health conditions observed in these communities include obesity, diabetes, high blood pressure, and painful, mottled, chipped, and missing teeth. In one area, she used mass media techniques, including radio announcements, posters, and leaflets. In a second area, she used lectures to deliver nutrition education involving six 1-hour sessions over 1 month at different sites. For a third area, she used demonstrations to deliver the nutrition education, involving six 1-hour sessions for 3 weeks. The educational sessions purposely were kept didactic, with minimum interaction. The second and third areas served as control groups. The control groups were able to receive the radio spots, but did not receive leaflets or posters. The face-to-face education groups also may have been exposed to radio broadcasts. Elon compared the impact of the program on a sample of mothers of children younger than 5 years of age in the control areas, the face-to-face education group, and the mass media group. She collected data about their dietary intake habits and frequency of food intake immediately after the educational programs, 3 months later, and 12 months later. Elon found that nutrition concepts were learned equally among the three groups; however, the control groups, which received radio spots, gained more nutrition knowledge than the other groups.

*(continues)*

## ⌕ CASE STUDY 16-1: The Impact of Using Different Nutrition Education Methods
*(continued)*

### Questions

1. What is nutrition education?
2. Elon considered the nature of learning by reviewing the cognitive, affective, and psychomotor domains of learning. What are the cognitive, affective, and psychomotor domains? Briefly describe each.
3. What are the six principles that can help Elon carry out effective nutrition education programs?
4. Identify and describe the adult learning stages.
5. What are the steps of a needs assessment when planning a nutrition education program that Elon must understand?
6. What is adult learning? Elon's audience will include this population; which nutrition intervention strategies have been proved effective in increasing adults' nutrition knowledge?
7. Children were also included in Elon's nutrition education program. What are some of the strategies that successful nutrition education programs have used for children?
8. What are some additional tips for providing an effective nutrition intervention to pregnant and lactating women that Elon needs to know?
9. A nutrition education lesson plan encourages advanced planning and organization. What is a lesson plan? What are the eight features Elon should include in the written format of the planned activities?
10. Elon utilized some of the communication guidelines for educational interaction presented in Table 16-5. Briefly describe four communication guidelines for educational interactions.
11. It is important to know the general ideas for designing nutrition and health messages that are presented in Table 16-6. What are the consumer-tested tips for communicating nutrition messages?
12. Work in small groups or individually to discuss the case study and practice using the Nutrition Care Process chart provided on the companion website. You can also add other nutrition and health-related conditions or assessments to the case study to make it more challenging and interesting.

## Think About It

**Answer:** Motivation and the performance of the educator.

## Key Terms

**adult learning:** Adults gaining knowledge and expertise.

**affective domain:** The domain of learning that includes the way individuals deal with things emotionally, such as feelings, values, appreciation, enthusiasm, motivation, and attitude. It also consists of changes in attitudes and the development of values.

**behavior:** The effects of nutrition education (such as the intake of specific foods) or actual behaviors (such as eating five fruits and vegetables per day).

**cognitive domain:** The domain of learning that involves knowledge and the development of intellectual skills. This includes the recall or recognition of specific facts, procedural patterns, and concepts that serve in the development of intellectual abilities and skills.

**learning:** The process of leading to relatively permanent behavioral change or potential behavioral change as a result of experience.

**lesson plan:** The blueprint for organizing a class. A well-designed lesson plan ensures a clear focus and articulates specific learning outcomes.

**nutrition education:** Any set of learning experiences designed to facilitate the voluntary adoption of eating and other nutrition-related behaviors conducive to health and well-being.

**objectives:** Written statements of intended outcomes. The expected outcomes need to be defined in measurable terms.

**participation:** When clients join others in health promotion activities.

**program identifier:** A statement or motto that succinctly defines or represents the aim of the program.

**psychomotor domain:** The domain of learning that includes the performance of skills that require some degree of neuromuscular coordination.

## References

1. Cowburn GG, Stockley LL. Consumer understanding and use of nutrition labelling: a systematic review. *Public Health Nutr.* 2005;8(1):21-28.
2. US Dept Health and Human Services. *Healthy People 2010: National Health Promotion and*

*Disease Prevention Objectives.* Washington, DC: US Dept of Health and Human Services; 2000.

3. Harrison K, Marskey AL. Nutritional content of foods advertised during the television programs children watch most. *Am J Public Health.* 2005;95(9):1568-1574.

4. Stanhope M, Lancaster J. *Community and Public Health Nursing: Population-Centered Health Care in the Community.* 9th ed. New York, NY: Elsevier; 2015.

5. Expert Learners. Cognitive information processing theory. http://www.expertlearners.com/cip_theory.php. Accessed March 16, 2017.

6. AllPsychOnline. Introduction to learning theory and behavioral psychology. https://allpsych.com/personalitysynopsis/learning/. Accessed March 16, 2017.

7. Dembo MH. *Applying Educational Psychology.* 5th ed. New York, NY: Longman; 1994.

8. Huitt WB. Taxonomy of the cognitive domain. In: Huitt WB, ed. *Educational Psychology Interactive.* Valdosta, GA: Valdosta State University; 2004.

9. Owen, L. Three domains of learning-cognitive, affective, psychomotor. http://thesecondprinciple.com/instructional-design/threedomainsoflearning/. Accessed March 16, 2017.

10. Denehy J. Health education: an important role for school nurses. *J Sch Nurs.* 2001;17(5):233-238.

11. Williams DP, LeBlanc H, Christensen NK. Diabetes stepping up to the plate: an education curriculum focused on food portioning skills. *J Extension.* 2004;42(3).

12. Knowles MS, Holton EF III, Swanson RA. *The Adult Learnier: The Definitive Classic in Adult Education and Human Resource Development.* 5th ed: Houston, TX: Gulf Publishing; 1998.

13. Contento I, Balch GI, Bronner YL, et al. Nutrition education for adults. *J Nutr Educ.* 1995;27:312-328.

14. Sims LS. Nutrition education research: reaching toward the leading edge. *J Am Diet Assoc.* 1987;87(suppl):S10-S18.

15. Steptoe A, Perkins-Porras L, Rink E, Hilton S, et al. Psychological and social predictors of changes in fruit and vegetable consumption over 12 months following behavioral and nutrition education counseling. *Health Psychol.* 2004;23(6):574-581.

16. Lanerolle PP. Nutrition education improves serum retinol concentration among adolescent school girls. *Asia Pacific J Clin Nutr.* 2006;15(1):43-49.

17. Assema P, Steenbakkers M, Rademaker C, Brug J. The impact of a nutrition education intervention on main meal quality and fruit intake in people with financial problems. *J Human Nutr Diet.* 2005;18:205-212.

18. Patterson R. *Changing Patient Behavior: Improving Outcomes in Health and Disease Management.* San Francisco, CA: Jossey-Bass, American Heart Association Press; 2001.

19. Stewart LL, Houghton J, Hughes A, Pearson D, et al. Dietetic management of pediatric overweight: development and description of a practical and evidence-based behavioral approach. *J Am Diet Assoc.* 2005;105(11):1810-1815.

20. Shafer L, Gillespie A, Wilkins L, Borra ST. Nutrition education for the public: position of the American Dietetic Association. *J Am Diet Assoc.* 1996;96:1183-1187.

21. Gaglianone CP, Taddei JA, Colugnati FA, Magalhaes CG,et al. Nutrition education in public elementary schools of Sao Paulo, Brazil: the reducing risks of illness and death in adulthood project. *Rev Nutr.* 2006;19(3):1-11.

22. Williamson D, Copeland A, Anton S, Champagne C, ct al. Wise mind project: a school-based environmental approach for preventing weight gain in children. *Obesity.* 2007;15:906-917.

23. Mullen PD, Green LW, Persinger GS. Clinical trials of patient education for chronic condition: a comparative meta-analysis of intervention types. *Prev Med.* 1985;14(6):753-781.

24. Sutton SM, Balch GI, Lefebvre RC. Strategic questions for consumer-based health communications. *Public Health Rep.* 1995;110(6):725-733.

25. Volker DL. Patient education: needs assessment and resource identification. *Oncol Nurs Forum.* 1991;18(1):119-123.

26. Anspaugh DJ, Dignan MB, Anspaugh SL. *Developing Health Promotion Programs.* 2nd ed. Long Grove IL: Waveland Press; 2006.

27. Radimer K. Dietary supplement use by US adults: data from the National Health and Nutrition Examination Survey, 1999-2000. *Am J Epidemiol.* 2004;160(4):339-349.

28. Dutta-Bergman MJ. Primary sources of health information: comparisons in the domain of health attitudes, health cognitions, and health behaviors. *Health Comm.* 2004;16(3):273-288.

29. Clark PG, Phillip G, Rossi JS, Joseph S. Intervening on exercise and nutrition in older adults: the Rhode Island SENIOR Project. *J Aging Health.* 2005;17(6):753-778.

30. Patacca DD, Rosenbloom CA, Kicklighter JR, Ball M. Using a focus group approach to determine older adults' opinions and attitudes toward a nutrition education program. *J Nutr Elder.* 2004;23(3):55-72.

31. International Food Information Council. Food for thought III: a quantitative and qualitative

content analysis of diet, nutrition and food safety reporting. 2001. http://www.foodinsight.org/topics. Accessed March 16, 2017.

32. Toner HM, Morris JD. A social-psychological perspective of dietary quality in later adulthood. *J Nutr Elderly.* 1992;11:35-53.

33. International Food and Information Council. Sharpen your skills. 2007. http://www.ific.org/. Accessed March 17, 2017.

34. Ghoneim EE. An intervention programme for improving the nutritional status of children aged 2-5 years in Alexandria. *East Med Health J.* 2004;10(6):828-843.

35. Adekunle LL. The effect of family structure on a sample of malnourished urban Nigerian children. *Food Nutr Bull.* 2005;26(2):230-233.

36. Tamborlane WV. *The Yale Guide to Children's Nutrition.* New Haven, CT: Yale Press; 1997.

37. Birch LL. Preschool children's preference and consumption paterns. *J Nutr Educ.* 1979(11):189-192.

38. Perry CL. A randomized school trial of environmental strategies to encourage fruit and vegetable consumption among children. *Health Educ Behav.* 2004;31(1):65-76.

39. Blom-Hoffman J, Kelleher C, Power TJ, Leff S. Promoting Healthy food consumption among young children: evaluation of a multi-component nutrition education program. *J Sch Psychol.* 2004;42(1):45-60.

40. Singleton JC, Achterberf CL, Shannon BM. Role of food and nutrition in the health perceptions of young children. *J Am Diet Assoc.* 1992;92:67-70.

41. Hitchcock J, Schubert PE, Thomas SA. *Community Health Nursing.* 2nd ed. Clifton Park, NY: Thomson Delmar Learning; 2003.

42. Saksvig BI, Gittelsohn J, Harris SB, Hanley AJG, et al. A pilot school-based healthy eating and physical activity intervention improves diet, food knowledge, and self-efficacy for native Canadian children. *J Nutr.* 2005;135(10):2392-2238.

43. Anderson S, Campbell DM, Shepherd RR. The influence of dietary advice on nutrient intake during pregnancy. *Br J Nutr.* 1995;73(2):163-177.

44. Hart AD, Azubuike CU, Barimalaa S, Achinewhu SC. Vegetable consumption pattern of households in selected areas of the Old Rivers State in Nigeria. *Afr J Food Agricult Nutr Dev.* 2005;5(1):57-62.

45. Kaiser L, McMurdo T, Block A. The Food Stamp Nutrition Education Program focuses on the learner *J Exension.* 2007;45(2): RIB5.

46. Gucciardi E, Demelo M, Lee RN, Sherry L. Assessment of two culturally competent diabetes education methods: individual versus individual plus group education in Canadian Portuguese adults with type 2 diabetes. *Ethn Health.* 2007;12(2):163-187.

47. McKenzie JF, Neiger BL, Smeltzer JL. *Planning, Implementing, and Evaluating Health Promotion Programs: A Primer.* 4th ed. San Francisco, CA: Benjamin Cummings; 2005.

48. Vella J. *Learning to Listen, Learning to Teach: The Power of Dialogue in Educating Adults.* San Francisco, CA: Jossey-Bass; 2002.

49. Norris J. *From Telling to Teaching.* North Myrtle Beach, SC: Learning by Dialogue; 2007.

50. Kim KH, Linnan L, Campbell MK, Brooks C, et al. The WORD (Wholeness, Oneness, Righteousness, Deliverance): a faith-based weight-loss program utilizing a community-based participatory research approach. *Health Educ Behav.* 2008;35(5):634-650.

51. Lefebvre CR, Flora JA. Social marketing and public health intervention. *Health Educ Q.* 1988;15(3):299-315.

52. Minkler M. Improving health through community organization. In: Glanz K, Lewis FM, Rimer BK, eds. *Health Behavior and Health Education: Theory, Research, and Practice.* San Francisco, CA: Jossey-Bass; 1990:257-287.

53. Kuczmarski MF, Aljadix L. Using food calendars to self-monitor: Got 5? nutrition for kids program. *J Nutr Educ.* 2003;35:269-270.

54. Struempler BJ, Cobrin, S. Feed your mind: an interactive nutrition evaluation for teenagers. *J Nutr Educ.* 2002;34(1):59-60.

55. Byrd-Bredbenner CF. Dietary fat and heart disease intervention strategies. *J Nutr Educ.* 2000;32(1):60-61.

56. Campbell D, Palm GF. *Group Parent Education: Promoting Parent Learning and Support.* London, UK: Sage; 2004.

57. Centers for Disease Control and Prevention. Five A Day mission and history. http://www.5aday.org/. Accessed March 17, 2017.

58. Boyle MA, Holben D. *Community Nutrition in Action: An Entrepreneurial Approach.* 4th ed. Belmont, CA: Thomson Wadsworth; 2013.

59. Rankin SH, Stallings KD. *Patient Education: Principles, and Practice.* 4th ed. Philadelphia, PA: J.B. Lippincott; 2001.

60. Farr AC, Witte C, Jarato K, Menard T. The effectiveness of media use in health education: evaluation of an HIV/AIDS radio [corrected] campaign in Ethiopia. *J Health Comm.* 2005;10(3):225-235.

61. Keller HH, Hedley H, Hadley M, Wong T, et al. Food workshops, nutrition education, and older adults: a process evaluation. *J Nutr Elder.* 2005;24(3):5-23.

62. Giger JN, Davidhizar, R. *Transcultural Nursing: Assessment and Intervention*. 7th ed. St. Louis, MO: Mosby; 2016.

63. Blanchette L, Brug J. Determinants of fruit and vegetable consumption among 6-12-year-old children and effective interventions to increase consumption. *J Human Nutr Diet*. 2005;18(6):431-443.

64. Dickin KL, Dollahite JS, Jean-Pierre H. Nutrition behavior change among EFNEP participants is higher at sites that are well managed and whose front-line nutrition educators value the program. *J Nutr*. 2005;135:2199-2205.

65. Lieberman L, Meana LL, Stewart D. Cardiac rehabilitation: gender differences in factors influencing participation. *J Womens Health*. 1998;7(6):717-723.

66. Person AL, Colby SE, Bulova JA, Eubanks JW. Barriers to participation in a worksite wellness program. *Nutr Res Pract*. 2010;4(2):149-154.

67. Lefebvre RCD, L Johnston C. Loughrey, et al. Use of database marketing and consumer-based health communication in a message design an example from the Office of Cancer Communication's "5 A Day for Better Health" Health Program. In: Maibach EW, Parrott RL, eds. *Designing Health Messages. Approaches from Communication Theory and Public Health Practice*. Thousand Oaks, CA: Sage; 1995:217-246.

68. International Food and Information Council. IFIC used the Marketing Model to develop quantitatively tested consumer messages regarding the. http://www.foodinsight.org/topics. Accessed March 16, 2017.

69. American Dietetic Association. *Nutrition Trend Survey: Executive Summary*. Chicago, IL: American Dietetic Assoiciation; 1997.

70. Darmon N, Briend A, Drewnowski. Energy-dense diets are associated with lower diet costs: a community study of French adults. *Public Health Nutr*. 2004;7:21-27.

71. McGee R. Analysis of poverty assessment (PPA) and household survey findings on poverty trends in Uganda. Institute of Development Studies. 2000. http://www.participatorymethods.org/resource/analysis-participatory-poverty-assessment-ppa-and-household-survey-findings-poverty-trends. Accessed March 16, 2017.

72. Food Marketing Institute. *Trends in the United States: Consumer Attitudes & the Supermarket*. Washington, DC: Food Marketing Institute; 1999.

73. Damroch S. General strategies for motivating people to change their behavior. *Nurs Clin North Am*. 1991;26(4):833-843.

74. Boyd NR, Richard AW. A formative evaluation in maternal and child health practice: the Partners for Life Nutrition Education Program for pregnant women. *Matern Child Health J*. 2003;7(2):137-143.

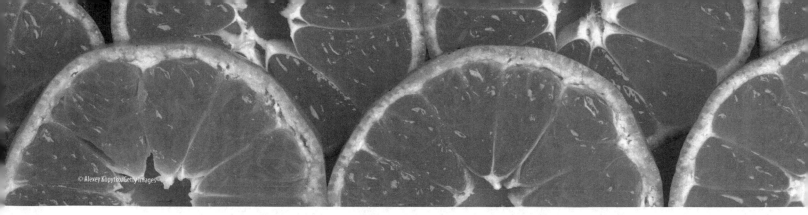

## CHAPTER 17

# Marketing Nutrition Programs and the Role of Food Industry in Food Choice

## CHAPTER OUTLINE

- Introduction
- Marketing Defined
- Developing a Marketing Plan
- Market Research and Situational Analysis
- Market Segmentation
- Communication Factor Analysis
- Social Marketing
- E-Professionalism
- Advertising the Program
- Food Industries, Advertising, and Food Choices
- The Role of Media in Childhood Obesity
- Public Health Approaches
- Approaches to Protecting Children
- Food and Nutrition Misinformation

## LEARNING OBJECTIVES

- Define marketing.
- Discuss the difference between social and business marketing.
- Define market segmentation.
- Discuss the 5 Ps of social marketing: product, price, place, promotion, and position.
- Discuss the different communication factors that may affect nutrition programs.
- Discuss how food industries influence food choice.
- Define advertising.

## ▶ Introduction

An effective marketing plan is necessary for any health promotion program to be successful. Marketing is not only an advertising campaign, a convenient package of low-fat foods and vegetables, or a $1 coupon for dairy products—marketing has a broader perspective in the context of nutrition. It focuses on all efforts to encourage and enable people to eat nutritiously.[1] Kotler and Zaltman[2] first used the term **social marketing** in 1971, referring to the application of marketing to solve social and health problems. **Marketing** involves the planned attempt to influence the market so there is a voluntary exchange of costs from that market with benefits to a provider.[3] Using media is one of the best marketing strategies to reach large segments of the population and can be used as a positive approach to communicate nutrition information and address related health issues. Community nutritionists and other healthcare practitioners need to understand the marketing strategies available for promoting nutrition messages. This chapter first discusses how to use marketing principles to modify individuals' behavior and promote health; then, it addresses how food industries use media to influence food choice and its effect on health. Finally, it discusses nutrition misinformation and how companies use marketing as a tool to promote unproven health products.

## ▶ Marketing Defined

Marketing is one of the techniques that community nutritionists, program administrators, and registered dietitians can use to promote and implement effective nutrition education programs. Marketing is directed at satisfying the needs and wants of the consumer through an exchange of processes or activities (goods, products, or programs).[4] But marketing is much more than just this. It encompasses everything the nutritionist does to provide services to the community, including creating, promoting, delivering, and finally consuming the product or service, such as the name for the nutrition program, the letterhead, and the services provided.

Marketing starts with the client's actual or perceived wants and needs.[5] The community will choose to work with the nutritionist based on the benefits to be gained. Few people will attend a workshop or planning session only out of curiosity.

## ▶ Developing a Marketing Plan

A marketing plan consists of specific goals and objectives, target groups, messages, the desires of the target population, channels, budgets, tracking and evaluation, and media selection factors.[6]

A formal marketing plan is a written statement of the marketing objectives, strategies, and all the specific actions that must be taken.[7] It explains how the nutrition and health information will be delivered to the targeted population. A marketing plan should contain the following: executive summary, situation analysis, objectives and goals, marketing strategy, action programs, budgets, and controls (see **BOX 17-1**).[8]

### Goals and Objectives

It is very important to be clear about the desired marketing outcomes and to state them in measurable terms. For instance, if the goal is to increase attendance over last year's weight management program, a specific objective might be to increase the community participation by 15 percent.[4]

### Target Groups

It is essential to define the target groups prior to marketing a nutrition program. For example, if the program is about diabetes, specify whether the target group is individuals in the community who have not yet developed diabetes, those who are already being treated for diabetes, or healthcare practitioners such as physicians, dietitians, and nurses who treat diabetes.[9] A secondary target audience could be the decision makers who influence the individual's choice to use the program (e.g., parents, spouses, friends, and coworkers). Another target group may be those who use a particular program, such as low-income pregnant or breastfeeding women and mothers of children younger than 5 years of age

## BOX 17-1   Contents of a Marketing Plan

**I.   Executive Summary**
- The main goals and recommendations
- The benefits to the consumers and needs of the target audience

**II.   Situation Analysis**
- Background (market description)
- Opportunities and threats (a review of competition)
- Strengths and weaknesses
- The nutritionist's position in the marketplace
- What health services he or she provides (a review of distribution)

**III.   Objectives and Goals**
- Defined marketing activities in measurable terms

**IV.   Marketing Strategy**
- Know:
  - The game plan
  - The target market
  - The tools and techniques appropriate to reach the target audience
  - The expenditure level
  - The advertising strategy and positioning

**V.   Action Programs**
- Have a month-by-month implementation timetable (specific marketing strategies that will accomplish specific actions)

**VI.   Budget**
- The cost of production, marketing, and administration
- The basis for marketing operations, financial planning, and personnel recruitment

**VII.   Controls**
- *Annual plan control:* Steps taken during the year to monitor and correct deviation from the plan
- *Profitability control:* Determining the actual profit or progress of different services or products, market segments, and distribution channels
- *Strategic control:* Systematic evaluation of the organization's market performance in relation to market opportunities

Modified from: Kotler P, Clark R. *Marketing for Healthcare Organizations: Steps in Market Segmentation, Targeting, and Positioning.* Englewood Cliffs, NJ: Prentice Hall; 1987.

participating in the Special Supplemental Nutrition Program for Women, Infants, and Children (WIC), elderly people participating in the Peace Meal Program, obese individuals participating in a weight-loss program, or postmenopausal women participating in a women's health program.

## Messages

Once the target group is determined, find out the beliefs, needs, and orientation of the target group. These will provide the types of marketing messages the target group needs and determine their sequence. In some cases, erroneous beliefs or information may need to be clarified first. Most programs use television, radio, and print (newspapers and magazines) to communicate their messages. However, word-of-mouth advertising is also important and effective. Referrals from satisfied participants of current or past programs may be the best source of new participants.[4]

## Channels

A good marketing plan must verify the communication channels the target groups use. If the target group is older individuals, for example, determine whether they read the Peace Meal Program newsletter, watch television, or listen to the radio. Use the target group's most popular communication channel to advertise the marketing message. One very good way to capture the target group's attention is through a story on a local cable television station (CNN local edition) or during the community segment of the local news.

Choose free or low-cost methods such as community bulletin boards, public service announcements, and fliers to reduce cost. Some printing businesses may donate fliers if the company can put their name, address, and phone number on each of the fliers.[4]

## Budget

It is important to extend the budget to provide media coverage throughout the entire program period. Be sure to include ideas for fundraising within the budget. It is important to budget wisely because advertising is expensive.[4]

Some related marketing costs include funds for logos, fliers, brochures, videos, and radio and/or TV public service announcements (PSAs).

A health promotion program budget may contain many facets and may use various formats. In health promotion, two budgeting formats are used most often—line item and functional. The line item format includes anticipated expenditures for the fiscal year.[3,10] Examples of line items are labor (full-time and part-time employees); the nutrition educator's, secretary's, and director's salaries; materials; supplies; travel (professional meetings, program sites, etc.); transportation; telephones; the Internet; computers; rent; and printing. In contrast, a functional budget is based on the specific functions each department provides and includes staff training, program evaluation, health screenings, educational materials, equipment, and facilities. These two budget formats must be considered when developing marketing strategies.[6,10,11]

## Marketing Evaluation

Monitoring the marketing program/plan will provide feedback on the success or relevance of the marketing strategy. An elaborate evaluation is not necessary; it could be as simple as asking the participants how they heard about the Heart Smart for Teens, menopause management, or bone density screening program. The nutritionist may desire to know who and what influenced the participant to enroll in the health promotion program. She or he may ask, "Did the cable show or the newspaper influence your interest in the program?" Evaluate whether the marketing channels used were effective or ineffective, whether they should be repeated, or whether they should be modified based on participants' feedback.[4]

## ▶ Market Research and Situational Analysis

Market research and situational analysis help the nutritionist identify whether the targeted community will be interested in the programs. Market attractiveness is based on the following[4,10]:

- Whether the market is large enough to support the program
- Whether the program has the potential to grow
- Whether the targeted community is aware of the program and whether they can afford the time or money to participate in the program
- Whether there is sufficient incentive to encourage private investment in the program
- Whether competitors are offering similar or related services

Market research is the systematic design, collection, analysis, and reporting of data and findings relevant to a specific marketing situation or problem facing an organization.[8] For example, Ling et al.[12] analyzed tobacco-industry marketing archives from August 2000 to February 2002 and found that the tobacco industry divided markets and defined targets according to consumer attitudes, aspirations, activities, and lifestyles. The tobacco industry marketing targeted smokers of all ages, especially young adults. The researchers recommended that public health professionals include people of all ages, though mainly young adults, instead of concentrating on teens and young children in smoking cessation programs.[13]

The initial step a nutritionist needs to take in the market research process is to determine the research objectives and define the problem. The objective may be to learn more about the different ethnic groups in the community or the impact of a marketing strategy or tool used in promoting a nutrition program or other programs. The next step is to conduct exploratory research.

## Exploratory Research

**Exploratory research** is carrying out preliminary research to learn more about the market before any formal research survey is conducted.[8] This includes collecting secondary data, observational research, competitive analysis, qualitative and quantitative data, and situation analysis by completing informal interviewing with individuals and groups in the community.[8]

## Secondary Data Research

Secondary data are information collected for another purpose (e.g., population census, National Health and Nutrition Examination Survey [NHANES], death certificates, demographic data, etc.). The secondary data need to be used with caution because they were collected for a purpose that may not be identical to the nutritionist's purpose; however, they may provide useful ideas and findings and reduce the cost of conducting primary research. They also may help the nutritionist define the problems and research objectives.[14]

## Observational Research and Analyzing the Environment

Observational research is the gathering of primary data by observing relevant situations, actions, environments, and people. For example, a nutritionist could collect data on postmenopausal women's actions after attending a Heart Smart for Women education program by calculating how many women signed up for a physical activity three times a week and by observing how often they exercised. In addition, the researcher will need to analyze the external forces and trends. Some examples of external situations that affect dietetics practice include recent trends in eating habits or behaviors of consumers, the availability of nutritious foods, the cost of foods, poverty, healthcare reform legislative and regulatory changes, and an increase in the number of older persons in the community.[14-16] In addition, he or she will need to evaluate the market trends both locally and nationally.

## Competitive Analysis

Market research also includes conducting a competitive analysis. The nutritionist will need to determine the competition's strengths and weaknesses, the distinctive characteristics that sets the nutritionist apart from other programs, and the short- and long-term trends that may affect program usage. Also, he or she should determine how the program can be positioned for the greatest degree of collaboration with competing programs.[8,14]

This analysis will help the nutritionist position the program as being different or better than programs that are similar in the services offered, consumer base (target market), or location. Market research can help the nutritionist identify the underserved or what the competitor is not providing.[4,8] The competitors in the field of nutrition could be other healthcare practitioners (physicians, chiropractors, alternative therapy practitioners, nurses, and others), businesses, health food stores, food industries, hospitals, or other public health organizations (e.g., American Heart Association, National Cancer Institute).

There are several methods of collecting information on the competition, including networking, speaking to colleagues in a dietetic practice group, reviewing secondary data, and establishing relationships with the consumer. In order to advertise the services, the dietitian must determine his or her competitive edge (area of expertise, professional image, screening equipment, etc.), establish a relationship with the consumer, build trust and rapport, understand the consumer's needs, and provide services that deliver the promised benefits.[15]

## Qualitative and Quantitative Data

In addition to collecting data through observation, focus groups, and surveys, the nutritionist needs to carry out some interviews during the exploratory stage of the market research project. The data collection should be qualitative in the exploratory stage. **Qualitative research** data typically come from small samples of the target audience, mainly through open-ended interviewing. The clients are asked leading questions that stimulate them to share their feelings and thoughts. The aim is to probe deeply into consumers' main needs, perceptions, preferences, and satisfactions with the program; understand the problems that could occur in marketing to this group; and generate ideas that can be used to conduct further studies using quantitative research.[8] The result of qualitative research cannot be generalized to the larger target audience because of the small sample size.[16,17]

In contrast, **quantitative research** utilizes selected samples to produce statistically reliable results that are expressed in numeric terms; for example, 10 percent of children living in an inner city reported skipping breakfast. Quantitative research involves interviewing or surveying a larger number of people than qualitative research and assumes that the interviewer knows the specific questions to ask prior to data collection.[18] Both

qualitative and quantitative data are used in the planning of social marketing strategies.[19]

## Situation Analysis

Observational research also includes conducting a situation analysis; for example, determine where the weight-loss class will be carried out. Observe whether the postmenopausal women mentioned earlier are working full time. Determine the cost of the weight-loss program.[14,20,21]

The step that is critical to the ultimate success of the entire marketing plan is sometimes referred to as SWOT analysis; SWOT is an acronym for strengths, weaknesses, opportunities, and threats.[14] SWOT is an exercise to analyze internal strengths and weaknesses and external opportunities and threats.[19]

The SWOT analysis is instrumental in strategy formulation and selection and provides information that is helpful for matching an agency's resources and capabilities to the competitive environment. It allows an agency's strengths, resources, and capabilities to be used as a basis for developing a competitive advantage. The absence of certain strengths may be viewed as an agency weakness. The analysis of external environmental factors may reveal certain new opportunities for profit and growth, whereas changes in the external environment may present threats to the agency. To develop strategies that take into account the SWOT profile, a matrix of these factors can be constructed[6,19]:

|  | Strengths | Weaknesses |
|---|---|---|
| Opportunities | S-O strategies | W-O strategies |
| Threats | S-T strategies | W-T strategies |

- *S-O strategies* pursue opportunities that are a good fit to the agency's strengths (e.g., a large number of older persons in the community).
- *S-T strategies* identify ways the agency can pursue opportunities (e.g., advertise to increase the number of Peace Meal Program participants in the community).
- *W-O strategies* identify ways the agency can use its strengths to reduce vulnerability to external threats (e.g., ask older individuals in the community to help recruit participants for the program).
- *W-T strategies* establish a defensive plan to prevent the agency's weakness from making it highly susceptible to external threats (e.g., involve community leaders, such as the mayor, church leaders, and others, to seek additional resources for the program and to avoid lack of Peace Meal Program participants).[19]

# ▶ Market Segmentation

**Market segmentation** is dividing a market or community into distinct groups of buyers or individuals who might require separate products or services or marketing mixes on the basis of needs, characteristics, or behavior.[22,23] The market is composed of many types of consumers, products and services, and needs and nutritionists must determine which segments provide the best opportunity for achieving the health promotion program's goals.[24] A **market segment** is a portion of a larger market; for example, African Americans or senior citizens represent a segment of the total U.S. market. Market segmentation is very valuable in identifying and choosing the target market instead of trying to reach everybody. **Market targeting** is the process of evaluating each market segment's attractiveness and selecting one or more segments to penetrate.[22,25] Market positioning is arranging for a product or program to take a clear, distinctive, and desirable place comparable to competing products or programs for nutrition and health services for the same clients or community; for example, physical activity could be repositioned as a form of relaxation, not exercise, to women age 55 years or older.

**FIGURE 17-1** presents the three major steps in market targeting. Once the nutritionist has defined the market segment, he or she can tailor the marketing mixes to the group's specific needs. The demographics, sociographics, behavioral aspects, and psychographics of the client base provide important information.[26] Some of the types of demographics are the size of the population for the program area, rate of change of the population, age or sex distribution, racial/ethnic composition, socioeconomic status, housing information, and fertility patterns.

Sociographics and psychographics are the sociology and psychology behind demographic analysis; they deduce the emotional needs, values, and lifestyles that can lead to good health.[4,27] Sociographics and psychographics also include the identification of behavior patterns of the individuals, which makes it easier for the nutritionist to predict their health conditions and market the program to the geographic areas that will benefit the community.[27] Also, data on health and nutrition behaviors may be helpful in determining the market segment. The nutritionist can analyze any of these sources of data to determine the needs of the population and gather ideas for planning a community health and nutrition promotion program. **TABLE 17-1** provides market segmentation categories. Examples of excellent sources of data are[20]:

- National Health Interview Survey (NHIS)
- National Health and Nutrition Examination Survey (NHANES)
- Behavioral Risk Factor Surveillance System (BRFSS)
- U.S. Census Bureau, National Center for Health Statistics (NCHS)
- Social Security Administration (SSA)
- U.S. Department of Agriculture (USDA)
- Youth Risk Behavior Survey (YRBS)

# ▶ Communication Factor Analysis

Communication involves everything that is carried out to market a community health and nutrition promotion program. The communication process includes identifying, engaging, and convincing the targeted community to collaborate with the nutritionist, and shaping the promotional program to obtain the desired audience response.[4] It also is important to analyze the communication factors when choosing methods of program promotion because these factors may significantly affect the success of the community health and nutrition program. The following are some of the communication factors that may affect a nutrition program[4,26,28]

- Perceptual distortions of information about the nutrition promotion program
- Differences in values and attitudes between the nutritionist and the target community
- Incorrect or improper use of words to convey specific information
- Lack of listening on the part of the targeted community
- Lack of explicit messages
- Lack of knowledge of what the target community needs or demands

Analyzing marketing segmentation can assist with developing market targeting and positioning strategies.

**Market Segmentation**
- Identify bases for segmenting the market.
- Develop segment profiles.

**Market Targeting**
- Develop measure of segment attractiveness.
- Select target segments.

**Market Positioning**
- Develop positioning for target segments.
- Develop a marketing mix for each segment.

**FIGURE 17-1** Steps in market segmentation, targeting, and positioning.

Modified from: Kotler P, Clark R. *Marketing for Healthcare Organizations*, 1987: *Steps in Market Segmentation, Targeting, and Positioning*. Englewood Cliffs, NJ: Prentice-Hall; 1987.

**TABLE 17-1** Segmentation Variables for Consumer Markets

| **Variables** |
|---|

*Geographic (regions, state, county size, city size, density, and climate)*

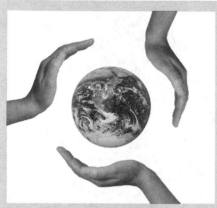

© Christoph Weihs/ShutterStock, Inc.

Consumer markets may be divided by the region, such as Pacific, Mid-Atlantic, New England, etc., and further subdivided by states within that region. Within that state are counties whose size is determined by census data. The counties are then subdivided into cities, whose size is also determined by census data, and are grouped by size ranges such as: under 5,000, 50,000-100,000, etc. Further geographic distinctions may be made by climate, such as southwest, southern, etc.

*Demographic (age, gender, family size, family life cycle, income, occupation, education, religion, race, nationality, social class, and generation)*

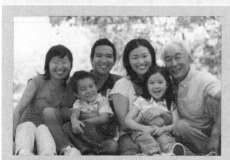

© Monkey Business Images/ShutterStock, Inc.

Divisions in age and gender are made along boundaries such as under 6, 6-11, 35-49, etc. and female, male, etc. Similarly, family size usually divides as 1 or 2, 3 or 4, or 5+. The individual's family life cycle also should be considered. Typical breaks include single, young; young, married, no children; young, married, youngest child under 6, etc. Sample income division breaks include under $2,500, $7,500-$10,000, $20,000-$30,000, etc. Concurrent with this is the individual's occupation: professional and technical; clerical; sales; postgraduate; managers; etc. and similarly education: grade school or less, high school, graduated from high school, etc. Categories such as religion, race, nationality, social class, and generation are also important to consider when assessing consumer markets.

*Psychographic (lifestyle and personality)*

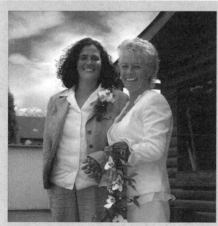

© Fleyeing/Dreamstime.com

Lifestyle and personality traits are often harder to categorize, but should still be taken into consideration if known. Examples of lifestyle choices are straight, swinger, conservative, liberal, etc. Personality traits might include ambitious, dependent, high or low achiever, gregarious, etc.

*(continued)*

| **TABLE 17-1** Segmentation Variables for Consumer Markets *(continued)* |
| --- |
| **Variables** |
| *Behavioral (occasions, benefits sought, user status, rate of status, loyalty status, readiness stage, and attitude toward health program)* |

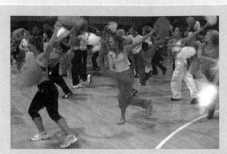

© nicepictures/ShutterStock, Inc.

Behavioral traits take into account how individuals react under certain circumstances and the motivations that drive consumerism. Whether individuals consume more on special occasions versus regular occasions should be considered. One should weigh the benefits that the individual seeks, such as health, comfort, safety, convenience, etc. Individuals often make choices based on their status as a user or not (ex-user, heavy user, first-time user) and how often that status occurs (light user, heavy users, infrequent user). Many consumers pride themselves on their loyalty to products, so that should be another trait to consider, as well as the individual's level of awareness of the message and feelings toward it.

Modified from: Kotler P, Clark RN. *Major Segmentation Variables for Consumer Markets*. Englewood Cliffs, NJ: Prentice Hall; 1999.

In order to communicate effectively, the nutritionist needs to understand the mechanism of communication. Kotler and Armstrong[22] recognized nine elements of communication (sender, receiver, message, media, decoding, encoding, noise, feedback, and response), which are presented in **FIGURE 17-2**. The sender and receiver are the major parties (the nutritionists and the community). The message and the media are the two major tools. Encoding, decoding, response, and feedback are the four major communication functions.[26]

The consumer or community will utilize cues from all aspects of the marketing provided to them to make a choice. It is imperative that the nutritionist/marketer knows 1) how the target consumer will likely respond to the appearance of the product or services and 2) that all aspects of communication are consistent with each other in communicating the messages.[29]

## ▶ Social Marketing

Many health promotion programs use marketing principles to guide their activities. Social marketing, the use of marketing principles for promoting social goods, was launched when Wiebe[30] said that radio and television could sell social objectives just as they sell soap. The significance of this principle is that **business marketing** focuses on fulfilling customers' needs and desires, but social marketing focuses on changing personal or social behaviors for the benefit of the public, even when the public neither recognizes their need nor desires the change. In 1971, Kotler and Zaltman[2] expanded Wiebe's

analysis by more fully applying marketing principles and theory. The theory was that the same marketing principles used to sell products to consumers could be used to "sell" ideas, attitudes, and behaviors. However, social marketing is sometimes less effective than its commercial counterpart because it aims to influence people's ideas and behaviors (e.g., eat less saturated fat) rather than steering existing patterns of thought and behavior in a certain direction (e.g., choose one fast-food restaurant instead of another).[31] Instead of telling people what they need, public health professionals are learning to listen to the needs and desires of the target audience by using focus groups and building programs based on those needs.[32]

It is difficult and expensive to reach every individual in a population with an individualized intervention. Social marketing programs reach a specific audience, satisfy clients' needs, and meet organizational objectives. For example, Reger et al.[33] used a 6-week media campaign to promote consumption of 1-percent-fat milk.[3] He found that 34 percent of high-fat milk drinkers reported switching to low-fat milk and that low-fat milk sales increased from 29 percent of overall milk sales to 46 percent. Social marketing affects the practice of dietetics by boosting clients' awareness of health issues and healthy foods and is able to help move consumers toward behavioral change.

### Social Marketing Components

The components of a business-marketing plan are known as the marketing mix or the 5 Ps of marketing: 1) **product** (what is being sold), 2) **price** (at what

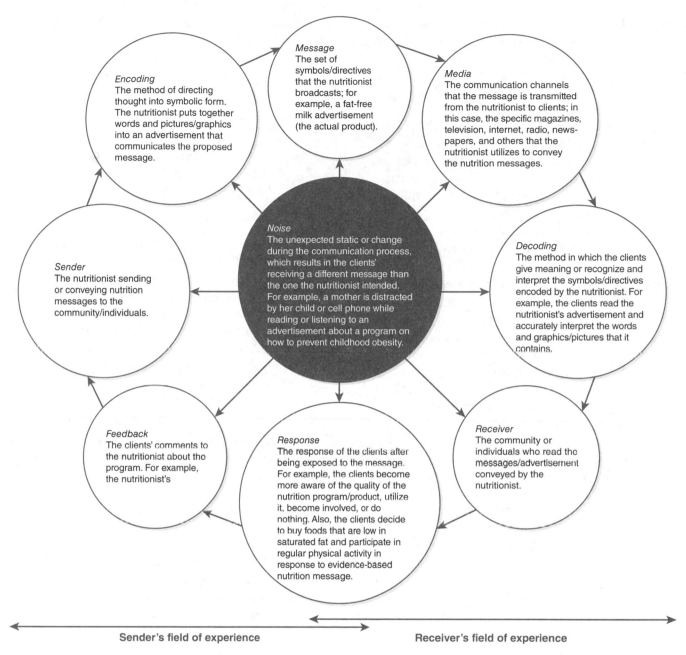

Noise
The unexpected static or change during the communication process, which results in the clients' receiving a different message than the one the nutritionist intended. For example, a mother is distracted by her child or cell phone while reading or listening to an advertisement about a program on how to prevent childhood obesity.

Message
The set of symbols/directives that the nutritionist broadcasts; for example, a fat-free milk advertisement (the actual product).

Encoding
The method of directing thought into symbolic form. The nutritionist puts together words and pictures/graphics into an advertisement that communicates the proposed message.

Media
The communication channels that the message is transmitted from the nutritionist to clients; in this case, the specific magazines, television, internet, radio, newspapers, and others that the nutritionist utilizes to convey the nutrition messages.

Sender
The nutritionist sending or conveying nutrition messages to the community/individuals.

Decoding
The method in which the clients give meaning or recognize and interpret the symbols/directives encoded by the nutritionist. For example, the clients read the nutritionist's advertisement and accurately interpret the words and graphics/pictures that it contains.

Feedback
The clients' comments to the nutritionist about the program. For example, the nutritionist's

Response
The response of the clients after being exposed to the message. For example, the clients become more aware of the quality of the nutrition program/product, utilize it, become involved, or do nothing. Also, the clients decide to buy foods that are low in saturated fat and participate in regular physical activity in response to evidence-based nutrition message.

Receiver
The community or individuals who read the messages/advertisement conveyed by the nutritionist.

Sender's field of experience          Receiver's field of experience

**FIGURE 17-2** The elements in the communication process.

Adapted from: Kotler P, Clark R. *Marketing for Healthcare Organizations: Steps in Market Segmentation, Targeting, and Positioning.* Englewood Cliffs, NJ: Prentice-Hall; 1987.

cost, both monetary and otherwise), 3) **place** (where and how it can be purchased), 4) **promotion** (how consumers learn about and are persuaded to use it), and 5) **positioning** (the way the consumer perceives the product or service relative to the nutritionist competition in the market).[23,34,35] The marketing mix can fit into the overall nutrition program plan.

Unlike the product of most businesses, the product in public health nutrition programs is not always concrete. In community nutrition, the product is a service to be delivered, such as nutrition information dissemination; diet counseling; food service consultation; food preparation demonstrations to different population groups,

including pregnant women, older persons, or college students; or provision of material such as low-fat cheese and soy milk.

Place is the second component of social marketing. It refers to the location where the exchange of service occurs. It also includes the distribution channels through which the product is made available to clients. Health departments, clinics, hospital outpatient departments, child daycare centers, Peace Meal Program sites, schools, and other similar facilities have served as distribution channels for nutrition programs and services. It is important to consider convenience so that clients can obtain products or services easily; for example, availability of transportation and access to parking such as handicapped parking. The service should be provided at an appropriate and convenient location.[35,36]

Price is the third component of social marketing. In business, price means setting a profitable price for a product that is acceptable to both consumers and the business. In social marketing, however, the interest is not financial gain, but instead the value of a service to society in terms of safety, health, or other social issues. There are three different pricing strategies in social marketing: 1) cost recovery, 2) market incentives, and 3) market disincentives.[36]

The request for donations for nutrition services could be considered a cost recovery strategy. Usually, the federal, state, or local government provides financial support for nutrition services, so a price may not need to be set for the product. Market incentives are used to stimulate the acceptance of a product. If the objective of a weight-control program is to increase the number of participants, the incentive could be $10 off the set price. The "buy-one-get-one-free" approach also appeals to many clients. Market disincentive pricing can be used to discourage clients from using a product. For instance, high taxes on cigarettes and liquor are attempts by the government to discourage their use. Another example of a market disincentive for a nutrition program could be higher prices for soft drinks rather than for fruit juices in vending machines on college campuses.[35,36]

The fourth social marketing perspective is promotion; this is the communication component of marketing. Promotion includes advertising, public relations, and consumer incentives. It informs the clients about the existence of a product or service.

**Advertising** is not a one-time activity. It involves a planned and continued series of activities known as an advertising campaign. To enhance the effectiveness of the promotion, the purpose of the campaign must be clear. The media used for advertising can include television, radio, newspapers, magazines, brochures, billboards, posters, booths at health fairs, and newsletters.[35,37]

The fifth perspective is position. The dietitian can position his or her services' strengths in relation to those of other providers. The benefits might include convenience, low cost, high credibility, guarantees, quick results, emotional support, or a high degree of control.[35,38] For instance, eating a variety of foods could be repositioned as an opportunity for choice instead of dieting. Serving low-fat meals to one's family could be positioned as an act of love.[39]

Taking into account each of the 5 Ps of marketing helps develop an action-oriented and effective nutrition program plan. A quality product offered in a convenient place at an economical price and promoted with an appealing message will be successful.[36]

In addition, each of the 5 Ps should be seen from the consumer's perspective. The 5 Ps concept considers only the seller's viewpoint of the market. The transformation of the 5 Ps to the consumer's perspective is accomplished by converting the Ps into the following Cs[22,29,35]:

| | |
|---|---|
| Product | Customer solution |
| Price | Customer cost |
| Place | Convenience |
| Promotion | Communication |
| Positioning | Change |

Hence, whereas marketers view themselves as selling a product or service, customers see themselves as buying value or a solution to their problems. Consumers are interested in more than the price; they are interested in the total costs of acquiring and utilizing a service. Consumers want the product and service to be as conveniently available as possible. They also want two-way communication and they want change, to experience something new and exciting. The change, however, must be relevant, slightly subtle, and not drastic.[22]

## Social Marketing at the Community Level

Community-based social marketing (CBSM) is a way to plan and communicate a message to achieve maximum impact with limited resources. One example of CBSM is the Honduran Ministry of Health's actions to reduce infant mortality in Honduras.[40] The ministry collaborated with the Academy for Educational Development (AED) to develop a comprehensive public education campaign. The project was designed to deliver information for the home treatment of infant diarrhea, to demonstrate the proper preparation and administration techniques of oral rehydration therapy (ORT), and to introduce a significant portion of Honduras' isolated rural populace to diarrhea-related prevention behaviors.

After considerable investigation of the medical and social issues being addressed and preparation of the instructional and training tools, the AED's Mass Media and Health Practices Program was launched.[40] The program operated in a site that included a representative population of 400,000 individuals. The campaign began by providing 900 healthcare workers with 4 to 8 hours of ORT training. The training program concentrated on teaching the proper mixing and administration of ORT salts and instructing other village assistants, who would finally have to conduct the same exercises directly with rural families. The program trainees used props and training dummies repeatedly to practice each step of the mixing and administration processes. The health workers and village trainees then began instructing mothers and grandmothers on ORT and other health behaviors such as breastfeeding, infant food preparation, and personal hygiene. When rural families completed their ORT training, a flag was posted at their house to let other mothers in the area know where they could obtain health advice and instruction.

A media campaign was implemented as the training program was being conducted to reinforce the healthcare instruction effort. The campaign developed print materials and radio advertisements to issue basic messages related to the diarrhea rehydration therapy and the AED training program. The messages emphasized the correct administration of oral rehydration salts (Litrosol) and the continuation of breastfeeding during infant diarrhea periods and encouraged mothers to seek medical assistance if a child's condition deteriorated. Posters and flipcharts were also created to illustrate ORT and to deliver supporting messages. The radio advertisements were placed in 30- to 60-second spot announcements and often included some form of jingle, slogan, or song. Many of the ads included a familiar announcer, the program's spokesman for technical information, who subsequently became a nationally known figure.

The tone of the campaign was serious, straightforward, and caring. It successfully promoted a mother-craft concept, where a mother's current actions and beliefs are supported and the program's health techniques become an added complement to her caregiving regimen. ORT training was presented as a new development in modern medicine: the latest remedy for lost appetite and a recovery aid.

One year after the implementation of the mass media program, an evaluation was conducted by Stanford University to chart the project's impact. A data sample was collected from 750 randomly selected families from more than 20 communities. The results were as follows[40]:

- The diarrhea rehydration project was very successful in both disseminating important health information and promoting specific changes in behavior related to treating infant diarrhea.
- The infant mortality rates for children under 5 years of age decreased from 47.5 to 25 percent.
- Ninety-three percent of the mothers sampled from rural Honduras knew that the program's radio campaign was promoting Litrosol, the brand name of the locally packaged ORS used to treat diarrhea.
- Seventy-one percent could recite the radio jingle used to promote the administration of liquids during diarrhea affliction.

In addition, Snow and Benedict[41] used social marketing to carry out a nutrition education program for teens in Nevada. The purpose of the program was to increase the teens' consumption of nutrient-dense foods, including fruits and vegetables, low-fat dairy foods, and whole grains. The researchers emphasized two concepts

of social marketing in their study: exchange theory and the 5 Ps of positioning product, price, place, and promotion. Exchange theory proposes that true marketing occurs when the provider and consumer voluntarily trade (or exchange) resources.[42-44]

A focus group interview was used to collect data from the participants. The teens described their perceptions about the benefits and barriers of consuming select nutrient-dense foods, such as dark-green leafy and deep-yellow vegetables, fruits, low-fat dairy foods, and whole grains, and their preferences for learning about foods and nutrition. The content was specific to nutrition education and Nevada youth, but it is applicable to a wide range of health behaviors and social conditions. It also has relevance for community and public health educators. See the Successful Community Strategies feature in this chapter for a description of a successful community marketing strategy.

Results showed that the participants named sodas, candies, chips, and sweets (the *products*) when they were asked what made it harder for them to consume nutrient-dense foods or beverages. Participants' perceptions about *place* included the belief that their food choices were limited to what parents and cafeteria workers purchased, prepared, and served to them. To reduce *price*, the participants suggested altering or disguising the taste of less favored foods by adding vegetables to soups, salads, and/or casseroles; serving cookies or quick breads with milk; and adding milk to cereal. The participants named several locations for *promotion* of nutrition information including cafeterias, schools, libraries, nurses' offices, classrooms, after-school programs, and walking routes to and from school. Also mentioned were community centers such as parks, gyms, swimming pools, public libraries, and Boys and Girls Clubs; retail and commercial outlets such as grocery and convenience stores, malls, and movie theatres; and public agencies, including health centers and clinics.

## ▶ E-Professionalism

**New media** is a general description of emerging technologies that allow for customization, interactivity, and a unique presentation of information. Community and public health nutritionists incorporating new media elements in electronic communications can be an effective method of increasing the impact of nutrition marketing and communication activities. Examples of interactive media include blogs, social networking, viral videos, Twitter, and Facebook. **E-professionalism** is the natural progression toward the use of electronic communication, including the Internet, cell phones and Blackberries, and social networking sites such as

Facebook, Twitter, and others, by professionals, including community and public health nutritionists.[45]

According to the Academy of Nutrition and Dietetics' (AND's) 2008 Nutrition Trends survey,[46] Americans obtain most of their food and nutrition information from television and magazines; however, there has been a substantial increase in the use of the Internet as a source of information. The Internet is the third most-often named source of information, replacing newspapers. In addition, new applications for the iPhone and iPad make it possible for diabetic clients to track their blood sugar levels and share that log with registered dietitians or physicians. The use of electronic communication such as Facebook and LinkedIn can make it easy to organize, promote, and share information; for example, the AND's current president used an election campaign page on Facebook. The AND also has a presence on Facebook and Twitter to provide the public with up-to-date evidence-based information.[46]

There is also evidence of increased client satisfaction and compliance online when that experience is interactive. For example, according to Deborah Tate et al.,[47] who conducted a research study at the University of North Carolina at Chapel Hill, clients lost more weight in on-line programs that offered e-mail support than clients simply directed to resources. Many professionals have embraced interactive websites, Facebook, Twitter, and blogs as convenient tools for this purpose.

Although these new technologies provide professionals another method of communicating and interacting with clients, it is important to consider the consequences, which may be personal, professional, or potentially legal, depending on the information and situation. The lines between personal and professional information shared electronically may become blurry, requiring caution. Maintaining a client's confidentiality is still essential.[45] It is vital that nutritionists review and abide by the AND Code of Ethics while using the new media to deliver effective nutrition programs.

## ▶ Advertising the Program

Advertising basics include advertising principles, developing attention-getting advertisements, collaborating with an agency to develop the advertisements, and choosing forms of media to use.[4] Advertising is one of the methods nutritionists can use to promote nutrition information to the targeted community. The direct effect of advertising on community participation in a nutrition program is not possible to determine. Despite this ambiguity, it is ~~important~~ to fulfill two advertising objectives: publicize [the] program and increase the demand for the program.[4]

The nutritionist needs to determine the best forms of advertising for the community nutrition promotion program and also determine the types of advertising that might best reach the community (newspapers, radio, television, magazines, direct mail, brochures, fliers, displays, or word of mouth).[4]

When advertising a health promotion program, consider the following principles[4,48,49]:

- Base the advertisement on the consumer's needs.
- Circulate the advertisement only to the target population.
- Provide background information about the program and update when the program changes.
- Request free public service announcements (PSAs) about the program. Ask public service directors to help raise awareness by airing them. (See more on PSAs later in this section.)
- Inform all media representatives as to why the story is timely and interesting (newsworthy), local (relates directly to the community), and important (the public needs to know this).
- Position the program as if you are the first to provide such services.

## Developing Attention-Getting Advertisements

Appropriate advertisement of a program is essential. The following are effective campaign techniques[4,34,50-52]:

- Use a slogan that is easily remembered, such as "Smoke-Free Forever" or "No More Dieting to Lose Weight."
- Test market the slogan on a sample population of the targeted group (e.g., the elderly, young adults, women of menopause age).
- Begin the headline of the advertisement with a question, such as "Which method to stop smoking do you prefer?" or "How would you like to lose weight?" Use a headline that will get the reader's attention.
- Put the program in perspective: 1) the time that is required, 2) the money or payment required, and 3) the effort the person will need to expend to get the desired reward.
- Describe the time commitment that will be required, such as "It will take 30 minutes a day for the next 10 weeks to stop smoking, but you will be free from smoking (or overeating, stress, arguing with your family) for the rest of your life. This could be the best 5-hour commitment you've ever made."
- Evaluate the advertisement periodically by asking people who enrolled how they heard about the program.

## Public Service Announcements

The nutritionist can communicate an important health promotion message fast to wide and diverse audiences or to a specific population using public service announcements (PSAs) for radio or television. Local TV or radio stations air PSAs during unsold blocks of advertising time or during station breaks. Contact station managers and public service directors after writing your PSAs.[4]

### PSAs

Radio PSAs are 10, 20, or 30 seconds long. It is important to note that broadcasters usually speak at the rate of 155 words per minute, so use that to gauge how long your message/copy should be. The following are examples of how to determine the lengths of PSAs[4]:

- 10-second PSA = 20 to 25 words
- 15-second PSA = 30 to 35 words
- 20-second PSA = 40 to 50 words
- 30-second PSA = 60 to 75 words

### Television PSAs

You will need to keep the message shorter for television PSAs than for radio PSAs. Television PSAs can be 8, 13, or 18 seconds long; 8- or 13-second spots are good for reminders. Keeping the message short will make it easier for you to obtain a time slot and prevent cutoff or mistimed PSAs. When writing a television PSA, use the same procedures as for radio, but add sight and additional sounds.[4] Including sound in radio ads may divert the listeners' attention from the main message and reduce the impact of the message. Prepare videotapes or slides with announcer copy that deliver action and include a soundtrack. See example at https://www.joe.org/joe/1986summer/iw1.php. Guidelines for developing television PSAs are as follows[4]:

- Repeat the main message as many times as possible and provide the main point at the end.
- Advocate a specific action; for example, make your ice cream cone a single, not a double dip.
- Express the problems, behaviors, or skills; for example, climb the stairs instead of riding the elevator.
- Be straightforward.
- Use music or sound effects to increase recall.
- Use only a few characters.

**BOX 17-2** presents the script for television public service announcement.

## ▶ Food Industries, Advertising, and Food Choices

It has been well established that food industries influence food choices through intensive advertising.[52] For

---

**BOX 17-2** Script for Television Public Service Announcement[4]

**Visual/Sound Idea**

Visual:–Picture of Protein-Energy Malnourished children with swollen abdomen and brittle hair

**Sound:** Whining cry
**Time:** 18 seconds
**Subject:** Effect of Hunger

**Voice Script**

Daily nutritious foods are essential to health and can prevent malnutrition.

---

the purposes of this chapter, food industries include companies that produce, process, manufacture, sell, and serve foods and beverages. They also include the food service sector, food carts, vending machines, restaurants, bars, fast food outlets, schools, hospitals, prisons, and workplaces. Food and food service companies spend more than $11 billion annually on direct media advertising (ads) in magazines, newspapers, radio, television, and billboards and twice as much on incentive coupons and fees paid to retailers for space on supermarket shelves.[53] The effectiveness of food and beverage advertising is attributed to its omnipresence as well as to the sophistication of the agencies that produce it.[54]

Research shows that approximately four of every five Americans think there is a relationship between diet and health,[55,56] and 57 percent are aware of the benefits of a healthy diet.[57] In addition, over half of shoppers reported actively seeking diet and nutrition information,[57] and 41 percent of Americans felt that they were doing their best to eat healthfully.[58]

Food companies' advertising costs for any single, nationally distributed food product are higher (often by 10 to 50 times) than federal expenditures for promotion of MyPlate or to encourage people to eat more fruits and vegetables. Therefore, it is very important for the federal government to provide more funds to encourage healthy eating habits. For example, McDonald's spent $627.2 million compared to $300 million that the USDA spends annually on nutrition education, most goes to research projects, the educational components of agricultural extension, and other activities that target relatively few people.[52]

## The Use of Advertising

Successful campaigns are carefully researched, targeted to specific groups, and repeated frequently. Food sales increase with the intensity, repetition, and visibility of the advertising messages.[59,60] A study that evaluated the preference, recall accuracy, and consumption behavior of boys ages 8 to 10 showed that their preferences were a result of advertising repetition.[61] The children were exposed to repetitive or varied 30-second television commercials for the same ice cream product during a half-hour show. Results indicated that a single exposure was sufficient to affect brand name recall in almost 50 percent of the children. Increasing exposure and varying the commercials also had a positive influence on the boys' product preference and consumer behavior.

The promotion of nutritional advantages (low-fat, no cholesterol, high-fiber, and calcium-added) and the use of health claims (lowers cholesterol, prevents cancer) can increase sales. When Kellogg's high-fiber cereals first added health claims about cancer prevention and dietary fiber to their package labels, sales escalated 47 percent within the first 6 months.[62] It is important for nutritionists to verify every health claim made by food companies because they may not be accurate or substantiated. For example, in March 2005, the Federal Trade Commission (FTC) reached a settlement with Tropicana Products about its advertisements that claimed its Healthy Heart orange juice could reduce blood pressure, cholesterol, and homocysteine levels. The advertisements appeared on television and in print publications including *Newsweek* and the *New York Times* between 2002 and early 2004. The FTC asserted that Tropicana's health claims were unproved and that it had no clinical support for the claims.[63]

Trade association programs also promote generic advertising, such as the "Got Milk?" campaign. One of the promotions features celebrities wearing milk mustaches. Analysis of sales data showed that these campaigns slowed or stopped the decreasing trend of milk consumption and that 47 pounds of milk were purchased for each advertising dollar spent on these campaigns.[64] Thus, consumers can change their perceptions of foods and food choices when given repeated and positive nutrition messages.

For every $4 spent on advertising, the food companies spend another $2 on discount incentives, for example, providing coupons for consumers and "slotting fees" for retailers to ensure space on supermarket shelves. In total, food companies spend more than $33 billion annually to advertise and promote their products to the public.[52]

There is a disproportionate distribution of marketing expenditures relative to dietary recommendations. Food industries spend more money on advertising to promote highly processed, elaborately packaged fast foods than the government does to market nutritious foods. About 70 percent of food advertising is for convenience foods, candy and snacks, alcoholic beverages, soft drinks, and desserts, whereas only 2.2 percent is for fruits, vegetables, grains, or beans.

In 2009, manufacturers introduced slightly more than 19,047 new products.[52] More than two thirds of those products were condiments, candies and snacks, baked goods, soft drinks, and dairy products (cheese products and ice cream novelties). Slightly more than one fourth were "nutritionally enhanced" and could be marketed as low in fat, cholesterol, salt, or sugar or as higher in fiber, calcium, or vitamins. Some of these products, such as no-fat cookies, vitamin-enriched cereals, and calcium-fortified juice drinks, were high in sugar content. Though these products contain some essential nutrients, it is important to note that a high intake of sugar promotes weight gain and contributes to long-term health and chronic disease risks.

## Successful Community Strategies

### National WIC Breastfeeding Promotion Project[40]

The National Special Supplemental Nutrition Program for Women, Infants, and Children (WIC) Breastfeeding Promotion Project created a marketing plan using the conceptual framework of the 4 Ps of marketing (product, price, place, and promotion) to reposition the product (breastfeeding). The program changed the traditional health benefits of breastfeeding to emphasize a new product, mothers' emotional bonding with the infant from breastfeeding.

A survey of pregnant women identified that embarrassment and conflicts with active lifestyles (price) were the constraints to breastfeeding. To reduce these constraints or price, a counseling program was developed to help mothers deal with the individual limitations. The place strategy targeted hospital environments as well as homes. It focused on the main intermediaries such as professional associations. The majority of the promotion strategy consisted of media and grassroots advocacy, with media stressing a congratulatory tone and by speaking to family spokespersons. Television and radio advertisements, billboards, posters, educational pamphlets, information booklets, and staff support kits with resource information and promotional materials were used for this program, which ran from August 1997 to August 2000. This program did not apply the 5th P (position) of social marketing in the project, but the nutritionist could position breastfeeding as an act of love instead of a type of infant feeding.

*(continues)*

## Successful Community Strategies *(continued)*

The four goals established for the program were increasing breastfeeding initiation rates, increasing the rate of breastfeeding duration among WIC participants, increasing referrals to the WIC program for breastfeeding support, and increasing the general public's knowledge of and support for breastfeeding.

In order to maximize the impact for each of the program's objectives, WIC clients were solicited to participate in the study. The targeted population for the campaign was organized into three separate audiences. The primary target audience was composed of pregnant European American, African American, and Hispanic American women who either were enrolled as WIC participants or met the income eligibility requirements (annual income below 185 percent of the U.S. poverty guidelines). The secondary audience consisted of individuals who might influence the primary target population, such as the mothers, husbands, and boyfriends of pregnant women; prenatal healthcare providers; and WIC staff. The general public were also included as the tertiary audience in order to change the established social norms and prevailing public perception regarding breastfeeding.

The campaign planners chose 10 pilot areas in which to conduct research and demonstrate the initial WIC Breastfeeding Promotion Project: Arkansas, California, the Chickasaw Nation, Iowa, Mississippi, Nevada, New Jersey, New York, Ohio, and West Virginia. Preliminary results from the Iowa study showed evidence of the program's success in both breastfeeding rates and changed attitude and awareness toward breastfeeding. The Iowa evaluation was based on the Ross Six Months Mothers' Infant Feeding Survey and a separate mail survey of WIC participants immediately before the campaign and 4 months afterward. Results showed:

- Breastfeeding rates for mothers while in the hospital increased from 57.8 to 64.4 percent, and a year after the promotion started they increased to 65.1 percent.
- The rates for women still nursing 6 months after birth increased from 20.4 to 29.3 percent and to 32.2 percent a year after the program started.

A major objective of the public information component of the National WIC Breastfeeding Promotion Project's Loving Support Campaign was to encourage the spouses, relatives, and friends of pregnant women to provide support for breastfeeding. A survey of the Iowa participants showed that support for breastfeeding increased in every relationship category:

- Support from the pregnant woman's mother increased from 35.2 to 53 percent.
- Support from the pregnant woman's husband or boyfriend increased from 47.7 to 53 percent.
- Support from the pregnant woman's friends or other relatives increased from 48.8 to 51.1 percent.
- Support from the pregnant woman's prenatal healthcare provider increased from 62.4 to 83.8 percent and from WIC employees from 81.9 percent to 92.5 percent.

## ▶ The Role of Media in Childhood Obesity

Childhood obesity is now an epidemic in the United States. The number of children who are overweight has doubled in the last two to three decades; currently one child in five is overweight. The increase is in both children and adolescents and in all age, race, and gender groups. According to the Centers for Disease Control and Prevention (CDC), since 1980, the proportion of overweight children ages 6 to 11 has more than doubled and the rate for adolescents has tripled.[65]

Children younger than 5 years view an average of more than 40,000 television commercials for food each year, or about 30 hours' worth.[66] Research studies show that viewing of television advertisements for foods of low nutritional quality is what leads to obesity, not television watching in isolation.[67] Consistent with expectations that children's cognitive ability to understand advertising differs by age approximately before

and after age 7 years, a slightly stronger association of commercial content with obesity before 7 years of age than after was reported.[67]

### Advertising to Children and Youth

There has been an explosion of media targeting children during the same period in which childhood obesity has increased. Children of all ages spend a large amount of their leisure time using a combination of various media, including broadcast television, cable networks, DVDs, video games, computers, the Internet, and cell phones. Children 6 years and under also spend as much time with screen media (TV, videos, video games, and computers) as they do playing outside.[68] Much of the media targeted to children is loaded with elaborate advertising campaigns, many of which promote foods such as candy, soda, and snacks. It is estimated that the typical child sees about 40,000 ads a year on TV alone.[7,69]

Exposure to these media affects children's choices and may have a strong influence on their tendency toward increased obesity and chronic disease risk. Television advertising can affect children's food and nutrition-related knowledge and purchase decisions, both those made directly and those made indirectly through parents. Annual sales of foods and beverages to young consumers exceeded $27 billion in 2002. Food and beverage advertisers collectively spend $10 billion to $12 billion a year to reach children and youth. Of that, more than $1 billion is spent on media advertising to children through television; more than $4.5 billion is spent on youth-targeted promotions such as premiums, coupons, sweepstakes, and contests; $2 billion is spent on youth-targeted public relations; and $3 billion is spent on packaging designed for children.[69]

The CDC launched the VERB campaign to encourage a more active lifestyle for teenagers ages 9 to 13. The campaign used advertising, marketing, online material, and on-the-ground events to get the message to youth, parents, and educators. The National Cancer Institute's Fruits and Veggies—More Matters program is designed to promote fruits and vegetables[70] and also includes a media component. However, these campaigns are very modest compared to those mounted by the food industry. The entire budget for the Fruits & Veggies—More Matters effort is $3.5 million a year, compared to $29 million in advertising for Pringles, $74 million for M&Ms, $209 million for Coke, and $665 million for McDonald's.[69]

## Exposure to Media

Although advertising has not been linked directly to childhood obesity, advertisements targeted to children through multiple media channels contribute to children's choices about foods, beverages, and a sedentary lifestyle. During the 1996 to 1997 school year, Stanford University researchers conducted a randomized controlled trial in which they reduced the amount of time a group of about 100 third and fourth graders in northern California spent with TV, videos, and video games.[71] Two matched elementary schools were selected to participate, one of which served as the control group. The intervention involved a "turnoff" period of no screen time for 10 days followed by limiting TV time to 7 hours per week as well as learning media literacy skills to teach selective viewing. At the end of a 6-month, 18-lesson classroom curriculum, students who received the intervention achieved a statistically significant reduction in their television viewing and number of meals eaten in front of the TV set, as well as decreases in body mass index (BMI), triceps skinfold thickness, waist circumference, and waist-to-hip ratio. Although these changes were not accompanied by reduced high-fat food intake or increased physical activity, the findings do seem to show

the feasibility of decreasing body weight by reducing time spent with screen media.[65]

The Kaiser Family Foundation report, "It's Child's Play: Advergaming and the Online Marketing of Food to Children," shows the increasing popularity of advergaming, a new type of advertising.[71] Advergaming is the use of online video games with embedded brand messages to engage a target audience. It is specifically designed to blur the boundary between advertising and entertainment.[72] The food industry is spending millions of dollars on this new form of advertising because it is very effective. The Kaiser Family Foundation reported in 2006 that there were an astonishing 12.2 million visits to advergaming sites in just 3 months by children ages 2 to 11.

Food companies know that children make highly lucrative customers, and their attention to this group has increased significantly. Children control increasing amounts of money, and society has granted them responsibility for purchasing decisions. It is difficult to know exactly how much money children now control from allowances, gifts, and jobs, but even small amounts add up to a very large amount when computed across the entire population. Studies in the late 1980s reported that children spent an average of $4.42 per week each, for a combined total of more than $6 billion a year, and that they influenced annual family spending decisions involving $50 billion in 1985, about $190 billion in 1997, and about $290 billion in 2000.[73] The amount controlled by children increases with age; children ages 7 to 12 have been reported to control $8.9 billion in spending money and teenagers $119 billion; in 2003 teens spent a projected $112.5 billion dollars. Overall, children ages 6 to 19 years were thought to have influenced $485 billion in purchase decisions in 1999.[73,74] Children also influence a substantial proportion of the total annual sales of certain foods: 25 percent of the total amount of salty snacks, 30 percent of soft drinks, 40 percent of frozen pizza, 50 percent of cold cereals, and 60 percent of canned pasta.[73,75]

One recent trend is an increase in programs designed especially for young children. Many of these children's television programs are linked directly to commercial products. For instance, Burger King first and later McDonald's sponsored *Teletubbies*, a public television program for toddlers. McDonald's distributed toys representing the show's four characters.

One study of the top-ranked prime-time shows (8 PM to 11 PM) in the 1988 TV season found that food references occurred almost 10 times per hour and that the majority (60 percent) were for low-nutrient beverages such as coffee, soft drinks, and alcohol. Most foods eaten were snacks (72 percent) and tended to be sweet (44 percent) or salty snacks (25 percent), with vegetables significantly behind (6 percent).[76] A decade later, by the 1998 TV season, a content analysis of the highest-ranked prime-time shows found little improvement. The highest-rated programs among 2- to 5-year-olds contained a reference to food in every episode, and one third had 16 or more references. At this rate, it was estimated that the average child viewer might see more than 500 food references per week, almost one third for empty-calorie foods high in fat, sugar, or salt and another one quarter for nutrient-rich foods also high in fat, sugar, and salt.[77]

Channel One is a 12-minute television program beamed into 12,000 schools throughout the United States and viewed daily by about 8.3 million students. Two minutes of every program is devoted to commercials. The private company responsible for Channel One provides television sets and installation of hardware estimated to be worth about $17,000 for the entire school. In exchange, the company requires students in 80 percent of the classrooms to watch the program on 90 percent of school days for the year.[78]

A study of advertisements appearing on Saturday morning TV in the United States found that 44 percent were for fats, oils, and sugar; 23 percent were for highly sugared cereals; and 11 percent were for fast food restaurants.[79,80] None were for fruits and vegetables. The authors concluded that the diet being presented on Saturday morning television does not support the recommendation for healthful eating for children. Similar findings were reported for Canadian TV.[81]

Based on children's commercial recall and because they lack the skills to understand the differences between information and advertising, there is not enough evidence of adverse impact of food, beverage, and entertainment advertising on children to support calling for a ban on all such advertising.

## Product Branding

Branding is an advertising technique designed to establish recognition and positive associations with a company name or product, and the aim is to create lifelong customers rather than generating immediate sales.[82] Brand recognition starts as early as 2 years of age, especially when cartoon (Tony the Tiger) or cartoonish (Ronald McDonald) licensed characters are used to market products that are mostly junk food. Promotional positions on advertisement-supported (Nickelodeon) and sponsor-supported (Public Broadcasting Service and Disney) networks use similar approaches and appeals, seeming to equate foods with fun and happiness.[70]

Although styles and approaches differed somewhat between the two sponsor-supported networks and the single advertisement-supported network, the overarching messages were the same. For example, the Chuck E. Cheese advertisements that appear on PBS,

with scenes of jumping, running, and laughing children, were not mainly about promoting an active lifestyle, but seemed to focus on creating warm feelings for parents about what a wholesome, child-oriented place Chuck E. Cheese is and helping children equate the restaurant and its licensed character with fun and happiness.[70]

In addition, the advertising industry plays an influential role in the growth and development of digital media content and services.[83] Advertising agencies, market research firms, and new media companies collaborate with major advertisers (with significant representation from food and beverage corporations) to develop technical standards for all new media delivery platforms, including mobile, online gaming, video, and social networks, to ensure the efficacy of these initiatives.[84] They combine research from a broad range of disciplines, including the following[85,86]:

- Semantics
- Artificial intelligence
- Action theory
- Social network and behavioral analysis
- Data mining and statistical modeling
- Neuroscience

Several of these research and development efforts are focused on interactive marketing technologies designed for adolescents and youth.[86] Hence, interactive marketing's ability to reach and influence consumers continues to grow as advertising industries incorporate knowledge from semantics, artificial intelligence, neuroscience, and many other scholarly fields.[87]

Constance Pechmann et al.[88] reviewed research within the fields of neuroscience, psychology, and marketing and identified several biological and psychosocial attributes of the adolescent experience that may make them more susceptible to certain kinds of marketing.[88] For example, scientists studying the development of the adolescent brain have found that the prefrontal cortex, which controls inhibitions, does not fully mature until late adolescence or early adulthood.[89-92] Children's bodies also experience hormonal changes as they reach puberty. This makes them more receptive to stressful environmental stimuli and at the same time experience intense urges they have not yet acquired the ability to control. Consequently, they are inclined to act impulsively when they are experiencing negative mood states.[93] This has made them vulnerable to a multitude of new marketing strategies (including viral marketing, brand engagement, and advergames) in which adolescents are increasingly subjected to implied subtle persuasion. For example, in games, food advertisers can direct personalized advertising messages at the most intense points in the games when users are in high states of encouragement, offering immediate gratification through online purchases and triggering mood-enhanced impulsive behaviors.[93] By using a growing array of sophisticated behavioral tracking tools, companies can forge intimate, ongoing relationships with individual teens.[93] The growing use of neuroscience by marketers suggests that digital advertising is increasingly designed to foster emotional and unconscious choices, rather than reasoned, thoughtful decision making.[91,92] In addition, through social media marketing, brands can insert themselves strategically into the complex web of adolescent social relationships, leveraging the power of peer pressure to promote their soft drinks, candies, and snack foods. Major food and beverage companies, including Kraft, Pepsi, and Taco Bell, are among the pioneers of this new marketing strategy. Also, Coca-Cola, McDonald's, Burger King, and Kentucky Fried Chicken have incorporated these elements into their interactive marketing strategies.[70]

## Barriers to the Prevention of Obesity

It is reported that Americans spend about half of their food budget and consume about one third of their daily energy on meals and drinks consumed outside the home, which makes it very difficult to estimate the energy content of the food.[94] About 170,000 fast-food restaurants[95] and 3 million soft-drink vending machines[96] help ensure that Americans are not more than a few steps from immediate sources of relatively nonnutritious foods.

Food eaten outside the home, on average, is higher in fat and lower in micronutrients than food prepared at home.[95] Many popular table-service restaurant meals for lunch or dinner provide 1,000 to 2,000 kcal each,[97] amounts equivalent to 35 to 100 percent of a full day's energy requirements for most adults.[98] Restaurants and movie theaters charge just a few cents more for larger orders of soft drinks, popcorn, and French fries, and the standard serving sizes of these and other foods have increased greatly in the past decade.[99] For example, in the 1950s, Coca-Cola was packaged only in 6.5-oz bottles; single-serving containers expanded first to 12-oz cans and, more recently, to 20-oz bottles. A 12-oz soft drink provides about 150 kcal, all from sugars, but contains no other nutrients of significance.[100]

Consequently, dietetics professionals must emphasize the need to select appropriate portion sizes. Nutrition education is critical because few consumers intuitively know that 3 oz of beef is considered an appropriate portion size. Choosing sensible portion sizes is a basic principle of the 2015 *Dietary Guidelines for Americans*.[101]

If a person thinks that a restaurant portion of broiled beef rib steak (8 oz) is the most appropriate portion size, he or she would be getting a caloric content that is far higher (500 kcal) than the 188 kcal from MyPlate's recommended 3-oz portion. Therefore, it is imperative that the message of appropriate portion sizes be incorporated into the total diet approach.

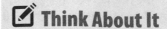

### Think About It

How can nutritionists use advertising to increase consumers' intake of healthy foods such as fruits and vegetables?

## ▶ Public Health Approaches

Effective interventions are needed to deal with the ways people make food choices. Such interventions require the implementation of policies, especially by the government. Health protection through legislative and fiscal means is more likely to make a greater impact.

The government has a variety of powers at its disposal that can be put into service. One approach, which relies entirely on voluntary cooperation, is to issue policy statements. However, these can easily amount to no more than hollow declarations, as is illustrated by government policies on tobacco in many countries. On the other hand, policy statements can serve as the basis for a call to action. For instance, British and U.S. government policy on diet and disease, in conjunction with the media and medical science, helped change the climate of opinion so that it is now widely accepted that diets should be much lower in fat and richer in fiber.[102] In March 2009, the U.S. Congress passed a federal appropriations bill that established an Interagency Working Group on Food Marketed to Children. With representatives from several federal agencies, the group is charged with studying and developing recommendations for standards for food marketing directed to youth under the age of 17 years.[87]

### The Effect of Price on Sales

The most common among available government powers are legislation and the use of taxation and subsidies. Action on tobacco control showed the necessity for using these powers as a tool of health promotion. Educational efforts over the last three decades have been very important in persuading millions of people to stop smoking, but smoking rates are still well above half of the level of 30 years ago.[103] There is convincing evidence that price hikes are an effective means to reduce smoking rates.[104] It was estimated that a 10 percent increase in price reduces tobacco consumption by about 5 percent, especially among lower socioeconomic groups.[105] In Canada, the prevalence of smoking in young Canadians was reduced by half during the 1980s due to the doubling of the price of cigarettes. This trend was reversed in the early 1990s when the price was decreased in an attempt to reduce smuggling from the United States.[106] Price increases appear to be a more effective means of tobacco control than education or media campaigns.[107]

## Government Policy and Food

It seems that government policies about food prices and, to a lesser extent, food advertising and labeling may be an effective means to induce desirable changes in eating patterns. The following are some specific suggestions as to how existing government policies can be modified to encourage diets higher in fruits and vegetables and lower in fat[48,108]:

- There is always the possibility for improved food labels to facilitate the purchase of foods with a low-fat content, especially saturated fat. In addition, labeling and nutrition information needs to be improved in areas presently outside the system, especially restaurant menus, fast foods (McDonald's, Burger King, etc.), and fresh meat.

- By means of regulations and rewards, schools could be encouraged to sell meals of superior nutritional value while restricting the sale of junk food (calorie-dense foods). Similar policies could be applied to other institutions under government control, such as the military, prisons, and cafeterias in government offices.

- Television advertising could be regulated so as to control the content, duration, and frequency of commercials for unhealthy food products, especially when the target audience is children.

**BOX 17-3** presents additional suggestions to encourage healthy diets. Also, see "Successful Community Strategies: The Aptos Middle School (San Francisco, California) Pilot Program" in Chapter 9 for an example of a cafeteria and vending machine success story from the San Francisco Unified School District.

## Successful Nutrition Education Campaigns

Mass media advertising needs to be a vital part of any campaign to reduce obesity through the promotion of positive changes in behavior, such as eating more fruits, vegetables, and whole grains; switching to lower fat meat or dairy products; eating fewer hamburgers and steaks; and drinking water instead of soda. Campaigns of this kind can be remarkably effective. For instance, the Center for Science in the Public Interest's 1 Percent or Less program doubled the market share of low-fat and fat-free milk in several communities through an intensive, 7-week paid advertising and public relations campaign that cost as little as 22 cents per person.[109] Those efforts demonstrate that advertising can be an affordable, effective method for promoting dietary change. Media motivational campaigns can be developed to encourage people to walk, jog, bicycle, and engage in other enjoyable activities that expend energy.

---

**BOX 17-3** Options for Controlling Unhealthy Food Advertisements

- Ban advertising to preschoolers.
- Provide federal funding to state public health departments for mass media health promotion campaigns that emphasize healthful eating and physical activity patterns.
- Declare and organize an annual national "No TV" week.
- Use a National Nutrition Summit to develop a national campaign to prevent obesity.
- Ban advertisements of junk food to children.
- Conduct an FTC investigation into marketing of junk food to children.
- Provide equal time for messages on nutrition or fitness to counteract food ads in children's shows.
- Include parental warnings about the nutritional value of advertised foods.
- Repeal tax deductions for company expenses associated with advertising junk food products to children.
- Forbid food advertising in school-based TV programs, such as Channel One.
- Increase the use of popular media characters and celebrities to promote nutritious foods.

---

## Barriers Against Public Health Policies

Although many might consider the policies discussed here to be worthy of implementation, it must be noted that barriers exist. In particular, industries profit significantly from the sale of highly processed food and are often resistant to change. Therefore, industries often secure government support.[110]

The history of attempts to enact legislative control over tobacco show how effective an industry can be when it utilizes a large budget in attempts to delay, dilute, or stop laws. If the tobacco industry can achieve so many successes, it will be much easier for the food industry to prevent interventions that threaten its profits. This is because the relationship between diet and disease is less clear than is the case with tobacco. There is evidence of how industry has successfully pressured governments to bend to their wishes on questions of nutrition policy. As discussed by Nestle,[110,111] the meat industry has been effective in rewriting dietary guidelines. In the late 1970s, the recommendation was to reduce the amount of meat consumed; then the emphasis moved to eating lean meat. By 1992, people were encouraged to consume at least two or three servings daily. There is also evidence that the 1992 version of Canada's Food Guide was similarly modified under pressure from the food industry.[112]

# ▶ Approaches to Protecting Children

Professionals, including community and public health nutritionists, need to use media histories or similar tools in well-child visits to help parents recognize the extent of their children's television exposure. Encourage parents and caregivers to consider carefully the advertising messages targeting children every day. Other suggestions include[70]:

- *Family control:* Make families responsible for monitoring their children's activities.
- *Coregulation of the advertisements:* Government-approved set of laws agreed to by industry; monitoring and sanctioning role maintained by an industry-sponsored body.
- *Industry performance indictors:* Targets for changes; in practice set by government but executed by the industry.
- *School rules:* Single-institution regulations to restrict marketing (e.g., beverage vending, gifts of branded equipment).
- *Local regulations:* City, county, or state regulations and by-laws.
- *National regulations:* Legislative acts and regulations set at the national level.
- *International rules:* Conferences and regulations agreed upon through U.N. bodies such as the World Health Assembly to monitor the marketers through an agency such as the World Trade Organization.
- *Private litigation:* Individual or class actions taken against specified companies.

# ▶ Food and Nutrition Misinformation

It is unethical to promote questionable products or images or manipulate results to satisfy the food industry. Community nutritionists working with the media or food industry must consider the accuracy of the product descriptions and claims, words, and images so they do not misinform the public. The past decade has seen an increase in the promotion and use of questionable health practices, many of which are nutrition related. The main factor has been the ease of acquiring misinformation through the Internet.[1]

According to the AND's *Complete Food and Nutrition Guide*, health **fraud** is falsely promoting a product or health remedy for financial gain that does not work or has not been proved to work in improving health and well-being.[113] **Quackery** applies to food and nutrition-related products and is defined as the promotion of an unproved health product or service, usually for personal gain. Nutrition misinformation, fraud, and quackery are impediments to optimal health habits and positive eating behaviors.[33,114] The health consequences of food quackery, faddism, misinformation, or the misuse or misinterpretation of emerging science may include delay or failure to seek legitimate medical care or to continue essential treatment, undesirable drug–nutrient interactions, nutrient toxicities or toxic components of products, and interference with sound nutrition education and practices.[112] Economic harm occurs when supposed remedies, treatments, and cures fail to work and when products are purchased needlessly.[114] The burden of proof is now on the federal government, so there are fewer roadblocks to developing expensive and ineffective products.[112]

Americans spend more than 30 billion annually on medical and nutritional health fraud and quackery, up from $1 to $2 billion in the early 1960s.[115] At the same time, the sale of weight-loss programs and products, as well as sports drinks to improve performance, has increased. Media attention to nutritional supplements has exacerbated the problem. Another problem is that foods are being supplemented with specific minerals and vitamins for their disease-preventing properties, and this has directed the marketing of many products as nutritional remedies. This practice may prevent the consumer from obtaining appropriate medical treatment.

## Consumer Protection Laws

The Food, Drug, and Cosmetics Act defines a **drug** as any article (except devices) intended for use in the diagnosis, cure, mitigation, treatment, or prevention of disease and articles (other than food) intended to affect the structure or function of the body.[1] This act permits the U.S. Food and Drug Administration (FDA) to stop the marketing of products with unsubstantiated drug claims on their labels. **Dietary supplements** are one area of concern because of the rapid expansion of the market and changing federal regulations.[116,117] No longer limited to vitamins and minerals, overabundances of herbal, botanical, and sport supplements, along with other products, now comprise over half the dietary supplement industry and have helped sales increase by over 60 percent to $13.9 billion each year.[113,114,117] Consumer spending on dietary supplements, natural/organic foods, natural personal care products, and functional foods totaled $128 billion in 2000.[116] Herbs and botanicals, sports and meal supplements, and other specialty products account for slightly more than half of these sales,[118,119] yet only 12 percent of people use herbal supplements.[117] Many supplements, such as herbs, remain largely uncontrolled and unregulated so long as their labels contain no health claims. Over 1,000 new dietary supplements are added annually to the already available 29,000.[120,121]

The most logical definition of a dietary supplement is that of a product made of one or more of the essential nutrients, such as vitamins, minerals, and protein. The Dietary Supplement Health Education Act of 1994 established specific guidelines for health claims and the labeling of dietary supplements, but it also shifted the burden of proving the accuracy of claims, safety, and quality from the manufacturer to the FDA.[122] This shift toward having to prove harm rather than safety can potentially affect consumers by creating a weak sense of credibility leading to misinformation or fraud, because the federal government has not yet discovered or taken action against it. Monitoring the claims made by marketers of those products creates an overwhelming task for the FDA, which further delays the time when information can be retracted or products removed from the marketplace.[123]

## Sources of Nutrition Misinformation

Consumers receive nutrition information from a variety of sources. According to the AND's Nutrition and You: Trends 2011 survey, the media are the major source of information for consumers.[123] The top three leading sources of nutrition information for consumers were television (67 percent), magazines (41 percent), Internet (40 percent) and newspapers (20 percent). Other sources cited were doctors (16 percent), family and friends (16 percent), radio (13 percent), and books (11 percent). Five percent cited registered dietitians, nurses, nutritionists, grocery stores package labels and USDA's MyPlate.[123]

Multilevel marketing companies promote nutrition misinformation of unproven health products such as dietary supplements. Manufacturers of weight-loss products and herbs also often disseminate nutrition misinformation.[123] These companies claim their products can prevent or cure diseases. Their product literature may contain illegal therapeutic claims, or product distributors may supply such information through anecdotes and independently published literature.[121]

The AND provides support for members through its Knowledge Center, a leading source of scientifically based, objective food and nutrition information for dietetics professionals, the media, other healthcare providers, and researchers. The Knowledge Center provides practical, positive nutrition information to professionals and consumers through recorded nutrition messages, other publications, and the AND website, http://www.eatright.org, which offers a gateway to government agencies and many allied professional organizations that focus on nutrition and health.

The following are strategies nutritionists can follow when communicating accurate nutrition information to consumers[112,124]:

- Keep advice simple to understand and implement. Be brief.
- Avoid contributing to the public's confusion by being too quick to support the latest nutrition theory.
- Avoid speaking in nutrition buzzwords.
- React continually to prevent misinformation.
- Keep your nutrition messages positive.
- Stay current with the latest literature.
- Avoid going against the tide. Tie your nutrition message to current lifestyle trends.
- Avoid being an alarmist. If you constantly proclaim the danger of certain foods, people will soon believe that they are not dangerous.
- Acknowledge possible ethical conflicts.
- Avoid arguing with other health professionals about subjects that have been discussed for years with no conclusion in sight.
- Stay inside your area of expertise.
- Know your subject area.

# Learning Portfolio

## Chapter Summary

- Marketing is directed at satisfying the needs and wants of the consumer through an exchange of processes or activities (e.g., goods, products, or programs).
- Social marketing focuses on behavior change instead of sales or funds raised.
- Marketing research is the systematic design, collection, analysis, and reporting of data and findings relevant to a specific marketing situation or problem facing an organization.
- SWOT is an acronym for strengths, weaknesses, opportunities, and threats. It analyzes internal strengths and weaknesses and external opportunities and threats.
- Market segmentation is dividing a market or community into distinct groups of individuals on the basis of needs, characteristics, or behavior.
- Community nutritionists can communicate important health promotion messages to wide and diverse audiences or to a specific population by developing public service announcements.

- Some of the communication factors that may affect a nutrition program are perceptual distortions of information about nutrition, incorrect or improper use of words to convey specific information, lack of listening on the part of the targeted community, and differences in values and attitudes between the nutritionist and the target community.

- Successful nutrition education campaigns are carefully researched, targeted to specific groups, and repeated frequently.

- For every $1 they spend on advertising, food companies spend $2 on discount incentives, for example, coupons for consumers and "slotting fees" for retailers to ensure space on supermarket shelves.

- The entire budget for the Fruits & Veggies—More Matters campaign is $3.5 million a year, compared to $29 million in advertising for Pringles, $74 million for M&Ms, $209 million for Coke, and $665 million for McDonald's.

- Although advertising has not been linked directly to childhood obesity, advertisements targeted to children through multiple media channels contribute to children's choices about foods, beverages, and a sedentary lifestyle.

- On average, food eaten outside the home is higher in fat and lower in micronutrients than food prepared at home.

- Americans spend more than $30 billion annually on medical and nutritional health fraud and quackery.

- Some marketing companies promote nutrition misinformation of unproven health products, such as dietary supplements, weight loss products, and herbs.

## Critical Thinking Activities

- Watch Saturday morning children's TV programs for 1 hour and determine the number of times food products were advertised and the types of products being advertised during the programs. Use the findings for an in-class discussion.

- Review and present two research articles on nutrition misinformation.

- List at least two ways, beyond those discussed in this chapter, that nutritionists can receive free advertising.

- Identify three media outlets in which to advertise a nutrition program.

- Develop a 30-second radio PSA for Building Better Bones.

## 🔍 CASE STUDY 17-1: The Challenges of Providing Community Nutrition Education

Marcea, a professor of nutrition at a local university, received grant money from the Department of Public Health's Office of Women's Health to increase women's knowledge of osteoporosis and its prevention. Studies show that about 30 percent of the women in her community have osteoporosis. Dietary analysis showed low calcium, fluoride, vitamin D, vitamin A, and magnesium intake. The grant also included funds for screening women for osteoporosis. The budget allowed only $250 for advertising, and she is required to reach 400 women age 55 or older by the end of the year. The university is located in a county with an estimated total population of 156,800 residents. Women make up 51.9 percent or more of the population, and 9.7 percent of the population is 65 years or older.

Marcea called the program "Building Better Bones." She spent the $250 promoting Building Better Bones, but had reached only 200 participants 6 months into the program. To increase the number of women in the program, she found the free public announcement section in one of the local newspapers and placed an ad in its calendar of events. She also convinced a local produce stand to provide a small fruit basket in exchange for giving the stand's business card to the first 50 people who came to the lecture. Finally, she obtained a list of potential consumers who were interested in osteoporosis from the local YWCA and sent a flier to each woman with a free packet of wildflower seeds. Marcea's university provided the funding for mailing the fliers.

### Questions

1. Marketing the nutrition education program is very important to Marcea. What is a marketing plan? What are the contents of a marketing plan?
2. What market research should Marcea conduct? Market research and situational analysis helped Marcea identify whether the targeted community will be interested in the program. What is market attractiveness, as discussed in this book?
3. Briefly describe the qualitative and quantitative research that Marcea may use to collect data for her program.
4. What are the steps in market segmentation, targeting, and positioning that helped Marcea?

*(continues)*

5. Marcea reviewed the nine elements of communication devised by Kotler and Armstrong[22] before designing the nutrition education program. Briefly describe them.
6. Marcea integrated the 5 Ps of marketing into her nutrition education program. What are the 5 Ps of marketing? Briefly describe each.
7. What are some of the things Marcea must consider when advertising a health promotion program?
8. List five of the options for controlling unhealthy food advertisements that may help Marcea.
9. Marcea's population is often a victim of fraud and quackery. What is fraud? What is quackery as it applies to food and nutrition-related products?
10. Marcea could use several different strategies to communicate accurate nutrition information. List five of the strategies Marcea can follow when communicating accurate nutrition information to consumers.
11. Work in small groups or individually to discuss the case study and practice using the Nutrition Care Process chart provided on the companion website. You can also add other nutrition and health-related conditions or assessments to the case study to make the case study more challenging and interesting.

## Think About It

**Answer:** Community nutritionists can use mass media to promote positive changes in behavior, such as an increase in fruit and vegetable consumption. They can also use Facebook, Twitter, or interactive games to provide nutrition education.

## Key Terms

**advertising:** The methods used to present health and nutrition promotion programs to targeted communities.

**business marketing:** The process of creating, distributing, promoting, and pricing goods, services, and ideas to facilitate satisfying exchange relationships with customers in a dynamic environment.

**dietary supplements:** Products made of one or more of the essential nutrients, such as vitamins, minerals, and protein. The Dietary Supplement Health and Education Act of 1994 (DSHEA) expanded the definition, stating that herbs or other botanicals (except tobacco) and any dietary substance that can be used to supplement the diet were to be included in the definition.

**drug:** A chemical compound intended for use in the diagnosis, cure, mitigation, treatment, or prevention of disease, and articles (other than food) intended to affect the structure or function of the body.

**E-professionalism:** The natural progression toward the use of electronic communication, including the Internet, cell phones and Blackberries, and social networking sites such as Facebook, Twitter, and others by professionals, including community and public health nutritionists.

**exploratory research:** Carrying out preliminary research to learn more about the market before any formal research survey is conducted.

**fraud:** Intentional deception or misrepresentation that an individual knows to be false or does not believe to be true with knowledge that the deception could result in some unauthorized benefit to himself or herself or some other person.

**marketing:** Directed at satisfying the needs and wants of the consumer through an exchange of processes or activities (goods, products, or programs).

**market positioning:** Arranging for a product or program to take a clear, distinctive, and desirable place comparable to competing products or programs for nutrition and health services for the same clients or community.

**market segment:** A portion of a larger market.

**market segmentation:** Dividing a market or community into distinct groups of individuals on the basis of needs, characteristics, or behavior who might require separate products or services or marketing mixes.

**market targeting:** The process of evaluating each market segment's attractiveness and selecting one or more segments to penetrate.

**new media:** A general description of emerging technologies that allow for customization, interactivity, and a unique presentation of information.

**place:** Where and how a product can be purchased.

**positioning:** Services' strengths in relation to those of other providers.

**price:** The cost of a product, both monetary and otherwise.

**product:** The item being sold, promoted, offered, or marketed.

**promotion:** How consumers learn about and are persuaded to use a product.

**quackery:** As it applies to food and nutrition-related products, the promotion of an unproved health product or service, usually for personal gain.

**qualitative research:** Acquired from a small sample of the target audience, mainly through open-ended interviewing.
**quantitative research:** Utilizes selected samples to produce statistically reliable results that are expressed in numeric terms.
**social marketing:** The application of marketing to solve social and health problems.

# References

1. Wansink B. *Marketing Nutrition: Soy, Functional Foods, Biotechnology, and Obesity.* Chicago, IL: University of Illinois Press; 2007.
2. Kotler P, Zaltman G. Social marketing: an approach to planned social change. *J Marketing.* 1971;35(3): 3-12.
3. Anspaugh DJ, Dignan MB, Anspaugh SL. *Developing Health Promotion Programs.* 2nd ed. Long Grove, IL: Waveland Press; 2006.
4. Clark CC. *Health Promotion in Communities: Holistic and Wellness Approaches.* New York, NY: Springer Publishing; 2002.
5. Bennett R, Barkensjo A. Relationship quality, relationship marketing, and client perceptions of the levels of service quality of charitable organisations. *Int J Serv Ind Manag.* 2005;16(1): 81-106.
6. Johnson JA, Breckon DJ. *Managing Health Promotion Programs: Leardship Skills for the 21st Century.* 2nd ed. Gaithersburg, MD: Aspen; 2007.
7. McDonald M. Strategic marketing planning: theory and practice. *Mark Rev.* 2006;6(4):375-418 (344).
8. Kotler P, Clark R. *Marketing for Healthcare Organizations.* 2nd ed. Englewood Cliffs, NJ: Prentice Hall; 2008.
9. Gombeski WR Jr. Better marketing through a principles-based model. *Healthc Leader Rev.* 1998;6.
10. Trouiller P, Olliaro P, Torreele E, Orbinski J, et al. Drug development for neglected diseases: a deficient market and a public-health policy failure. *Lancet* 2002;359(9324):2188-2194.
11. Tassonyi A. Municipal budgeting. *Can Tax J.* 2002;50(1):181-198.
12. Ling PM, Glantz SA, Stanton A. Using tobacco-industry marketing research to design more effective tobacco-control campaigns. *JAMA.* 2002;287(22):2983-2989.
13. Ling S, Chow C, Chan A, Tse K, et al. Lead poisoning in new immigrant children from the mainland of China. *Chin Med J.* 2002;115(1):17-20.
14. Boyle MA, Holben D. *Community Nutrition in Action: An Entrepreneurial Approach.* 4th ed. Belmont, CA: Thomson Wadsworth; 2013.
15. Escott-Stump S. *Nutrition and Diagnosis-Related Care.* 8th ed. New York, NY: Wolters Kluwer Lippincott Williams & Wilkins; 2015.
16. Harmon AH, Gerald BL; American Dietetic Association. Position of the American Dietetic Association: food and nutrition professionals can implement practices to conserve natural resources and support ecological sustainability. *J Am Diet Assoc.* 2007;107(6):1033-1043.
17. Levinson JC. *The Guerrilla Marketing Handbook.* New York, NY: Houghton Mifflin; 1994.
18. Kotler P, Fox KFA. *Strategic Marketing for Educational Institutions.* 2nd ed. Englewood Cliffs, NJ: Prentice-Hall; 1995.
19. QuickMBA. Strategic management: SWOT analysis. http://www.quickmba.com/strategy/swot/. Accessed March 17, 2017.
20. Edelstein S. *Nutrition in Public Health: A Handbook for Developing Programs and Services.* 3rd ed. Sudbury, MA: Jones & Bartlett; 2011.
21. Helm KK. *The Competitive Edge: Advanced Marketing for Dietetics Professionals.* 2nd ed. Chicago, IL: American Dietetic Association; 1995.
22. Kotler P, Armstrong G. *Principles of Marketing.* 16th ed. Upper Saddle River, NJ: Prentice Hall; 2015.
23. Barbeau E, Leavy-Sperounis AA, Balbach ED. Smoking, social class, and gender: what can public health learn from the tobacco industry about disparities in smoking? *Tob Control.* 2004;13(2):115-120.
24. Zikmund WG, d'Amico M. *Effective Marketing: Creating and Keeping Customers.* New York, NY: West; 1995.
25. Randolph W, Viswanath K. Lessons learned from public health mass media campaigns: marketing health in a crowded media world. *Annu Rev Public Health.* 2004;25:419-437.
26. American Dietetic Association. Position: Breaking the barrier of breastfeeding. *J Am Diet Assoc.* 2001;101(10).
27. Gerson R. *Marketing Health/Fitness Services.* Champaign, IL: Human Kinetics Book; 1989.
28. Peregrin T. Getting into the media spotlight: the ADA's public relations team promotes the Association as the most recognized source for nutrition information. *J Am Diet Assoc.* 2001;101(7):738-739
29. Lauterborn R. New marketing litany: 4 P's passe: C-words take over. *Advert Age.* 1990:61(41)26.
30. Wiebe G. Merchandising commodities and citizenship on television. *Public Opin Q.* 1951/52; 15:679-691.
31. Hampl JS, Hill R. Dietetic approaches to US hunger and food insecurity. *J Am Diet Assoc.* 2002;102(7): 919-923.

32. Hampl J, Sass S. Focus groups indicate that vegetable and fruit consumption by food stamp-eligible Hispanics is affected by children and unfamiliarity with non-trational foods. *J Am Diet Assoc.* 2001; 101:685-687.

33. Reger B, Wootan MG, Booth-Butterfield S, Smith H. Using mass media to promote health eating: a community-base demonstration project. *Prev Med.* 1999;29(5):414-421.

34. Stead M. A systematic review of social marketing effectiveness. *Health Educ.* 2007;107(2):126-191.

35. Kotler R, Roberto E. *Social Marketing: Strategies for Changing Public Behavior.* New York, NY: Free Press; 1989.

36. Kaufman M. *Nutrition in Public Health: A Handbook for Developing Programs and Services.* Rockville, MD: Aspen; 2007.

37. Kaufman M. *Nutrition in Promoting the Public's Health: Strategies, Principles, and Practice.* Burlington, MA: Jones and Bartlett; 2009.

38. Parks SC, Moody D. A marketing model: applications for dietetic professionals. *J Am Diet Assoc.* 1986; 86(1):37-40.

39. Center for Advanced Studies in Nutrition and Social Marketing. Social marketing. http://socialmarketing-nutrition.ucdavis.edu. Accessed May 23, 2016.

40. Social Marketing Institute. Success stories: mass media and health practices project. http://www.social.-marketing.org. Accessed May 17, 2017.

41. Snow G, Benedict J. Using social marketing to plan a nutrition education program targeting teens. *J Nutr Educ Behav.* 2003;41(6):6Γ.

42. Andreason AR. *Marketing Social Change: Changing Behavior to Promote Health, Social Development, and the Environment.* Washington, DC: Jossey-Bass; 1995.

43. Kotler P, Zaltman G. Social marketing: an approach to planned social change. *J Market.* 1971;35(3):3-12.

44. Lefebvre RC, Flora JA. Social marketing and public health intervention. *Health Educ Q.* 1988;15(3):299-315.

45. Aase S. Toward E-professionalism: thinking through the implications of navigating the digital world. *J Am Diet Assoc.* 2010;110(10):1442-1449.

46. American Dietetic Association. Nutrition and you: 2008 trend survey. http://www.eatright.org. Accessed March 17, 2017.

47. Tate DF, Jackvony EH, Wing RR. Effects of internet behavioral counseling on weight loss in adults at risk for type 2 diabetes: a randomized trial. *JAMA.* 2003;289(14):1833-1836.

48. Caraher M, Landon J, Dalmeny K. Television advertising and children: lessons from policy development. *Public Health Nutr.* 2006;9(5): 596-605.

49. Lee M, Johnson C. *Principles of Advertising: A Global Perspective.* 2nd ed. New York, NY: Haworth Press; 2005.

50. DiLima SN, Schust C. *Publicizing Your Program: Community Health Education and Promotion Manual.* Gaithersburg, MD: Aspen; 1997.

51. Friedman RJ, Altman P. *Marketing Your Seminar: How To Design, Develop, And Market Healthcare Seminars.* Sarasota, FL: Professional Resource Press; 1997.

52. US Dept of Agriculture. Economic research service food marketing system in the U.S. new product introductions. https://www.ers.usda.gov/webdocs/publications/aer811/31184_aer811b_002.pdf. Accessed March 16, 2017.

53. Gallo AE. Food advertising in the United States. In: Frazao E, ed. *America's Eating Habits: Changes and Consequences.* Washington, DC: US Dept of Agriculture; 1999:173-180.

54. American Dietetic Association. *Nutrition Trends Survey: Executive Summary.* Chicago IL: American Dietetic Association; 1997.

55. Cartera SJ, Roberts MB, Saltera J. Relationship between mediterranean diet score and atherothrombotic risk: findings from the Third National Health and Nutrition Examination Survey (NHANES III), 1988–1994. *Atherosclerosis.* 2010;210(2):630-636.

56. Mangalam KS. Nutrition and lung health. *Proc Nutr Soc.* 1999;58:303-308.

57. Food Marketing Institute. *Trends in the United States: Consumer Attitudes & the Supermarket.* Washington, DC: Food Marketing Institute; 1999.

58. American Dietetic Association. *Nutrition and You: Trends 2000.* Chicago, IL: American Dietetic Association; 2000.

59. Novelli WD. Applying social marketing to health promotion and disease prevention. In: Glanz K, Lewis FM, Rimer BK, eds. *Health Behavior and Health Education: Theory, Research, and Practice.* San Francisco, CA: Jossey-Bass; 1990:342-369.

60. Kelly B, Smith B, King L, Flood V, et al. Television food advertising to children: the extent and nature of exposure. *Public Health Nutr.* 2007:1-7.

61. Gorn GJ, Goldberg ME. Children's responses to repetitive television commercials. *J Cons Res.* 1980;6(4):421-424.

62. Levy AS, Stokes RC. Effects of a health promotion advertising campaign on sales of ready-to-eat cereals. *Public Health Rep.* 1987;102:398-403.

63. Beverage Daily. Breaking news on beverage technology & markets. 2005. http://www.beveragedaily.com/news/news-ng.asp?n=60451-ftc-quashes-tropicana. Accessed March 17, 2017.

64. Blisard N. Advertising and what we eat: the case of dairy products. In: Frazao E, ed. *America's Eating*

*Habits: Changes & Consequences.* Washington, DC: US Dept of Agriculture; 1999:181-188.

65. Centers for Disease Control and Prevention. Overweight among U.S. children and adolescents. http://www.cdc.gov. Accessed March 17, 2017.

66. Gantz W, Schwartz N, Angelini JR, Rideout V. *Television Food Advertising to Children in the United States.* Menlo Park, CA: Kaiser Family Foundation; 2007.

67. Zimmerman F, Bell J. Associations of television content type and obesity in children. *Am J Public Health.* 2010;100:334-340.

68. Rideout V, Vandewater E, Wartella E. *Zero to Six: Electronic Media in the Lives of Infants, Toddlers and Preschoolers.* Menlo Park, CA: Henry J. Kaiser Family Foundation; 2003.

69. Kaiser Family Foundation. The role of media in childhood obesity. http://www.kff.org/. Accessed May 30, 2016.

70. Connor SM. Food-related advertising on preschool television: building brand recognition in young viewers. *Pediatrics.* 2006;118(4):1478-1485.

71. Moore ES. It's child's play: advergaming and the online marketing of food to children http://www.kff.org/. Accessed March 17, 2017.

72. Salber P. Is the food industry playing games with our children? *MedGenMed.* 2006;8(4):37.

73. Mediamark Research. Teen market profile. http://www.magazine.org/content/files/teenprofile04.pdf. Accessed March 17, 2017.

74. Stipp H. New ways to reach children. *Am Demogr.* 1993;15:51-56.

75. Pollack J. Foods targeting children aren't just child's play: shape-shifting foods, interactive products chase young consumers. *Advert Age.* 1999:16.

76. Story M, Faulkner P. The prime time diet: a content analysis of eating behavior and food messages in televison program content and commercials. *Am J Public Health.* 1990;80(6):738-740.

77. Byrd-Bredbenner C, Finckenor M, Grasso D. Health related content in prime-time televison programming. *J Health Commun.* 2003;8:329-341.

78. Hoynes W. News for a captive audience: an analysis of Channel One. *Extra!* 1997:11-17.

79. Kotz K, Story M. Food advertisements during children's Saturday morning television programming: are they consistent with dietaey recommendations? *J Am Diet Assoc.* 1994;94:1296-1300.

80. Christakis DA, Dimitri A. The hidden and potent effects of television advertising. *JAMA.* 2006;295(14):1698-1699.

81. Chester J. *Digital Destiny: New Media and the Future of Democracy.* New York, NY: New Press; 2007.

82. Booth FW, Gordon SE, Carlson CJ, Hamilton MT. Waging war on modern chronic diseases: primary prevention through exercise biology. *J Appl Physiol.* 2000;88(2):774-787.

83. Interactive Advertising Bureau. Platform status reports. http://www.iab.net/media/file/IAB-Games-PSR-Update_0913.pdf. Accessed March 17, 2017.

84. Microsoft. About Microsoft adCenter labs. http://www.adlab.msn.com. Accessed August 2, 2016.

85. Association for Computing Machinery. Special interest group on knowledge discovery and data mining (SIGKDD). http://www.acm.org/publications. Accessed August 2, 2016.

86. Montgomery S, Wells W. Fiscal year 2005 impact and review of the Expanded Food and Nutrition Education program. 2006. http://www.csrees.usda.gov/nea/food/efnep. Accessed July 23, 2016.

87. Pechmann C, Levin L, Loughlin S. Impulsive and self-conscious: adolescents' vulnerability to advertising and promotion. *J Public Pol Market.* 2005;24:202-221.

88. Giedd JN. The teen brain: development—forging new links. *J Adolesc Health.* 2008;42:335-343.

89. McAnarney ER. Adolescent brain development: forging new links. *J Adolesc Health.* 2008;42:321-333.

90. Steinberg L. A social neuroscience perspective on adolescent risk taking. *Dev Rev.* 2008;28(1):78-106.

91. Steinberg L. Risk taking in adolescence: new perspectives from brain and behavioral science. *Curr Dir Psychol Sci.* 2007;16:55-59.

92. Collins RL, Ellickson PL, McCaffrey D. Early adolescent exposure to alcohol advertising and its relationship to underage drinking. *J Adolesc Health.* 2007;40:527-534.

93. Ostbye T, Pomerleau WM. Food and nutrition in Canadian "prime time" television commercials. *Can J Public Health.* 1993;84:370-374.

94. Lin BH, Frazao E, Guthrie J. *Away-from-Home Foods Increasingly Important to Quality of the American Diet.* Washington, DC: US Dept of Agriculture; 1999:749.

95. US Census Bureau. *Statistical Abstract of the United States.* 110th ed. Washington, DC: US Census Bureau; 1990.

96. Postlewaite K. Vended bottled drinks. *Vending Times.* 1998;38:21-22.

97. Burros M. Losing count of calories as plates fill up. *New York Times.* April 2, 1997;C1,4.

98. National Research Council. *Recommended Dietary Allowances.* Washington, DC: National Academies Press; 1989.

99. Young LR, Nestle M. Portion sizes in dietary assessment: issues and policy implications. *Nutr Rev.* 1995;53(6):149-158.

100. Zimlichman E, Ilan K, Mimouni FB, Shochat T, et al. Smoking habits and obesity in young adults. *Addiction*. 2005;100(7):1021-1025.

101. US Dept of Agriculture, US Dept of Health Human Services. *Nutrition and Your Health: Dietary Guidelines for Americans*. 8th ed. Home and Garden Bulletin. US Dept of Agriculture, US Dept of Health Human Services; 2015.

102. US Dept of Health and Human Services. *Healthy People 2000: National Health Promotion and Disease Prevention Objectives*. PHS 91-50213. US Dept of Health and Human Services.

103. Wilson T, Temple NJ. *Nutritional Health: Strategies for Disease Prevention*. Totowa, NJ: Humana Press; 2001.

104. Meier KJ, Licari MJ. The effect of cigarette taxes on cigarette consumption, 1995 through 1994. *Am J Public Health*. 1997;87(7):1126-1130.

105. Townsend J. Price and consumption of tobacco. *Br Med J*. 1998;316:1220.

106. Stephens T, Pederson LL, Koval JJ, Kim C. The relationship of cigarette prices and no-smoking bylaws to the prevalence of smoking in Canada. *Am J Public Health*. 1997;87:1519-1521.

107. Townsend J, Roderick P, Cooper J. Cigarette smoking by socioeconomic group, sex, and age effects of price income, and health publicity. *Br Med J*. 1994;309:923-927.

108. Razzouk N. Marketing to the heart: a practical approach to dealing with health care quackery. *Clin Res Regul Aff*. 2003;20(4):469-478.

109. Nestle M. Toward more healthful dietary patterns-a matter of policy. *Pub Health Rep*. 1998;113(5):420-423.

110. Nestle M. Food lobbies, the food pyramid and U.S. nutrition policy. *Int J Health Serv*. 1993;23(3):483-496.

111. Nestle M. The politics of dietary guidance a new opportunity. *Am J Public Health*. 1994;84(5):713-715.

112. Kant AK, Schatzkin A, Harris TB, Ziegler RG, et al. Dietary diversity and subsequent mortality in the first NHANES epidemiological follow-up study. *Am J Clin Nutr*. 1993;57(3):434-440.

113. Duffy V, Backstrand JR, Ferris AM. Olfactory dysfunction and related nutritional risk in free-living elderly women. *J Am Diet Assoc*. 1995;95:879-884.

114. Pepper C. *Quackery: A $10 Billion Scandal*. Subcommittee on Health and Long Term Care of the Selected Committee on Aging U.S. House of Representatives. Washington, DC: US Government Printing Office; 1984:698.

115. Hathcock J. Recent advances on the nutritional effects associated with the use of garlic as a supplement dietary supplements: how they are used and regulated. *J Nutr*. 2001;131(suppl):1114S-1117S.

116. Sarubin A. *The Health Professional's Guide to Popular Dietary Supplements*. Chicago, IL: American Dietetic Assoc; 2000.

117. DeAngelis CD, Fontanarosa PB. Drugs alias dietary supplements. *JAMA*. 2003;290(11):1519-1520.

118. Buettner C, Phillips RS, Davis RB, Gardiner P, et al. Use of dietary supplements among United States adults with coronary artery disease and atherosclerotic risks. *Am J Cardiol*. 2007;99(5):661-666.

119. Klotzbach-Shimomura K. Project Healthy Bones: an osteoporosis prevention program for older adults. *J Extension*. 2001;39(3).

120. Cassileth BR, Vickers AJ. High prevalence of complementary and alternative medicine use among cancer patients: implications for research and clinical care. *J Clin Oncol*. 2005;23(12):2590-2592.

121. The Dietary Supplement Health and Education Act. Pub L No.103-417 (S784) (codified at 42 USC 287C-11). 1994.

122. Gurley BJ. Clinical Pharmacology and dietary supplements: an evolving relationship. *Clin Pharmacol Ther*. 2010;87:235-238.

123. Settings M. Position of the American Dietetic Association: food and nutrition misinformation. *J Am Diet Assoc*. 2006;106(4):601-607.

124. O'Malley R, MacMunn A. Where did you hear that? Do you believe it? American Dietetic Association survey reveals popularity and perceived credibility of sources of nutrition information. https://www.eatrightpro.org/~/media/eatrightpro%20files/media/trends%20and%20reviews/nutrition%20and%20you/where_did_you_hear_that_ada_trends_2011.ashx. Accessed March 16, 2017.

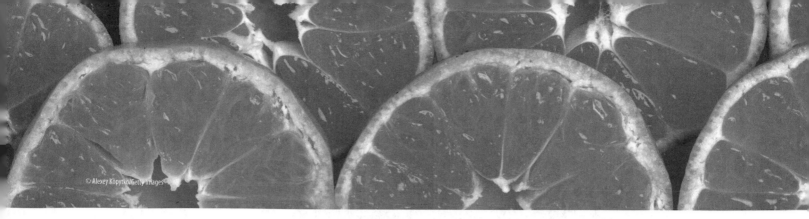

# CHAPTER 18

# Private and Government Healthcare Systems

## CHAPTER OUTLINE

- Introduction
- Healthcare Coverage Versus Uninsured
- Private Health Insurance
- Government Health Insurance and Public Insurance
- The U.S. Healthcare Reform Bill

## LEARNING OBJECTIVES

- Differentiate between private and government healthcare systems in the United States.
- Discuss the eligibility and services criteria for Medicare and Medicaid.
- Discuss the different types of group insurance.
- List the different types of current health coverage status.
- Discuss the impact of the Personal Responsibility and Work Opportunity Reconciliation Act (PRWORA).

## ▶ Introduction

In the United States, a wide variety of healthcare providers are available to give comprehensive health care to individuals who can afford it. In 2009, total U.S. expenditure on health care was $2 trillion and increased to $3.2 trillion in 2015[1] However, healthcare services are unevenly distributed. Even some individuals who have access to employer-sponsored **health insurance** are unable to obtain coverage due to the high cost of premiums and rising healthcare costs.[2]

In 2006, employer health insurance **premiums** were 7.7 percent, and increased significantly to 14 percent in 2010, which may be one of the reasons why approximately 47 million Americans are uninsured.[3,4] In 2014, 32 million nonelderly were uninsured, a decrease of 9 million from 2013 due to the expansion of the Affordable Care Act (ACA). The reasons for being uninsured were high cost of health insurance, poor adults in states that did not expand Medicaid through the ACA, plus ineligibility of undocumented immigrants for Medicaid or ACA Marketplace health insurance coverage.[5] The United States spends a great deal of money on acute care and insufficient amounts on the promotion of health and prevention of diseases. One of the major goals of Healthy People 2010 and 2020 is to increase the quality and years of healthy life. This goal can be accomplished by increasing funding for health promotion, disease prevention, and care for people with chronic illnesses and by providing health insurance to the poor. See Chapter 1 for more information on Healthy People 2010 and 2020.

Poverty limits access to health care, leading to poorer health status. People in the lowest income households are more likely than those in higher income households to report their **health status** as fair or poor.[6] Poor health and physical and mental disabilities can lead to food insecurity by limiting the ability to acquire and prepare food and by affecting nutrient needs.[6] For instance, research shows a higher incidence of iron-deficiency anemia in low-income children[7] and that the incidence of heart disease, cancer, hypertension, and obesity increases with decreasing income.[8-10] In the United States, health insurance coverage is generally classified as either private (nongovernment) coverage or government-sponsored coverage. The following discussion highlights healthcare economics terms that community nutritionists should be able to recognize.

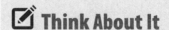

## Think About It

Why are some people uninsured?

## ▶ Healthcare Coverage Versus Uninsured

The National Center for Health Statistics defines health **insurance** as a broad term that includes both public and private payers who cover medical expenditures incurred by a defined population in a variety of settings.[10] The total number of people with health insurance in the United States in 2009 was 255.1 million; in 2015 approximately 90.9 percent had health insurance coverage.[5,11] In the United States, the risk for becoming uninsured increases significantly for those earning low wages (the working poor); for the unemployed, especially young adults because they have higher rates of unemployment; and when employers are unable to provide or offer insurance to workers. These people generally do not qualify for Medicaid because it is for the low-income elderly, children, blind and disabled people, pregnant women, single parents, or unemployed parents (in some states). Employed adults are not eligible for Medicaid regardless of income unless they are blind, disabled, or pregnant.[10] **TABLE 18-1** presents the rates of healthcare coverage in 2014 and 2015.

## ▶ Private Health Insurance

The majority of private healthcare expenses are incurred by individuals receiving treatment and are paid by private insurers making payments on behalf of the client/enrollee.[10] But is not a rare event. For instance, it was reported that during 2015, an estimated 922.6 million individuals visited physicians' offices in the United

| **TABLE 18-1** The Rate of Healthcare Coverage in 2013 to 2014[12,13] | | |
|---|---|---|
| **Health Insurance Coverage** | **2014 (percent)** | **2015 (percent)** |
| People without health insurance coverage | 10.4 | 9.1 |
| People covered by employment-based health insurance | 55.4 | 56 |
| People covered by government health insurance programs | 36.5 | 37.1 |
| People covered by Medicaid | 19.5 | 19.6 |
| People covered by Medicare | 16.0 | 16.3 |
| Insured Caucasian Americans | 92.4 | 91.3 |
| Insured African Americans | 88.2 | 88.9 |
| Insured Hispanics | 80.1 | 83.6 |
| Insured Asian Americans | 90.7 | 92.5 |

Reproduced from: U.S. Census Bureau. Health insurance coverage in 2005. Available at: https://www.census.gov/content/dam/Census/library/publications/2015/demo/p60-253.pdf, August 03, 2016.

States, an overall rate of 296.7 visits per 100 persons. In contrast, uninsured persons (as measured by self-pay and charity visits) had a much lower number of visits to physicians' offices, placing them at a disadvantage for disease prevention and early diagnosis.[13]

The concept of insurance is to combine the health-care experiences of many enrollees in order to reduce expenses for any one individual to a manageable pre-payment amount. There are different types of insurance plans and organizations. This section will discuss some of the plans and organizations clients may enroll.

## Employment-Based Plans

**Employment-based health insurance** is coverage offered through one's own employment or a relative's employment. It may be offered by an employer or by a union. Traditionally, a person is enrolled in the healthcare delivery system by contracting directly with a healthcare provider for individual care based on fee for service, also known as direct-purchase plans.[13] However, in recent years, more physicians are contracting for all or part of their practices with managed healthcare organizations, mainly independent practice associations (IPAs), health maintenance organizations (HMOs), and preferred provider organizations (PPOs). These are all prepaid group practice plans that offer healthcare services through groups of medical practitioners.

## Direct-Purchase or Fee-for-Service Plans

**Fee-for-service plans** are the traditional type of healthcare policy. The physician sets a price for each type of service delivered, and then the client or insurance company pays the fee. This type of health insurance provides the most preference to doctors and hospitals. The client can choose any doctor he or she wishes and can change doctors at any time. The client can use any hospital in any part of the country. With fee-for-service, the insurer pays for only part of the doctor and hospital bills. The client pays a monthly fee called a premium. The main concern about the fee-for-service plan is that it encourages unnecessary care (laboratory tests, procedures, etc.).

The **Medicare** system is based on fee-for-service for paying physicians. The physician payment mechanism for Medicare has been modified. Medicare pays an individual physician an amount that does not exceed the 75th percentile of charges by all physicians in a community. (This is termed the *prevailing* fee.[14])

There are two kinds of fee-for-service coverage: basic and major medical. Basic covers some hospital services and supplies, such as x-rays and prescribed medicine. Basic coverage also pays the cost of surgery, whether it is performed in or out of the hospital, and for some doctor visits. Major medical insurance covers the cost of long-term, high-cost illnesses or injuries plus whatever basic did

not cover. Some policies combine basic and major medical insurance coverage into one plan. This is sometimes called a comprehensive plan. It is important for clients to check their policy to make sure they have both kinds of protection. Insurance coverage can be purchased from commercial insurance companies such as Blue Cross Blue Shield.[10]

## Group Contract Insurance

The group contract health insurance system was developed because of the need for hospitals and physicians to make their products and services affordable to ordinary people in the United States. With unmanaged care (fee-for-service) payments, healthcare providers had the opportunity to increase the number of single services they delivered in order to increase their profit. The more fees paid, the greater the revenue generated for the provider (physician, hospital, etc.) and the greater the cost is to the insurer (private or public). This was a cause for concern because of rising health service costs in the last quarter of the twentieth century. Unmanaged care also caused employers to reduce their coverage and shift costs to employees by making the employees pay a larger share of the premiums, higher deductibles, and higher copayments.[14] This was a concern to the government (Medicare and Medicaid) and to employers because they typically used fee-for-service as their primary payment approach. Increasingly, however, they are using managed care in the hope that it will provide the quality and quantity of care needed to ensure people's health and well-being as well as control costs.[15]

## Managed Care

**Managed care** is a system that manages the cost and delivery of healthcare services, the quality of that health care, and access to care. It is based on the belief that healthcare costs can be controlled by "managing" the way in which health care is delivered. Enrollees have a financial incentive to use participating providers that agree to provide a wide range of services. Providers may be paid on a pre-negotiated basis (as with HMOs, point-of-service plans [POSs], and PPOs).[16]

Managed care influences how much health care clients can use. Almost all plans have some type of managed care program to help control costs. For example, if a client needs to go to the hospital, one form of managed care requires that the client receive approval from the insurance company before being admitted because the insurance company wants to make sure that the hospitalization is needed. The hospital cost may not be covered if approval is not obtained.[17]

## Health Maintenance Organizations

**Health maintenance organizations (HMOs)** are prepaid health plans. The goal of an HMO is to provide affordable, well-organized health care by allowing clients to prepay (**capitation** payment) on a regular monthly basis for all services provided by the practice, including physicians' visits, hospital stays, emergency care, surgery, laboratory tests, x-rays, and therapy for all members and their families. The HMO arranges for this care either directly in its own group practice or through physicians and other healthcare professionals under contract.[18] Typically, the client's choice of physicians and hospitals is limited to those that have agreements with the HMO to provide care. However, exceptions are made in emergencies or when medically necessary.

There may be a small copayment for each office visit, such as $25 for a doctor's visit or $200 for hospital emergency room treatment. The client's total medical costs will likely be lower and more predictable in an HMO than with fee-for-service health insurance. Because HMOs receive a fixed fee for the coverage of medical care, it is in their interest to make sure the client receives basic health care for problems before they become serious. HMOs typically provide preventive care, such as office visits, immunizations, well-baby checkups, mammograms, and physicals. The range of services covered varies among HMOs, so it is important to compare available plans. In 2010, President Obama signed the Equal Coverage Laws that require insurers to provide the same level of benefits for mental illness, serious mental illness, or substance abuse as the insurers would other diseases, such as diabetes or cancer, so outpatient services are no longer limited for the mentally ill.

Conventional HMOs employ a staff of physicians, nurses, and other healthcare professionals who earn a salary and consequently have no incentive to provide unnecessary expensive treatments.[14] They can be located at one or more locations in the client's community as part of a prepaid group practice known as the **staff model**. Another type, known as the **group model**, consists of independent groups of physicians who contract with an HMO to provide services to enrollees.

**Individual practice associations (IPAs)** are made up of private physicians in private offices who provide services to HMO members as well as clients with other forms of insurance. The HMO clients can select a physician from a list of participating physicians that make up the IPA network. In the IPA network type, the HMO contracts with a number of multispecialty physician groups to provide services to enrollees. Often, these physician groups also deliver services to non-HMO clients.[10,19]

## Point-of-Service Plans

Many HMOs offer an option known as a **point-of-service (POS) plan**. It offers enrollees the option of receiving

services from participating or nonparticipating providers. The benefits package is designed to encourage the use of participating providers through higher **deductible**s and/or partial reimbursement for services provided by nonparticipating providers. The primary care physicians in a POS plan usually make referrals to other providers in the plan. However, members can refer themselves outside the plan and still get some coverage.[10] If the physician makes a referral out of the network, the plan pays all or most of the bill. However, if the client refers himself or herself to a provider outside the network (and the service is covered by the plan), the **copayment** and deductibles would increase significantly.[10]

## Preferred Provider Organizations

A **preferred provider organization (PPO)** is a combination of traditional fee-for-service and an HMO. Similar to an HMO, clients use the physicians and hospitals that have agreed to give discounts to their insurer. The incentive is either a lower insurance premium or a waiver of cost-sharing requirements. Like an HMO, a PPO requires that clients choose a primary care physician to monitor their health care. Most PPOs also cover preventive care. This typically includes visits to the physician, well-baby care, immunizations, and mammograms. If the client decides to choose a physician that is not part of the plan, the client will pay a larger portion of the bill (and also fill out claims forms to be reimbursed for medical expenses). Some people like this option because it does not require network care. For example, if the client's physician is not a part of the network, he or she will not be required to change physicians to join a PPO.[10]

## ▶ Government Health Insurance and Public Insurance

Government health insurance includes plans funded by governments at the federal, state, or local level. The major categories of government health insurance are Medicare, Medicaid, and the State Children's Health Insurance Program (SCHIP). The Center for Medicare and Medicaid Services (CMS), a federal agency, administers these programs. These plans provide a medical safety net for the poor, elderly, disabled, and some uninsured individuals.[20]

## The Medicare Program

Medicare, Title XVIII of the Social Security Act, is the designated health insurance for the aged and disabled. Part of the Social Security Amendments of 1965, the

Medicare legislation provides hospital and medical insurance to elderly persons, permanently and totally disabled persons, and people with end-stage renal disease (ESRD). The Medicare program is administered by the CMS, a division of the U.S. Department of Health and Human Services (DHHS). The following groups also are eligible for Medicare benefits: persons entitled to Social Security or Railroad Retirement disability cash benefits for at least 23 months and certain noncovered aged persons who elected to pay a premium for Medicare coverage.[21] The Medicare, Medicaid, and SCHIP Benefits Improvement and Protection Act of 2000 (Public Law 106-554) allowed persons with amyotrophic lateral sclerosis (Lou Gehrig's disease) to waive the 24-month waiting period.

Medicare has traditionally consisted of two parts: hospital insurance (HI), also known as Part A, and supplementary medical insurance (SMI), also known as Part B. A third part of Medicare, sometimes known as Part C, is the Medicare Advantage program, which was established as the Medicare+Choice program by the Balanced Budget Act (BBA) of 1997 (Public Law 105-33). Later, it was renamed and modified by the Medicare Prescription Drug, Improvement, and Modernization Act (MMA) of 2003.[22] The MMA also established a fourth part of Medicare: a prescription drug benefit known as Part D, which became available in 2006. Part D activities are handled within the SMI trust fund, but in an account separate from Part B. The purpose of the two separate accounts within the SMI trust fund is to ensure that funds from one part are not used to finance the other.[22]

When Medicare began on July 1, 1966, approximately 19 million people were enrolled. In 2015, almost 53.3 million people were enrolled in one or both of Parts A and B of the Medicare program, and about 5 million of them chose to participate in a Medicare Advantage plan.[23,24]

In 2015, total federal spending was approximately $632 billion. The projected Medicare spending is expected to increase from $551 billion to $903 billion in 2020 (including offsets). Spending on Social Security totaled ($750 billion), and defense spending accounted for 20 percent ($598.5 billion). **FIGURE 18-1** presents Medicare spending as part of the federal budget, and **FIGURE 18-2** (later) presents the historical and projected average annual growth rate in Medicare per capita.[23-25]

## Part A Coverage

Part A is generally provided automatically, and free of premiums, to persons age 65 or over who are eligible for Social Security or Railroad Retirement benefits, whether they have claimed these monthly cash benefits or not. Also, workers and their spouses with a sufficient

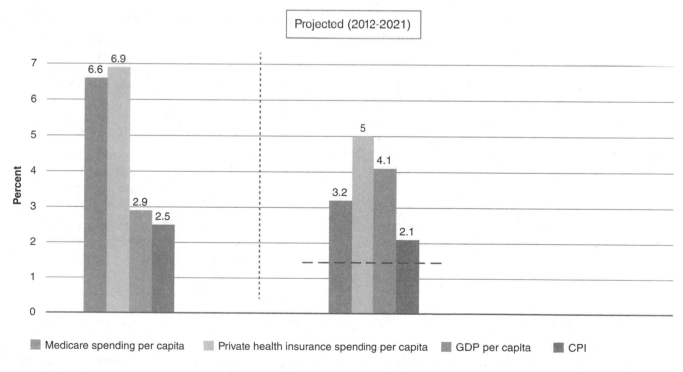

**FIGURE 18-1** Historical and projected average annual growth rate in Medicare spending per capita and other measures sources.

Sources: Kaiser Family Foundation analysis of data from Boards of Trustees, Congressional Budget Office, Centers for Medicare & Medicaid Services, U.S. Census Bureau. Available at: http://kff.org/health-costs/slide/historical-and-projected-average-annual-growth-rate-in-medicare-spending-per-capita-and-other-measures/. Accessed, August 04, 2016.

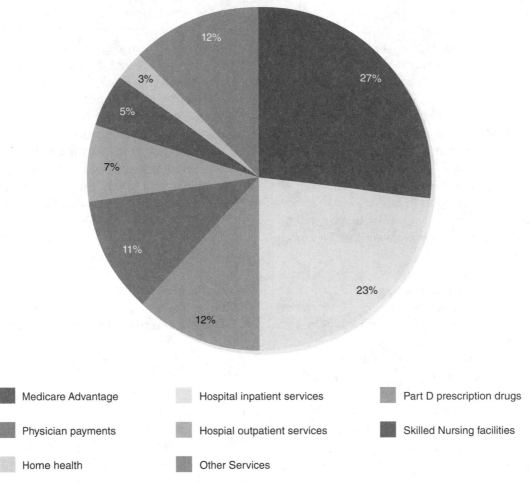

**FIGURE 18-2** Medicare benefit payments by type of service for 2015.

Note: *Consists of Medicare benefit spending on hospice, durable medical equipment, Part B drugs, outpatient dialysis, ambulance, laboratory services, and other Part B services; also includes the effect of sequestration on spending for Medicare benefits and amounts paid to providers and recovered.

Source: Congressional Budget Office, 2016 Medicare Baseline (March, 2016). Available at: http://kff.org/health-costs/slide/historical-and-projected-average-annual-growth-rate-in-medicare-spending-per-capita-and-other-measures/. Accessed August 04, 2016

period of Medicare-only coverage in federal, state, or local government employment are eligible beginning at age 65. Equally, individuals who have been entitled to Social Security or Railroad Retirement disability benefits for at least 24 months, and government employees with Medicare-only coverage who have been disabled for more than 29 months, are entitled to Part A benefits.[23-25]

Part A coverage also is provided to insured workers with ESRD (and to insured workers' spouses and children with ESRD), as well as ineligible aged and disabled beneficiaries who voluntarily paid a monthly premium for their coverage.[25,26]

## Part B Coverage

Part B covers physicians' and surgeons' services, including some covered services furnished by chiropractors, podiatrists, dentists, and optometrists. Also covered are the services provided by the following Medicare-approved practitioners who are not physicians: certified registered nurse anesthetists, clinical psychologists, clinical social workers (other than in a hospital), physician assistants,

and nurse practitioners and clinical nurse specialists in collaboration with a physician.[26]

In 2002, Medicare started to pay qualified dietitians who enrolled in the Medicare program as providers, whether they provide medical nutrition therapy (MNT) services in an independent practice setting, hospital outpatient department, or any other setting. Medicare does not pay dietitians for hospital inpatients or individuals in a skilled nursing facility.[27,28] Medicare will pay dietitians (enrolled as Medicare MNT providers) for services to Medicare beneficiaries with type 1 diabetes, type 2 diabetes, gestational diabetes, nondialysis kidney disease, and post–kidney-transplant status using specified codes. Referral from a physician for MNT is required.[29-31]

The insurance coverage for MNT services plays a significant role in the primary, secondary, and tertiary levels of prevention and in the maintenance of diabetes, cardiovascular diseases, and other diet-related health conditions. For example, primary prevention addresses lifestyle risk factors; the control of blood cholesterol levels is a secondary preventive measure that can slow the onset and progression of heart disease. As for tertiary prevention, heart disease becomes more manageable with intense MNT. Sheils et al.[3] estimated the costs and savings associated with providing the entire Medicare population with coverage for MNT. Results showed that MNT was associated with reduced utilization of hospital services by 9.5 percent for patients with diabetes and 8.6 percent for patients with cardiovascular disease. In addition, utilization of physician services decreased by 23.5 percent for MNT users with diabetes and 16.9 percent for MNT users with cardiovascular disease.[3] The researchers concluded that, overall, after an initial period of implementation, coverage for MNT can result in a net reduction in health services utilization and cost. Also, research studies show that diet and exercise can prevent or delay the development of diabetes.[32,33] See Box 6-1 in Chapter 6 for highlights of the success of the American Dietetic Association in obtaining Medicare coverage for some MNT services.

## Part D

The Medicare Prescription Drug Improvement and Modernization Act added a prescription drug benefit that became available in 2006. Part D provides subsidized access to prescription drug insurance coverage on a voluntary basis, upon payment of a premium, to individuals entitled to Part A or enrolled in Part B, with premium and cost-sharing subsidies for low-income enrollees. Beneficiaries may enroll in either a stand-alone prescription drug plan (PDP) or an integrated Medicare Advantage plan that offers Part D coverage.[34] Part D coverage includes most U.S. Food and Drug Administration (FDA)–approved prescription drugs.[35]

## Coverage Gaps

Although Medicare provides extensive benefits, there are significant gaps in coverage. These gaps include Medicare deductibles, copayments, excess charges by doctors who do not accept Medicare assignments, and medical services and supplies that Medicare does not cover. Services not covered by Medicare include long-term nursing care, custodial care, and certain other healthcare needs, such as dentures and dental care, eyeglasses, and hearing aids. Medicare Supplemental Insurance, also known as **Medigap**, was developed to provide extra protection beyond Medicare by filling some of the gaps in Medicare coverage.[36] Medigap is a type of private insurance coverage that may be purchased by an individual enrolled in Medicare to cover some needed services not covered by Medicare.

## The Medicaid Program

Title XIX of the Social Security Act is a federal and state entitlement program that pays for medical assistance for certain low-income individuals and families. This program, known as **Medicaid**, became law in 1965 as a cooperative venture jointly funded by the federal and state governments (including the District of Columbia and the Territories) to assist states in providing medical assistance to eligible low-income persons. Medicaid is the largest source of funding for medical and health-related services for poor people. Within broad national guidelines established by federal statutes, regulations, and policies, each state must do the following[37]:

- Establish its own eligibility standards
- Determine the type, amount, duration, and scope of services
- Set the rate of payment for services
- Administer its own program

Medicaid policies for eligibility, services, and payment are complex and vary among states of similar size or geographic proximity. Therefore, a person who is eligible for Medicaid in one state may not be eligible in another state, and the services provided by one state may differ considerably in amount, duration, or scope from services provided in a similar or neighboring state. In addition, state legislatures may change Medicaid eligibility, services, and/or reimbursement during the year.[38]

## Basis of Eligibility

Medicaid does not provide medical assistance for all poor persons. Under the broadest provisions of the federal statute, Medicaid does not provide healthcare services even for very poor persons unless they are in one of the following designated groups. Individuals are usually eligible for Medicaid if they meet the following criteria[38]:

- Are 6 years old or younger and have a family income at or below 133 percent of the Federal Poverty Level (FPL). See Table 4-9 in Chapter 4 for the Federal Poverty Guidelines.
- Are pregnant with a family income below 133 percent of the FPL. (Services to these women are limited to those related to pregnancy, complications of pregnancy, delivery, and postpartum care.)
- Are Supplemental Security Income (SSI) recipients. (Some states use more restrictive Medicaid eligibility requirements that predate SSI.)
- Are recipients of adoption or foster care assistance under Title IV of the Social Security Act.
- Belong to a special protected group (typically individuals who lose their cash assistance due to earnings from work or from increased Social Security benefits, but who may keep Medicaid for a time).

## The Personal Responsibility and Work Opportunity Reconciliation Act (PRWORA)

The Personal Responsibility and Work Opportunity Reconciliation Act of 1996 (Public Law 104-193) is known as the "welfare reform" bill. It made restrictive changes regarding eligibility for SSI coverage that have an impact on the Medicaid program. For example, legal resident aliens and other qualified aliens who entered the United States on or after August 22, 1996, are ineligible for Medicaid for 5 years. Medicaid to resident aliens can continue only if these persons can be covered for Medicaid under some other eligibility status (with the exception of emergency services, which are mandatory).[38,39]

In addition, welfare reform repealed the open-ended federal entitlement program known as Aid to Families with Dependent Children (AFDC) and replaced it with Temporary Assistance for Needy Families (TANF), which provides states with grants to be spent on time-limited cash assistance. TANF generally limits a family's lifetime cash welfare benefits to a maximum of 5 years and permits states to impose a wide range of other requirements as well, in particular those related to employment.[39] However, welfare reform had a significant negative impact on Medicaid coverage before pregnancy among eligible participants, which resulted in a small decline in participants' first-trimester prenatal care initiation.[40] Under welfare reform, persons who would have been eligible for AFDC generally are still eligible for Medicaid.[37,41]

## State Children's Health Insurance Program

The **State Children's Health Insurance Program (SCHIP)**, Title XXI, was initiated by the BBA of 1997. The federal government created the SCHIP program to cover individuals who have incomes too high to qualify for state medical assistance but who cannot obtain private insurance. All states participate, but some do not cover dental. In addition to allowing states to design or expand an existing state insurance program, SCHIP provides more federal funds for states to expand Medicaid eligibility to include children who are currently uninsured. With certain exceptions, those who qualify are as follows[37,41,42]:

- Children in low-income families who would not qualify for Medicaid (based on the plan that was in effect on April 15, 1997)
- Eligible children under the age of 19 whose state provides 12 months of continuous Medicaid coverage (without reevaluation)

- Inpatient hospital services
- Outpatient hospital services
- Prenatal care
- Vaccines for children
- Physician services
- Nursing facility services for persons age 21 or older
- Family planning services and supplies
- Rural health clinic services
- Home healthcare for persons eligible for skilled-nursing services
- Laboratory and x-ray services
- Pediatric and family nurse practitioner services
- Nurse-midwife services
- Early and periodic screening, diagnosis, and treatment services for children under age 21

## Medicaid, Title XIX of the Social Security Act

Title XIX of the Social Security Act allows considerable flexibility within the states' Medicaid plans. However, some federal requirements are mandatory if federal matching funds are to be received. A state's Medicaid program must offer medical assistance for certain basic services to most categorically needy populations. **BOX 18-1** presents services generally provided by the state Medicaid programs. This chapter's Successful Community Strategies feature presents a success story of lowering infant mortality by integrating WIC and Medicaid.

## Balanced Budget Act

The Balanced Budget Act (BBA) includes a state option known as Programs of All-Inclusive Care for the Elderly (PACE). PACE provides an alternative to institutional care for individuals age 55 or older who require a nursing facility level of care. The PACE team (an interdisciplinary team consisting of professional and paraprofessional staff) offers and manages all health, medical, and social services and mobilizes other services as needed to provide preventive, rehabilitative, curative, and supportive care. This care, provided in day health centers, homes, hospitals, and nursing homes, helps the person maintain independence, dignity, and quality of life. Regardless of source of payment, PACE providers receive payment only through the PACE agreement and must make available all items and services covered under both Titles XVIII and XIX, without amount, duration, or scope limitations and without application of any deductibles, copayments, or other cost sharing. The individuals enrolled in PACE receive benefits solely through the PACE program.[26,37] Total Medicare benefit payments in 2015 was $632 billion. **FIGURE 18-2** presents the payments by type of service.

# ▶ The U.S. Healthcare Reform Bill

The main function of the Affordable Care Act (ACA) is to produce private health insurance exchanges in every state. These exchanges will serve as a marketplace for consumers, offering local, standardized healthcare plans from a variety of providers. The aims were as follows[43]:

- Expand health insurance coverage to include uninsured Americans
- Improve the quality of coverage and health care
- Serve as a cost-saving mechanism
- Improve affordability and stability of insurance for those who already have it

The ACA specified many benefits to be included in exchanges; however, the official rulemaking process by the DHHS is in progress. The ACA stated that health plans must offer a minimum level of benefits to qualify for inclusion in state exchanges, including inpatient, outpatient, emergency, and maternity care; mental health and substance abuse treatment; oral and vision care; and prescription drugs and lab tests.[43] The law also emphasizes coverage for preventive services and a reformed delivery system that includes more primary care providers, medical homes, and community-based health centers. In addition, healthcare providers must offer these services with no patient cost sharing. The new structure focuses on preventive care and wellness and a client-centered approach to treating and managing various chronic diseases. It is important to recognize that this setup will provide several opportunities for community and public health nutritionists to influence the services available in their states or regions through inclusion of nutrition services in the benefit package.[44] Visit https://www.nwica.org/blog/aca-basics-for-the-wic-community#.VCHVqitdX6Y and http://www.catrightpro.org/resource/advocacy/disease-prevention-and-treatment/cardiovascular/rdns-and-prevention-strategic-investments-for-long-term-health-cost-savings for healthcare reform that is relevant to dietetic practice.

## Successful Community Strategies

### Integrating WIC with Medicaid and Reducing Infant Mortality in Illinois[45]

In 2002, the Illinois infant mortality rate was 7.4 deaths for every 1,000 live births. The Illinois Department of Human Services designed a program to reduce the state's infant mortality rate by merging federal and state funds. It integrated the Special Supplemental Nutrition Program for Women, Infants, and Children (WIC) with two state-funded programs: Family Case Management (FCM) and Targeted Intensive Prenatal Case Management (TIPCM). The WIC (federal) funds and the state funds were used to leverage federal matching funds through the Medicaid program. These programs serve more than 40 percent of all infants born in Illinois every year and approximately 90 percent of Medicaid-eligible infants. The department supplements these statewide programs with targeted initiatives for women who have a higher chance of giving birth prematurely. Integration of these programs allowed them to operate more efficiently. For example, staff members of many local health departments were trained to provide both WIC and FCM services. The success of the coordinated program can be summarized as follows:

- The proportion of WIC-eligible children with health insurance increased to 89.9 percent.
- The proportion of fully immunized 1-year-olds in WIC increased to 86.8 percent.
- The proportion of fully immunized 2-year-olds in WIC increased to 76.4 percent.
- The proportion of infants in WIC who were breastfed increased to 61.4 percent.
- The proportion of infants in WIC who continued to breastfeed through 6 months of age increased to 30.5 percent.
- The proportion of children in FCM who received at least three well childcare visits during the first year of life increased to 57.9 percent.
- For 6 years in a row, infants born to Medicaid-eligible pregnant women who participated in WIC or FCM were in better health than those born to Medicaid-eligible women who did not participate in either program:
  - The rate of premature birth was 60 to 70 percent lower.
  - The rate of infant mortality was 50 to 70 percent lower.
  - Medicaid expenditures for healthcare in the first year of life were 30 to 50 percent lower.
- Participation in WIC and FCM saved Illinois an average of $200 million each year in Medicaid expenses.

# Learning Portfolio

## Chapter Summary

- Private health insurance is coverage by a health plan provided through an employer or union or purchased by an individual from a private health insurance company.
- Traditionally, a person can enroll in a healthcare delivery system by contracting directly with a healthcare provider for individual care based on fee-for-service, also known as direct-purchase plans.
- Medicare pays individual physicians an amount that does not exceed the 75th percentile of charges by all physicians in a community (termed the prevailing fee). The main concern about fee-for-service plans is that they encourage unnecessary care (laboratory tests, procedures, etc.).
- Managed care influences how much health care clients use.
- In some HMOs, physicians are salaried and they all have offices in an HMO building at one or more locations in the client's community as part of a prepaid group practice. This is known as a staff model.
- Although Medicare provides extensive benefits, there are gaps in coverage. Some of these gaps include Medicare deductibles, copayments, long-term nursing care, custodial care, and certain other healthcare needs, such as dentures and dental care.
- Medicaid became law in 1965 as a cooperative venture jointly funded by the federal and state governments (including the District of Columbia and the Territories) to assist states in providing medical assistance to eligible low-income persons.
- Welfare reform repealed the open-ended federal entitlement program known as Aid to Families with Dependent Children (AFDC) and replaced it with Temporary Assistance for Needy Families

(TANF), which provides states with grants to be spent on time-limited cash assistance.
- The federal government created the State Children's Health Insurance Program (SCHIP) to cover individuals whose families have incomes too high to qualify for state medical assistance but who cannot obtain private insurance.
- The main function of the Affordable Care Act (ACA) is to produce private health insurance exchanges in every state.

## Critical Thinking Activities

- The United States does not yet have a universal health insurance that ensures access to health care to all Americans. Therefore, many people are without health insurance or are underinsured. Which level of prevention and segment of the population (e.g., children, older adults, pregnant and lactating women, etc.) should the government guarantee healthcare services for, and why?
- Discuss as a group the aspect of managed care that should be of the most concern to a consumer and why.
- Evaluate two research articles about nutrition services covered through Medicare and/or Medicaid.
- Determine the eligibility criteria for Medicare and Medicaid.
- Evaluate the nutritional status of older persons participating in a congregate meal program.
- Determine the types of nutrition-related health conditions that can qualify for Medicare.
- Plan a nutrition education class for older persons on how to reduce the incidence of cancer, osteoporosis, and heart disease using current research information/articles.
- Teach older individuals who are not enrolled in the Medicare program about the eligibility criteria for Medicare and Medicaid.

## 🔍 CASE STUDY 18-1: Lifestyle Interventions and Long-Term Benefits for Medicare

Justina, a community dietitian in Chicago, was asked to evaluate the nutritional status of and provide nutrition counseling to older persons in a community health center program in which the majority of clients were experiencing nutrition-related health conditions such as hypertension and diabetes. Before carrying out the activities, she read a research article by Ackermann et al.[46] that explored whether lifestyle interventions could be offered in a way that allows a return on investment for private health insurers while remaining attractive for consumers, employers, and Medicare.

*(continues)*

## CASE STUDY 18-1: Lifestyle Interventions and Long-Term Benefits for Medicare
*(continued)*

The results of the research showed that providing a lifestyle intervention at age 50 years could prevent 37 percent of new cases of diabetes before age 65, at a cost of $1,288 per quality-adjusted life year (QALY; a way of measuring both the quality and the quantity of life lived) gained. The researchers concluded that cost-sharing strategies for offering lifestyle interventions for eligible people between ages 50 and 64 could provide financial return on investment for private payers and long-term benefits for Medicare.[46] Justina conducted the nutrition assessment, which showed that:

- 30 percent of the participants were underweight (BMI > 17), had poor appetites, and had fluid intakes of less than 1 liter per day with symptoms of dry skin and dry mouth
- Many participants had chapped, red, swollen lips
- 60 percent of the participants' fruit and vegetable intake was below the recommended amount
- 80 percent of the participants consumed less than 1,000 kcal daily
- 60 percent of the participants qualified for Medicare
- 40 percent had managed care health insurance

Justina provided diet instruction to help the clients improve their nutrients and fluid intake. She also suggested they enhance their diet with dietary supplements and keep a record of food intake. On follow-up about 3 weeks later, the food records showed improved dietary intake. At the 6-week follow-up, the clients had gained more than 10 pounds. Their fruit and vegetable intake increased by two to three servings daily. Justina's services were paid for by Medicare and managed care because Justina was a Medicare medical nutrition therapy provider.

### Questions

1. What are the different types of private health insurance in which the participant might have enrolled?
2. Some of the participants had Medicare coverage. What are the different types of Medicare coverage? What are some of the gaps in the Medicare programs that Justina may observe?
3. Some of the participants had health insurance coverage gap. What is Medicare Supplemental Insurance or Medigap?
4. Justina explained to the participants that some of them might qualify for Medicaid. What is the Medicaid program, and who is eligible for the program?
5. The participants wanted to know the difference between the Medicare and Medicaid programs. What are the similarities and differences in the Medicare and Medicaid programs?
6. Justina needed to know more about Medicare and Medicaid. In what settings would a Registered Dietitian see clients with Medicare? What are some nutrition-related health conditions that can qualify for Medicare?
7. Justina also needed to know more about SCHIP. What is the State Children's Health Insurance Program (SCHIP)? Who qualifies for this program?
8. Justina needed to know if the health conditions of her participants will be covered by Medicare. What are the types of nutrition-related health conditions that can qualify for Medicare?
9. Work in small groups or individually to discuss the case study and practice using the Nutrition Care Process chart provided on the companion website. You can also add other nutrition and health-related conditions or assessments to the case study to make the case study more challenging and interesting.

## Think About It

**Answer:** Many people are uninsured because of low wages (working poor) or unemployment (especially young adults because they have higher rates of unemployment) and when employers are unable to provide or offer insurance to workers.

## Key Terms

**capitation:** A payment method in which each provider, such as an HMO, receives a flat annual fee for each individual, regardless of how often services are used.

**copayment:** A specified amount that an insured individual must pay for a specified service or procedure (e.g., $20 for an office visit).

**deductible:** The amount an individual must pay out-of-pocket, usually yearly on a calendar-year basis, before insurance will begin to cover expenses.

**employment-based health insurance:** Coverage offered through one's own employment or the employment of a relative.

**fee-for-service plans:** The traditional type of healthcare policy; the physician sets a price for each type of service delivered, and then the patient or his or her insurer pays this price.

**group model:** An HMO that contracts with a medical group for the provision of healthcare services.

**health insurance:** A broad term that includes both public and private payers who cover medical expenditures incurred by a defined population in a variety of settings.

**health maintenance organization (HMO):** A managed care company that organizes and provides health care for its enrollees for a fixed prepaid premium.

**health status:** The condition of an individual's physiological and psychological state, and his or her interaction with the environment.

**individual practice association (IPA):** A type of healthcare provider organization composed of a group of independent practicing physicians who maintain their own offices and band together for the purpose of contracting their services to HMOs. An IPA may contract with and provide services to both HMO and non-HMO plan participants.

**insurance:** A plan in which individuals and organizations who are concerned about potential risks will pay premiums to an insurance company, who subsequently will reimburse them if there is loss.

**managed care:** A system that seeks to manage the cost of health care, the quality of that health care, and access to care; it is based on the belief that healthcare costs can be controlled by "managing" the way in which health care is delivered.

**Medicaid:** A joint federal/state/local program of health care for individuals whose income and resources are insufficient to pay for their care; it is governed by Title XIX of the federal Social Security Act and is administered by the states. Medicaid is the major source of payment for nursing home care of the elderly.

**Medicare:** A federal entitlement program of medical and healthcare coverage for the elderly, disabled, and persons with end-stage renal disease, governed by Title XVIII of the federal Social Security Act and consisting of four parts: Part A for institutional and homecare, Part B for medical care, Part C Medicare advantage program, and Part D drug prescription program.

**Medigap:** A type of private insurance coverage that may be purchased by an individual enrolled in Medicare to cover some needed services that are not covered by Medicare Parts A and B (i.e., "gaps").

**point-of-service (POS) plan:** A healthcare plan that offers enrollees the option of receiving services from participating or nonparticipating providers.

**preferred provider organization (PPO):** A network of providers who agree to deliver services for a reduced fee; the providers generally incur no financial risk. The financial burden is on the patient rather than the providers.

**premium:** A periodic payment required to keep an insurance policy requirement.

**staff model:** An HMO that employs providers directly and the providers see members/enrollees in the HMO's own facilities.

**State Children's Health Insurance Program (SCHIP):** A federal program that covers individuals who have incomes too high to qualify for state medical assistance but who cannot obtain private insurance. All states participate, but some do not cover dental.

## References

1. Catlin A, Cowan S, Heffler S, et al. National health spending in 2005. *Health Aff.* 2006;26(1):142-153.
2. Baicker K, Chandra A, Skinner JS. Geographic variation in health care and the problem of measuring racial disparities. *Perspect Bio Med.* 2005;48(1):S42-S53.
3. Sheils JF, Ruben R, Stapleton DC. The estimated costs and savings of medical nutrition therapy: the Medicare population. *J Am Diet Assoc.* 1999;99(4):428-435.
4. The Henry J. Kaiser Family Foundation. Employee health benefit: annual survey. http://www.nchc.org/. Accessed March 17, 2017.
5. The Henry J. Kaiser Family Foundation. Key facts about the unisured population. http://kff.org/uninsured/fact-sheet/key-facts-about-the-uninsured-population/. Accessed March 17, 2017.
6. Heflin C, Seifert K, Williams D. Food insufficiency and women's mental health: findings from a 3-year panel of welfare recipients. *Soc Sci Med.* 2005;61(9):1971-1982.
7. Ali NS. The relationship of socio-demographic factors with iron deficiency anaemia in children of 1-2 years of age. *J Pakistan Med Assoc.* 2001;51(3):130-132.
8. Massing MW. Income, income inequality, and cardiovascular disease mortality: relations among county populations of the United States, 1985 to 1994. *South Med J.* 2004;97(5):475-484.
9. Cohen S, Signorello L, Gammon M, Blot W. Obesity and recent mammography use among black and white women in the Southern Community Cohort Study (United States). *Cancer Causes Control.* 2007;8(7):765-773.

10. Kovener A, Jonas S. *Healthcare Delivery in the United States.* 11th ed. New York, NY: Springer; 2016.

11. U.S. Census Bureau. People with or without health insurance coverage by selected characteristics: 2002 and 2003. https://www.census.gov/topics/health/health-insurance.html. Accessed March 17, 2017.

12. National Center for Health Statistics. http://www.cdc.gov/nchs/datawh/nchsdefs/healthinsurancecov.htm. Accessed March 17, 2017.

13. National Center for Health Statistics. Ambulatory health care data. 2007. http://www.cdc.gov/nchs/about/major/ahcd/adata.htm#Physician. Accessed March 17, 2017.

14. Schneider MJ. *Introduction to Public Health.* Sudbury, MA: Jone and Bartlett; 2006.

15. Hitchcock J, Schubert PE, Thomas SA. *Community Health Nursing.* 2nd ed. United States: Clifton Park, NY: Thomson Delmar Learning; 2003.

16. Relman AS. Restructuring the U.S. health care system. http://www.issues.org/19.4/relman.html. Accessed March 17, 2017.

17. National Center for Health Statistics. Health insurance coverage. http://www.cdc.gov/nchs/. Accessed March 17, 2017.

18. National Center for Health Statistics. Health maintenance organization (HMO). http://www.cdc.gov/nchs. Accessed March 17, 2017.

19. The Henry Kaiser Family Foundation. Medicare expenditure. 2005. http://www.kff.org/medicare/upload/medicare-chart-Book-3rd-Edition-summer-2005-section-pdf.6. Accessed March 17, 2017.

20. Henry J. Kaiser Family Foundation. Medicare at a glance fact sheet. http://www.kff.org/medicare/1066.cfm. Accessed March 17, 2017.

21. Center for Medicare and Medicaid Services, US Dept of Health and Human Services. Medicare and Medicaid programs programs of all-inclusive care for the elderly (PACE) program revisions: final rule. *Fed Reg.* 2016;71(236):71243-71337.

22. Social Security Act. Entitlement to hospital insurance benefits. 2007. Sec. 226. [42 U.S.C. 426]. http://www.ssa.gov/OP_Home/ssact/title02/0226.htm. Accessed March 17, 2017.

23. Cox EE. Medicare beneficiaries' management of capped prescription benefits. *Med Care.* 2001;39(3):296-301.

24. Center for Medicare and Medicaid Services. Overview. http://www.cms.hhs.gov/MedicaidGenInfo/01_Overview.asp#TopOfPage. Accessed March 17, 2017.

25. Center for Medicare and Medicaid Services. Research, statistic, data, system. http://www.cms.gov/home/rsds.asp. Accessed March 17, 2017.

26. Center for Medicare and Medicaid. Brief summaries of Medicare & Medicaid. http://www.cms.hhs.gov/MedicareProgramRatesStats/02_SummaryMedicareMedicaid.asp. Accessed March 17, 2017.

27. Michael P. Impact and components of the Medicare MNT benefits. *J Am Diet Assoc.* 2001;101:1140-1141.

28. Hager MH. Medicare reform opens door for preventive nutrition services. *J Am Diet Assoc.* 2004;104(6):887-889.

29. Troyer JL, McAuley WJ, McCutcheon ME. Cost-effectiveness of medical nutrition therapy and therapeutically designed meals for older adults with cardiovascular disease. *J Am Diet Assoc.* 2010;110(12):1840-1851.

30. Philipson T, Dai C, Helmchen L, Jayachandran NV. The economics of obesity: a report on the workshop held at USDA's Economic Research Service. https://www.ers.usda.gov/publications/pub-details/?pubid=43451. Accessed March 17, 2017.

31. Ochs M. New Medicare changes to expand MNT access in 2002. *J Am Diet Assoc.* 2002;102:30.

32. Boyle MA, Holben D. *Community Nutrition in Action: An Entrepreneurial Approach.* 4th ed. Belmont, CA: Thomson Wadsworth; 2013.

33. Harvard Medical School. Simple changes in diet can protect you against friendly fire: what you eat can fuel or cool inflammation, a key driver of heart disease, diabetes, and other chronic conditions. *Harv Heart Lett.* 2007;17(5):3.

34. Daubenmier JJ, Weidner G, Sumner MD, et al. The contribution of changes in diet, exercise, and stress management to changes in coronary risk in women and men in the multisite cardiac lifestyle intervention program. *Ann Behav Med.* 2007;33(1):57-68.

35. Rice TT. Does open enrollment control premiums? A case study from the Medigap market. *Inquiry.* 2004;41(3):291-300.

36. US Dept of Health and Human Services, Center for Medicare and Medicare Services. https://www.cms.gov/medigap/. Accessed August 3, 2016.

37. Kilian JJ. Medicare part D: selected issues for pharmacists and beneficiaries in 2007. *J Manage Care Pharm.* 2007;13(1):59-65.

38. Center for Medicare and Medicaid Services. Medicare and Medicaid. https://www.cms.gov/medicareprogramratesstats/02_summarymedicaremedicaid.asp. Accessed March 17, 2017.

39. Berkowitz EE. Medicare and Medicaid: the past as prologue. *Health Care Financ Rev.* 2005;27(2):11-23.

40. Gavin NI, Adams EK, Manning WG, Raskind-Hood C, et al. The impact of welfare reform on insurance coverage before pregnancy and the timing

of prenatal care initiation. *Health Serv Res.* 2007;42(4):1564-1588.

41. Ozawa MM. Leavers from TANF and AFDC: how do they fare economically? *Soc Work.* 2005;50(3):239-249.

42. American Academy of Pediatrics. AAP agenda for children. 2006. https://www.aap.org/en-us/about-the-aap/aap-facts/AAP-Agenda-for-Children-Strategic-Plan/pages/AAP-Agenda-for-Children-Strategic-Plan-Medical-Home.aspx. Accessed March 17, 2017.

43. Dubay L, Guyer J, Mann C, Odeh M. Medicaid at the ten-year anniversary of SCHIP: looking back and moving forward. *Health Aff (Millwood).* 2007;26(2):370-381.

44. American Dietetic Association. Proposed insurance exchnages alter health care landscape. *J Am Diet Assoc.* 2011;9(12):1-3.

45. Illinois Department of Human Services. The reduction of infant mortality in Illinois. http://www.dhs.state.il.us/page.aspx?item=54927. Accessed March 17, 2017.

46. Ackermann RT, Morrero DG, Hicks KA, Hoerger TJ, et al. An evaluation of cost sharing to finance a diet and physical activity intervention to prevent diabetes. *Diabetes Care.* 2006;29(6):1237-1241.

# Appendix A

## Intervention Messages

---

**BOX A-1** Eat More Fiber

---

Eat five cups of fruits and vegetables a day.

- Use vegetables for main dishes, soups, salads, or snacks.
- Use fruits for breakfast, as salads, as desserts, or as snacks.

Eat more high-fiber cereal every day.

- Whole-grain bread products
- Brown rice
- Dried beans, peas, or lentils

# Appendix B

## Nutrition Assessment and Screening

### ▶ Purpose

Appendix B instructs community nutritionists and healthcare providers on how to use and interpret the Centers for Disease Control and Prevention (CDC) growth charts to assess physical growth in children and adolescents. Nutritionists can use these charts to compare growth in infants, children, and adolescents with a nationally representative reference based on children of all ages and racial or ethnic groups. Comparing body measurements with the appropriate age- and gender-specific growth chart enables nutritionists to monitor growth and identify potential health or nutrition-related problems.

Community nutritionists can assess the physical growth of children using the child's weight, stature, length, and head circumference during routine screening. Although one measurement plotted on a growth chart can be used to screen children for nutritional risk, it does not provide adequate information to determine the child's growth pattern. When plotted correctly, a series of accurate weights and measurements of stature or length provide important information about a child's growth pattern, which may be influenced by such factors as gestational age, birth weight, and parental stature. It is important to consider parental stature before assuming there is a health or nutrition concern. Other factors, such as the presence of a chronic illness or special healthcare need, must be considered, and additional evaluation may be required.

### ▶ How Is Body Mass Index Calculated and Interpreted?

Body mass index (BMI) is calculated the same way for both adults and children. The calculation is based on the formulas shown in **TABLE B-1**.

It is necessary to convert the weight and stature measurements to the appropriate decimal value. See **TABLE B-2**.

| TABLE B-1 Formulas for Calculating BMI | |
|---|---|
| **Measurement Units** | **Formula and Calculation** |
| Kilograms and meters (or centimeters) | Formula: weight (kg) ÷ [height (m)]$^2$<br>With the metric system, the formula for BMI is weight in kilograms divided by height in meters squared. Because height is commonly measured in centimeters, divide height in centimeters by 100 to obtain height in meters.<br>**Example: Weight = 68 kg, height = 165 cm (1.65 m)**<br>**Calculation: 68 ÷ (1.65)$^2$ = 24.98** |
| Pounds and inches | Formula: weight (lb) ÷ [height (in)]$^2$ × 703<br>Calculate BMI by dividing weight in pounds by height in inches squared and then multiplying by a conversion factor of 703.<br>**Example: Weight = 150 lb, height = 5'5" (65")**<br>**Calculation: [150 ÷ (65)2] × 703 = 24.96** |

## TABLE B-2  Decimal Conversions

| Fraction | Ounces | Decimal |
|----------|--------|---------|
| 1/8 | 2 | 0.125 |
| 1/4 | 4 | 0.25 |
| 3/8 | 6 | 0.375 |
| 1/2 | 8 | 0.5 |
| 5/8 | 10 | 0.625 |
| 3/4 | 12 | 0.75 |
| 7/8 | 14 | 0.875 |

*Examples:* 40 lb 4 oz = 40.25 lb; 44½ in = 44.5 in

## ▶ Aids for Calculation

### Length

1 meter (m) = 39 in

1 centimeter (cm) = 0.4 in

1 inch (in) = 2.5 cm

1 foot (ft) = 30 cm

This information is from the Centers for Disease Control and Prevention. CDC growth chart training. http://www.cdc.gov/nccdphp/dnpa/growthcharts /resources/growthchart.pdf and http://www.cdc.gov /nccdphp/dnpa/bmi/adult_BMI/about_adult_BMI.htm. Accessed October 30, 2008.

### Weight

1 kilogram (kg) = 1,000 g or 2.2 lb

1 gram (g) = 1/1,000 kg, 1,000 mg, or 0.035 oz

1 milligram (mg) = 1/1,000 g or 1,000 mcg

1 microgram (μg) = 1/1,000 mg

1 pound (lb) = 16 oz, 454 g, or 0.45 kg

1 ounce (oz) = about 28 g

## ▶ Assessing a Child's Growth Status

1. *Obtain accurate weights and measures.* When weighing and measuring children, follow procedures that yield accurate measurements and use equipment that is well maintained.
   - *Recumbent length:* Distance from the crown of the head to the bottom of the feet while the child is lying down
   - *Stature:* Height
2. *Select the appropriate growth chart.* Select the correct growth chart based on the age and gender of the child being weighed and measured.
   Use the following information when measuring boys and girls in the *recumbent* position (should be limited to those younger than 36 months):
   - Length-for-age
   - Weight-for-age
   - Head circumference-for-age
   - Weight-for-length
   Use the following information when determining the *stature* (standing height) of boys and girls ages 2 to 20 years:
   - Weight-for-age
   - Stature-for-age
   - BMI-for-age
3. *Record data.* After selecting the appropriate chart and entering the client's name and record number, if appropriate, complete the data entry table.
   First, record information about factors obtained at the initial visit that influenced growth:
   - Enter mother's and father's stature as reported.
   - Enter the gestational age in weeks.
     For children under 2 years of age, it is important to reserve a line for recording the child's birth data. (Omit this step when using growth charts for children ages 2 to 20 years.)
   - Enter the date of birth.
   - Enter birth weight, length, and head circumference.
   - Add notable comments (e.g., breastfeeding).
   Record information obtained during the current visit, including today's date.
   Determine the child's age to the nearest month for infants and quarter year for children 2 to 20 years.
4. *Plot measurements.* On the appropriate growth chart, plot the measurements recorded in the data entry table for the current visit.
   - Find the child's age on the horizontal axis. When plotting weight-for-length, find the length on the horizontal axis. Use a straight edge or right-angle ruler to draw a vertical line up from that point.

- Find the appropriate measurement (weight, length, stature, head circumference, or BMI) on the vertical axis. Use a straight edge or right-angle ruler to draw a horizontal line across from that point until it intersects the vertical line.
- Make a small dot where the two lines intersect.

## Overview of the CDC Anthropometric Indices

Weight, stature, length, and head circumference are used most often to assess size and growth (see **TABLE B-3**). When any of these measures is combined with age or length/stature, the result is an anthropometric index (e.g., weight-for-age). The CDC growth charts reflect five anthropometric indices that are gender-specific:

- *BMI-for-age* is an anthropometric index of weight and height combined with age. BMI-for-age is used to classify children and adolescents as underweight, overweight, or at risk for overweight.
- *Stature- or length-for-age* describes linear growth relative to age. Stature- or length-for-age is used to define shortness or tallness.
- *Weight-for-age* reflects body weight relative to age and is influenced by recent changes in health or nutritional status. It is not used to classify infants, children, and adolescents as underweight or overweight. However, it is important in early infancy for monitoring weight and helps explain changes in weight-for-length and BMI-for-age in older children.

- *Weight-for-length or stature* reflects body weight relative to length and requires no knowledge of age. It is an indicator to classify infants and young children as overweight and underweight.
- *Head circumference-for-age* is critical during infancy and can be charted up to 36 months of age. Head circumference measurements reflect brain size.

An appropriate reference population, accurate measurements, and age calculations are important factors when assessing childhood growth. Comparing body measurements to the appropriate age- and gender-specific growth chart enables community nutritionists and other healthcare professionals to monitor growth and identify potential health or nutrition-related problems.

## Assessment of Overweight Children and Adolescents

### Screening

The growth chart in **TABLE B-4** shows the BMI-for-age pattern of a boy who became overweight early in his preschool years. On the BMI-for-age chart at age 2, he was at the 50th percentile; his BMI-for-age increased rapidly, crossing the 75th and 85th percentiles to become at risk for overweight at 3 and 4 years old. His BMI-for-age continued to increase to above the 95th percentile at ages 7, 11, and 13 years.

**TABLE B-3** Anthropometric Indices

| Anthropometric Index | Percentile Cutoff Value | Nutritional Status Indicators |
|---|---|---|
| BMI-for-age | ≥ 95th percentile | Overweight |
| BMI-for-age | ≥ 85th and <95th percentile | At risk for overweight |
| Weight-for-length/stature | > 95th percentile | Overweight |
| BMI-for-age Weight-for-length | < 5th percentile | Underweight |
| Stature or length-for-age | < 5th percentile | Short stature |
| Head circumference-for-age | < 5th percentile > 95th percentile | Developmental problems |

Reproduced from: Centers for Disease Control and Prevention. Anthropometric indices. https://www.cdc.gov/nccdphp/dnpao/growthcharts/training/overview/page5_1.html. Accessed March 17, 2017.

**2 to 20 years: Boys**
**Body mass index-for-age percentiles**

NAME _____

RECORD # _____

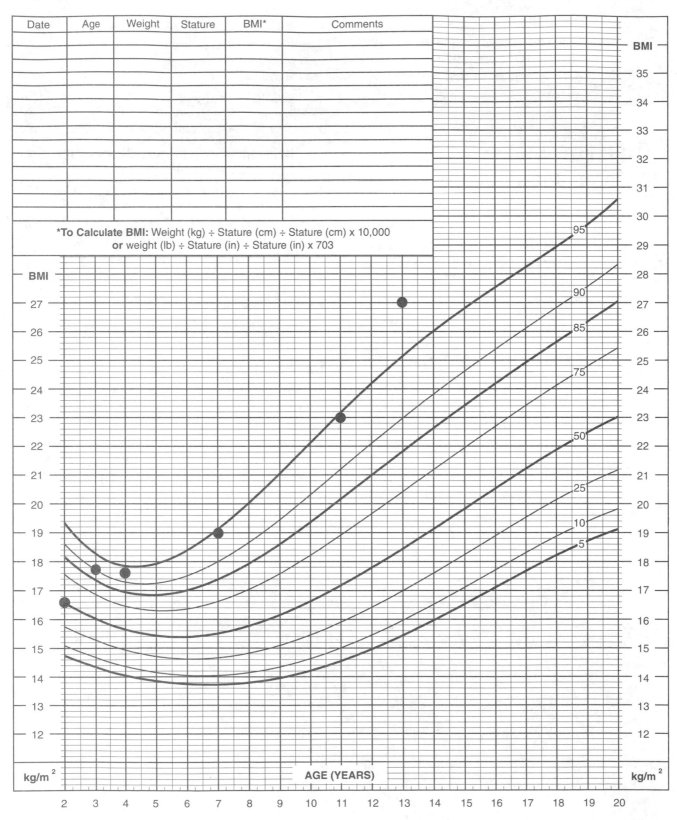

| Date | Age | Weight | Stature | BMI* | Comments |
|------|-----|--------|---------|------|----------|
| | | | | | |

***To Calculate BMI:** Weight (kg) ÷ Stature (cm) ÷ Stature (cm) x 10,000*
**or** weight (lb) ÷ Stature (in) ÷ Stature (in) x 703

AGE (YEARS)

Published May 30, 2000 (modified 10/16/00).

SOURCE: Developed by the National Center for Health Statistics in collaboration with
the National Center for Chronic Disease Prevention and Health Promotion (2000).
http://www.cdc.gov/growthcharts

SAFER • HEALTHIER • PEOPLE™

**TABLE B-4**  Sample BMI-for-Age Pattern Showing Early Onset of Overweight

| Age | Weight (lb) | Stature (in) | BMI |
|---|---|---|---|
| 2 | 28¼ | 34¾ | 16.4 |
| 3 | 38¼ | 38⅞ | 17.8 |
| 4 | 43½ | 41⅝ | 17.6 |
| 7 | 69¼ | 50⅜ | 19.2 |
| 11 | 111 | 58⅛ | 23.1 |
| 13 | 166¼ | 65¾ | 27 |

**TABLE B-5**  Weight- and Stature-for-Age for the Same Child

| Weight- and Stature-for-Age for the Same Child | | | |
|---|---|---|---|
| Age | Weight (lb) | Stature (in) | BMI |
| 2 | 28¼ | 34 3/4 | 16.4 |
| 3 | 38¼ | 38 7/8 | 17.8 |
| 4 | 43½ | 41 5/8 | 17.6 |
| 7 | 69¼ | 50 3/8 | 19.2 |
| 11 | 111 | 58 1/8 | 23.1 |
| 13 | 166¼ | 65 3/4 | 27 |

To understand how changes in weight and stature contributed to this boy's increase in BMI-for-age, it is helpful to review the weight-for-age and stature-for-age curves (see **TABLE B-5**). His stature-for-age at 2 years was above the 50th percentile, and it increased to above the 90th percentile by age 13. However, his weight-for-age increased more rapidly than stature (from the 50th percentile at age 2 to greater than the 95th percentile at age 13), which contributed to the increase in BMI-for-age.

## Assessment

When this boy was identified as at risk for overweight on the BMI-for-age chart at age 3, he should have received a medical assessment, as well as additional nutrition and physical activity assessments. The information from the assessments could have been used to target efforts for appropriate weight management goals to prevent the development of overweight.

## ▶ Management of Overweight Children and Adolescents

Strategies used in a management plan are based on information obtained from the assessment. Weight loss is recommended if complications such as hyperlipidemia or hypertension are identified, and for children 7 years or older with a BMI-for-age ≥ 95th percentile. Otherwise, weight maintenance is recommended.

| Age (Years) | BMI (Percentile) | Complication | Action |
|---|---|---|---|
| 2–7 | 85th–94th | N/A | Weight maintenance |
| | ≥ 95th | Yes | Weight loss |
| | | No | Weight maintenance |
| 7 and older | 85th–94th | Yes | Weight loss |
| | | No | Weight maintenance |
| | ≥ 95th | N/A | Weight loss |

Recommendations for weight management for children and adolescents 2–20 years old.

Modified from: Barlow SE, Dietz WH. Obesity evaluation and treatment: expert committee recommendations. *Pediatrics*. 1998; 102;e29, Figure 2, © 1998.

**2 to 20 years: Boys**

**Stature-for-age and Weight-for-age percentiles**

NAME _____

RECORD # _____

| Mother's Stature _____ Father's Stature _____ | | | | |
|---|---|---|---|---|
| Date | Age | Weight | Stature | BMI* |
| | | | | |
| | | | | |
| | | | | |
| | | | | |
| | | | | |

*To Calculate BMI: Weight (kg) ÷ Stature (cm) ÷ Stature (cm) x 10,000
or weight (lb) ÷ Stature (in) ÷ Stature (in) x 703

AGE (YEARS)

12  13  14  15  16  17  18  19  20

STATURE

WEIGHT

AGE (YEARS)

2  3  4  5  6  7  8  9  10  11  12  13  14  15  16  17  18  19  20

Published May 30, 2000 (modified 11/21/00).

SOURCE: Developed by the National Center for Health Statistics in collaboration with
the National Center for Chronic Disease Prevention and Health Promotion (2000).

http://www.cdc.gov/growthcharts

SAFER • HEALTHIER • PEOPLE™

# Appendix C

## Complementary and Alternative Practices

The use of complementary and alternative medicine (CAM) has increased significantly. The World Health Organization (WHO) classified 65 to 80 percent of the world's healthcare services as "traditional medicine."[1] According to this information and looking at CAM from a worldwide perspective, more people use CAM than modern Western medicine.[2]

The National Center for Complementary and Alternative Medicine (NCCAM), a part of the National Institutes of Health, defines CAM as "a group of diverse medical and healthcare systems, practices, and products that are not currently considered to be a component of conventional medicine [scientific medicine]."[3] Conventional medicine relies on modern scientific principles, modern technologies, and scientifically proven methods to prevent, diagnose, and treat health conditions.[4] The list of what is considered CAM changes as the therapies that are proved to be safe and effective are implemented into conventional health care. *Complementary medicine* is nonconventional treatment used in addition to conventional therapies; for example, a physician may ask a patient to use tai chi or massage therapy in addition to prescribing medicine for anxiety or arthritis. *Alternative medicine* replaces conventional therapies; for instance, a patient with cancer may use diets, supplements, herbs, and antioxidants instead of undergoing surgery, radiation, or chemotherapy that a conventional doctor recommended.

As stated by Gagne et al.[5]:

"Over the past decade, the magnitude and quality of the CAM evidence base has increased, to the point where several dozen meta-analyses and systematic reviews have been conducted. Examples include systematic reviews of acupuncture for postoperative nausea, massage for low back pain, and ginkgo for dementia. Because of the large number of CAM therapies, and the wide range of conditions for which these therapies are used, a great deal of additional research is needed that can provide a comprehensive basis for establishing dependable information CAM's safety and efficacy."

Herbal supplements are a type of dietary supplement that contains herbs either individually or in a blend. An herb (also called a botanical) is a plant or plant part used for its perfume, flavor, and/or therapeutic properties. In the United States, herbal and other dietary supplements are regulated by the U.S. Food and Drug Administration (FDA) as foods. This means that herbs do not have to meet the same standards as drugs and over-the-counter medications for proof of safety, effectiveness, and what the FDA calls Good Manufacturing Practices.[6] **TABLES C-1** and **C-2** present common alternative medical practices and popular herbal supplements.

| **TABLE C-1**  Common Alternative Medical Practices | | |
| --- | --- | --- |
| **Type** | **Claims and Principles of Practice** | **Results of Scientific Research** |
| Acupuncture | Used to treat a variety of common ailments. Based on an ancient Chinese medical practice in which thin needles are inserted into the skin or underlying muscles at specific places and stimulated to regulate the flow of "chi," the life force. | Although testing acupuncture is difficult, most studies fail to support its usefulness when not combined with conventional therapies. It may relieve nausea and vomiting associated with morning sickness and cancer chemotherapy. Acupuncture may stimulate the body to release natural pain-relieving compounds. |

*(continues)*

**TABLE C-1**  Common Alternative Medical Practices (*continued*)

| Type | Claims and Principles of Practice | Results of Scientific Research |
|---|---|---|
| Ayurvedic medicine | According to ancient Hindu religious beliefs, people can achieve good health by meditating; eating grains, *ghee* (a form of butter), milk, fruits, and vegetables; and using herbs. Lack of balance between "energies" causes health problems. Fasting and enemas are used to treat severe ailments. | Meditation relieves stress; fruits, vegetables, and dairy products are nutritious foods; and some herbs have medicinal value. Ghee, however, can be fattening, and fasting is not a healthy practice. Enemas are unnecessary for good health and should be used only under a physician's instructions. |
| Chiropractic medicine | According to some chiropractors, misaligned spinal bones cause disease. Spinal manipulation prevents or cures disease by correcting the spine. Other practitioners use spinal manipulation, but accept the germ theory of disease. | Can be effective in treating certain types of back pain, but some spinal conditions require medications and surgery that only a physician can provide. There is no scientific evidence that all diseases can be treated by spinal adjustment. |
| Homeopathy | Use of extremely dilute solutions of natural substances to treat specific illness symptoms. The U.S. Congress passed a law in 1938 declaring that homeopathic remedies are to be regulated by the FDA in the same manner as nonprescription, over-the-counter (OTC) drugs, which means that they can be purchased without a physician's prescription. | Studies do not indicate that homeopathy is effective. |
| Naturopathy or natural medicine | Practice based on natural healing. Practitioners believe diseases occur as the body rids itself of wastes and toxins. Treatments include fasting, enemas, acupuncture, and "natural" drugs. | There is no standardized training for practitioners, who are called naturopaths. They may recommend patients ignore conventional medical advice and practices, which can be harmful. |
| Reflexology or zone therapy | Specific areas of the hands and feet correspond to certain organs. To alleviate pain or treat certain diseases, practitioners press on the area that is related to the affected tissues. | Scientific evidence does not indicate that pressing on body parts is an effective method for diagnosing or treating ailments. |
| Biofield therapies | These practices aim to affect energy fields that surround and penetrate the human body. Some of these therapies use manipulation such as touch, reiki, and qi gong. | The existence of such fields has not been scientifically proven. |
| Bioelectromagnetic | This therapy uses unconventional electrical energy, magnetic energy, or alternating-current or direct-current fields to stimulate wound and bone healing. | The efficacy of this treatment has not been scientifically proven. |

| Type | Claims and Principles of Practice | Results of Scientific Research |
|------|-----------------------------------|-------------------------------|
| Mind–body medicine | These practices use a variety of techniques to improve mind capacity, and thus to affect the symptoms and functions of the body. They include behavioral therapy, mental healing (prayer, hypnosis, meditation, imagery, humor, yoga), and creative outlets (music, art, dance, tai chi). | Some of the practices, such as support groups and cognitive improvement, are considered CAM. There is evidence that mind–body interventions can be effective in the treatment of coronary artery disease, cardiac rehabilitation, chronic pain management, and quality of life. They also improve individuals' mood and immune system and relieve stress. |
| Chelation therapy | Chelation therapy is an investigational therapy using a manmade amino acid, ethylenediaminetetraacetic acid (EDTA). It is added to the blood through a vein to treat heart disease. | An international research study is now testing whether chelation therapy is safe and effective for treating heart disease. However, this has not been scientifically proven. |
| Orthomolecular medicine | This practice is based on the premise that many diseases and abnormalities result from varying biochemical and/or chemical needs specific to each individual. It holds that they can be prevented, treated, or sometimes cured by achieving optimum levels for that individual's body of various natural chemical substances. It normally employs such dietary elements as vitamins, minerals, amino acids, trace elements, and essential fatty acids. | There is not sufficient evidence for clinical use; scientific foundations are weak, and studies that have been performed are too few. |
| Aromatherapy | This is a generic term that refers to any of the various traditions' use of essential oils and other scented compounds from plants to improve a person's mood or health. It is sometimes used in combination with other alternative medical practices and spiritual beliefs. | The consensus among most medical professionals in the United States and England is that although pleasant scents can improve relaxation, there is currently insufficient scientific proof of the effectiveness of aromatherapy in general. |

## TABLE C-2  Popular Herbal Supplements

| Supplement | Common Claims | Uses | Risks |
|------------|---------------|------|-------|
| St. John's wort | Relieves depression. | Can reduce mild to moderate depression symptoms; no value for major depression. | Can interfere with birth control pills and other prescribed medicines, increase sensitivity to sunlight, and cause stomach upset. |
| Saw palmetto | Improves urine flow. | May reduce symptoms of prostate enlargement that are not caused by cancer. | May interfere with PSA test to detect prostate cancer. |

(continues)

**TABLE C-2** Popular Herbal Supplements *(continued)*

| Supplement | Common Claims | Uses | Risks |
|---|---|---|---|
| Feverfew | Relieves headaches, fever, and arthritis pain. | Contains a chemical that may prevent migraines or reduce their severity. | May cause dangerous interactions with aspirin or warfarin (Coumadin; a prescription drug). |
| Echinacea | Prevents colds and influenza. | Does not prevent colds or reduce their severity. | May cause allergic response and may be a liver toxin. |
| Ginkgo biloba | Enhances memory and sense of well-being; prevents dementia. | May mildly improve mental performance but is ineffective as a treatment for Alzheimer's disease. | May interfere with normal blood clotting, cause intestinal upset, and increase blood pressure. |
| Ginseng | Enhances sexual, mental, and exercise performance; increases energy; relieves stress and depression. | Has no mood-enhancing effect. Asian ginsengs may improve immune system functioning and reduce fatigue. Lack of scientific findings to support benefits in humans. | Can cause "jitters," insomnia, hypertension, and diarrhea and can be addictive; can be contaminated with pesticides and the toxic mineral lead. |
| Yohimbe | Enhances muscle development and performance. | Dilates blood vessels but has no beneficial effects on muscle growth or sex drive of humans, prevention of erectile dysfunction, or reduction of adipose tissues. | Can produce abnormal behavior, high blood pressure, and heart attacks. Large amount can cause anxiety reactions. |
| Ma huang (ephedra) | Enhances weight loss and muscle growth. | Increases heart rate and blood pressure; contains the stimulant ephedrine. | Has been linked to headaches, heart attacks, strokes, and death. |
| Guarana | Boosts energy and enhances weight loss. | Acts as a stimulant drug. | May cause nausea, anxiety, and irregular heartbeat. |
| Kava | Relieves anxiety and induces sleep. | Acts as a depressant drug. | May cause serious liver damage; do not use when driving. |
| Aloe | Heals damaged skin. | Used externally to relieve skin discomforts and internally as a laxative. | Research suggests it can negatively affect healing. |
| Black cohosh | Remedies the symptoms of premenstrual tension, menopause, and other gynecological problems. | Reduces gynecological problems. | Inhibits iron absorption; may increase or prolong bleeding. |
| Chaparral leaves | Allegedly cures cancer, venereal disease, arthritis, tuberculosis, bowel cramps, rheumatism, and colds. | Chaparral tea is an old Indian remedy for cancer. | Risk of liver and kidney problems. |

| Supplement | Common Claims | Uses | Risks |
|---|---|---|---|
| Garlic bulbs | Prevent heart disease and cancer, lower blood cholesterol and blood pressure. | Used for cardiovascular and cancer benefits. | Excessive amounts can thin the blood similar to the effect of aspirin, and cause diarrhea, nausea, and indigestion. |
| Valerian | A sedative anticonvulsant. It sedates agitated persons and stimulates fatigued persons. | Used for migraine treatment and pain. | Large doses or chronic use may result in stomachaches, apathy, and feelings of mental dullness or mild depression. |
| Ginger | Used for colic and nausea. It is classified as a stimulant. | It is used to control the nausea associated with cancer caused by chemotherapy; it may be directly involved in the treatment of cancer. | Allergic reactions to ginger can result in a rash. It is generally recognized as safe. |
| Goldenseal | Used as an antimicrobial, antiinflammatory, muscle stimulant, and laxative. | Used for atonic dyspepsia, chronic constipation, hepatic congestion, urinary infection, and cirrhosis of the liver. | Taking goldenseal over a long period can reduce absorption of B vitamins. It should not be used if an infection is at an early stage or there are more chills than fever. |

Modified from: Alters S, Schiff W. *Essential Concepts for Health Living,* 4th ed. Sudbury, MA: Jones & Bartlett; 2006; and National Institutes of Health, National Center for Complementary Alternative Medicine. Understanding CAM. http://nccam.nih.gov/health. Accessed December 17, 2007.

There are several reasons why CAM is popular among consumers. The following are some of the factors responsible for the increased use of CAM[2]:

- It is familiar and easy to understand.
- It is noninvasive, with few side effects.
- Conventional modern medicine does not fully correspond to the individual's demands.
- The trend is toward a more holistic medical approach.
- Medical expenses are increasing.
- Many health conditions have no cure.
- It is harder for people to access conventional medicine.

One of the major roles and responsibilities of dietetics nutritionists is to advocate eating a wide variety of foods. Low levels of nutrients that do not exceed the Recommended Dietary Allowance (RDA) are recommended for clients who choose to use supplements. The use of dietary supplements should be based on well-accepted scientific evidence, and they should be recommended by physicians or dietitians. Also, consider the following recommendations when dealing with clients[7]:

- Appreciate the individuality of clients and that they have the right to be involved in decision making about their treatment.
- Learn from clients, all members of the primary health-care team, and other resources in the community.
- Realize the importance of clear communication between different individuals involved in patient care.
- Recognize the importance of consulting with complementary therapists, including those utilizing therapeutic touch.
- Maintain an open mind about alternative approaches to client care.

- Understand that not all clients will disclose their use of complementary therapies to a conventional practitioner, and understand why this may be.
- Respect the rights of clients to choose different forms of therapy or to attend a range of practitioners.

## References

1. Jonas WB. Researching alternative medicine. *Nat Med.* 1997;3:824-882.
2. Suzuki N. Complementary and alternative medicine: a Japanese perspective. *Evid Based Complement Alternat Med.* 2004;1(2)113.
3. National Center for Complementary and Alternative Medicine. What is CAM? http://nccam.nih.gov/health/whatiscam. Accessed November 14, 2008.
4. Alters S, Schiff W. *Essential Concepts for Health Living*, 4th ed. Sudbury, MA: Jones and Bartlett; 2006.
5. Gagne L, Schnurr J, Star B, Premkumar K, et al. *Complementary and Alternative Medicine: Description of Vertical Theme.* Saskatoon, SK: College of Medicine, University of Saskatchewan; 2006.
6. National Center for Complementary and Alternative Medicine. Herbal Supplements. Consider safety, too. https://nccih.nih.gov/health/herbsataglance.htm. Accessed March 17, 2017.
7. Molassiotis A, Fernandez-Ortega P, Pud D, Ozden G, et al. Use of complementary and alternative medicine in cancer patients: a European survey. *Ann Oncol.* 2005;16(4):655-663.

# Appendix D

## MyPlate

**10 tips**
*Nutrition Education Series*

# liven up your meals with vegetables and fruits

**10 tips to improve your meals with vegetables and fruits**

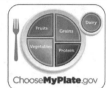

ChooseMyPlate.gov

**Discover the many benefits of adding vegetables and fruits to your meals.** They are low in fat and calories, while providing fiber and other key nutrients. Most Americans should eat more than 3 cups—and for some, up to 6 cups—of vegetables and fruits each day. Vegetables and fruits don't just add nutrition to meals. They can also add color, flavor, and texture. Explore these creative ways to bring healthy foods to your table.

**1 fire up the grill**
Use the grill to cook vegetables and fruits. Try grilling mushrooms, carrots, peppers, or potatoes on a kabob skewer. Brush with oil to keep them from drying out. Grilled fruits like peaches, pineapple, or mangos add great flavor to a cookout.

**2 expand the flavor of your casseroles**
Mix vegetables such as sauteed onions, peas, pinto beans, or tomatoes into your favorite dish for that extra flavor.

**3 planning something Italian?**
Add extra vegetables to your pasta dish. Slip some peppers, spinach, red beans, onions, or cherry tomatoes into your traditional tomato sauce. Vegetables provide texture and low-calorie bulk that satisfies.

**4 get creative with your salad**
Toss in shredded carrots, strawberries, spinach, watercress, orange segments, or sweet peas for a flavorful, fun salad.

**5 salad bars aren't just for salads**
Try eating sliced fruit from the salad bar as your dessert when dining out. This will help you avoid any baked desserts that are high in calories.

**6 get in on the stir-frying fun**
Try something new! Stir-fry your veggies—like broccoli, carrots, sugar snap peas, mushrooms, or green beans—for a quick-and-easy addition to any meal.

**7 add them to your sandwiches**
Whether it is a sandwich or wrap, vegetables make great additions to both. Try sliced tomatoes, romaine lettuce, or avocado on your everday sandwich or wrap for extra flavor.

**8 be creative with your baked goods**
Add apples, bananas, blueberries, or pears to your favorite muffin recipe for a treat.

**9 make a tasty fruit smoothie**
For dessert, blend strawberries, blueberries, or raspberries with frozen bananas and 100% fruit juice for a delicious frozen fruit smoothie.

**10 liven up an omelet**
Boost the color and flavor of your morning omelet with vegetables. Simply chop, saute, and add them to the egg as it cooks. Try combining different vegetables, such as mushrooms, spinach, onions, or bell peppers.

Go to www.ChooseMyPlate.gov for more information.

# Appendix E

## Canada's Food Guide

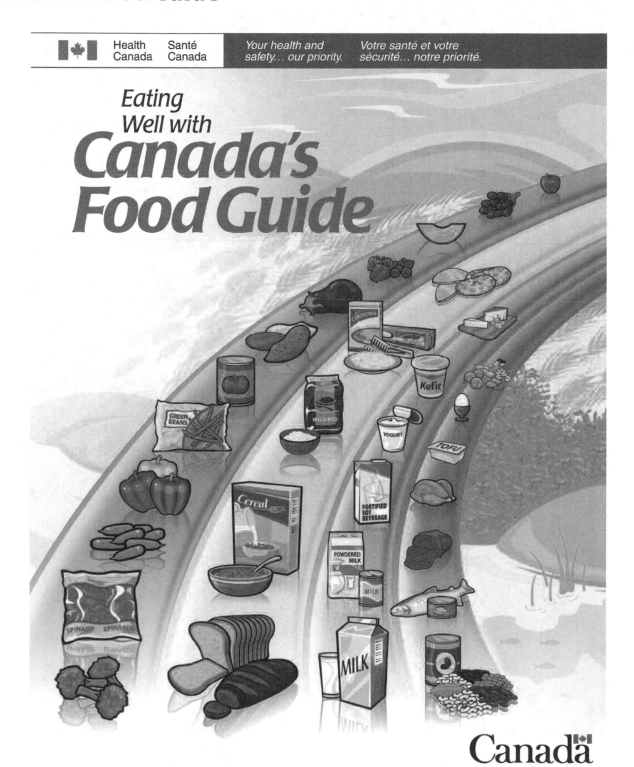

# Recommended Number of *Food Guide Servings* per Day

| | Children | | | Teens | | Adults | | | |
|---|---|---|---|---|---|---|---|---|---|
| **Age in Years** | **2-3** | **4-8** | **9-13** | **14-18** | | **19-50** | | **51+** | |
| **Sex** | **Girls and Boys** | | | **Females** | **Males** | **Females** | **Males** | **Females** | **Males** |
| **Vegetables and Fruit** | 4 | 5 | 6 | 7 | 8 | 7-8 | 8-10 | 7 | 7 |
| **Grain Products** | 3 | 4 | 6 | 6 | 7 | 6-7 | 8 | 6 | 7 |
| **Milk and Alternatives** | 2 | 2 | 3-4 | 3-4 | 3-4 | 2 | 2 | 3 | 3 |
| **Meat and Alternatives** | 1 | 1 | 1-2 | 2 | 3 | 2 | 3 | 2 | 3 |

The chart above shows how many Food Guide Servings you need from each of the four food groups every day.

Having the amount and type of food recommended and following the tips in *Canada's Food Guide* will help:

- Meet your needs for vitamins, minerals and other nutrients.
- Reduce your risk of obesity, type 2 diabetes, heart disease, certain types of cancer and osteoporosis.
- Contribute to your overall health and vitality.

## *What is One Food Guide Serving?*
*Look at the examples below.*

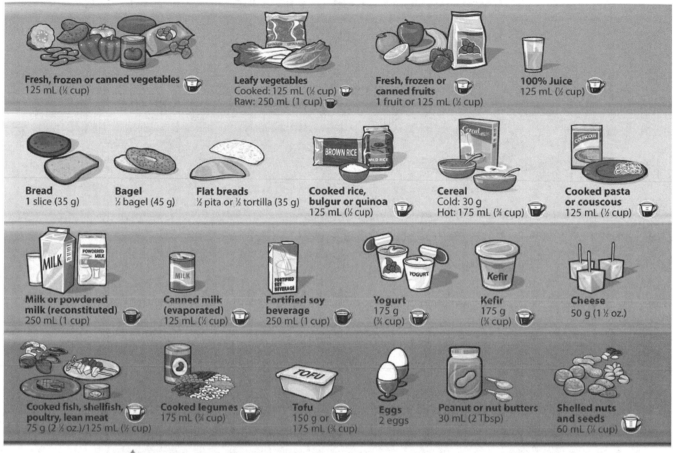

**Fresh, frozen or canned vegetables**
125 mL (½ cup)

**Leafy vegetables**
Cooked: 125 mL (½ cup)
Raw: 250 mL (1 cup)

**Fresh, frozen or canned fruits**
1 fruit or 125 mL (½ cup)

**100% Juice**
125 mL (½ cup)

**Bread**
1 slice (35 g)

**Bagel**
½ bagel (45 g)

**Flat breads**
½ pita or ½ tortilla (35 g)

**Cooked rice, bulgur or quinoa**
125 mL (½ cup)

**Cereal**
Cold: 30 g
Hot: 175 mL (¾ cup)

**Cooked pasta or couscous**
125 mL (½ cup)

**Milk or powdered milk (reconstituted)**
250 mL (1 cup)

**Canned milk (evaporated)**
125 mL (½ cup)

**Fortified soy beverage**
250 mL (1 cup)

**Yogurt**
175 g
(¾ cup)

**Kefir**
175 g
(¾ cup)

**Cheese**
50 g (1 ½ oz.)

**Cooked fish, shellfish, poultry, lean meat**
75 g (2 ½ oz.)/125 mL (½ cup)

**Cooked legumes**
175 mL (¾ cup)

**Tofu**
150 g or
175 mL (¾ cup)

**Eggs**
2 eggs

**Peanut or nut butters**
30 mL (2 Tbsp)

**Shelled nuts and seeds**
60 mL (¼ cup)

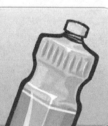

**Oils and Fats**
- Include a small amount – 30 to 45 mL (2 to 3 Tbsp) – of unsaturated fat each day. This includes oil used for cooking, salad dressings, margarine and mayonnaise.
- Use vegetable oils such as canola, olive and soybean.
- Choose soft margarines that are low in saturated and trans fats.
- Limit butter, hard margarine, lard and shortening.

# Make each Food Guide Serving count...
## wherever you are – at home, at school, at work or when eating out!

▸ **Eat at least one dark green and one orange vegetable each day.**
- Go for dark green vegetables such as broccoli, romaine lettuce and spinach.
- Go for orange vegetables such as carrots, sweet potatoes and winter squash.

▸ **Choose vegetables and fruit prepared with little or no added fat, sugar or salt.**
- Enjoy vegetables steamed, baked or stir-fried instead of deep-fried.

▸ **Have vegetables and fruit more often than juice.**

▸ **Make at least half of your grain products whole grain each day.**
- Eat a variety of whole grains such as barley, brown rice, oats, quinoa and wild rice.
- Enjoy whole grain breads, oatmeal or whole wheat pasta.

▸ **Choose grain products that are lower in fat, sugar or salt.**
- Compare the Nutrition Facts table on labels to make wise choices.
- Enjoy the true taste of grain products. When adding sauces or spreads, use small amounts.

▸ **Drink skim, 1%, or 2% milk each day.**
- Have 500 mL (2 cups) of milk every day for adequate vitamin D.
- Drink fortified soy beverages if you do not drink milk.

▸ **Select lower fat milk alternatives.**
- Compare the Nutrition Facts table on yogurts or cheeses to make wise choices.

▸ **Have meat alternatives such as beans, lentils and tofu often.**

▸ **Eat at least two Food Guide Servings of fish each week.***
- Choose fish such as char, herring, mackerel, salmon, sardines and trout.

▸ **Select lean meat and alternatives prepared with little or no added fat or salt.**
- Trim the visible fat from meats. Remove the skin on poultry.
- Use cooking methods such as roasting, baking or poaching that require little or no added fat.
- If you eat luncheon meats, sausages or prepackaged meats, choose those lower in salt (sodium) and fat.

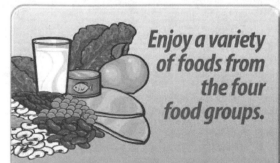

## Enjoy a variety of foods from the four food groups.

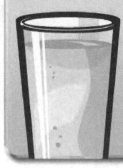

## Satisfy your thirst with water!

Drink water regularly. It's a calorie-free way to quench your thirst. Drink more water in hot weather or when you are very active.

\* Health Canada provides advice for limiting exposure to mercury from certain types of fish. Refer to www.healthcanada.gc.ca for the latest information.

## *Advice for different ages and stages...*

### Children

Following *Canada's Food Guide* helps children grow and thrive.

Young children have small appetites and need calories for growth and development.

- Serve small nutritious meals and snacks each day.

- Do not restrict nutritious foods because of their fat content. Offer a variety of foods from the four food groups.

- Most of all... be a good role model.

### Women of childbearing age

All women who could become pregnant and those who are pregnant or breastfeeding need a multivitamin containing **folic acid** every day. Pregnant women need to ensure that their multivitamin also contains **iron**. A health care professional can help you find the multivitamin that's right for you.

Pregnant and breastfeeding women need more calories. Include an extra 2 to 3 Food Guide Servings each day.

**Here are two examples:**
- Have fruit and yogurt for a snack, or

- Have an extra slice of toast at breakfast and an extra glass of milk at supper.

### Men and women over 50

The need for **vitamin D** increases after the age of 50.

In addition to following *Canada's Food Guide*, everyone over the age of 50 should take a daily vitamin D supplement of 10 µg (400 IU).

## *How do I count Food Guide Servings in a meal?*

### Here is an example:

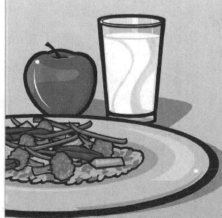

| Vegetable and beef stir-fry with rice, a glass of milk and an apple for dessert | | |
|---|---|---|
| 250 mL (1 cup) mixed broccoli, carrot and sweet red pepper | = | 2 **Vegetables and Fruit** Food Guide Servings |
| 75 g (2 ½ oz.) lean beef | = | 1 **Meat and Alternatives** Food Guide Serving |
| 250 mL (1 cup) brown rice | = | 2 **Grain Products** Food Guide Servings |
| 5 mL (1 tsp) canola oil | = | part of your **Oils and Fats** intake for the day |
| 250 mL (1 cup) 1% milk | = | 1 **Milk and Alternatives** Food Guide Serving |
| 1 apple | = | 1 **Vegetables and Fruit** Food Guide Serving |

# Eat well and be active today and every day!

## The benefits of eating well and being active include:
- Better overall health.
- Lower risk of disease.
- A healthy body weight.
- Feeling and looking better.
- More energy.
- Stronger muscles and bones.

## Be active

To be active every day is a step towards better health and a healthy body weight.

*Canada's Physical Activity Guide* recommends building 30 to 60 minutes of moderate physical activity into daily life for adults and at least 90 minutes a day for children and youth. You don't have to do it all at once. Add it up in periods of at least 10 minutes at a time for adults and five minutes at a time for children and youth.

*Start slowly and build up.*

## Eat well

Another important step towards better health and a healthy body weight is to follow *Canada's Food Guide* by:

- Eating the recommended amount and type of food each day.
- Limiting foods and beverages high in calories, fat, sugar or salt (sodium) such as cakes and pastries, chocolate and candies, cookies and granola bars, doughnuts and muffins, ice cream and frozen desserts, french fries, potato chips, nachos and other salty snacks, alcohol, fruit flavoured drinks, soft drinks, sports and energy drinks, and sweetened hot or cold drinks.

## Read the label

- Compare the Nutrition Facts table on food labels to choose products that contain less fat, saturated fat, trans fat, sugar and sodium.
- Keep in mind that the calories and nutrients listed are for the amount of food found at the top of the Nutrition Facts table.

### Nutrition Facts
Per 0 mL (0 g)

| Amount | % Daily Value |
|---|---|
| Calories 0 | |
| Fat 0 g | 0 % |
| Saturates 0 g | 0 % |
| + Trans 0 g | |
| Cholesterol 0 mg | |
| Sodium 0 mg | 0 % |
| Carbohydrate 0 g | 0 % |
| Fibre 0 g | 0 % |
| Sugars 0 g | |
| Protein 0 g | |
| Vitamin A 0 % | Vitamin C 0 % |
| Calcium 0 % | Iron 0 % |

## Limit trans fat

When a Nutrition Facts table is not available, ask for nutrition information to choose foods lower in trans and saturated fats.

## Take a step today...

✓ Have breakfast every day. It may help control your hunger later in the day.

✓ Walk wherever you can – get off the bus early, use the stairs.

✓ Benefit from eating vegetables and fruit at all meals and as snacks.

✓ Spend less time being inactive such as watching TV or playing computer games.

✓ Request nutrition information about menu items when eating out to help you make healthier choices.

✓ Enjoy eating with family and friends!

✓ Take time to eat and savour every bite!

*For more information, interactive tools, or additional copies visit Canada's Food Guide on-line at:*
**www.healthcanada.gc.ca/foodguide**

or contact:

Publications
Health Canada
Ottawa, Ontario K1A 0K9
E-Mail: publications@hc-sc.gc.ca
Tel.: 1-866-225-0709
Fax: (613) 941-5366
TTY: 1-800-267-1245

Également disponible en français sous le titre : Bien manger avec le Guide alimentaire canadien

This publication can be made available on request on diskette, large print, audio-cassette and braille.

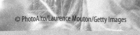

# Appendix F

## The Research Process

In community and public health nutrition, research, nutrition, and epidemiological processes are used to solve health-related problems. These processes involve assessment, planning, implementation, evaluation, and action. The action stage involves a continuous assessment of the community's needs coupled with planning, implementation, and evaluation. The epidemiological and research processes develop knowledge.[1] The nutrition process uses nutrition knowledge to provide nutrition-related services to individuals, families, groups, communities, and the public. The community nutritionist must consider several stages when planning or conducting nutrition research. These stages are presented in **BOX F-1**.

---

**BOX F-1** Stages of the Research Process

### Assessment and Conceptual Stage
- Identify and choose the problem or issue that is important to the community.
- Review related literature.
- Contact people in the field and discuss the problem with them.
- Identify available resources (personnel, equipment, data process capabilities, nutrient database, and other collaborative opportunities).
- Identify the purpose of the research (*what*, such as body weight, iron levels, calcium levels, or sodium intake).
- Determine the direct and indirect costs for conducting the research.
- Choose the population to be studied.

### Planning and Designing Stage
- State the research problem (*who*, such as gender, age, or ethnicity).
- Continue the review of related literature.
- Select an appropriate theoretical framework.
- Select a research design and appropriate methodology (*how*, such as alterations in food selection, physical activity level, or eating habits).
- Design the data collection plan (*when*, such as the starting and ending of the research).
- Select appropriate statistical methods and data analysis methods.
- Finalize and review the research plan.
- Implement the human subject approval process obtained from the local institutional review board, or boards can be included to support the research study.
- Implement pilot studies and revisions in design. (The results from the pilot studies may be used to support an application for funding for the study.)

### Implementation and Empirical Stage
- Invite and select community members to participate (key informants, focus group, community forum, etc.).
- Implement the data collection plan (collected by questionnaire using 24-hour recall or food frequency checklist, interviews, physical examination such as anthropometric measurements, and laboratory evaluation such as blood for iron status, bone density measurement, and blood pressure measurement).
- Prepare data for analysis. (If unavoidable, only minimal necessary individually identifiable information should be used.)

*(continues)*

**BOX F-1** Stages of the Research Process *(continued)*

### Evaluation/Analytical Stage
- Analyze the data using the appropriate statistical method.
- Interpret the results. (Consider limitations to the study methodology such as low response rate.)
- Draw conclusions.

### Action and Dissemination Stage
- Present the research findings to the target community.
- Use the results in practice (nutrition education programs).
- Present the results to the funding agency, if applicable.

Modified from Stanhope M, Lancaster J. Community and Public Health Nursing. 5th ed. New York: Mosby; 2000.

The research process requires a great deal of time and patience. Therefore, the researcher must first select the health problem that is important to the community and then work through each stage of the research process to find a solution to that problem. The researcher can start from the first stage (assessment and conceptual) and progress from stage to stage. Each stage must be consistent with the objective of the research project, and all must reflect the total study. Sometimes the researcher may go back and forth among the different stages of the research process, but it is important to start with the first stage.

## ▶ Assessment and Conceptual Stage

During the conceptual stage, the researcher must translate the abstract concept into a measurable outcome. This stage is driven by the nutritionist's curiosity, interest, or the results of the community's needs assessment. It also stimulates or generates research questions that typically narrow the problem to a more specific issue that must be addressed.[2] For example, a nutritionist may wonder why some African American older persons experience high rates of hypertension. The nutritionist would then critically review related research literature to gain more knowledge of the nutrition problem and how the results from the various studies relate to the nutrition problem. It is important for the nutritionist to evaluate the quality of the literature being reviewed—for example, the appropriateness of the methodology used. It is also important to note that in some situations the concept for the research study may not have been tested in published literature.

This initial literature review helps the nutritionist select a hypothesis or purpose and scope for the study. In the example given, the nutritionist would have learned from the review of literature that high sodium intake and obesity are linked to hypertension in some individuals.[3] The hypothesis then could be stated in this way: There will be a significant decrease in the sodium, fat, and caloric intake of those African American older persons in a particular community who participate in a nutrition intervention program. Another example of a community-based research study might be to increase bone density in postmenopausal women. The hypothesis could be that there will be a significant increase in the level of physical activity and the intake of calcium and vitamin D for postmenopausal women employees in 10 worksites who received a nutrition intervention program compared with postmenopausal women employees in 10 control worksites who did not receive the intervention program.

Once the research question (hypothesis) has been developed, the next step is to clearly define the characteristics of the study population. For example, the study population may include older African American people in a particular community or postmenopausal women of different ethnic backgrounds within a specific age range who live in a specified geographic area served by a particular community or public health agency. Strategies for collecting the data will vary with the community and the health issues to be addressed. Some suggested strategies that have been used successfully include community surveys (both self-administered and assisted questionnaires), focus groups, direct interviews, community forums, and collection of health services data.[4,5]

## ▶ Planning and Designing Stage

After the researcher has reviewed the related literature and determined the purpose, scope, and characteristics of the study, he or she needs to plan or design the study. Planning is a logical, organized process that proceeds step by step. It involves determining the procedure for collecting the data and making the concept of the study clear to the community, staff, and funding agency. In the planning stage, the specific research focus is stated and important terms are defined.[1,6]

Designing a research project for the community is a problem-solving process. After the nutritionist has conducted the community needs assessment, he or she selects the most pressing nutrition problem for the study and decides on a methodology consistent with the research question. The researcher can use the information obtained from the literature review to define terms and develop a scientific body of knowledge for the research study.

The nutritionist must also select a theoretical framework that is appropriate for the problem to be investigated. In the fictitious examples provided earlier, the nutritionist could select the Health Belief Model, which can be used for an intervention for persons with clinical nutrition–related risk factors, such as cardiovascular disease, hypertension, or osteoporosis.[6-9] Such individuals are faced with important and often overriding concerns about health. However, the Health Belief Model is of limited use for studies on subjects such as the primary prevention of cancer.[6] See Chapter 13 for details on the Health Belief Model and other models.

After selecting the theoretical framework, the nutritionist determines the important variables of the study, such as the dependent and independent variables. A variable is a characteristic of a person, object, or phenomenon that can take on different values.[10] These may be in the form of numbers (e.g., age, weight, height, income) or nonnumeric characteristics (e.g., gender, ethnicity, religion, and geographic location). Dependent variables are the outcomes measured in an experiment. They are expected to change as a result of an experimental manipulation of the independent variable(s). Independent variables are the conditions of an experiment that are methodically manipulated by the investigator. The state of the problem and the objective of the study determine whether a variable is dependent or independent. Therefore, when designing a research study, it is important to state which variable is dependent and which is independent.

Another variable to consider is the confounding variable. A variable that is associated with a health problem and with a possible cause of the problem (e.g., cigarette smoking causes cancer) may be a confounding variable.[11] Confounding variables may strengthen or weaken the relationship between the health problem being studied and the potential cause. For example, a confounding variable may influence the outcome of a research study. The following figure presents dependent, independent, and confounding variables. The figure shows the relationship between bottle-feeding and diarrhea in infants, but a confounding variable (such

as the mother's level of education, income, or age) may be related to bottle-feeding and diarrhea. Therefore, the mother's education level, income, and age should be considered in determining the cause of diarrhea. The researcher may consider this variable in the research design (e.g., selecting only mothers with a specific level of education, income, and age) or separate mothers according to education level, income, and age during data analysis to determine the relationship between bottle-feeding and the incidence of diarrhea.[11,12]

After determining the variables for the study, the nutritionist next selects a research procedure that is appropriate to the incident being investigated. The technique may be historical, observational, surveys, or experimental. The researcher must consider the different requirements a research design creates, determine whether the data will be collected at one point in time or longitudinally, and decide whether the data will be collected from a single group or across various groups in the population. The nutritionist may decide that a survey is the most appropriate procedure for investigating dietary habits and for intervention studies because it permits collecting data during one time period.

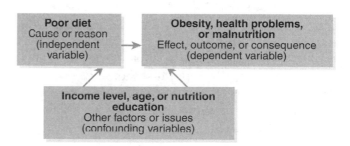

Examples of dependent, independent, and confounding variables.

## Selecting a Data-Gathering Method

Once the researcher has considered the preferred methodology, the next stage involves selecting a data-gathering method, such as observing, measuring, or interviewing. The researcher should identify specific techniques or instruments that are consistent with the research design. For example, if a questionnaire is considered for data collection, a specific instrument can be selected, such as a food frequency questionnaire, 24-hour recall, or 3-day food record (see Chapter 2).

Because decisions need to be made about a data-gathering method for each of the major variables in the research study, the researcher may decide to use more than one instrument. In the examples described previously about investigating African American sodium and caloric intake and increasing postmenopausal women's calcium and vitamin D intake, the researcher may decide to use both focus groups and interviewing methods. An interview (using 24-hour recall or a food frequency checklist) may be used to determine the nutrient intake and eating habits of these individuals.

## Protecting the Subjects and Researcher

An important aspect of the design phase is research approval by the institutional review board (IRB). IRBs are groups of representatives of various related disciplines or departments organized to review research proposals. Their major concerns are protecting human research participants from physical or mental harm and protecting the researcher from unnecessary complaints. This process also satisfies a number of funding agencies and federal, state, and institutional regulations. If the research is being conducted in a university setting, every university has a committee that reviews research proposals involving health services.

The nutritionist must obtain approval from the committee before the research begins. The first step is to communicate clearly to the review committee, in writing, what is planned, how participants will be involved in the research, and whether their participation will put them at risk for physical or mental harm. The researcher is ethically responsible for carrying out these plans as directed or approved by the committee. Changes that occur in the plans need to be reported to the committee for further authorization. In situations in which there is no existing IRB, a committee should be organized, consisting of experts in the area of the research study who will review and approve the research design before data collection begins.

## Performing a Pilot Study

Pilot studies can be used to test data-gathering methods and verify the data analysis plan. A pilot study is very important when the data-gathering technique is unfamiliar to the researcher or has not been used by other researchers. It is also necessary when the instrument is new or has not been used with the population being studied, or when the study is being conducted in an unfamiliar environment.[1] In addition, the data and results obtained from the pilot study can be used to increase support and funding for a major research project.

In the fictitious example using African American older persons, the researcher might decide to pilot test the study with 20 older African Americans from a neighboring county, after obtaining permission from both the IRB and the participants.

Next, the assumptions and limitations of research need to be identified. Assumptions are characteristics of the research situation that will not be explored in the study.[1] The assumption may be determined from the findings in the literature the researcher reviewed. For

example, in the fictitious scenario, it is assumed that some older African Americans are consuming foods high in sodium. Limitations are unmanageable elements of the research study. These elements limit the certainty of the findings or their applicability to the population in general. In the fictitious examples, a limitation is that deliberate sampling does not ensure that all older African American persons or postmenopausal women are equally represented. As a result, the study findings may not be applicable beyond the study sample.

## ▶ Implementation and Empirical Stage

The implementation phase of the research plan is when the researcher actually carries out the research procedures. The researcher must comply with the objectives or the hypothesis of the project and must invest enough time to obtain longitudinal data and breadth of information. The implementation stage includes carrying out the following activities[1,13]:

- Inviting the sample group or community members to participate in the project or research
- Obtaining informed consent from the participants
- Collecting and verifying the data
- Analyzing the data

The researcher may recruit participants by sending a letter of invitation to potential participants, composing a radio announcement, or providing information to churches, local community centers, schools, men's and women's associations, and so on. Many factors can affect the recruitment process, such as the sample size, exclusion criteria for participation, perceived benefits, length of the study, and location of the study.[1,14]

After the participants have been recruited, the next step is to obtain informed consent for participation in the study. The researcher and the participants must sign consent forms after a detailed explanation of the research protocol.

The nutritionist then collects data using focus groups and interviews or any other appropriate method. Information collected in qualitative studies is validated with participants by analyzing the results for completeness. If the method is qualitative, the nutritionist may carry out the data analysis concomitantly with data collection. If the method is quantitative, analysis would be performed at the conclusion of the data collection phase.

Regardless of the type of method utilized for the study, the researcher must consider several data collection and analysis guidelines that must be observed throughout the study period. These include, but are not limited to the following[15-17]:

- *Awareness:* The researcher and staff must understand the guidelines of all methodologies used.
- *Management plan:* This should include the responsibilities of each staff member, contingency plans, a written work plan that includes specific objectives, an action plan, and a time line. A regular meeting schedule also must be established.
- *Recruitment and retention goal:* The researcher must make a significant effort to meet the targeted sample size and must have a retention strategy in place (such as follow-up telephone calls, continuous social support, conducting raffles, paying attention to details, making the study area comfortable, etc.).
- *Data collection:* The researcher needs to gather data from all the participants at the appropriate times.
- *Reexamining the procedures:* The researcher needs to make sure the data collection procedure(s) corresponded with the research objective(s).

## ▶ Evaluation and Analytical Stage

In the evaluation stage, the researcher analyzes the data collected during the implementation stage. The researcher must familiarize himself or herself with the data through repeated reading and listening to the staff and study participants. Evaluation methods can vary greatly depending on the theoretical focus (i.e., qualitative or quantitative research) and methods. This stage includes the following[15,17]:

- Coordinating and coding the collected data
- Transcribing interviews and other material
- Choosing a data entry and analysis program (e.g., the Statistical Package for the Social Sciences [SPSS] available at http://www.spss.com)
- Reviewing data (e.g., surveys, questionnaires) for completeness
- Entering the data into a secured computer for statistical analysis
- Controlling access to the data to ensure confidentiality
- Storing the data in a secured area using a consistent method for storage

The last step of data analysis consists of interpreting and comparing the results with previous research; seeing whether the findings support the research study's hypotheses, theory, or research questions; and then drawing conclusions. The researcher then writes a report to present the findings. A research report is a carefully structured piece that clearly states the purpose, findings, relevance, and implications of the research activity.[17] Research reports should provide clear documentation of what, how, why, and when the study was conducted.

A combination of visual and literary description will help make the information presented precise. The researcher must include all the findings. Hypotheses that were not supported also need to be reported. Within the report, the researcher should make recommendations for further research that is consistent with the findings of the research study. The researcher also may indicate whether there is a need to replicate the study with other populations or communities.

## ▶ Action and Dissemination Stage

The results of nutrition research should be used in practice. The research findings must be presented to as wide a range of people as possible, such as in professional journals and to professional colleagues at their annual meeting; to persons in decision-making positions such as administrators, policy makers, and legislators; and even to reporters for articles in a local newspaper. Consistent with primary healthcare and health promotion approaches, relevant research findings also must be reported to community groups. This information can become part of the community's educational experience and help the community make appropriate decisions based on local needs.[1,17] The nutritionist must make specific recommendations for improving the health of the community based on the research findings.

## References

1. Stanhope M, Lancaster J. *Community and Public Health Nursing.* 5th ed. New York, NY: Elsevier; 2000.
2. Trochim WMK. Research methods knowledge base. http://www.socialresearchmethods.net/kb/strucres.htm. Accessed November 26, 2011.
3. Roberts WC. High salt intake, its origins, its economic impact, and its effect on blood pressure. *Am J Cardiol.* 2001;88(11):1338-1346.
4. Huff R, Kline M. *Promoting Health in Multicultural Populations: A Handbook for Practitioners.* Thousand Oaks, CA: Sage; 1999.
5. Abramson JJ. *Survey Methods in Community Medicine: Epidemiological Research Programme Evaluation Clinical Trials.* 5th ed. London, UK: Churchill Livingstone 1999.
6. Ueland A. Colorectal cancer prevention and screening: a Health Belief Model-based research study to increase disease awareness. *Gastroenterol Nurs.* 2006;29(5):357-363.
7. Abood D. Nutrition education worksite intervention for university staff: application of the health belief model. *J Nutr Educ Behav.* 2003;35(5):260-267.

8. Tussing L. Osteoporosis prevention education: behavior theories and calcium intake. *J Am Diet Assoc*. 2005;105(1):92-97.

9. Grant MM. Women's health beliefs regarding hypertension. *West Indian Med J*. 1993;42(4):158-160.

10. Anderson E, McFarlane J. *Community as Partner: Theory and Practice in Nursing*. 3th ed. Philadelphia, PA: Lippincott; 2000.

11. Varkevisser CM, Brownlee B. *Designing and Conducting Health Systems Research*. Ottawa, ON, Canada: World Health Organization, International Development Research Centre; 2003.

12. Frank K. The impact of a confounding variable on the inference of a regression coefficient. *Sociol Methods Res*. 2002;29(2):147-194.

13. DeLeeuw E. Reducing missing data in surveys: an overview of methods. *Qual Quant*. 2001; 35(2):147-160.

14. Monsen ER. *Research: Successful Approaches*. 2nd ed. Chicago, IL: American Dietetic Association; 2003.

15. Gibson RS. *Principles of Nutritional Assessment*. 2nd ed. Dunedin, New Zealand: Oxford University Press; 2005.

16. Munhall PL, Boyd, CO. *Nursing Research: A Qualitative Perspective*. New York, NY: National League for Nursing; 1993.

17. RD Direct. Your research project how and where to start? https://www.noexperiencenecessarybook.com/mVmMm/research-process-flow-chart.html. Accessed March 17, 2017.

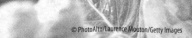

# Appendix G

## Guidelines for Assessing Evidence of Causation

| TABLE G-1 | |
|---|---|
| **Criteria** | **Association** |
| Strength | The cause and effect should not be dismissed easily because the observed association seems minor. This means that a small association does not imply that a causal effect does not exist. |
| Consistency | Consistent findings observed by different individuals in different places with different samples strengthen the likelihood of cause and effect. For example, several research studies established that there is an association between cigarette smoking and lung cancer. |
| Specificity | Causation is likely if a very specific population at a specific site has a disease with no other likely explanation. This means that the health condition is limited to specific individuals at a particular location. |
| Temporality | The effect has to occur after the cause (and if there is an expected delay between the cause and expected effect, the effect must occur after that delay). The investigator may consider this question: Does a high-fat diet lead to heart disease or do the early stages of heart disease lead to poor dietary habits? |
| Biological gradient | Greater exposure should lead to greater incidence of the effect. For example, the evidence that the death rate from lung cancer increases linearly with the number of cigarettes smoked every day adds significantly to the simpler evidence that cigarette smokers have a higher lung cancer death rate than nonsmokers. |
| Plausibility | A credible mechanism between cause and effect is helpful. However, an association that is not biologically credible at one time may eventually prove to be so in the future. Implausible associations may be the beginning of the advancement of knowledge. |
| Coherence | Coherence between epidemiological and laboratory findings increases the likelihood of an effect. However, lack of such laboratory evidence cannot nullify the epidemiological findings. |
| Experiment | Sometimes it is possible to request experimental evidence. The investigator may ask this question: Does increased consumption of diets high in calcium prevent colon cancer or osteoporosis? |
| Analogy | The effects of similar substances may be considered supportive of causality. The investigator may ask this question: Can parallels be drawn with examples of other well-established cause-and-effect relationships (e.g., the relationship between obesity and heart disease)? |

Data from: Hennekens CH, Buring JE. *Epidemiology in Medicine.* In: Mayren SL, ed. Boston, MA: Little, Brown; 1965; and Hill AB. The environment and disease: association or causation? *Proc Royal Soc Med.* 1965;58:295-300.

# Appendix H

## Dietary Reference Intakes (DRI)

| Life stage group | Vitamin A (µg/d)[1] | Vitamin D (IU/d)[2] | Vitamin E (mg/d)[3] | Vitamin K (µg/d) | Thiamin (mg/d) | Riboflavin (mg/d) | Niacin (mg/d)[4] | Pantothenic Acid (mg/d) | Biotin (µg/d) | Vitamin B$_6$ (mg/d) | Folate (µg/d)[5] | Vitamin B$_{12}$ (µg/d) | Vitamin C (mg/d) | Choline (mg/d) | Sodium (g/d) |
|---|---|---|---|---|---|---|---|---|---|---|---|---|---|---|---|
| **Infants** | | | | | | | | | | | | | | | |
| 0-6 mo | 400* | 400* | 4* | 2.0* | 0.2* | 0.3* | 2* | 1.7* | 5* | 0.1* | 65* | 0.4* | 40* | 125* | 0.12* |
| 6-12 mo | 500* | 400* | 5* | 2.5* | 0.3* | 0.4* | 4* | 1.8* | 6* | 0.3* | 80* | 0.5* | 50* | 150* | 0.37* |
| **Children** | | | | | | | | | | | | | | | |
| 1-3 y | 300 | 600 | 6 | 30* | 0.5 | 0.5 | 6 | 2* | 8* | 0.5 | 150 | 0.9 | 15 | 200* | 1.0* |
| 4-8 y | 400 | 600 | 7 | 55* | 0.6 | 0.6 | 8 | 3* | 12* | 0.6 | 200 | 1.2 | 25 | 250* | 1.2* |
| **Males** | | | | | | | | | | | | | | | |
| 9-13 y | 600 | 600 | 11 | 60* | 0.9 | 0.9 | 12 | 4* | 20* | 1.0 | 300 | 1.8 | 45 | 375* | 1.5* |
| 14-18 y | 900 | 600 | 15 | 75* | 1.2 | 1.3 | 16 | 5* | 25* | 1.3 | 400 | 2.4 | 75 | 550* | 1.5* |
| 19-30 y | 900 | 600 | 15 | 120* | 1.2 | 1.3 | 16 | 5* | 30* | 1.3 | 400 | 2.4 | 90 | 550* | 1.5* |
| 31-50 y | 900 | 600 | 15 | 120* | 1.2 | 1.3 | 16 | 5* | 30* | 1.3 | 400 | 2.4 | 90 | 550* | 1.5* |
| 51-70 y | 900 | 600 | 15 | 120* | 1.2 | 1.3 | 16 | 5* | 30* | 1.7 | 400 | 2.4[7] | 90 | 550* | 1.3* |
| >70 y | 900 | 800 | 15 | 120* | 1.2 | 1.3 | 16 | 5* | 30* | 1.7 | 400 | 2.4[7] | 90 | 550* | 1.2* |
| **Females** | | | | | | | | | | | | | | | |
| 9-13 y | 600 | 600 | 11 | 60* | 0.9 | 0.9 | 12 | 4* | 20* | 1.0 | 300 | 1.8 | 45 | 375* | 1.5* |
| 14-18 y | 700 | 600 | 15 | 75* | 1.0 | 1.0 | 14 | 5* | 25* | 1.2 | 400[6] | 2.4 | 65 | 400* | 1.5* |
| 19-30 y | 700 | 600 | 15 | 90* | 1.1 | 1.1 | 14 | 5* | 30* | 1.3 | 400[6] | 2.4 | 75 | 425* | 1.5* |
| 31-50 y | 700 | 600 | 15 | 90* | 1.1 | 1.1 | 14 | 5* | 30* | 1.3 | 400[6] | 2.4 | 75 | 425* | 1.5* |
| 51-70 y | 700 | 600 | 15 | 90* | 1.1 | 1.1 | 14 | 5* | 30* | 1.5 | 400 | 2.4[7] | 75 | 425* | 1.3* |
| >70 y | 700 | 800 | 15 | 90* | 1.1 | 1.1 | 14 | 5* | 30* | 1.5 | 400 | 2.4[7] | 75 | 425* | 1.2* |
| **Pregnancy** | | | | | | | | | | | | | | | |
| ≤18 y | 750 | 600 | 15 | 75* | 1.4 | 1.4 | 18 | 6* | 30* | 1.9 | 600 | 2.6 | 80 | 450* | 1.5* |
| 19-30 y | 770 | 600 | 15 | 90* | 1.4 | 1.4 | 18 | 6* | 30* | 1.9 | 600 | 2.6 | 85 | 450* | 1.5* |
| 31-50 y | 770 | 600 | 15 | 90* | 1.4 | 1.4 | 18 | 6* | 30* | 1.9 | 600 | 2.6 | 85 | 450* | 1.5* |
| **Lactation** | | | | | | | | | | | | | | | |
| ≤18 y | 1,200 | 600 | 19 | 75* | 1.4 | 1.6 | 17 | 7* | 35* | 2.0 | 500 | 2.8 | 115 | 550* | 1.5* |
| 19-30 y | 1,300 | 600 | 19 | 90* | 1.4 | 1.6 | 17 | 7* | 35* | 2.0 | 500 | 2.8 | 120 | 550* | 1.5* |
| 31-50 y | 1,300 | 600 | 19 | 90* | 1.4 | 1.6 | 17 | 7* | 35* | 2.0 | 500 | 2.8 | 120 | 550* | 1.5* |

This table presents Recommended Dietary Allowances (RDA) and Adequate Intakes (AI). An asterisk (*) indicates AI. RDAs and AIs may both be used as goals for individual intake.

[1] As retinol activity equivalents (RAE).

[2] As cholecalciferol.

[3] As α-tocopherol.

[4] As niacin equivalents (NE).

[5] As dietary folate equivalents (DFE).

[6] In view of evidence linking folate intake with neural-tube defects in the fetus, it is recommended that all women capable of becoming pregnant consume 400 µg of folic acid from supplements or fortified foods in addition to intake of food folate from a varied diet.

[7] Because 10 to 30% of older people may malabsorb food-bound vitamin B$_{12}$, it is advisable for those older than 50 years to meet their RDA mainly by consuming foods fortified with vitamin B$_{12}$ or a supplement containing vitamin B$_{12}$.

[8] The AI for water represents total water from drinking water, beverages, and moisture from food.

The Food and Nutrition Board of the National Academy of Sciences determines recommended nutrient intakes that apply to healthy individuals. Beginning in 1997, the Food and Nutrition Board (with the involvement of Health Canada) began releasing updated recommendations under a new framework called the Dietary Reference Intakes (DRI). In these revisions, target intake levels for healthy individuals in the U.S. and Canada are listed as either Adequate Intake (AI) levels or Recommended Dietary Allowances (RDA). Also, the DRI values include a set of Tolerable Upper Intake Levels (UL) which are levels of nutrient intake that should not be exceeded due to the potential for adverse effects from excessive consumption. For more on the Dietary Reference Intakes, see Chapter 2.

| Life stage group | Potassium (g/d) | Chloride (g/d) | Calcium (mg/d) | Phosphorus (mg/d) | Magnesium (mg/d) | Iron (mg/d) | Zinc (mg/d) | Selenium (µg/d) | Iodine (µg/d) | Copper (µg/d) | Manganese (mg/d) | Fluoride (mg/d) | Chromium (µg/d) | Molybdenum (µg/d) | Water (L/d)[8] |
|---|---|---|---|---|---|---|---|---|---|---|---|---|---|---|---|
| **Infants** | | | | | | | | | | | | | | | |
| 0-6 mo | 0.4* | 0.18* | 200* | 100* | 30* | 0.27* | 2* | 15* | 110* | 200* | 0.003* | 0.01* | 0.2* | 2* | 0.7* |
| 6-12 mo | 0.7* | 0.57* | 260* | 275* | 75* | 11 | 3* | 20* | 130* | 220* | 0.6* | 0.5* | 5.5* | 3* | 0.8* |
| **Children** | | | | | | | | | | | | | | | |
| 1-3 y | 3.0* | 1.5* | 700 | 460 | 80 | 7 | 3 | 20 | 90 | 340 | 1.2* | 0.7* | 11* | 17 | 1.3* |
| 4-8 y | 3.8* | 1.9* | 1,000 | 500 | 130 | 10 | 5 | 30 | 90 | 440 | 1.5* | 1* | 15* | 22 | 1.7* |
| **Males** | | | | | | | | | | | | | | | |
| 9-13 y | 4.5* | 2.3* | 1,300 | 1,250 | 240 | 8 | 8 | 40 | 120 | 700 | 1.9* | 2* | 25* | 34 | 2.4* |
| 14-18 y | 4.7* | 2.3* | 1,300 | 1,250 | 410 | 11 | 11 | 55 | 150 | 890 | 2.2* | 3* | 35* | 43 | 3.3* |
| 19-30 y | 4.7* | 2.3* | 1,000 | 700 | 400 | 8 | 11 | 55 | 150 | 900 | 2.3* | 4* | 35* | 45 | 3.7* |
| 31-50 y | 4.7* | 2.3* | 1,000 | 700 | 420 | 8 | 11 | 55 | 150 | 900 | 2.3* | 4* | 35* | 45 | 3.7* |
| 51-70 y | 4.7* | 2.0* | 1,000 | 700 | 420 | 8 | 11 | 55 | 150 | 900 | 2.3* | 4* | 30* | 45 | 3.7* |
| >70 y | 4.7* | 1.8* | 1,200 | 700 | 420 | 8 | 11 | 55 | 150 | 900 | 2.3* | 4* | 30* | 45 | 3.7* |
| **Females** | | | | | | | | | | | | | | | |
| 9-13 y | 4.5* | 2.3* | 1,300 | 1,250 | 240 | 8 | 8 | 40 | 120 | 700 | 1.6* | 2* | 21* | 34 | 2.1* |
| 14-18 y | 4.7* | 2.3* | 1,300 | 1,250 | 360 | 15 | 9 | 55 | 150 | 890 | 1.6* | 3* | 24* | 43 | 2.3* |
| 19-30 y | 4.7* | 2.3* | 1,000 | 700 | 310 | 18 | 8 | 55 | 150 | 900 | 1.8* | 3* | 25* | 45 | 2.7* |
| 31-50 y | 4.7* | 2.3* | 1,000 | 700 | 320 | 18 | 8 | 55 | 150 | 900 | 1.8* | 3* | 25* | 45 | 2.7* |
| 51-70 y | 4.7* | 2.0* | 1,200 | 700 | 320 | 8 | 8 | 55 | 150 | 900 | 1.8* | 3* | 20* | 45 | 2.7* |
| >70 y | 4.7* | 1.8* | 1,200 | 700 | 320 | 8 | 8 | 55 | 150 | 900 | 1.8* | 3* | 20* | 45 | 2.7* |
| **Pregnancy** | | | | | | | | | | | | | | | |
| ≤18 y | 4.7* | 2.3* | 1,300 | 1,250 | 400 | 27 | 12 | 60 | 220 | 1,000 | 2.0* | 3* | 29* | 50 | 3.0* |
| 19-30 y | 4.7* | 2.3* | 1,000 | 700 | 350 | 27 | 11 | 60 | 220 | 1,000 | 2.0* | 3* | 30* | 50 | 3.0* |
| 31-50 y | 4.7* | 2.3* | 1,000 | 700 | 360 | 27 | 11 | 60 | 220 | 1,000 | 2.0* | 3* | 30* | 50 | 3.0* |
| **Lactation** | | | | | | | | | | | | | | | |
| ≤18 y | 5.1* | 2.3 | 1,300 | 1,250 | 360 | 10 | 13 | 70 | 290 | 1,300 | 2.6* | 3* | 44* | 50 | 3.8* |
| 19-30 y | 5.1* | 2.3 | 1,000 | 700 | 310 | 9 | 12 | 70 | 290 | 1,300 | 2.6* | 3* | 45* | 50 | 3.8* |
| 31-50 y | 5.1* | 2.3 | 1,000 | 700 | 320 | 9 | 12 | 70 | 290 | 1,300 | 2.6* | 3* | 45* | 50 | 3.8* |

**Sources:** Data compiled from *Dietary Reference Intakes for Calcium, Phosphorus, Magnesium, Vitamin D, and Fluoride.* Washington, DC: National Academies Press; 1997. *Dietary Reference Intakes for Thiamin, Riboflavin, Niacin, Vitamin B$_6$, Folate, Vitamin B$_{12}$, Pantothenic Acid, Biotin, and Choline.* Washington, DC: National Academies Press; 1998. *Dietary Reference Intakes for Vitamin C, Vitamin E, Selenium, and Carotenoids.* Washington, DC: National Academies Press; 2000. *Dietary Reference Intakes for Vitamin A, Vitamin K, Arsenic, Boron, Chromium, Copper, Iron, Manganese, Molybdenum, Nickel, Silicon, Vanadium, and Zinc.* Washington, DC: National Academies Press; 2000. *Dietary Reference Intakes for Water, Potassium, Sodium, Chloride, and Sulfate.* Food and Nutrition Board. Washington, DC: National Academies Press; 2005. *Dietary Reference Intakes for Calcium and Vitamin D.* Washington, DC: National Academies Press; 2011. These reports may be accessed via http://nap.edu.

## Tolerable Upper Intake Levels (UL[1])

| Life stage group | Vitamin A[2] (µg/d) | Vitamin D (µg/d) | Vitamin E[3,4] (mg/d) | Niacin[4] (mg/d) | Vitamin B$_6$ (mg/d) | Folate[4] (µg/d) | Vitamin C (mg/d) | Choline (g/d) | Calcium (g/d) | Phosphorus (g/d) | Magnesium[5] (mg/d) | Sodium (g/d) |
|---|---|---|---|---|---|---|---|---|---|---|---|---|
| **Infants** | | | | | | | | | | | | |
| 0-6 mo | 600 | 25 | ND[7] | ND | ND | ND | ND | ND | ND | ND | ND | ND |
| 7-12 mo | 600 | 25 | ND | ND | ND | ND | ND | ND | ND | ND | ND | ND |
| **Children** | | | | | | | | | | | | |
| 1-3 y | 600 | 50 | 200 | 10 | 30 | 300 | 400 | 1.0 | 2.5 | 3 | 65 | 1.5 |
| 4-8 y | 900 | 50 | 300 | 15 | 40 | 400 | 650 | 1.0 | 2.5 | 3 | 110 | 1.9 |
| **Males, females** | | | | | | | | | | | | |
| 9-13 y | 1,700 | 50 | 600 | 20 | 60 | 600 | 1,200 | 2.0 | 2.5 | 4 | 350 | 2.2 |
| 14-18 y | 2,800 | 50 | 800 | 30 | 80 | 800 | 1,800 | 3.0 | 2.5 | 4 | 350 | 2.3 |
| 19-70 y | 3,000 | 50 | 1,000 | 35 | 100 | 1,000 | 2,000 | 3.5 | 2.5 | 4 | 350 | 2.3 |
| >70 y | 3,000 | 50 | 1,000 | 35 | 100 | 1,000 | 2,000 | 3.5 | 2.5 | 3 | 350 | 2.3 |
| **Pregnancy** | | | | | | | | | | | | |
| ≤18 y | 2,800 | 50 | 800 | 30 | 80 | 800 | 1,800 | 3.0 | 2.5 | 3.5 | 350 | 2.3 |
| 19-50 y | 3,000 | 50 | 1,000 | 35 | 100 | 1,000 | 2,000 | 3.5 | 2.5 | 3.5 | 350 | 2.3 |
| **Lactation** | | | | | | | | | | | | |
| ≤18 y | 2,800 | 50 | 800 | 30 | 80 | 800 | 1,800 | 3.0 | 2.5 | 4 | 350 | 2.3 |
| 19-50 y | 3,000 | 50 | 1,000 | 35 | 100 | 1,000 | 2,000 | 3.5 | 2.5 | 4 | 350 | 2.3 |

| Life stage group | Iron (mg/d) | Zinc (mg/d) | Selenium (µg/d) | Iodine (µg/d) | Copper (µg/d) | Manganese (mg/d) | Fluoride (mg/d) | Molybdenum (µg/d) | Boron (mg/d) | Nickel (mg/d) | Vanadium[6] (mg/d) | Chloride (g/d) |
|---|---|---|---|---|---|---|---|---|---|---|---|---|
| **Infants** | | | | | | | | | | | | |
| 0-6 mo | 40 | 4 | 45 | ND | ND | ND | 0.7 | ND | ND | ND | ND | ND |
| 7-12 mo | 40 | 5 | 60 | ND | ND | ND | 0.9 | ND | ND | ND | ND | ND |
| **Children** | | | | | | | | | | | | |
| 1-3 y | 40 | 7 | 90 | 200 | 1,000 | 2 | 1.3 | 300 | 3 | 0.2 | ND | 2.3 |
| 4-8 y | 40 | 12 | 150 | 300 | 3,000 | 3 | 2.2 | 600 | 6 | 0.3 | ND | 2.9 |
| **Males, females** | | | | | | | | | | | | |
| 9-13 y | 40 | 23 | 280 | 600 | 5,000 | 6 | 10 | 1,100 | 11 | 0.6 | ND | 3.4 |
| 14-18 y | 45 | 34 | 400 | 900 | 8,000 | 9 | 10 | 1,700 | 17 | 1.0 | ND | 3.6 |
| 19-70 y | 45 | 40 | 400 | 1,100 | 10,000 | 11 | 10 | 2,000 | 20 | 1.0 | 1.8 | 3.6 |
| >70 y | 45 | 40 | 400 | 1,100 | 10,000 | 11 | 10 | 2,000 | 20 | 1.0 | 1.8 | 3.6 |
| **Pregnancy** | | | | | | | | | | | | |
| ≤18 y | 45 | 34 | 400 | 900 | 8,000 | 9 | 10 | 1,700 | 17 | 1.0 | ND | 3.6 |
| 19-50 y | 45 | 40 | 400 | 1,100 | 10,000 | 11 | 10 | 2,000 | 20 | 1.0 | ND | 3.6 |
| **Lactation** | | | | | | | | | | | | |
| ≤18 y | 45 | 34 | 400 | 900 | 8,000 | 9 | 10 | 1,700 | 17 | 1.0 | ND | 3.6 |
| 19-50 y | 45 | 40 | 400 | 1,100 | 10,000 | 11 | 10 | 2,000 | 20 | 1.0 | ND | 3.6 |

[1] UL = The maximum level of daily nutrient intake that is likely to pose no risk of adverse effects. Unless otherwise specified, the UL represents total intake from food, water, and supplements. Due to lack of suitable data, ULs could not be established for vitamin K, thiamin, riboflavin, vitamin B$_{12}$, pantothenic acid, biotin, or carotenoids. In the absence of ULs, extra caution may be warranted in consuming levels above recommended intakes.

[2] As preformed vitamin A (retinol) only.

[3] As $\alpha$-tocopherol; applies to any form of supplemental $\alpha$-tocopherol.

[4] The ULs for vitamin E, niacin, and folate apply to synthetic forms obtained from supplements, fortified foods, or a combination of the two.

[5] The ULs for magnesium represent intake from a pharmacological agent only and do not include intake from food and water.

[6] Although vanadium in food has not been shown to cause adverse effects in humans, there is no justification for adding vanadium to food and vanadium supplements should be used with caution. The UL is based on adverse effects in laboratory animals and these data could be used to set a UL for adults but not children or adolescents.

[7] ND = Not determinable due to lack of data on adverse effects in this age group and concern with regard to lack of ability to handle excess amounts. Source of intake should be from food only to prevent high levels of intake.

**Sources:** Data compiled from *Dietary Reference Intakes for Calcium, Phosphorus, Magnesium, Vitamin D, and Fluoride.* Washington, DC: National Academies Press; 1997. *Dietary Reference Intakes for Thiamin, Riboflavin, Niacin, Vitamin B$_6$, Folate, Vitamin B$_{12}$, Pantothenic Acid, Biotin, and Choline.* Washington, DC: National Academies Press; 1998. *Dietary Reference Intakes for Vitamin C, Vitamin E, Selenium, and Carotenoids.* Washington, DC: National Academies Press; 2000. Institute of Medicine, Food and Nutrition Board. *Dietary Reference Intakes for Vitamin A, Vitamin K, Arsenic, Boron, Chromium, Copper, Iron, Manganese, Molybdenum, Nickel, Silicon, Vanadium, and Zinc.* Washington, DC: National Academies Press, 2000. *Dietary Reference Intakes for Water, Potassium, Sodium, Chloride, and Sulfate.* Washington, DC: National Academies Press; 2005. These reports may be accessed via http://nap.edu.

## Daily Values for Food Labels

The Daily Values are standard values developed by the Food and Drug Administration (FDA) for use on food labels.

| Nutrient | Amount |
|---|---|
| Protein[1] | 50 g |
| Thiamin | 1.5 mg |
| Riboflavin | 1.7 mg |
| Niacin | 20 mg |
| Pantothenic Acid | 10 mg |
| Biotin | 300 µg |
| Vitamin $B_6$ | 2 mg |
| Folate | 400 µg |
| Vitamin $B_{12}$ | 6 µg |
| Vitamin C | 60 mg |
| Vitamin A[2] | 5,000 IU |
| Vitamin D[2] | 400 IU |
| Vitamin E[2] | 30 IU |
| Vitamin K | 80 µg |
| Chloride | 3,400 mg |
| Calcium | 1,000 mg |
| Phosphorus | 1,000 mg |
| Magnesium | 400 mg |
| Iron | 18 mg |
| Zinc | 15 mg |
| Selenium | 70 µg |
| Iodine | 150 µg |
| Copper | 2 mg |
| Manganese | 2 mg |
| Chromium | 120 µg |
| Molybdenum | 75 µg |

[1] The Daily Values for protein vary for different groups of people: pregnant women, 60 g; nursing mothers, 65 g; infants under 1 year, 14 g; children 1 to 4 years, 16 g.

[2] The Daily Values for fat-soluble vitamins are expressed in International Units (IU), an old system of measurement.

| Food Component | Amount | Calculation Factors |
|---|---|---|
| Fat | 65 g | 30% of kcalories |
| Saturated fat | 20 g | 10% of kcalories |
| Cholesterol | 300 mg | Same regardless of kcalories |
| Carbohydrate (total) | 300 g | 60% of kcalories |
| Fiber | 25 g | 11.5 g per 1000 kcalories |
| Protein | 50 g | 10% of kcalories |
| Sodium | 2,400 mg | Same regardless of kcalories |
| Potassium | 3,500 mg | Same regardless of kcalories |

**Note:** Daily Values were established for adults and children over 4 years old. The values for energy-yielding nutrients are based on 2,000 kcalories a day.

## Dietary Reference Intakes (DRI) for Carbohydrates, Fiber, Fat, Fatty Acids, and Protein

| Life stage group | Carbohydrate (g/d) | Fiber (g/d) | Fat (g/d) | Linoleic Acid (g/d) | α-Linolenic Acid (g/d) | Protein[1] (g/d) |
|---|---|---|---|---|---|---|
| **Infants** | | | | | | |
| 0-6 mo | 60* | ND[2] | 31* | 4.4* | 0.5* | 9.1* |
| 7-12 mo | 95* | ND | 30* | 4.6* | 0.5* | 11 |
| **Children** | | | | | | |
| 1-3 y | 130 | 19* | ND | 7* | 0.7* | 13 |
| 4-8 y | 130 | 25* | ND | 10* | 0.9* | 19 |
| **Males** | | | | | | |
| 9-13 y | 130 | 31* | ND | 12* | 1.2* | 34 |
| 14-18 y | 130 | 38* | ND | 16* | 1.6* | 52 |
| 19-30 y | 130 | 38* | ND | 17* | 1.6* | 56 |
| 31-50 y | 130 | 38* | ND | 17* | 1.6* | 56 |
| 51-70 y | 130 | 30* | ND | 14* | 1.6* | 56 |
| > 70 y | 130 | 30* | ND | 14* | 1.6* | 56 |
| **Females** | | | | | | |
| 9-13 y | 130 | 26* | ND | 10* | 1.0* | 34 |
| 14-18 y | 130 | 26* | ND | 11* | 1.1* | 46 |
| 19-30 y | 130 | 25* | ND | 12* | 1.1* | 46 |
| 31-50 y | 130 | 25* | ND | 12* | 1.1* | 46 |
| 51-70 y | 130 | 21* | ND | 11* | 1.1* | 46 |
| > 70 y | 130 | 21* | ND | 11* | 1.1* | 46 |
| **Pregnancy** | | | | | | |
| ≤ 18 y | 175 | 28* | ND | 13* | 1.4* | 71 |
| 19-30 y | 175 | 28* | ND | 13* | 1.4* | 71 |
| 31-50 y | 175 | 28* | ND | 13* | 1.4* | 71 |
| **Lactation** | | | | | | |
| ≤ 18 y | 210 | 29* | ND | 13* | 1.3* | 71 |
| 19-30 y | 210 | 29* | ND | 13* | 1.3* | 71 |
| 31-50 y | 210 | 29* | ND | 13* | 1.3* | 71 |

This table presents Recommended Dietary Allowances (RDA) and Adequate Intakes (AI). An asterisk (*) indicates AI. RDAs and AIs may both be used as goals for individual intake.

[1] Based on 1.52 g/kg/day for infants 0-6 mo, 1.2 g/kg/day for infants 7-12 mo, 1.05 g/kg/day for 1-3 y, 0.95 g/kg/day for 4-13 y, 0.85 g/kg/day for 14-18 y, 0.8 g/kg/day for adults, and 1.3 g/kg/day for pregnant women (using pre-pregnancy weight) and lactating women.

[2] ND = Not determinable due to lack of data on adverse effects in this age group and concern with regard to lack of ability to handle excess amounts. Source of intake should be from food only to prevent high levels of intake.

**Source:** Data compiled from *Dietary Reference Intakes for Energy, Carbohydrate, Fiber, Fat, Fatty Acids, Cholesterol, Protein, and Amino Acids.* Food and Nutrition Board. Washington, DC: National Academies Press; 2005. This report may be accessed via http://nap.edu.

# Glossary

**24-hour recall** A method of dietary assessment in which the individual is asked to remember everything eaten during the past 24 hours.

**5-year survival rate** The number of individuals who are alive and without recurrence of cancer 5 years after diagnosis.

## A

**acculturation** Repeated exposure to influences from a different culture. The process is related to age, education, frequency of interaction, and income and occurs on a continuum.

**action plan** A concise statement of the methods, activities, or intervention strategies to be undertaken.

**activities of daily living (ADLs)** Performing personal care, either independently or with help. Determining whether an older person can perform ADLs helps evaluate ability to care for himself or herself.

**adenomas** Cancers that arise from glandular tissues.

**adolescence** The period of life between 12 and 19 years of age.

**adult learning** Adults gaining knowledge and expertise.

**advertising** The methods used to present health and nutrition promotion programs to targeted communities.

**affective domain** The domain of learning that includes the way individuals deal with things emotionally, such as feelings, values, appreciation, enthusiasm, motivation, and attitude. It also consists of changes in attitudes and the development of values.

**after-school snack program** Gives children a nutritional enhancement and encourages them to participate in supervised activities that are safe and filled with learning opportunities.

**Alzheimer's disease (AD; senile dementia of the Alzheimer's type)** A disease that results in the relentless and irreversible loss of mental function.

**android obesity** Excess storage of fat, mainly in the abdominal area.

**anorexia nervosa** An eating disorder characterized by extreme weight loss, poor body image, and irrational fears of weight gain and obesity.

**anorexia of aging** The loss of appetite and wasting associated with old age.

**anthropometry** The measurement of human body size, weight, and proportions.

**antioxidants** Vitamins C and E and beta-carotene, which neutralize free radicals and other reactive chemicals and terminate harmful chemical reactions.

**assessment** Determining nutritional status by analyzing clinical, dietary, and social history; anthropometric data; biochemical data; and drug–nutrient interactions.

**atherosclerosis** A common form of arteriosclerosis in which plaque forms within the intima of medium and large arteries; a group of diseases characterized by thickening and loss of elasticity of arterial walls.

## B

**balance sheet approach** The most common method of estimating per capita food availability at the national level. Food exports, nonfood use (e.g., livestock feed, seeds, and industrial use), and year-end inventories are subtracted from data on beginning-year inventories, total food production, and imports to arrive at an estimate of per capita food availability.

**basal metabolic rate (BMR)** The minimum amount of energy that an awake, fasted, resting body needs to maintain itself; often used interchangeably with resting metabolic rate (RMR). BMR measurements are performed in a warm room in the morning before the individual rises, and at least 12 hours after the last food intake and activity.

**basic ethical principles** General judgments that serve as a basic justification for the particular ethical prescriptions and evaluations of human actions.

**behavior** The effects of nutrition education (such as the intake of specific foods) or actual behaviors (such as eating five fruits and vegetables per day).

**behavior modification** A process used to gradually and permanently change habitual behaviors.

**beneficence** Ethical principle stating that one should do good and prevent or avoid doing harm.

**binge eating** A disorder characterized by consuming large quantities of food in a very short period until the individual is uncomfortably full, which normally is not followed by vomiting or the use of laxatives. The individual typically feels out of control during a binge episode, followed by feelings of guilt and shame. People must experience eating binges twice a week on average for over 6 months to qualify for this diagnosis.

**block grant** A sum of money the federal government gives to a state or local government. The federal government suggests a general purpose for the use of the money (e.g., community services or social services) as authorized by legislation, but permits the state or local area to spend the money without meeting specific conditions.

**body mass index (BMI)** Weight (kg)/height (m²); an index calculated by a ratio of height to weight, used as a measure of obesity.

**budget** A financial plan that shows expenses and income related to a specific service.

**bulimia nervosa** An eating disorder characterized by recurrent episodes of rapid, uncontrolled eating of large amounts of food in a short period. Purging often follows episodes of binge eating.

**business marketing** The process of creating, distributing, promoting, and pricing goods, services, and ideas to facilitate satisfying exchange relationships with customers in a dynamic environment.

# C

**capitation** A payment method in which each provider, such as an HMO, receives a flat annual fee for each individual, regardless of how often services are used.

**carcinogen** An agent that can cause cancer.

**carcinogenic** Producing cancer; a substance that can produce or enhance the development of cancer.

**case-control study** Exposure and other characteristics of cases of the disease under investigation are compared with a control group of persons unaffected by the disease. The results are analyzed to acquire effect estimates.

**cesarean section** Surgical childbirth in which the infant is delivered through an incision in the woman's abdomen and uterus.

**Child and Adult Care Food Program (CACFP)** Serves nutritious meals and snacks to eligible children and adults who are enrolled for care at participating childcare centers, daycare homes, and adult daycare centers.

**childhood disability** Children and adolescents who have or are at increased risk for a chronic physical, developmental, behavioral, or emotional condition and who require health and related services.

**chronic condition** An occurrence of a disease that cannot be cured and extends over a period of time.

**code of ethics** A set of statements encompassing rules that apply to people in professional roles.

**Code of Federal Regulations (CFR)** A comprehensive summary of all federal regulations currently in force.

**cognitive domain** The domain of learning that involves knowledge and the development of intellectual skills. This includes the recall or recognition of specific facts, procedural patterns, and concepts that serve in the development of intellectual abilities and skills.

**cohort study** Groups of individuals, defined in terms of their exposures, are followed over time to see if there are differences in the development of new cases of the disease of interest (or other health outcome) between the groups with and without exposure.

**collaboration** Working with others toward a common goal.

**colostrum** The first fluid secreted by the breast during late pregnancy and the first few days after birth. This thick fluid is rich in immune factors and protein.

**Commodity Supplemental Food Program (CSFP)** Provides food and administrative funds to states to supplement the diets of low-income pregnant and breastfeeding women, infants, children up to age 6, and elderly people at least 60 years of age.

**communication** A process of information sharing in which those involved in the communication share a common set of rules.

**community** A group of people who share a common geographic location, values, culture, or languages.

**community assessment** The process of getting to know and understanding the community as a client. It helps to identify community needs, clarify problems, and identify strengths and resources.

**community nutrition assessment** An attempt to evaluate the nutritional status of individuals or populations through measurements of food and nutrient intake and evaluation of nutrition-related health indicators.

**community nutrition** An area of nutrition that addresses the entire range of food and nutrition issues related to preventing disease and improving the health of individuals, families, and the community.

**community nutrition research** Organized study of a trend at both the basic and more applied levels that focuses on social, structural, and physical environmental inequities through active involvement of community members.

**competitive foods** Any foods sold in competition with U.S. Department of Agriculture school meals and that are considered as foods of minimal nutritional value, available at concession stands, vending machines, and fundraisers that are in direct competition with the Child Nutrition Program during meal services anywhere on campus.

**compression of morbidity** The postponement of the onset of chronic disease such that disability occupies a smaller and smaller proportion of the life span.

**conceptual framework** A visual way of demonstrating relationships that are known and ones that have not been investigated but that may be the focus of the project.

**contract** A written agreement between a grantee and a third party to acquire routine goods and services. The contract could stipulate any number of things, such as that the grantee must submit a quarterly and/or final report when the project is completed, that there was a reduction in the amount requested, or that the president of the organization must sign the contract.

**coordination** Efficient management of services without gaps or overlaps.

**copayment** A specified amount that an insured individual must pay for a specified service or procedure (e.g., $20 for an office visit).

**cost–benefit analysis** The analytic process whereby the costs and benefits of a program are identified and measured in monetary (dollar) terms.

**cross-sectional study** Measures the prevalence of disease and measures exposure and effect at the same time.

**cultural competence** Understanding the importance of social and cultural influences on individuals' health beliefs and behaviors, considering how these factors interact at multiple levels of the healthcare delivery system, and devising interventions that take these issues into account ensure quality of care.

**cultural sensitivity** Planning interventions that are relevant and acceptable within the cultural framework of the population to be reached.

**culture** The customary beliefs, social forms, and material traits of a racial, religious, or social group.

# D

**deductible** The amount an individual must pay out-of-pocket, usually yearly on a calendar-year basis, before insurance will begin to cover expenses.

**deliberate sampling** Inviting specific people to participate in a study.

**demography** An analytic tool used to measure a population by recording births, deaths, age distribution, and other vital statistics.

**demonstration grant** A grant given to show a new approach to delivering a community health program or demonstrating a technique.

**dental caries** Tooth decay.

**developed countries** Countries that have reached a stage of economic development characterized by the growth of industrialization. The amount of money made by the population (national income) is enough to pay for schools, hospitals, and other services (domestic savings).

**developing countries** Countries that have not reached the stage of economic development characterized by the growth of industrialization. The amount of money made (national income) is less than the amount of money needed to pay for schools, hospitals, and other services (domestic savings).

**diabetes mellitus** A disease caused by insufficient insulin secretion by the pancreas or insulin resistance by body tissues causing high blood glucose level.

**diet history** A detailed dietary assessment, which may include a 24-hour recall, food frequency questionnaire, and additional information such as weight history, previous diet changes, use of supplements, and food intolerances.

**dietary acculturation** The process that occurs when members of a minority group adopt the eating patterns or food choices of the majority group.

**dietary supplements** Products made of one or more of the essential nutrients, such as vitamins, minerals, and protein. The Dietary Supplement Health and Education Act of 1994 (DSHEA) expanded the definition, stating that herbs or other botanicals (except tobacco), and any dietary substance that can be used to supplement the diet were to be included in the definition.

**drug** A chemical compound intended for use in the diagnosis, cure, mitigation, treatment, or prevention of disease, and articles (other than food) intended to affect the structure or function of the body.

# E

**eclampsia** Advanced pregnancy-induced hypertension that is characterized by seizures.

**ecological study** Involves the investigation of a group of people, such as those living within a geographic area such as a region or state.

**Elderly Nutrition Program (ENP)** Provides grants to support nutrition services to older people throughout the country. It provides for congregate and home-delivered meals programs.

**electronic benefit transfer (EBT) system** An electronic system that allows a recipient to authorize transfer of their government benefits from a federal account to a retailer.

**employment-based health insurance** Coverage offered through one's own employment or the employment of a relative.

**entitlement programs** Programs funded by Congress for any person who qualifies due to level of income or other eligibility requirements; SNAP is an entitlement program.

**epidemiology** The study of the determinants, occurrence, and distribution of health and disease in a defined population. It studies scientifically the factors that affect the health of individuals in the community.

**E-professionalism** The natural progression toward the use of electronic communication including the Internet, cell phones and Blackberries, and social networking sites such as Facebook, Twitter, and others by professionals, including community and public health nutritionists.

**equipment grant** A grant for small instruments for a start-up fund.

**ethical decision making** Making decisions in an orderly process that considers ethical principles, individual values, and professional obligations.

**ethics** The study of the nature and justification of principles that guide human behaviors. They are applied when moral problems arise. Also the science of moral values and a code of principles and ideals that guides actions.

**ethnic** The commonality of a group expressed by its nationality, language, or race.

**ethnicity** Implies one or more of the following: shared origins or social background; shared, distinctive culture and traditions that are maintained between generations; and shared culture that contributes to a sense of identity and group.

**ethnocentrism** The belief that one's own group view of the world is superior to that of others.

**evaluation** The systematic comparison of current program results/outcomes with previous status, interventions, goals, or a reference standard.

**evidence-based practice** Using the highest quality available information to make practice decisions.

**exploratory research** Carrying out preliminary research to learn more about the market before any formal research survey is conducted.

**exposure** Characteristics or agents (e.g., food, medications, sunlight) that the participant comes in contact with that may be related to disease risk.

# F

**failure to thrive (FTT)** When a child's weight for age falls below the fifth percentile of the standard National Center for Health Statistics growth chart.

**famine** Widespread lack of access to food due to a disaster or war that causes a collapse in the food production and marketing systems.

**Federal Register** A weekly publication that contains all regulations, proposed regulations, and the Code of Federal Regulations (CFR).

**fee-for-service plans** The traditional type of healthcare policy; the physician sets a price for each type of service delivered, and then the patient or his or her insurer pays this price.

**ferritin** A complex of iron and apoferritin that is a major storage form of iron.

**fetal alcohol syndrome** The cluster of symptoms seen in an infant or a child whose mother consumed excessive alcohol during pregnancy.

**fetus** The developing infant from 8 weeks after conception until birth.

**food distribution disaster assistance programs** Distribute commodity foods directly to households in need as a result of an emergency. Such direct distribution takes place when normal commercial food supply channels, such as grocery stores, have been disrupted, damaged, or destroyed or cannot function (e.g., lack of electricity).

**Food Distribution Program on Indian Reservations (FDPIR)** The U.S. Department of Agriculture purchases commodities and ships them to Indian Tribal Organizations to help low-income American Indian and non-Indian households living on a reservation to maintain a nutritionally balanced diet.

**food frequency questionnaire (FFQ)** A method of dietary assessment in which the questions relate to how often foods are consumed.

**food insecurity** The inability to obtain sufficient food for any reason.

**food record** A written record of the amounts of all foods and liquids consumed during a period, usually 3 to 7 days; often includes information on time, place, and situation of eating.

**food security** To have access to an adequate amount of food at all times that is safe, nutritious, and culturally appropriate for an active and healthy life.

**formula grant** Noncompetitive awards based on a predetermined formula provided to grantees. The amount is established by a formula based on certain criteria (e.g., population, per capita income, poverty, service needs, or number of substandard housing units in a community) that are written into the legislation and program regulations. These are directly awarded and administered in a department's program offices. These programs are sometimes referred to as state-administered programs.

**frameworks** Schemes that specify the steps in a process.

**Frankfurt horizontal plane** An imaginary plane intersecting the lowest point on the margin of the orbit (the bony socket of the eye) and the tragion (the notch above the tragus, the cartilaginous projection just anterior to the external opening of the ear). This plane should be horizontal with the head and in line with the spine.

**fraud** Intentional deception or misrepresentation that an individual knows to be false or does not believe to be true with knowledge that the deception could result in some unauthorized benefit to himself or herself or some other person.

**free radicals** Atoms or molecules that have lost an electron and vigorously pursue its replacement. Free radicals can damage normal cell constituents.

# G

**galactosemia** Lack of the enzyme needed to metabolize galactose.

**gestational diabetes mellitus** Diabetes that appears during pregnancy.

**grant** Money given to an individual or an organization for a need and that does not require repayment. Grants can be given out by foundations, governments, and the like. Grants to individuals can be either scholarships or donations.

**grant proposal** A written request for money (and occasionally for other resources).

**grantee** The organization or individual awarded a grant or cooperative agreement by the grantor and who is legally responsible and accountable for the use of the funds provided and for the performance of the grant-supported project or activities.

**grassroots liaison (GRL)** A position in the Academy of Nutrition and Dietetics (AND) that is appointed or elected by the state affiliate to serve as the primary communicator between AND members and the congressperson.

**ground truthing** A verification process that uses data gathered by direct observation to corroborate data gathered from secondary sources.

**group model** A health maintenance organization that contracts with a medical group for the provision of healthcare services.

**growth chart** Charts that plot the weight, length, and head circumference of infants and children as they grow.

**growth spurt** A period of peak growth rate that begins at about ages 10 to 13 years in girls and 12 to 15 years in boys.

**gynoid obesity** Excess storage of fat, mainly in the buttocks and thigh. Also called gynecoid obesity.

# H

**head circumference** Measurement of the largest part of an infant's head to determine brain growth.

**Head Start program** A comprehensive child development program for low-income preschool children and their families.

**health insurance** A broad term that includes both public and private payers who cover medical expenditures incurred by a defined population in a variety of settings.

**health maintenance organization (HMO)** A managed care company that organizes and provides health care for its enrollees for a fixed prepaid premium.

**health promotion** The process of enabling people to increase control of and improve their health.

**health status** The condition of an individual's physiological and psychological state, and his or her interaction with the environment.

**Healthy People Objectives** A tool to help a community create a vision for its future. It is designed to serve as a roadmap for improving the health of people in the United States.

**homeless people** Individuals who do not have a fixed, regular, and adequate nighttime residence.

**housing wage** The amount a person working full time must earn to pay for a two-bedroom rental unit at fair market rent.

**human subject** A living individual about whom an investigator (e.g., professional or student) is conducting research to obtain data through intervention or interaction with the individual or to obtain identifiable private information.

**hypercholesterolemia** Elevated cholesterol level in the blood.

**hyperemesis gravidarum** Excessive vomiting that produces weight loss and dehydration during pregnancy.

**hypertension** A condition in which blood pressure remains persistently elevated.

**hypothesis** A supposition or question that is raised to explain an event or guide investigation.

# I

**immunization** Injection of a killed or inactivated organism into the body to stimulate the immune system to develop antibodies against an active disease-causing organism.

**individual practice association (IPA)** A type of healthcare provider organization composed of a group of independent practicing physicians who maintain their own offices and band together for the purpose of contracting their services to HMOs. An IPA may contract with and provide services to both HMO and non-HMO plan participants.

**infancy** The period between birth and 1 year of age.

**infant mortality rate** The death of an infant under 1 year of age, expressed as a rate per 1,000 live births.

**informed consent** When an individual agrees to a treatment plan after receiving sufficient information concerning the proposal, its incumbent risks, and the acceptable alternatives.

**in-kind** Contribution of equipment, supplies, or other tangible resources, as distinguished from a monetary grant. Some organizations also may donate the use of office space or staff time as an in-kind contribution.

**insensible water losses** The continual loss of body water by evaporation from the respiratory tract and diffusion through the skin, as well as a higher overall metabolic rate.

**instrumental activities of daily living (IADLs)** Performing housekeeping chores and other activities that are required for a person to remain independent.

**insurance** A plan in which individuals and organizations who are concerned about potential risks will pay premiums to an insurance company, who subsequently will reimburse them if there is loss.

**interdisciplinary team** Collaborating personnel representing different disciplines (e.g., nurses, social workers, physicians, daycare workers, dietitians, and dietetic technicians).

**iron deficiency** Absent bone marrow iron stores, an increase in hemoglobin concentration of less than 1.0 g/dl after treatment with iron, or other abnormal laboratory values, such as serum ferritin concentration.

# J

**justice** Ethical principle that claims people should be treated equally. It is the standard of fairness served when an individual is given what is due, owed, or deserved.

# K

**ketone bodies** The compounds, such as acetone and diacetic acid, formed when fat is metabolized incompletely.

**ketosis** The physical state of the human body when ketone bodies are elevated in the blood and present in the urine; one example is diabetic ketoacidosis.

# L

**lactogenesis** The transition from pregnancy to lactation. The growth and proliferation of the ductal tree and further formation of lobules after birth is lactogenesis stage II (days 2 or 3 to 8 postpartum). During lactogenesis II, milk volume increases rapidly from 38 to 98 hours postpartum and then abruptly levels off.

**learning** The process of leading to relatively permanent behavioral change or potential behavioral change as a result of experience.

**legislative network coordinator (LNC)** An elected state affiliate member of the Academy of Nutrition and Dietetics (AND) who organizes and mobilizes AND members at the state level to become involved in federal public policy issues.

**length**  The proper measurement method of infants and children not yet able to stand.

**lesson plan**  The blueprint for organizing a class. A well-designed lesson plan ensures a clear focus and articulates specific learning outcomes.

**life expectancy**  The average length of life span for a population of individuals.

**linoleic acid**  An essential omega-6 fatty acid that contains 18 carbon atoms and 2 carbon–carbon double bonds (18:2).

**longevity**  A measure of life's duration in years.

**low birth weight (LBW)**  A birth weight less than 2.5 kg (5.5 lb) at birth; mostly due to preterm birth (born before 37 weeks of gestation).

**low-risk individual**  An individual without diabetes or cardiovascular disease and with systolic blood pressure less than 160 mm Hg and diastolic blood pressure less than 100 mm Hg.

# M

**malnutrition**  Poor nutritional status due to dietary intake either above or below the optimal level.

**managed care**  A system that seeks to manage the cost of health care, the quality of that health care, and access to care; it is based on the belief that healthcare costs can be controlled by "managing" the way in which health care is delivered.

**market positioning**  Arranging for a product or program to take a clear, distinctive, and desirable place comparable to competing products or programs for nutrition and health services for the same clients or community.

**market segment**  A portion of a larger market.

**market segmentation**  Dividing a market or community into distinct groups of individuals on the basis of needs, characteristics, or behavior who might require separate products or services or marketing mixes.

**market targeting**  The process of evaluating each market segment's attractiveness and selecting one or more segments to penetrate.

**marketing**  Directed at satisfying the needs and wants of the consumer through an exchange of processes or activities (goods, products, or programs).

**matching grant**  The amount of project costs that the organization, other sponsors, or the institution will contribute toward the project. Support may consist of money, equipment needed for the project, personnel (in-kind), or supplies.

**Medicaid**  A joint federal/state/local program of health care for individuals whose income and resources are insufficient to pay for their care; it is governed by Title XIX of the federal Social Security Act and is administered by the states. Medicaid is the major source of payment for nursing home care of the elderly.

**medical nutrition therapy**  A service provided by a Registered Dietitian or nutrition professional that includes counseling, nutrition support, and nutrition assessment and screening to improve people's health and quality of life.

**Medicare**  A federal entitlement program of medical and healthcare coverage for the elderly, disabled, and persons with end-stage renal disease, governed by Title XVIII of the federal Social Security Act and consisting of four parts: Part A for institutional and homecare, Part B for medical care, Part C Medicare advantage program, and Part D drug prescription program.

**Medigap**  A type of private insurance coverage that may be purchased by an individual enrolled in Medicare to cover some needed services that are not covered by Medicare Parts A and B (i.e., "gaps").

**menarche**  The onset of menstruation (monthly bleeding); normally happens between 10 and 15 years of age.

**metastasize**  To spread cancer by the movement of cancer cells from one part of the body to another.

**models**  Physical, symbolic, or mental ways of viewing a real object.

**moral obligation**  Duty to act in a particular way in response to moral norms.

# N

**National School Lunch Program**  Child nutrition program started in 1946 that provides cash reimbursement to schools so they can provide a free or reduced price lunch that meets specified nutritional requirements.

**neural tube defect (NTD)**  Developmental abnormality resulting in anencephaly (absence of a brain) or spina bifida (spinal-cord or spinal-fluid bulge through the back); related to folic acid deficiency.

**new media**  A general description of emerging technologies that allow for customization, interactivity, and a unique presentation of information.

**nonentitlement programs**  Programs that compete for funds through the congressional appropriation process and establish eligibility requirements for recipients.

**nonstandard work schedule**  Working irregular hours, irregular days, rotating hours or days, weekend days, and regular evening or night hours.

**nutrification**  The process of adding one or more nutrients to commonly consumed foods in an attempt to increase their nutrient content.

**nutrition care indicators**  Signs that can be observed and measured; they are used to quantify the changes that occurred due to nutrition intervention.

**Nutrition Care Process and Model (NCPM)**  A four-step approach to nutrition problem solving and care designed to guide and clarify the work of the nutritionist. It is a standardized process for providing nutrition care.

**nutrition counseling**  The nutritionist provides direction or advice pertaining to a decision or course of action.

**nutrition diagnosis**  Determining a nutrition problem that will be resolved with the dietitian's intervention.

**nutrition education** Any set of learning experiences designed to facilitate the voluntary adoption of eating and other nutrition-related behaviors conducive to health and well-being.

**nutrition implementation** The action phase of the nutrition intervention. The nutritionist carries out and communicates the plan of care/program to the clients.

**nutrition intervention** A specific nutrition-related action that resolves a nutrition diagnosis and consists of two components: planning and implementation.

**nutrition monitoring** An ongoing description of nutrition conditions in the population with particular attention to subgroups defined in socioeconomic terms, for purposes of planning, analyzing the effects of policies and programs on nutrition problems, and predicting future trends.

**nutrition monitoring and evaluation** A procedure that determines whether the goals/expected outcomes were achieved and whether the nutrition intervention resolved the nutrition problem.

**nutrition prescription** Recommended dietary intake of selected foods or nutrients for an individual or a community based on current reference standards and dietary guidelines and the client's or community's condition and nutrition diagnosis.

**Nutrition Services Incentive Program (NSIP)** Provides incentives to states and tribes for the effective delivery of nutritious meals to older adults. The U.S. Department of Agriculture provides cash and/or commodities to supplement meals provided under the authority of the Older Americans Act.

**nutrition transition** A shift in dietary habit from a diet high in complex carbohydrates and fiber to a diet higher in fat, saturated fat, and sugar; this occurs as incomes increase.

**nutritional epidemiology** Study of dietary intake and the occurrence of disease in human populations.

**nutritional status** A measurement of the extent to which an individual's physiological needs for nutrients are being met.

**nutritionist** A professional with academic credentials in nutrition; also may be a Registered Dietitian.

# O

**obesity** A condition characterized by excess body fat. It is defined as a body mass index of 30 kg/m² or greater or a body weight that is 20 percent or more above the healthy body weight standard.

**obesogenic environments** The sum of influences that the surroundings, opportunities, or conditions of life have on promoting obesity in individuals or populations.

**objective data analysis** The collection and analysis of available demographic and health statistics to prepare a community diagnosis and problem list.

**objectives** Written statements of intended outcomes. The expected outcomes need to be defined in measurable terms.

**osteopenia** Low bone density, or thinning of the bones, but at a lower rate than osteoporosis. This stage of bone loss occurs before osteoporosis develops.

**osteoporosis** Porous bone due to reduction in bone mass.

**overweight** A body mass index of 25 to 29.9 kg/m² or a body weight 10 to 19 percent above the healthy body weight standard.

# P

**parallax error** The apparent difference in the reading of a measurement scale (e.g., a skinfold caliper's needle) when viewed from various points not in a straight line with the eye.

**participation** When clients join others in health promotion activities.

**percentile** Classification of a measurement of a unit into divisions of 100 units.

**phenylketonuria (PKU)** An inherited error in phenylalanine metabolism, most commonly caused by a deficiency of phenylalanine hydroxylase, which converts the amino acid phenylalanine to tyrosine.

**phytochemicals** Nonnutrient compounds found in plant-derived foods that produce biological activity in the body.

**pica** The practice of eating nonfood items such as dirt, laundry starch, or clay.

**place** Where and how a product can be purchased.

**placenta** An organ that forms inside the uterus early in pregnancy. The placenta transfers oxygen and nutrients from the mother's blood to the fetus; fetal wastes are removed through the placenta, and it releases hormones that maintain the pregnancy.

**point-of-service (POS) plan** A healthcare plan that offers enrollees the option of receiving services from participating or nonparticipating providers.

**policy** A framework for making decisions that guide actions to help the public.

**political action committee (PAC)** A group of individuals united by similar interests or issues.

**polypharmacy** The use or prescription of two or more different drugs to treat one or more health problems.

**position** Services' strengths in relation to those of other providers.

**preferred provider organization (PPO)** A network of providers who agree to deliver services for a reduced fee; the providers generally incur no financial risk. The financial burden is on the patient rather than the providers.

**premium** A periodic payment required to keep an insurance policy requirement.

**prenatal (antenatal)** Occurring before childbirth.

**preventive nutrition** Dietary practices and interventions directed toward reducing disease risk and/or improving health outcomes.

**price** The cost of a product, both monetary and otherwise.

**primary prevention** Activities designed to prevent a problem or disease before it occurs.

**principle of autonomy** The freedom of an individual to act as he or she chooses.

**principles** The foundations for rules.

**product** The item being sold, promoted, offered, or marketed.

**program evaluation** An ongoing process from the beginning of the planning phase until a program ends.

**program identifier** A statement or motto that succinctly defines or represents the aim of the program.

**program implementation** The process of putting a program into action.

**program paradigms** Representations of approaches to programming that offer explanations of the processes involved.

**program planning** The process of exploring a situation, deciding on a more desirable situation, and designing actions to create the desired situation.

**program** A collection of activities intended to produce particular results.

**promotion** How consumers learn about and are persuaded to use a product.

**psychomotor domain** The domain of learning that includes the performance of skills that require some degree of neuromuscular coordination.

**public health** The science and art of preventing disease, prolonging life, developing policy, and promoting health through organized community effort.

**public health nutrition** Focuses on the community and society as a whole and aims at optimal nutrition and health status. Public health nutritionist positions require dietetic registration by the Commission on Dietetic Registration and a graduate-level science degree that includes study of environmental sciences, health promotion, and disease prevention programs.

# Q

**quackery** As it applies to food and nutrition-related products, the promotion of an unproved health product or service, usually for personal gain.

**qualitative research** Acquired from a small sample of the target audience, mainly through open-ended interviewing.

**quantitative research** Utilizes selected samples to produce statistically reliable results that are expressed in numeric terms.

# R

**race** A social classification that relies on physical markers, such as skin color, to identify group membership.

**random sampling** When every case or participant has an equal opportunity to be included in a study.

**Registered Dietitian (RD)** A dietitian meeting eligibility requirements (education, experience, and a credentialing examination) of the Commission on Dietetic Registration.

Some RDs possess additional certifications in specialized areas of practice, such as diabetes, pediatrics, geriatrics, or renal nutrition.

**reliability** The consistency or repeatability and reproducibility of test results.

**research** A systematic investigation, including development, testing, and evaluation, designed to develop or contribute to generalizable knowledge.

**research grant** Grant money to support an ongoing research study, develop new hypotheses, or improve existing ideas. Normally there are no, or only very few, conditions associated with the award. The researcher is free to decide on the course of his or her research and to use the funds accordingly, subject only to the general conditions of the sponsor and the policies of the university or organization.

**rule of utility** Derived from the principle of beneficence; this includes a moral duty to weigh and balance benefits against harms in order to increase benefits and reduce the occurrence of harms.

# S

**School Breakfast Program** Provides a nutritious breakfast to children in participating schools or institutions.

**screening** An effort to detect unrecognized health conditions among individuals.

**secondary legislation** The action of administrative bodies such as the U.S. Department of Agriculture interpreting the law and providing the detailed regulations or rules that set a policy into effect after a law is passed.

**secondary prevention** Activities related to early diagnosis and treatment, including screening for diseases.

**self-efficacy** The belief in one's capabilities of making a behavior change.

**Senior Farmers' Market Nutrition Program (SFMNP)** Provides low-income older persons coupons to purchase locally grown fresh, unprepared fruits, vegetables, and herbs at farmers' markets, roadside stands, and community-supported agriculture programs.

**sensitivity** The ability to correctly identify individuals or a proportion of persons with a disease or condition.

**sensory-specific satiety** The change in palatability of a food once an individual begins to eat it.

**service grant** Grant money that supports activities and services to the community over and above those outreach programs already funded. This also could be accomplished through a block grant.

**small for gestational age (SGA)** Full-term newborns who weigh less than 2.5 kg (5.5 lb).

**social marketing** The application of marketing to solve social and health problems.

**Special Milk Program (SMP)** Provides milk to school-age children in childcare centers and in schools or institutions where there is no School Lunch Program.

**specificity** The ability to correctly identify individuals or a proportion of persons without a disease or condition, as confirmed by a test.

**stadiometer** A device capable of measuring stature in children over 2 years of age and in adults in a standing position.

**staff model** A health maintenance organization (HMO) that employs providers directly and the providers see members/enrollees in the HMO's own facilities.

**standing committees** Permanently established committees that create and approve legislation, authorize programs, and oversee program implementation.

**State Children's Health Insurance Program (SCHIP)** A federal program that covers individuals who have incomes too high to qualify for state medical assistance but who cannot obtain private insurance. All states participate, but some do not cover dental.

**stimulus control** Altering the environment to minimize the stimuli for eating; for example, removing foods from sight and storing them in kitchen cabinets.

**stunting** A decrease in linear growth rate that is an indicator of inadequate nutrient intake in children.

**subjective data analysis** The collection and analysis of data on various clients that are observable and measurable, such as listening to radio stations, watching local television coverage, and interviewing key informants/community leaders.

**successful aging** Slowing the number and rate of aging changes through positive lifestyle choices or health-related interventions.

**Summer Food Service Program** Provides nutritious meals to children during summer as a substitute for the National School Lunch and School Breakfast Programs.

**Supplemental Nutrition Assistance Program (SNAP)** A federal entitlement program established in 1964 as the Food Stamp Program and administered by the U.S. Department of Agriculture to give more food-buying power to low-income persons or families through monthly allotments of stamps.

**Supplemental Nutrition Assistance Program Nutrition Education (SNAP-Ed)** Provides educational programs that help all SNAP recipients make healthy food choices consistent with the most recent dietary advice as reflected in the Dietary Guidelines for Americans and MyPlate.

# T

**Temporary Assistance for Needy Families (TANF)** A program created by 1996 welfare reform to replace Aid to Families with Dependent Children. It is the major source of funding for cash welfare for needy families with children.

There are federal requirements about work and time limits for families receiving assistance.

**tertiary prevention** Activities designed to treat a disease state or injury and to prevent it from further progression.

**The Emergency Food Assistance Program (TEFAP)** Distributes commodities to state agencies (food banks), which distribute the foods to the public, including homeless people via soup kitchens and food pantries.

**theory** A construct that accounts for or organizes events.

**training grant** Grant money to learn how to prepare a grant proposal and/or learn new techniques.

**travel grant** Grant money funding travel and related expenses outside of the state, community, or local area for the purposes of research, both basic and applied; to attend conferences; or to attend a workshop on how to write a grant proposal.

**trophoblast** The outer layer of embryonic ectoderm that nourishes the embryo or develops into fetal membranes with nutritive functions.

# U

**undernutrition** A health condition caused by a deficiency of one or more nutrients.

# V

**validity** The ability of the test instrument to accurately measure what it is supposed to measure.

# W

**WIC** The Special Supplemental Nutrition Program for Women, Infants, and Children was established in 1972 to improve the nutritional status of medically high-risk pregnant and lactating women as well as children up to 5 years of age from low-income families. WIC is funded through the U.S. Department of Agriculture.

**WIC Farmers' Market Nutrition Program** Provides fresh, unprepared, locally grown fruits and vegetables to WIC participants; also expands the awareness, sales, and use of farmers' markets.

**working poor** Those who spent at least 27 weeks in the labor force (working or looking for work), but whose income is below the official poverty threshold.

# Index